ACE
Personal Trainer
Manual

**The Ultimate Resource for
Fitness Professionals**

Third Edition

American Council on Exercise®

Cedric X. Bryant, Ph.D.

Daniel J. Green

Editors

AMERICAN COUNCIL ON EXERCISE

Library of Congress Control Number: 2003106913

Third edition
ISBN 13: 978-1-890720-14-8   ISBN 10: 1-890720-14-3
Copyright © 2003, 1996 American Council on Exercise®(ACE®)
Printed in the United States of America.

I J K L M

Distributed by:
American Council on Exercise
P. O. Box 910449
San Diego, CA92191-0449
800-825-3636
www.acefitness.org

Third Edition:
Managing Editor: Daniel J. Green
Technical Editor: Cedric X. Bryant, Ph.D.
Publications Director: Christine J. Ekeroth
Cover Design & Art Direction: Karen McGuire
Editorial Assistant: Jennifer Schiffer
Production: Nancy Garcia
Photography: Dennis Dal Covey
Anatomical Illustrations: James Staunton
Index: Bonny McLaughlin
Proofreader: Mariapaz Ramos Englis
Chapter Models: Tricia Baglio, Doug Balzarini, Richard T. Cotton, Cara Dawson, Todd Durkin, Kafi Espy, Scott Fischer, Karen Kay Francis, James Freeman, Brian Friedman, Rebecca Galavan, Barnaby Hall, Vanessa C. Langer, Michael Martinez, Stefanie Moody, Tony Ordas, Beckie Page, Kristie Paterson, Stacey Penney, Carolyn Rhyba, Jennifer Schiffer, Opal Teague, Jim Trageser, David Weck, Jennifer Weck
Cover Models: Barnaby Hall, Carolyn Rhyba

Acknowledgements:
Thanks to the entire American Council on Exercise staff for their support and guidance through the process of creating this manual.

NOTICE

The fitness industry is ever-changing. As new research and clinical experience broaden our knowledge, changes in programming and standards are required. The authors and the publisher of this work have checked with sources believed to be reliable in their efforts to provide information that is complete and generally in accord with the standards accepted at the time of publication. However, in view of the possibility of human error or changes in industry standards, neither the authors nor the publisher nor any other party who has been involved in the preparation or publication of this work warrants that the information contained herein is in every respect accurate or complete, and they are not responsible for any errors or omissions or the results obtained from the use of such information. Readers are encouraged to confirm the information contained herein with other sources.

P09-016

REVIEWERS

Diane Buchta, B.A., is an ACE-certified Personal Trainer and the owner of Tri Fitness, a personal training and consulting company. She is also the former strength coach for the United States triathlon team.

Karen J. Calfas, Ph.D., is a licensed clinical psychologist and the assistant clinical professor in the family and preventative medicine department at the University of California, San Diego. She is also the director of health promotion at San Diego State University and conducts research in exercise adherence.

J. E. Lindsay Carter, Ph.D., is a professor emeritus of exercise and nutritional science at San Diego State University. He is an international consultant and workshop presenter as well as the author and editor of several books and chapters. He conducts research in physique and performance and is an international examiner for anthropometry certification courses.

Larry Gettman, Ph.D., is a renowned exercise physiology researcher, speaker, and author. He served as Board Chairman for the American Council on Exercise, received the prestigious Healthy American Fitness Leader Award from the President's Council on Physical Fitness, and is a Certified Program Director and Fellow in the American College of Sports Medicine.

Louis Horwitz, M.D., F.A.C.E.P., is the director of the University Hospital Health System at Bedford Medical Center Emergency Department. He is board certified in Emergency Medicine.

Gwen Hyatt, M.S., is president and director of education for Desert Southwest Fitness, Inc., and served as the chairperson of the ACE Aerobic Instructor Certification Examination and Accreditation Committees.

W. Larry Kenney, Ph.D., F.A.C.S.M., is a professor of physiology and kinesiology at Pennsylvania State University where he has received the prestigious Faculty Scholar Medal. He is a Fellow of the American Academy of Kinesiology and Physical Education and is president (2003-04) of the American College of Sports Medicine.

He also served as the senior editor of the 5th edition of *ACSM's Guidelines for Exercise Testing and Prescription.*

Brian E. Koeberle, J.D., is a sports/entertainment attorney and the president of Koeberle & Associates, a sports and entertainment marketing agency based in Pittsburgh, Penn. He is the author of *Legal Aspects of Personal Fitness Training,* and is on the faculty of Robert Morris University, teaching courses in sports and recreation law.

Karen P. Nelson, M.A., former director of certification for the American Council on Exercise, has worked for more than 20 years in the fitness field as an aerobics instructor, personal trainer, clinician in spine and joint rehabilitation, and exercise physiologist for Canyon Ranch Spa in Tucson, Ariz.

George Salem, Ph.D., is an assistant professor in the University of Southern California's department of biokinesiology and physical therapy. He is also the co-director of the USC Musculoskeletal Biomechanics Research Laboratory (MBRL). Dr. Salem is a fellow of the American College of Sports Medicine and a member of the American Society of Biomechanics, the International Society of Biomechanics, and the National Strength and Conditioning Association.

Barbara Scott, M.P.H., R.D., is an associate professor in the nutrition education and research program and the department of pediatrics and family and community medicine at the University of Nevada School of Medicine in Reno, Nev.

Mitch Sudy is the former vice president of programs and services for the American Council on Exercise and past assistant executive director for the Lockheed Employee Recreation Association, Sunnyvale, Calif. He was the editor of the first edition of the ACE Personal Trainer Manual and is a 13-year fitness industry veteran.

Stephen J. Tharrett, M.S., is senior vice president of strategic operations, with responsibility for athletics, tennis, and golf, for ClubCorp, a Dallas-based company that owns and operates more than 200 private clubs and resorts worldwide. He has been involved in the fitness and sport industry for more than 22 years, during which he served as president of the International Health, Racquet and Sportsclub Association, on several committees for the American College of Sports Medicine, and on the advisory boards for Star Trac, StairMaster, and Intelligent Health, Inc. Tharrett is the editor of *ACSM's Health/Fitness Facility Standards and Guidelines,* 2nd edition.

Steven P. Van Camp, M.D., is a cardiologist at the Alvarado Medical Group in San Diego, Calif., and has served as the president of the American College of Sports Medicine (1995-1996).

Larry S. Verity, Ph.D., F.A.C.S.M., is a professor of exercise physiology for the department of exercise and nutrition sciences at San Diego State University, and is a preventive and rehabilitation exercise specialist certified by the American College of Sports Medicine.

Denise Wiksten, Ph.D, A.T.C., is an associate professor of athletic training in the department of exercise and nutrition sciences at San Diego State University. She also serves as the undergraduate program director of the athletic training accredited program. Dr. Wiksten is a member of the National Athletic Trainers' Association and serves as a board member on NATA's Education Council.

CONTENTS

FOREWORD

With the "modern" fitness industry approaching its fourth decade, the role of certified fitness professionals has never been more important than it is today. Physical activity is now recognized as a means of preventing or treating obesity, type 2 diabetes, hypertension, and countless other ailments so common in our largely sedentary society. The need for fitness leadership is clear. The challenge ahead of you is reaching and motivating potential clients and positively affecting their lives.

The need for reliable, research-based exercise protocols and procedures has never been more critical. Educators are competing in an infomercial world of believable fiction that cuts to the core of their profession. With a more educated—and litigious—consumer, it is paramount that your level of expertise and commitment to continuing education be second to none.

This manual and the decision that you have made to become an ACE-certified Personal Trainer are the first steps on your journey as a fitness expert recognized the world over. ACE has certified more than 100,000 individuals and has more than 40,000 currently certified professionals in 77 countries connecting with millions of consumers. In addition, ACE averages more than 450 million media impressions each year citing our research and content. Fitness professionals and consumers both recognize ACE certification as a mark of distinction.

To achieve these high standards, you must make an internal commitment to continue your education and remain on the cutting edge of physical activity in delivering quality service, information, and ultimately results to your clients. You must also make an ethical commitment to stay within your professional "scope of practice" as defined by the American Council on Exercise and the certification that you will earn. Misinformation is rampant in this industry and there are many consumers who will depend on your knowledge and professionalism to lead them in the right direction. ACE is here to support your efforts.

Lastly, your commitment to your community as a fitness leader and professional should drive initiatives concerning the physical activity and health of our nation. Obesity and inactivity claim more than 300,000 American lives annually and the financial impact on the country is staggering. I urge you, ACE urges you, to get involved with organizations and activities to help make our nation more active and healthier.

In closing, I wish you good luck on your quest for health and fitness knowledge and Personal Trainer certification. Make good use of this manual and all it has to offer and please don't hesitate to utilize our website, www.acefitness.org, or contact our in-house professionals if you need help in your quest. Study materials are also available that can walk you chapter-by-chapter through the material. In case you feel you need additional help learning the material, ACE offers an exam preparation course (live or online) and practical training workshops that will be valuable throughout your career. As a committed fitness professional, you have a great challenge ahead, but together with ACE you can help our nation move forward and reach new levels of health and fitness.

Scott Goudeseune
President and CEO

INTRODUCTION

The first edition of the *ACE Personal Trainer Manual* was published in 1991 and was a major step in defining the scope of a personal trainer's responsibilities and in bringing professionalism to a young industry. The second edition of the manual was introduced in 1996 and was an entirely new text, written by 18 of the leading experts in a flourishing and widely respected fitness industry. This, the third edition of the *ACE Personal Trainer Manual,* is a revision of the second, with all research and guidelines updated and new topics added to reflect the new directions that the profession is traveling.

We worked with the same 18 experts to update each of their chapters, asked a 19th to provide new material on health behavior and psychology, and added an appendix covering the role that mind-body fitness is playing in one-on-one training. Modalities such as yoga and tai chi, once relegated to the fringes of the fitness world, are now as well-known as kickboxing and step training and are beginning to make the move from the group fitness room to the training floor. Personal trainers can no longer rely on their ability to train clients using traditional resistance equipment. In the new environment of educated fitness consumers, trainers are now likely to face questions on balancing a client's chi (covered in the new Appendix C) or may need to incorporate the concept of behavioral chains (covered in the new Chapter 15) into their motivational repertoire. From more knowledgeable consumers come higher expectations. It is the goal of this book and the ACE Personal Trainer Certification Examination to help you meet those expectations.

The foundation upon which your personal training career must be built is found in the four chapters that make up Part I of this manual. Chapter 1 covers not only how the body functions while at rest, but also how it responds to the added stress of exercise in all its forms. New material has been added to reflect current research on the

effects of exercise duration, and the section on neuromuscular anatomy and physiology has been revised to better meet the needs of a personal trainer. Chapter 2 explains the structure of the human body, including the cardiovascular, respiratory, nervous, skeletal, and muscular systems. Chapter 3 presents the essential information you will need to understand the principles of biomechanics and how they can be applied to the design of a safe and effective training program. Substantial changes have been made throughout this chapter, particularly to the photographs, in an effort to better illustrate proper lifting, stretching, and movement technique. Chapter 4 presents an introduction to nutrition and offers the fundamental knowledge you will need to effectively advise your clients without overstepping your bounds and operating outside of a personal trainer's scope of practice. A discussion of the ongoing development of Dietary Reference Intakes has been added to this chapter, along with updated information regarding the glycemic index and sports nutrition facts and fallacies. Also included are new sections on phytochemicals and probiotics.

Part II addresses screening and evaluation, which together represent an essential but sometimes overlooked aspect of a successful fitness career. Not only must you be able to work safely and effectively with a wide variety of clients, but you must also know when exercise is not appropriate for a given individual. Chapter 5 covers the health-screening process, which will help you determine when there are potential contraindications to exercise. The Physical Activity Readiness Questionnaire, or PAR-Q, a common screening tool, has been updated from the 1994 to the 2002 edition. A new section on angiotensin-II receptor antagonists and their effect on physical activity has been added here as well. Some substantial changes have been made to Chapter 6, which will help you better assess a client's ability and level of readiness to participate in a regular exercise program. More specifically, the protocols and norms of all YMCA tests have been updated wherever appropriate to match that organization's most recent publications, including the replacement of the "curl-up test" with the newer "half sit-up test," which is a safer variation on the traditional sit-up.

Part III, Principles and Methods of Training, provides you with the practical knowledge needed to develop comprehensive fitness programs. Chapter 7 covers cardiorespiratory fitness and exercise, with topics ranging from the components of a traditional aerobic exercise program to a new section presenting guidelines for incorporating mind-body fitness into your personal-training programming. Other new material in this chapter includes the American Heart Association's classification of exercise intensity, a discussion of recent research questioning the validity of the "220 – age" prediction formula for estimating maximum heart rate, and a section on pedometer walking. Chapters 8 and 9 cover muscular strength and endurance and strength-training program design. The biggest change to Chapter 8 is a new section on strength training–related ergogenic aids and supplements, which includes the current research on protein supplements, steroids, androstenedione (andro), creatine, and DHEA. Chapter 9 underwent an extensive revision based on research advancements and industry programming trends. A new section has been added on core training and the material on functional training and periodization have been expanded to reflect the increased interest in these areas. In addition, the sample exercise program has been completely revamped and now includes exercises using resistance machines, stability balls, and free weights, as well as three exercises geared toward stabilizing the core. Chapter 10, which discusses flexibility training, was augmented with new material on active isolated stretching and the effects of pregnancy

on flexibility training. Some photographs have also been added to show advances in stretching technique.

Part IV of this new edition of the *ACE Personal Trainer Manual* covers individualized program design, both for healthy adults in Chapter 11 and special populations in Chapter 12. The primary changes in Chapter 11 come in the form of revised tables from the American College of Sports Medicine and U.S. Department of Health and Human Services, which summarize updated guidelines and new nationwide fitness goals. Information on how to help clients manage stress through exercise has also been added. The case studies in Chapter 11 have been revised to reflect new industry guidelines. Changes have been made throughout Chapter 12 to include breakthroughs in our understanding of the causes and effects of various disabilities and diseases.

Part V, Leadership and Implementation, was expanded with the addition of a new chapter covering the basics of behavior change and health psychology. Chapter 13 will walk you through the difficult process of motivating new clients and keeping experienced exercisers on the path to improved health and fitness. New information on assessing clients' motivational readiness to change has been added throughout this chapter. Chapter 14, which will help you perfect your teaching techniques, features a new section on the various stages of learning and how recognizing and understanding those stages will improve your clients' chances for fitness success. Chapter 15 was added to this edition to improve ACE-certified Professionals' abilities to recognize and understand the behavioral and adherence challenges of each individual client and better prepare themselves for challenging situations. The chapter covers determinants of behavior, principles of behavior change, behavioral strategies, implementing behavior change, a basic teaching method, and when a personal trainer should ask for help from more qualified health professionals.

Finally, Parts VI and VII cover injury prevention and first aid, and personal trainers' legal responsibilities, respectively. Chapter 16 discusses how to prevent musculoskeletal injuries and how to treat them should they occur. The biggest change concerning emergency procedures, which are discussed in Chapter 17, is the use of automated external defibrillators, or AEDs. The use of AEDs is becoming more widespread in the fitness industry. For this reason, the legal issues surrounding their use are discussed in Chapter 18. This chapter also features an expanded definition of personal trainers' scope of practice, which is an issue that arises often with newly certified trainers. In addition, updates were made throughout concerning recent court cases and judgments that affect the fitness industry.

Some substantial changes were made to the Appendices of this new edition as well. Appendix A, which covers the ACE Code of Ethics, has been expanded to further clarify what was previously simply a list of principles, each of which is now accompanied by a lengthy discussion of its meaning and importance. Appendix B, the ACE Personal Trainer Certification Examination Content Outline, has been updated to match the role delineation study that was conducted in the summer of 2001. This material has also been made more reader-friendly in that we have added chapter numbers to help individuals preparing for the certification exam more easily find material in the manual. Three new Appendices have also been added, the first of which (Appendix C) is an extensive overview of

mind-body exercise and its importance to the personal-training industry moving forward. Appendix D is a list of commonly prescribed medications by class. Finally, Appendix E presents ACE's position statement on nutritional supplements, the sale of which are becoming more and more widespread in health clubs, making this an increasingly important issue in the fitness industry.

Over the past 12 years since ACE first introduced this manual, the fitness industry has grown at an incredible pace and the amount of information (and misinformation) that consumers have at their fingertips is frequently overwhelming. One of your many roles as a personal trainer will be to help clients sort through all of this material, find what works for each of them as an individual, and design a customized program that will help them safely and effectively achieve their goals.

The American Council on Exercise is proud to have certified more than 60,000 personal trainers since our first examination back in May of 1990, making us the largest certifying agency of personal trainers in the world.

We hope that you enjoy a long and successful fitness career. And we hope that the improvements made in this new, third edition of the *ACE Personal Trainer Manual* serve you well as you move toward your own goals, both personal and professional.

Cedric X. Bryant, Ph.D.
Chief Exercise Physiologist/Vice President
of Educational Services

Daniel J. Green
Managing Editor

PART I

Exercise
Science

CHAPTER 1

Exercise
Physiology

*Daniel Kosich, Ph.D., is
president of EXERFIT
Consulting in Denver,
Colorado, and was formerly
on the faculty in exercise
science at the University of
Maine. He is the author of*

**Daniel
Kosich**

GET REAL:
A Personal
Guide to
Real Life Weight
Management, *an
international presenter,
former contributing exercise
science editor for* SHAPE *and*
New Woman *magazines,
and has developed numerous
fitness and nutrition
education programs for
fitness center personnel and
the general public.*

Individuals involved with designing or supervising exercise programs must have a basic understanding of the principles of human physiology and anatomy. Physiology is the study of the myriad functions in a living organism, and exercise physiology is the study of the ways cells and tissues of the body function during exercise. The study of exercise physiology challenges you, as a personal trainer, first to be familiar with how the body functions at rest and then to understand how the body responds and adapts to many different types of exercises.

How does the body respond to a gradually increasing exercise pace? Does the body respond differently to a dramatic increase in pace compared with a gradual increase? What are the differences between responses to lifting weights and running or cycling? Why is a slow, sustained stretch held with no pain safer and generally more effective than rapid, bouncing stretches? These are all questions that you must be able to easily answer.

This chapter presents the fundamental concepts of exercise physiology that you must understand to design a safe and effective exercise program that will enable a healthy adult to achieve optimum fitness.

OPTIMUM FITNESS

There are many ways to define physical fitness. It may be helpful for you to think about physical fitness in relation to "specificity of training," which means that physiological adaptations to exercise are specific to the system worked during the stress of exercise. In other words, the type of exercise that develops **cardiovascular endurance** is not very effective for developing an optimum balance of muscular strength. **Flexibility** training usually increases the **range of motion** about a specific joint, such as the hip, but it is not effective for improving cardiovascular endurance or muscle strength. Resistance training, such as weight lifting, is the best way to increase strength, but it is not the most effective way to improve cardiovascular fitness.

Optimum physical fitness is often defined as the condition resulting from a lifestyle that leads to the development of an optimal level of cardiovascular endurance, muscular strength, and flexibility, as well as the achievement and maintenance of ideal body weight. Because training is specific, as described above, an individual must participate in cardiovascular (cardiorespiratory), strength, and flexibility exercise to achieve optimum (balanced) physical fitness.

DEFINITIONS

Cardiovascular, or cardiorespiratory, endurance, also referred to as aerobic fitness, describes the ability of the cardiovascular/cardiorespiratory system (heart, lungs, blood vessels) to deliver an adequate supply of oxygen to exercising muscles. [Some exercise physiologists prefer to use the term cardiorespiratory rather than cardiovascular, because cardiorespiratory includes the reference to the lungs (respiratory). These terms are used interchangeably in this chapter.] Blood must flow from the heart through blood vessels (vascular) to the lungs to pick up oxygen that can be delivered to exercising muscles.

Muscular strength is the maximum amount of force a muscle or muscle group can develop during a single contraction. Muscular endurance is the number of repeated contractions a muscle or muscle group can perform against a resistance without fatiguing, or the length of time a contraction can be held without fatigue.

Flexibility describes the amount of movement that can be accomplished at a joint (an articulation), such as the knee or shoulder, and is usually referred to as the "range of motion about a joint." Maintaining flexibility may help reduce the risk of injury and can also help improve performance in many activities.

Healthy body weight represents a healthy **body composition.** An individual's weight on a scale consists of two dimensions: (1) body fat (adipose tissue); and (2) **fat-free weight** (muscle, bones, blood, organs, etc.). Body fat, which is the body's primary reserve of stored energy, is stored as **triglycerides** both in fat (adipose) cells located between the skin and muscles all over the body, as well as within skeletal muscles. While the energy available from fat is used throughout the body, exercising muscles can utilize a tremendous amount of fat to produce the energy necessary for muscle contraction. Percent body fat represents the percentage of total body weight that is carried as fat. In general, the body-fat percentage of a fit individual falls in the range of 21 to 24% for women and 14 to 17% for men. Fat-free weight represents all the rest of the body's weight, excluding fat—muscles, bones, organs, and nervous tissue. Achieving and maintaining a healthy body composition is an important part of health and fitness.

Fitness Testing

It is possible to measure one's level of fitness in each of the areas of optimum fitness using a variety of fitness tests. The most important value of fitness testing, which is discussed in detail in Chapter 6 and referred to throughout this manual, is to establish a baseline against which improvements can be measured over time.

Fitness testing can be done in a controlled laboratory environment, which usually involves expensive, precision instruments. Gas analyzers for measuring true oxygen consumption, hydrostatic tanks with nitrogen or helium washout apparatus for measuring body composition, and calibrated static gauges on isokinetic machines for measuring strength are typical examples of laboratory testing devices.

Fitness testing also can be done with less sophisticated equipment using what are often referred to as "field tests." Field tests, which typically use prediction equations developed by comparing data with laboratory tests, give personal trainers the opportunity to perform accurate assessments without the need for expensive equipment. The 1.5-mile run/walk for estimating aerobic capacity and the skinfold caliper and circumference measurements for estimating body composition are examples of field tests that are specific to your client's training (e.g., walking, running) and are often more accurate than submaximal lab tests such as stationary bike and step tests.

PHYSIOLOGY OF THE CARDIOPULMONARY (CARDIOVASCULAR) SYSTEM

The cardiopulmonary system is primarily a transport network in the body. Blood serves as the vehicle to carry gases (such as oxygen) and nutrients (such as **fats, amino acids,** and **glucose**) from where they are taken into the body to the cells where they are needed. Blood also picks up by-products (such as **lactic acid** and carbon dioxide) from the cells where they are made and carries them to where they can be expelled or metabolized.

Cardio (as well as cardiac, coronary, and myocardial) refers to the heart. Pulmonary, as mentioned earlier, refers to the lungs. In the lungs, blood gives up carbon dioxide and picks up oxygen. Blood is transported in the body through an incredible network of blood vessels. Therefore, the cardiopulmonary system is composed of the heart, which pumps the blood; the lungs, where the blood picks up oxygen; and the blood vessels, which transport the blood throughout the body. Vascular refers to the blood vessels: arteries, veins, and capillaries. The cardiovascular system, therefore, refers to the heart and all the vessels through which blood flows.

There are three basic kinds of blood vessels: arteries, capillaries, and veins. Generally, **arteries** carry blood with a fresh oxygen (O_2) supply away from the heart to be delivered to the various cells and tissues. (An exception to this is the pulmonary arteries and veins. Pulmonary arteries have a low O_2 content and pulmonary veins have a high O_2 content.) **Capillaries** are very narrow, thin-walled vessels across which the exchange of gases, nutrients, and cellular waste products occurs between the blood and the cells of the body. After passing through the capillaries, blood enters the **veins.** The systemic venous system provides the network of vessels through which the blood, now lower in oxygen content than arterial blood but with a much higher content of carbon dioxide, flows back to the heart to continue the cyclic blood flow.

The Heart

The heart muscle is divided into right and left sides, and each side is further divided into upper and lower chambers,

Physiology of the Cardiopulmonary (Cardiovascular) System

making a total of four separate chambers. The upper chambers are called **atria;** the lower chambers are called **ventricles.** As depicted in Figure 1.1, the right side of the heart receives the venous blood (blood coming back to the heart through the veins), then pumps this blood to the lungs. All of the blood from the venous system enters the right atrium, then flows to the right ventricle. When the heart muscle contracts, the right ventricle squeezes against the volume of blood that has filled into the chamber and sends this blood to the lungs through the pulmonary arteries.

In the lungs, the blood picks up a fresh supply of oxygen and gives off carbon dioxide (CO_2) in the pulmonary capillaries. Oxygen and, to a limited extent, carbon dioxide are carried in red blood cells on a protein called hemoglobin. The freshly oxygenated blood returns to the left atrium through the pulmonary veins, then flows to the left ventricle. While the right ventricle contracts, the left ventricle also contracts and pumps the blood in its chamber through the largest artery in the body—the aorta—to be delivered to the rest of the body.

In essence, the cardiovascular system has two circulatory patterns: one is pulmonary circulation—from the heart to the lungs and back; the other, often referred to as systemic circulation, is the flow of blood from the left ventricle to the rest of the body and back. Remember, the right and left ventricles contract at the same time, and each side pumps the same amount of blood per contraction.

The two phases in the rhythmic pattern of cardiac contraction and relaxation constitute the cardiac cycle: systole and diastole. **Systole** refers to the contraction phase of the cardiac cycle; **diastole** refers to the relaxation phase. During systole, the atria contract first, pumping blood to the ventricles. A fraction of a second later, the ventricles contract, pumping blood to the lungs and the body.

Remember, the left and right sides of the heart contract simultaneously, so at the same time blood from the right ventricle is pumped (ejected) to the lungs through the pulmonary arteries, blood from the left ventricle is ejected to the rest of the body through the aorta.

As the heart muscle relaxes during diastole, blood fills the left and right chambers of the heart in preparation for the next contraction. Note that during diastole, the heart muscle itself is supplied with its blood flow (therefore, its oxygen supply) through the coronary arteries. One of the many benefits of having a high level of cardiopulmonary fitness is that the heart spends more time resting (in diastole) at any submaximal exercise intensity, including rest, than when the system is poorly trained. The reasons for this are discussed later in the chapter.

Cardiac Output

Cardiac output (Q) is the amount of blood that flows from each ventricle in one minute. The cardiac output from the left and right ventricles is exactly the same. However, the blood in the left ventricle is ejected with significantly greater force than the blood in the right ventricle. This is because the blood from the right ventricle goes just to the lungs and back, whereas the blood from the left ventricle has to be pumped with enough force to send it throughout the rest of the body.

Cardiac output is a product of two factors. One is heart rate (HR), the number of times the heart beats per minute (bpm). The other is **stroke volume** (SV), the amount of blood pumped from each ventricle each time the heart beats. Stroke volume is measured in milliliters (mL) per beat (1 ounce = 29.6 mL). If heart rate is multiplied by stroke volume, or the number of beats per minute is multiplied by the amount of blood pumped from each ventricle per beat, the resulting volume represents the cardiac output. Cardiac output

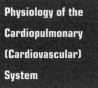

Physiology of the Cardiopulmonary (Cardiovascular) System

Superior vena cava

Pulmonary veins

Right atrium

Pulmonary valve

Tricuspid valve

Right ventricle

Inferior vena cava

Aorta

Right and left pulmonary arteries

Pulmonary trunk

Left atrium

Aortic valve

Mitral (bicuspid) valve

Left ventricle

Interventricular septum

FIGURE 1.1
Anatomy of the heart and pattern of blood flow through it.

can be expressed by the following equation:

$$Q = HR \times SV$$

For example, if the heart beats 60 times per minute (HR = 60), and 70 milliliters of blood are pumped each beat (SV = 70 mL), the cardiac output would be

60 bpm x 70 mL/beat = 4200 mL/min

This equals about one gallon of blood per minute, a fairly typical cardiac output at rest.

Ejection Fraction

The amount of blood that fills the ventricles during diastole is not always completely ejected (pumped out) during systole. The percentage of the total volume of blood in the ventricle at the end of diastole that is subsequently ejected during contraction is called the **ejection fraction.**

The ejection fraction at rest is only about 50% because there is minimal need for oxygen in the muscle cells at rest; the heart can supply adequate oxygen with minimal effort. But during work, when

there is an increase in the need for oxygen in the muscles, the heart is able to completely empty the ventricles during contraction. During exercise, the ejection fraction can increase to 100% of the blood in the ventricles at the end of diastole. The importance of the increase in ejection fraction (which clearly increases cardiac output) as one goes from rest to increasingly higher exercise intensities will be clarified later in the chapter.

Oxygen Extraction at the Muscles

As mentioned earlier, a primary purpose of the cardiovascular system during exercise is to deliver oxygen and other nutrients to the exercising muscle cells and to carry carbon dioxide and other waste products away from the muscles. Cardiac output represents the volume of blood (therefore, oxygen) flowing toward the muscles each minute. But another critically important factor, especially in exercise performance, is the amount of oxygen taken from the hemoglobin (remember, this occurs in the capillaries of the muscles) and subsequently used in the exercising

muscle cells. This process is referred
to as **oxygen extraction.**

Normally, all of the oxygen delivered to
the cells via the arteries is not extracted
in the capillaries. So, while the amount
of oxygen in venous blood is certainly less
than the amount of oxygen in arterial
blood, there is some oxygen in the blood
that returns back to the heart. In other
words, we are able to load the blood with
more oxygen in the lungs than our body is
able to use at the cellular level. Therefore,
in a healthy person, the inability to breathe
fast enough is not the limiting factor in
performance. A significant limitation to
exercise performance is the capacity of the
muscles to extract oxygen from the blood-
stream to produce energy.

ENERGY PRODUCTION IN THE CELLS

Why is oxygen so important? An
understanding of the functions
of the cardiopulmonary system
in oxygen delivery and extraction can help
explain energy production in the cells,
particularly in muscle cells.

ATP—The Energy Molecule

When a muscle fiber contracts and exerts force, the energy used to drive the
contraction comes primarily from a special substance in the cell known as **adenosine triphosphate,** or **ATP.** For our purposes,
ATP is the body's energy source, just as
gasoline is the energy source in an auto-
mobile engine. How quickly and efficiently a muscle cell produces ATP determines
how much work the cell can do before it
fatigues. While there is some ATP stored
in a muscle cell, the supply is limited.
Therefore, muscle cells must produce
more ATP to continue working. Muscle
cells replenish the ATP supply using three
distinct biochemical pathways, or separate
series of chemical reactions: the **aerobic
system, anaerobic glycolysis,** and the **creatine
phosphate system.**

Aerobic and Anaerobic Energy Systems

The word "**aerobic**" means "with oxygen."
The first system for producing ATP, the
aerobic energy system, is dominant when
adequate oxygen is delivered into the cell
to meet energy production needs, such as
when the muscle is at rest. Most cells, including muscle cells, contain structures
called **mitochondria.** The mitochondria are
the site of aerobic energy (ATP) production. The greater the number of mitochondria in a cell, the greater the aerobic
energy production capability of that cell.

The other two energy systems, anaerobic
glycolysis and the creatine phosphate system, are the primary sources of ATP when
an inadequate supply of oxygen is available
to the cell to meet its energy needs. In the
absence of sufficient oxygen, as when a
muscle needs to generate force quickly
(e.g., to lift a heavy weight), the muscle
relies primarily on the anaerobic systems,
which provide a rapidly available source
of ATP. "**Anaerobic**" means "without oxygen." The anaerobic production of ATP
occurs inside the cell, but outside the
mitochondria.

Most cells, such as those in the heart,
brain, and other organs, have little or no
anaerobic capability. Therefore, these cells
must be continuously supplied with oxygen
or they will die. For example, if a coronary
artery (which supplies blood and oxygen to
the heart muscle) becomes clogged with a
build-up of cholesterol deposits, there will
be a diminished flow of blood through that
artery. The decreased blood flow can lead
to an insufficient oxygen supply to the
heart muscle (known as **ischemia**), during
rest or exercise, which often leads to a sensation of pain and/or pressure in the chest
called **angina pectoris.**

If the oxygen supply is cut off, such as
when a blood clot forms where the coronary artery has become clogged, the area
of the heart muscle (myocardium) beyond
the blockage suffers a **myocardial infarction,**
often called a heart attack. If enough of

the myocardium is involved, the result is a fatal heart attack. In the brain, ischemia can lead to a **stroke.**

Unlike the heart and the brain, skeletal muscles such as the triceps and quadriceps have a significant anaerobic capability. You must understand aerobic and anaerobic energy production in relation to what substances are used to produce ATP, as well as to exercise intensity, with rest and maximum effort representing the two extremes of possible intensity. The body uses an extremely complex chemical process to produce ATP. However, just a basic understanding of the process will assist you in designing effective exercise programs.

Fat (fatty acids) and carbohydrate (glucose) are the two substances the body's cells use to produce most of the ATP supply. Proteins, which are composed of various combinations of amino acids, are not a preferred energy source. In an adequately nourished client, proteins play a minor role in energy production. However, when a diet does not supply sufficient calories, the body is capable of using amino acids stored in tissues such as muscle to produce the energy it needs. This is certainly not an ideal process.

When the body is at rest, and the cardiopulmonary system is easily able to supply adequate oxygen to the mitochondria of muscle cells, both fatty acids and glucose are used to produce ATP. In other words, at rest, most of the needed ATP is produced aerobically, using both fatty acids and glucose. In fact, the body produces about one calorie per minute at rest. (The actual number is related to lean body mass.) About 50% of this one calorie per minute comes from fatty acids, even in an untrained person. In a well-trained endurance athlete, fatty acids provide as much as 70% of the resting caloric expenditure.

With increasing exercise intensity, the cardiovascular system makes every attempt to increase its delivery of oxygen into the mitochondria of exercising muscles to aer-obically produce enough ATP. At some point in increasing intensity, determined both by a client's level of aerobic fitness and by genetics, the cardiovascular system becomes unable to supply enough oxygen to the exercising muscles, so they call on the anaerobic systems to rapidly produce ATP. The intensity at which adequate oxygen is unavailable is referred to as the **anaerobic threshold.** (The terms respiratory and lactate threshold also are used.) The anaerobic threshold corresponds to the upper limit of sustainable aerobic exercise and it generally occurs in the range of 50 to 85% of maximum effort (Figure 1.2).

The anaerobic systems cannot predominate for a prolonged period. The primary source of anaerobic ATP production is glucose, which is carried in the blood and also is stored in muscles and the liver as **glycogen** (a large molecule made up of chains of glucose). A second source of anaerobic ATP production is **creatine phosphate,** a molecule that can be quickly broken apart to help produce ATP. However, as with the muscles' store of ATP, there is an extremely limited supply of creatine phosphate. Research done more than 30 years ago demonstrated that even in a well-trained athlete, the muscles store only enough creatine phosphate and ATP, together referred to as **phosphagens,** to last for about 10 seconds of maximal effort (Bergstrom et al., 1971).

The unit of energy most often used in exercise science is the kilocalorie (kcal). One kcal is the amount of heat that will raise the temperature of 1 kilogram of water 1 degree centigrade.

To summarize, as long as a muscle cell is aerobic, it uses both fatty acids and glucose to produce ATP. The aerobic system produces much more ATP than the anaerobic systems, primarily because fat yields nine calories of energy per gram, while carbohydrate (glucose) and protein yield only four calories of energy per gram. Further, the end products of aerobic ATP production are

Energy Production in the Cells

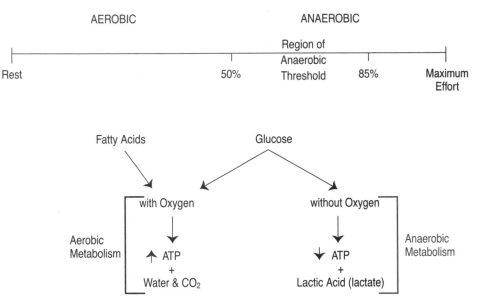

FIGURE 1.2
Energy production and relative intensity in an exercising muscle.

water and carbon dioxide (CO_2). Both are relatively easy for the body to deal with, so that aerobic energy production does not lead to muscle fatigue.

When an exercising muscle becomes anaerobic, it relies on glucose (and to a limited extent the phosphagen system) to produce ATP. However, not only is much less ATP produced anaerobically than aerobically per molecule of substrate used, the by-products of anaerobic ATP production include **lactic acid,** heat, and hydrogen ions. As the level of lactic acid and other by-products increases in a muscle, continued contraction of that muscle is soon inhibited. Lactic acid is thought to be the principal cause of the immediate soreness (the "burn") in an exercising muscle.

In addition to lactic acid build-up, muscles give other signals when they can no longer produce enough ATP aerobically. One is **hyperventilation,** defined as "breathing faster than is necessary at a given pace," an indication that anaerobic ATP production is predominating. When inadequate oxygen is available, the muscle signals the brain to increase the rate and depth of breathing. However, the limiting factor is not usually the ability to increase the rate and depth of breathing. It is primarily the ability to extract and use oxygen at the muscle. Therefore,

hyperventilation is a futile process. Table 1.1 summarizes the essential elements of the biochemical mechanisms used to produce the ATP needed for contraction.

The chemistry that the body uses to produce ATP depends on proteins in the body called **enzymes.** Enzymes are needed to start and carry out the chemical reactions that produce ATP both aerobically and anaerobically. The fat-metabolizing enzymes are different from the carbohydrate-metabolizing enzymes. Further, separate enzymes are used to metabolize carbohydrate aerobically than are used to metabolize carbohydrate anaerobically. When we exercise at an intensity below the anaerobic threshold, the aerobic enzymes that metabolize fat and carbohydrate are dominating in the production of ATP. But when exercise is done above the anaerobic threshold, the anaerobic enzymes take over the dominant role in producing ATP.

Aerobic training will lead to an increased capacity in the aerobic system, but has little effect on anaerobic enzymes. Aerobic training significantly increases our ability to burn fat. Anaerobic training, on the other hand, will lead principally to an improved function in the anaerobic enzyme system—another application of the principle of specificity of training.

Table 1.1
Energy Systems Available to an Exercising Muscle

Energy System	Substance(s) Used	Limitation to Produce ATP	Primary Use
Anaerobic			
1. Phosphagen	Creatine phosphate (CP) Stored ATP	Muscle stores very little CP and ATP	High-intensity, short-duration activities; less than 10 seconds to fatigue
2. Breakdown of glucose	Glucose and glycogen	Lactic acid buildup causes rapid fatigue	High-intensity, short-duration activities; from 1 to 3 minutes to fatigue
Aerobic	Fatty acids, glucose, and glycogen	Depletion of muscle glycogen and sugar; insufficient oxygen delivery	Long-duration, subanaerobic threshold activities; longer than 3 minutes to fatigue

Aerobic Capacity (Maximal Oxygen Consumption)

The total capacity to consume oxygen at the cellular level is referred to as **maximal oxygen consumption,** or $\dot{V}O_2$ **max.** This phrase represents an individual's maximum aerobic capacity. $\dot{V}O_2$ max depends on two factors: (1) the delivery of oxygen to the working muscle by the blood, or the cardiac output; and (2) the ability to extract the oxygen from the blood at the capillaries and use it in the mitochondria. Maximum oxygen consumption is represented by the following formula:

$$\dot{V}O_2\,max = (cardiac\ output\ max)\ x$$
$$(oxygen\ extraction\ max)$$

$\dot{V}O_2$ (the volume of oxygen consumed) is measured as either milliliters of oxygen consumed per kilogram of body weight per minute (mL O_2/kg/min), or as liters of oxygen consumed per minute (L O_2/min).

We can illustrate how much oxygen is actually used at rest when compared with a hypothetical* maximum aerobic capacity of a client who weighs 70 kilograms (154 pounds). If his resting heart rate is 60 beats per minute (bpm), stroke volume is 70 mL/beat (remember: cardiac output = heart rate x stroke volume), and oxygen extraction is 6 mL O_2/100 mL of blood, then his resting $\dot{V}O_2$ is

$$\dot{V}O_2 = (60\ bpm\ x\ 70\ mL/beat)$$
$$x\ (6\ mL\ O_2/100\ mL\ blood)$$
$$= 252\ mL\ O_2/min$$

Divided by 70 kg, his resting $\dot{V}O_2$ is about 3.6 mL/kg/min. During maximal exercise this man has a heart rate of 180 bpm, a stroke volume of 115 mL/beat, and an oxygen extraction of 15 mL O_2/100 mL blood. So his maximum $\dot{V}O_2$ is

$$\dot{V}O_2\ max = (180\ bpm\ x\ 115\ mL/beat)$$
$$x\ (15\ mL\ O_2/100\ mL\ blood)$$
$$= 3,105\ mL\ O_2/min$$

This can be expressed in mL O_2/kg/min by dividing by the man's weight (70 kg)

3105 mL O_2/min divided by 70 kg= 44.4 mL/kg/min

While the example represents a hypothetical client in moderate condition, it clearly illustrates that our bodies have a

---

* Personal trainers are typically unable to directly measure these values.

tremendous capacity to increase oxygen consumption, in this case by more than 12.5 times. While increases in both heart rate and stroke volume account for the increased cardiac output during exercise, the increase in **oxygen extraction** (referred to as arteriovenous oxygen difference, or a–$\bar{v}$ O$_2$ diff) results from different stimuli. During exercise, several changes occur that make it easier for oxygen to be taken off the hemoglobin molecule for use in aerobic energy production in the muscles. The changes include increases in temperature, acidity, and level of carbon dioxide in muscles.

The resting $\dot{V}O_2$ of 3.5 mL/kg/min is often referred to as one **metabolic equivalent,** or 1 **MET.** Activities are sometimes described in terms of METs; for example, volleyball has a range of about 3 to 6 METs, and high- or low-impact and step aerobics classes have a range of about 6 to 10 METs. To determine the $\dot{V}O_2$ equivalent of any MET value, simply multiply the MET value by 3.5. Physicians often prescribe exercise by MET values for patients in cardiac rehabilitation programs and reevaluate the MET capacity of the patient as the rehabilitation progresses.

Not only does $\dot{V}O_2$ max increase with aerobic training, the percentage of maximum effort at which the anaerobic threshold occurs also increases. Practically speaking, this means that a client is able to aerobically produce ATP at increasingly greater intensities in response to aerobic training. Further, the aerobically trained person generally can perform more intense activities than the untrained person, while still working aerobically.

CARDIOVASCULAR/CARDIOPULMONARY RESPONSES TO EXERCISE

Since maximal aerobic capacity is actually a function of cardiac output times oxygen extraction, you must understand how these factors change in response to aerobic training, as well as the guidelines for effective cardiovascular (aerobic) training.

Changes in Oxygen Delivery

As one begins an exercise session, heart rate and stroke volume (cardiac output) increase in order to increase the delivery of oxygen to working muscles. Blood flow is shunted from the abdominal area to the exercising muscles. This redistribution results from a **vasodilation,** or an increase in diameter, in the arterial vessels that supply blood to the exercising muscles, along with a **vasoconstriction,** or decrease in diameter, of the vessels that supply blood to the abdominal area. Breathing rate also increases.

In addition, blood pressure changes. **Systolic blood pressure** (SBP) generally refers to the amount of pressure generated by the contraction of the left ventricle (systole). Systolic pressure provides the force that propels blood through the system. **Diastolic blood pressure** represents the amount of pressure left in the system when the heart muscle relaxes between beats (diastole). Blood pressure of 120/80 means that the left ventricle generates 120 millimeters of pressure (mercury) during contraction and 80 millimeters of pressure remain in the vascular system when the heart is relaxing between beats. The driving force for blood flow is called pulse pressure, which is the difference between the systolic and diastolic pressures.

Blood pressure response is one of the important measures taken during a clinical stress test to evaluate cardiovascular fitness and health. During exercise, systolic pressure should increase as the cardiovascular system attempts to increase oxygen delivery to the muscles. A drop in SBP, or failure of SBP to increase, with increased exercise intensity is considered an abnormal response.

Diastolic pressure, on the other hand, should stay the same or even decrease a little, because the dilation of blood vessels in the muscles (and in the skin to help get rid of heat as exercise continues) decreases the amount of peripheral resistance in the vascular system.

All of these changes occur in an attempt to deliver more oxygen to the exercising muscles. It is clear that when the muscles need to produce more ATP to meet the increased energy needs of exercise, oxygen consumption also increases. As long as enough oxygen can be delivered into the mitochondria to meet this increased energy need, ATP production will proceed primarily through the aerobic system.

Changes in Cardiac Output

In response to proper aerobic training, several adaptations occur in the cardiopulmonary system that lead to a significantly increased aerobic capacity. Resting heart rate decreases, in part because the interior dimensions of the ventricles increase; that is, the ventricles can hold more blood as the heart gets larger inside. Since the ventricles can fill with a greater volume of blood during diastole, stroke volume at rest also increases. The same cardiac output can be maintained at a lower heart rate. Because a given intensity of activity requires a given amount of oxygen, the cardiac output at a given intensity is essentially the same whether one is trained or untrained. Since more blood is pumped with each contraction, the heart beats fewer times per minute to achieve the necessary oxygen delivery. This increased efficiency is certainly a benefit to the heart.

In response to aerobic training, the stroke volume during exercise also becomes greater. Since a given intensity requires a given amount of oxygen, the heart rate at any given submaximal intensity will be lower following as few as three months of regular aerobic exercise. If a given work effort (say, a 10-minute-mile pace) raised the heart rate to 150 bpm before training, then the same work effort after training may raise the heart rate to only 125 bpm. To get to 150 bpm, the trained client will need to exercise at a greater intensity, perhaps an 8-minute mile.

Maximum cardiac output is significantly greater following training because of the increase in stroke volume. Maximum heart rate is determined by age, not by state of training, but a greater maximum stroke volume multiplied by the same maximum heart rate yields a greater maximal cardiac output.

Changes in Oxygen Extraction

In addition to increased stroke volume and maximum cardiac output, other changes occur that enable individuals to sustain exercise at a much greater intensity and still be "aerobic" following training (Table 1.2). Recall that the other factor responsible for $\dot{V}O_2$ is the extraction of oxygen from the blood and its subsequent use in the mitochondria of muscle cells. The exchange of gases and nutrients between blood and tissues occurs in the capillaries. One change in response to aerobic training is that new capillaries are produced in the active skeletal muscles, increasing the area for the exchange of oxygen. The other major change in response to aerobic training is a significant increase in the mitochondrial density, which means more of the muscle cell is occupied by mitochondria. This also leads to a significant increase in the amount of aerobic enzyme activity in the cell, since the mitochondria are the site of aerobic ATP production. The increased aerobic enzyme capacity allows for a greater use of oxygen; thus, exercising at greater intensities can still be accomplished "aerobically." The increased ability to use O_2 also is part of the reason why resting and submaximal heart rates decrease with training.

The increased maximum cardiac output combined with the increased extraction capability yields not only a greater maximum aerobic capacity, but also an elevated anaerobic threshold. The greater the ability to aerobically make ATP at higher exercise intensities, the more "fit" a client becomes, and the greater the ability to "burn" fat.

Guidelines for Cardiovascular Fitness

Table 1.2
Summary of Adaptations to Cardiovascular Training

Cardiac Output Factors	Oxygen Extraction Factors
1. Decreased HR at any submaximal effort, including rest	1. Increased capillary density
2. Increased SV at rest, and at all intensities	2. Increased number of mitochondria
3. Increased maximum cardiac output	3. Increased activity of mitochondrial (aerobic) enzymes

$$\uparrow \text{cardiac output} + \uparrow \text{oxygen extraction yields} \uparrow \dot{V}O_2 \text{ max}$$

Aerobic training also produces a number of other changes that influence performance during submaximal exercise. First, the body uses more fatty acids for ATP production at any submaximal intensity. Second, during submaximal exercise, the body stores more glycogen in trained muscles and produces less lactic acid, both of which lead to improved endurance. Aerobic training also increases the body's tolerance to the lactic acid that is produced during exercise. It is clear that aerobic exercise is beneficial. What follows are some specific guidelines for cardiovascular training.

GUIDELINES FOR CARDIOVASCULAR FITNESS

Any type of fitness training, whether it is aerobic training, strength training, or flexibility training, is based on what exercise physiologists call the **overload principle.** Overload means that to train one of the body's systems, such as the cardiopulmonary system or the skeletal muscle system, that system must be made to work harder than it is accustomed to working. The overload to cause significant improvement in the cardiovascular system is an increased **venous return** sustained for a prolonged period. In simpler terms, the exercise(s) must cause a sustained increase in the amount of blood returning to the heart.

To maximize overload, aerobic training should follow four rules. The exercise should

(1) be the correct type, (2) be done at the proper intensity, (3) be of sufficient duration, and (4) occur with adequate frequency. Please refer to Chapter 7 for a detailed discussion of the variables to consider when developing a cardiovascular-training program.

Type of Exercise

The type of exercise chosen is related to the **principle of specificity of training.** For maximum effectiveness, aerobic exercises need to be rhythmic and continuous and involve the large muscle groups. Generally, the hip flexors (iliopsoas, rectus femoris) and extensors (gluteus maximus, hamstrings) and the knee flexors (hamstrings) and extensors (quadriceps) should be involved. Walking, jogging, cycling, cardiokickboxing, and stair climbing are examples of activities that use these muscle groups. Activities combining upper- and lower-extremity movements, such as cross-country skiing, rowing, and swimming, can lead to high levels of aerobic capacity. However, for those with physical challenges, such as spinal cord problems that prohibit lower-extremity movement, using large upper-body muscles—such as in upper-body ergometry—will clearly enhance aerobic fitness.

Rhythmic, large muscle movements are essential for an effective increase in blood flow back to the heart. The rhythmic squeezing action of the large muscles against the veins within them is called the "muscle pump." This muscle pump leads to a significant increase in venous return, which is required for effective aerobic conditioning.

Intensity of Exercise

The intensity rule is critical. The principles of aerobic and anaerobic energy production make it clear that exercise at too great an intensity for a client's level of fitness will rely on the anaerobic systems, not the aerobic systems. Research shows that optimum exercise intensity for fitness improvement is in the range of about 50 to 85% of maximum oxygen consumption. This corresponds to about 60 to 90% of maximum heart rate. The ranges are broad because of the effects of the level of fitness, as well as genetic factors. The higher a client's level of fitness, the higher the appropriate exercise intensity. Research also shows that untrained individuals will begin to improve aerobic fitness at intensities as low as 40% of $\dot{V}O_2$max ($\cong 50\%$ HR max) (Pollock et al., 1998).

Heart rate during exercise can provide an excellent monitor of intensity. Keep in mind that many factors will cause an increase in heart rate and that an elevated heart rate is not necessarily an indication of an effective aerobic training pace. However, if the increased heart rate is accomplished by the correct type of activity, then the cardiovascular training potential is substantial.

Monitoring a **target heart rate (THR)** training zone provides an excellent indication of correct exercise intensity. Clients also monitor intensity by learning to recognize their anaerobic (lactate, respiratory) threshold. Exercising above this threshold leads to hyperventilation, lactic acid build-up, and rapid fatigue. The **talk test** utilizes the hyperventilation response to monitor intensity. The client should be able to carry on a comfortable conversation while exercising. If breathing is labored and difficult, the intensity is too great. Hyperventilation during exercise is normally accompanied by a burning, sometimes painful sensation in the active muscles because of lactic acid accumulation.

Another excellent way to monitor intensity is to use Borg's **Rating of Perceived Exertion (RPE).** Clients can use this scale as a subjective way of measuring how hard they are exercising. For most people, exercising at a "moderate to hard" level (12 to 15 on the 6 to 20 scale, or 3 to 5 on the 0 to 10 scale) correlates well with an appropriate training heart rate. Please refer to pages 219–223 for a discussion of these and other intensity monitoring techniques.

Duration of Exercise

The third rule is that an aerobic exercise bout should last for a minimum of 10 minutes per session with a goal of at least 20 minutes of aerobic activity accumulated over the course of a day to lead to substantial fitness improvements over time (American College of Sports Medicine, 2000). (This is distinct from the Surgeon General's recommendation to accumulate at least 30 minutes of moderate physical activity on most days of the week.) Once a client reaches the proper intensity, the activity must be sustained for the minimum time to cause adequate aerobic overload. Research has shown that three 10-minute sessions will lead to the same improvements as one 30-minute session if they are done at the same relative intensity (Franklin, 1999; Murphy & Hardman, 1998; Jakicic et al., 1995).

Because aerobic training is related to the oxygen cost of activity, there is an inverse relationship between intensity and duration. If intensity is increased, the duration can be decreased and a similar training effect will be achieved. Conversely, if the intensity is decreased, the duration must be increased to elicit the same training effect. In general terms, when the cells of the body consume 1 liter (about 1 quart) of oxygen per minute, about 5 **calories** per minute have been expended (1 liter O_2/min $\cong$ 5 calories/min). If 2 liters per minute are consumed, the expenditure would rise to about 10 calories per minute. For example, walking costs approximately 5 cal/min; jogging costs approximately 10 cal/min. So jogging for

Guidelines for Cardiovascular Fitness

30 minutes would use about 300 calories (10 x 30 = 300), the same as 60 minutes of walking (5 x 60 = 300). Therefore, walking for twice as long as jogging will result in approximately the same training effect. This is an especially important consideration for the untrained client.

A method of training that is increasingly being applied to the general public is interval exercise. There are two types of **interval training:** (1) performance interval training, which is a very high-intensity effort designed to enhance competitive performance in a specific sport, and (2) fitness interval training, a modest-to-vigorous intensity effort designed to improve general fitness.

Interval training has been used for many years by competitive athletes. In performance training, interval training often involves periods of maximal or near-maximal effort followed by short periods of rest. Such a method of training leads to significant performance benefits, largely because of an increased tolerance to the build-up of lactic acid. Performance intervals are generally recommended only for well-trained athletes. Because of the high intensity, an untrained person is at an increased risk for injury, not to mention quick fatigue, if performance intervals are attempted.

You can, however, encourage clients to perform fitness intervals. In fitness interval exercise, the client periodically increases intensity throughout a workout. The intervals are not rigidly defined as in performance interval training. Most importantly, the increase in intensity is capped when the anaerobic threshold is reached. At this point, the intensity is decreased. Figure 1.3 illustrates how interval exercise might look in a fitness-training application.

Frequency of Exercise

The fourth rule for cardiovascular training is that the proper type of activity, done at the correct intensity and continued for a sufficient length of time, must be performed at least three days per week. While training three days per week may be sufficient, especially for those just beginning an exercise program, more frequent exercise, such as a brisk, daily walk, is certainly acceptable. It also will lead to more rapid improvements. Keep in mind that it is important to allow adequate rest and recovery to minimize the risks associated with overtraining. Most experts encourage even competitive athletes to take at least one day per week for rest or a low-intensity recreational activity, like a round of golf.

Warm-up and Cool-down

Warm-up and cool-down periods are essential parts of any exercise session (not just aerobic exercise). Warming up brings about important physiologic changes that reduce the risk of injury, as well as make the exercise session more comfortable. First, it causes an actual increase in the temperature of the muscle and connective tissue, thereby reducing the risk of soft tissue injury. Second, it allows the cardiovascular system to effectively adjust blood flow from the abdominal area to the active muscles where the need for oxygen is increasing in response to the exercise, while maintaining adequate venous return. This blood shunt is accomplished by constriction in arteries that supply blood to the gut, and dilation in arteries that deliver blood to the active muscles. Heart rate will quickly rise to near maximum in an attempt to supply adequate oxygen if the necessary three to five minutes of warm-up are not performed, especially if an intense pace is attempted too soon. Cool down to 18 to 20 beats per 10 seconds (108 to 120 bpm) to allow the system to reverse the blood shunt.

It may be difficult for you to convince a client of the need for warm-up and cool-down. The best activities for both are simply to work at a much lower pace in whatever activity the client is using for training. Examples include slow cycling for cycling, walking for jogging, and slow

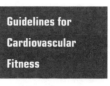

Guidelines for
Cardiovascular
Fitness

FIGURE 1.3
Fitness interval
training.

swimming for swimming. You should remind your clients that adequate warm-up and cool-down periods not only reduce the potential for fatigue, but they also reduce the risk of exercise-related injuries.

Benefits of Regular Aerobic Exercise

Research has shown that regular aerobic exercise has a number of significant health benefits, both for those who are apparently healthy and for those who suffer from various health problems. In addition to the positive body composition benefits, aerobic exercise has been reported to actually decrease appetite in many people. But even if it does not decrease appetite, the calorie-burning effects of regular aerobic exercise allow for a substantial daily calorie intake. In fact, competitive endurance athletes often consume 3,000 to 5,000 or more calories per day, and yet remain lean. Clearly, long-term aerobic training (combined with a sensible diet) is critical to achieving and maintaining a healthy body composition.

Weightbearing exercises, such as jogging and brisk walking, have been shown to help strengthen the skeletal system. This not only helps reduce the risk for developing osteoporosis, but for those with physician approval to exercise, it may help stop further progress of the condition.

Since cardiovascular training increases the sensitivity of the cells to insulin, aerobic exercise is often part of the treatment program for diabetics whose blood sugar is well controlled. Berger (1995) reported that less insulin is required to regulate blood sugar levels effectively in diabetics who exercised regularly. In several reported cases, people with **type 2 diabetes** who were medicated with drugs other than insulin were able to significantly reduce, or completely eliminate, medications by following a prudent course of exercise and healthy diet. The American Diabetes Association recommends that any diabetic considering beginning an exercise program consult with a physician to learn how to carefully monitor blood glucose levels before, during, and after exercise. Eating a carefully designed diet is equally essential in the management of diabetes.

Aerobic exercise is often part of the therapy for reducing the risk of **coronary artery disease** in high-risk individuals, as well as for those who have suffered a heart attack. Four primary risk factors for developing coronary artery disease are: (1) lack of adequate aerobic exercise, (2) high blood pressure (**hypertension**), (3) smoking, and (4) high blood cholesterol levels (American Heart Association, 2002). Aerobic exercise is effective in minimizing these primary **risk factors** for several reasons. First, many of those with high blood pressure also are overweight. Aerobic exercise assists in reducing excess body fat and lowering blood pressure in those with hypertension. Second, many smokers find that regular aerobic exercise provides a great incentive to quit smoking. Third, regular, moderate-intensity aerobic exercise often leads to an increase in the level of **high-density lipoprotein (HDL),** or "good" cholesterol.

Aerobic exercise is frequently part of the therapy for those with arthritis. It helps maintain aerobic fitness, as well as a healthy body weight, but most importantly, it increases joint range of motion.

When working with clients with significant health risks, your role as a personal trainer is to help implement the physician's recommendations. It is illegal, unethical, and certainly not in the client's interest for you to attempt to diagnose a problem or suggest an exercise prescription for high-risk clients. See Chapter 12 for a discussion of considerations for working with clients' physicians to implement exercise programs for those with specific health problems.

Environmental Concerns

Altitude. Because there is less oxygen in the air at progressively higher altitudes, even well-trained athletes need to work at reduced intensity levels until they become acclimated to higher than their normal training altitude. While the length of the acclimatization process depends on a comparison of the new altitude and the altitude the person is accustomed to, it takes about two weeks to acclimate significantly to altitudes up to about 8,000 feet, but can take up to four to five weeks to fully adapt to altitudes over 12,000 feet. However, noticeable improvements are generally observed within four to five days.

Since there is less oxygen in the air at higher altitudes, the heart will beat faster at any given submaximal intensity to deliver adequate oxygen to the muscles, even at rest. During exercise, the heart rate at any given intensity may be as much as 50% higher than normal, so pay particularly close attention to the onset of hyperventilation when beginning an exercise program at a high altitude. Decrease exercise pace to an intensity that allows the client to complete the session without becoming exhausted.

A number of potential problems are associated with high altitude, including headache, insomnia, irritability, weakness, and dizziness. Be sure to report any such symptoms to a physician to reduce the risk of more severe complications. It might seem reasonable to assume that training at higher altitudes would enhance aerobic capacity upon return to a lower altitude. While it may be true in the short term, the changes the body makes to enhance oxygen carrying and delivery capacity to muscles due to the lower pressure at higher altitudes are lost within three to four weeks upon return to lower altitudes.

Heat. When exercising in an environment that is hotter than the body is accustomed to, blood vessels near the skin open to facilitate the transfer of body heat to the environment. This is so the body's internal temperature can be maintained. This causes a reduction in both venous return and stroke volume. At any given exercise pace, heart rate will be higher than usual as the cardiovascular system attempts to maintain cardiac output to meet oxygen needs in the muscles.

Because sweating is one of the most effective means of regulating internal body temperature, exercising in hot, humid conditions is especially stressful to the unacclimated person. For sweat to dissipate heat, it must evaporate. When the humidity is high, sweat does not evaporate. So even though your client may be sweating profusely, there is a risk of severe heat problems. See Chapter 17 for a discussion of the signs and symptoms of heat-related problems.

The main concerns of exercising in the heat and humidity are replenishment of water and allowing the maximum amount of sweat to evaporate. To replenish fluids, drink at least 7 to 10 ounces every 10 to 20 minutes during exercise—the cooler the water the better, because cooler water empties more rapidly than warm water from the stomach into the intestines where it can be absorbed. Drink 17–20 ounces of fluid two hours before exercise, and another 16 to 24 ounces of fluid for every pound of body weight lost following the exercise session, whether thirsty or not. To allow evaporation of sweat, wear lightweight clothing. Light colors (white is best) reflect heat better than darker colors. Wear a light-colored hat to keep from absorbing heat through the top of the head. Never wear rubberized or waterproof garments that prevent the evaporation of sweat. Such a practice could lead to severe heat stress. Experts often recommend 100% cotton garments for exercising in the heat. In addition, a number of specialized fabrics are now available that wick perspiration away from the body more effectively. Be sure to advise your clients to use sunscreen to reduce their risk of skin cancer.

Cold. It surprises some to learn that replenishment of body fluids is just as im-

portant when exercising in a cold environment as it is when exercising in the heat. Not only is water lost as vapor in exhaled air, but the kidneys increase urine production in the cold. Exercising in the cold generally produces enough body heat so that few problems occur during the exercise session. However, risks can become apparent when exercise is stopped and the possibility of losing too much body heat increases.

The easiest way to be certain that the body does not overheat during exercise or lose too much heat during a rest period is to dress in layers. As the body temperature increases during high-intensity exercise, successive layers of clothing can be removed to allow the heat to dissipate. Layers can be replaced during rest or periods of low-intensity effort to help maintain body heat.

Be certain that the layers near the client's skin are made from fabrics that allow sweat to pass through, such as wool, polypropylene, or any synthetic material that wicks moisture away from the skin. During a period of rest or low-intensity effort, a layer of wet clothing next to the skin will cause the body to lose heat. If the day is windy, the outer layer should provide wind protection to reduce chilling during a rest period. It is important to wear a hat when exercising in the cold, especially during periods of rest, since a significant amount of heat can be lost through the scalp.

BASIC NEUROMUSCULAR ANATOMY AND PHYSIOLOGY

In addition to acquiring a basic knowledge of function and training of the cardiopulmonary system, you must give similar attention to the skeletal muscle system. There are three primary types of muscle cells in the body:

1. Cardiac cells are muscle cells unique in structure and function and are found only in the heart.

2. Smooth muscle cells are found in the walls of arteries and in the walls of the intestines and allow for the shunting of blood (the constriction and dilation in blood vessels) to redistribute blood flow.

3. Skeletal muscle cells are bound together to form skeletal muscles, which attach to bones across one or more joints. Coordinated contraction of the skeletal muscles, which are the only type of muscle under voluntary control, causes movement at the joint(s), and, therefore, of the body.

Muscle Fiber Types

There are two primary types of skeletal muscle fibers (cells): **slow-twitch (Type I) fibers** and **fast-twitch (Type II) fibers.** The determination of the type of muscle fiber is possible through a laboratory technique known as a muscle biopsy. In a muscle biopsy, a sample of muscle tissue is extracted (taken out) using a needle that is inserted directly into the muscle. The section of tissue that is taken is mounted on a slide and stained for microscopic analysis. With an acidic stain, slow-twitch fibers have a dark appearance because they have a rich blood supply, while fast-twitch fibers have a white appearance.

As their name implies, slow-twitch fibers contract more slowly than fast-twitch fibers. Slow-twitch fibers, also called slow-oxidative, have a smaller cross-section than fast-twitch fibers, have many mitochondria and a high aerobic capacity and, therefore, are most resistant to fatigue. Fast-twitch fibers are divided into two types: IIa and IIb. Type IIa fibers are called fast oxidative and have more mitochondria than type IIb, which are referred to as fast glycolytic. Although type IIa fibers have some oxidative properties, they do not have nearly the endurance or aerobic capability of slow-twitch fibers.

In terms of the distribution of fast- and slow-twitch fibers, there are two general considerations. First, in a given individual, the distribution of fast- and slow-twitch fibers varies in different muscles. For example, there is a different percentage of fast- and

slow-twitch fibers in the biceps compared to the quadriceps and in the deltoids compared to the triceps.

Second, the percentage of fast- and slow-twitch fibers of a given muscle varies from person to person. For example, one person may have a high percentage of fast-twitch fibers in the quadriceps muscles, whereas another person will have a lower percentage. These differences influence the person's ability to successfully perform speed and power events versus endurance events.

World-class power athletes, such as power weight lifters, have a distribution of approximately 60 to 90% fast-twitch fibers in those muscles that are used in their activity. In comparison, world-class endurance athletes, such as long-distance runners and cross-country skiers, would likely have 60 to 90% slow-twitch fibers in the muscles used in their events.

Endurance training does not change fast-twitch fibers (type II) to slow-twitch fibers (type I). Similarly, power training does not change slow-twitch fibers to fast-twitch fibers. However, research shows that it is possible to increase either the oxidative capacity or glycolytic capacity, especially in the type IIa fibers, depending on the specificity of training. Because a client's fiber type distribution is genetically predetermined, training will not change one fiber type to the other; however, you can design individual programs and understand the reasons why different clients respond differently to the same training program.

There are no differences between males and females with respect to fiber-type distribution. A muscle fiber is a muscle fiber, and fast- and slow-twitch fibers are found in both females and males, with the same general distribution and fiber performance characteristics.

Neuromuscular Anatomy

Functionally, fast-twitch fibers contract to maximal force more rapidly than the slow-twitch fibers, but the physiology behind muscle contraction is exactly the

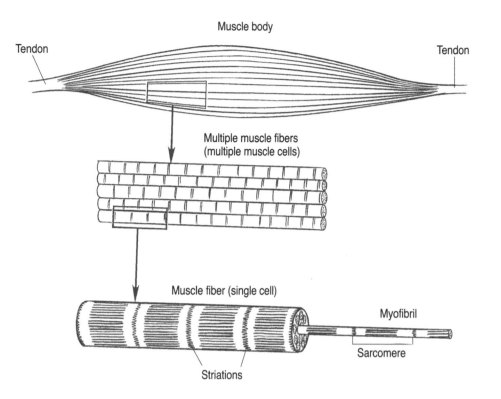

Basic Neuromuscular Anatomy and Physiology

FIGURE 1.4
Anatomy of skeletal muscle: muscle, muscle fiber, myofibrils, and sarcomere.

same. Refer to Figure 1.4 for an illustration of basic skeletal muscle anatomy.

Muscle contraction originates as nerve impulses from the brain to the muscle fiber are conducted through **motor neurons.** Neurons are the main type of nervous tissue cells that make up the brain and spinal cord. Each motor neuron stores a **neurotransmitter** called **acetylcholine,** which chemically transmits nerve impulse to muscle fibers. The junction at which a motor neuron and a myofibril meet is known as the **neuromuscular junction.**

Running the length of each muscle fiber are strands of protein known as **myofibrils.** There are several proteins in a myofibril. The proteins **actin** and **myosin,** also known as contractile proteins, are the two primary proteins related to the process of muscle contraction.

Looking at a muscle fiber under a microscope shows it is made of several repeating units called **sarcomeres** along the length of the muscle cell. Each sarcomere is surrounded by a membrane called the **sarcolemma** and a gelatin-like tissue called the **sarcoplasm.** Within the sarcoplasm can be found mitochondria

and **sarcoplasmic reticulum,** which functions to store and release calcium. Running through all the sarcomeres, from one end of the cell to the other, are the myofibrils (of which actin and myosin are a part). Within each sarcomere of the muscle cells, the proteins actin and myosin are located in different areas. The myosin protein is located in the middle of each sarcomere; each actin portion of the myofibril overlaps a portion of one end of the myosin and extends through the sarcomere boundary into the adjacent sarcomere, where it overlaps one end of the myosin in that sarcomere.

Muscle Contraction

For muscle contraction to occur, there must be sufficient ATP near the actin and myosin proteins, and there must be a nervous impulse from the central nervous system. According to the **sliding filament theory** of muscle contraction, when these two factors are present, the tiny projections from the myosin (myosin heads) attach to the actin, forming an actin-myosin cross bridge. Figure 1.5 illustrates this process.

The energy from ATP causes the myosin heads on each end of the myosin to swivel toward the center of the sarcomere, pulling on the attached actin filament so that the actin slides inward toward the center of the sarcomere. This process causes each sarcomere along the entire length of the muscle fiber to shorten. Since all of the sarcomeres shorten at the same time, the overall length of the muscle fiber is decreased. When a multitude of fibers contract, the result is muscle contraction, which is really nothing more than the simultaneous shortening of many of the fibers in the muscle.

Muscle contraction summary

1. A nervous impulse from the brain causes motor neurons to release acetylcholine into the neuromuscular junction.

2. The acetylcholine is detected and the nerve impulse continues to spread across the sarcolemma and deep into the sarcoplasmic reticulum.

3. The sarcoplasmic reticulum releases calcium into the sarcoplasm of the muscle fiber.

4. The calcium binds with the proteins (troponin and tropomyosin) along the actin filament and exposes the binding sites for the myosin filament.

5. With sufficient ATP, myosin binds with the actin filaments to form cross-bridges.

6. The myosin pulls the actin toward the center and the sarcomere shortens.

7. Once a nervous impulse ceases, calcium is returned to the sarcoplasmic reticulum and the linkages between myosin and actin are broken.

Even though individual fibers attempt to shorten when they contract, muscle contraction does not always involve a shortening in the length of the whole muscle. A **concentric** (positive) **contraction** shortens the muscle. However, an **eccentric** (negative) **contraction** lengthens the muscle. An eccentric contraction occurs when individual fibers contract, but the external resistance to the muscle's major action is greater than the force generated, so the muscle actually lengthens. **Isometric contraction** describes a contraction of individ-

---

FIGURE 1.5
Anatomy of a muscle:

Resting myofibril.

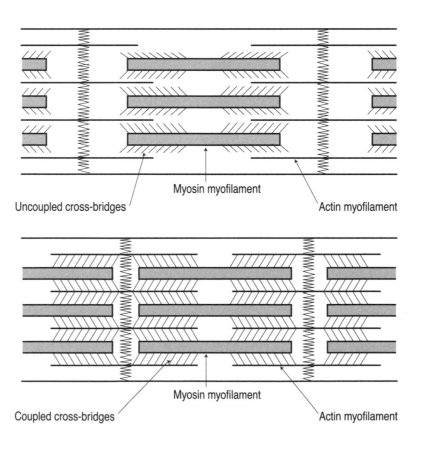

Myosin myofilament

Uncoupled cross-bridges

Actin myofilament

Contracted myofibril.

Myosin myofilament

Coupled cross-bridges

Actin myofilament

ual fibers but no change in the length of the whole muscle.

To review, muscle contraction is an interaction between the actin and myosin proteins that causes an attempted shortening of individual muscle fibers. If the force of contraction is greater than the external resistance, a concentric contraction occurs. If the external resistance is greater than the force of contraction, an eccentric contraction occurs. It is important to remember that sufficient ATP (energy) must be present, as well as a continued nervous impulse, to sustain this contraction process.

Force of Contraction (Strength). When a muscle fiber contracts, it exerts force. Skeletal muscle tissue functions according to an all-or-none principle. This means that when a single muscle fiber shortens, it generates its maximum force capability. A skeletal muscle fiber has no inherent ability to grade its force of contraction (as cardiac muscle cells do); when it is stimulated to contract, it does so maximally. The amount of force that is generated during contraction in the whole muscle depends on two factors: (1) the size of the individual fibers contracting (a larger fiber is a stronger fiber) and (2) the number of muscle fibers that contract simultaneously (to generate more force, more fibers are recruited).

The force generated by muscle contraction is related to the speed of movement at the associated joint, as well as the initial length of the muscle belly. The "force-velocity" relationship suggests that, in general, the faster the speed of movement, the lower the force generated by the contracting muscle. For example, the biceps muscle will generate more force during a maximal contraction when the elbow joint is flexing at 60 degrees of movement per second than when the elbow is flexing at 180 degrees of movement per second.

The "length-tension" relationship demonstrates that a muscle generates maximum force when it begins its contraction at 1.2 times its resting length. This rela-

tionship helps explain why athletes such as baseball players and golfers slightly stretch the appropriate muscles before beginning the swinging movement.

Muscle Fiber Size. The force the fiber generates is related to its cross-sectional area. A larger fiber exerts more force than a smaller one. Note that the strength of a given cross-sectional area of muscle tissue from males and females is the same. Males are generally stronger because of a greater amount of muscle tissue. Women respond to a strength-training program in many of the same ways men do. Therefore, strength training is an important part of a physical fitness program for both genders.

Motor Units. In a given muscle, muscle fibers are stimulated in units or groups. A single motor nerve (from the spinal cord) and all the muscle fibers it stimulates together are called a **motor unit.** Motor units come in different sizes. Those made up of a single nerve stimulating just 5 to 10 fibers are responsible for fine, delicate movements like moving the eye, blinking the eyelid, and drawing intricate detail in a picture. On the other hand, motor units consisting of one motor nerve and 500 to 1,000 fibers are called on for forceful tasks like lifting, kicking, or jumping. Regardless of the size, motor units are made of either all fast-twitch fibers or all slow-twitch fibers. When the fibers of a motor unit are called on to contract, all of the muscle fibers in the unit contract together, and they contract with maximum force (remember the all-or-none principle). So the amount of force generated at any one time depends on how many motor units are called on to contract simultaneously.

To exert minimal force—like picking up a pencil—only a few motor units in the forearm muscles are recruited. To pick up a dumbbell, many more motor units in these muscles would be stimulated to contract. To exert maximum muscle force, the nervous system will attempt to contract as many motor units in the muscle as possible. Since the number of motor units (fibers) and the size of the fibers in those contraction motor units determine how much force will be generated on contraction, you need to understand how muscle fibers respond to a strength-training program.

ADAPTATIONS TO STRENGTH TRAINING

Describing adaptations to strength training is not as straightforward as the discussion of adaptations to aerobic training. There are many variables that influence strength-training adaptations, including the relationship of resistance and repetitions in the lifting program, the distribution of fast- and slow-twitch fibers in the muscles being trained, and the level of the hormone testosterone. It is important to understand that individual differences in the above-mentioned variables can dramatically influence specific response in a given client.

The specific overload to cause strength gains is a progressive increase in the amount of resistance (weights, elastic bands, air, electromechanical) used in the training program. To continue to increase strength, one must continue to increase overload. This section describes the changes that occur in the body as a result of strength training that account for an increased ability to generate force.

Muscle Fiber Adaptation

The most obvious adaptation to strength training is usually an increase in the size of the muscle. This is known as muscle **hypertrophy.** Hypertrophy is an increase in the number and size of myofibrils inside muscle fibers. More simply, it is an increased amount of actin, myosin, and related proteins that are responsible for force generation. Within the muscle, this is probably the most important adaptation leading to an increase in strength. When men and women are exposed to the same

strength-training program, men will generally hypertrophy to a greater extent than will women. This is primarily because of higher levels of the hormone testosterone (which plays an important role in the production of the contractile proteins such as actin and myosin) in men than in women. Greater muscle size is one reason most men are capable of greater absolute strength than most women.

While hypertrophy will generally result as an adaptation to strength training, the relationship of repetitions (reps) and resistance to hypertrophy is clear. A high-resistance (6 to 10 RM) program will usually lead to significant hypertrophy in most males. Most females, because of naturally lower levels of testosterone, will not generate significant hypertrophy even with this type of program. Conversely, a low-resistance, high-rep program will generally lead to little hypertrophy even in males. Many women shy away from strength training because of a fear of the "body-builder" hypertrophy. You can allay their fears by using lower resistance (12 to 15 RM) programs.

Besides increasing fiber size, training also will increase the number of sarcomeres in trained fibers. The increase in size enhances the amount of contractile protein in the fibers as well, adding to the strength potential of the fiber. Further, some research with animals suggests that the use of extremely high resistance might possibly increase the number of muscle fibers (hyperplasia) in the muscle. Evidence for muscle fiber hyperplasia in humans is lacking. The prevailing thought is that the change in the muscle size is due to an increase in protein content, and often in the diameter, of existing fibers, not an increase in the number of muscle fibers.

Connective Tissue Adaptation

In addition to changing muscle tissue itself, training also changes the **connective tissues** of the body. There are three basic types of connective tissue: **cartilage,** which serves as padding between the bones that meet at a joint in the skeleton; **ligaments,** which connect bones to bones at a joint; and **tendons,** which connect skeletal muscles to the bones, transmitting the force of muscle contraction to the bones. The tendons are an extension of tendinous connective tissue, which weaves a network of support around and between the muscle fibers of a muscle, giving strength and stability to the belly of the muscle by holding the fibers of the motor units together.

In response to strength training, the connective tissues (i.e., ligaments and tendons) associated with muscle become stronger by becoming thicker and are thus able to withstand the increase in force of contraction generated by the strength-trained muscle. The increased strength of connective tissue is thought to play a highly significant role in the total strength gain that results from a regular resistance-training program.

Increased Nervous System Activity

A third change in response to strength training is the stimulation of motor units that were previously inactive. Part of strength generation depends on the number of motor units contracting. When untrained and not working against much resistance, some fibers (motor units) are never used. But the need to generate more force in a strength-training program stimulates activation of some inactive fibers (motor units).

When an untrained client begins a carefully designed strength program, gains in strength can often be noted in just a couple of weeks. Clearly, there will not be noticeable hypertrophy in such a short period. What accounts for the initial gains? Most likely, the recruitment of previously inactive motor units is responsible for much of the initial increase in strength. In addition, the brain increases its ability to coordinate the recruitment of individual motor units.

Decreased Nervous Inhibition

One of the most important adaptations to strength training is that we can overcome, or decrease, nervous inhibition to the muscles. Nervous inhibition is both psychological and physiological. In a psychological sense, confidence increases, allowing lifts never before thought possible. This is especially true in nonathletes who think themselves weaker than they actually are.

Physiological (functional) adaptation also is important. In the tendons, which connect the muscle to the bones, there is a sensor called a muscle tendon organ, or a **Golgi tendon organ.** This tendon organ is a part of the nervous system, a protection against generating too much contractile force. When the muscle tendon organ is stimulated by too much contractile force, its associated muscle will relax to prevent injury to the muscle itself or to its associated connective tissues. Under normal circumstances, maximal contraction is prevented; that is, all of the motor units in a muscle will not contract simultaneously because of the inhibitory protection of the muscle tendon organ.

It is possible, however, to override the physiological Golgi protective inhibition. Two examples can illustrate the consequences of overriding the Golgi inhibition. The first is that of a woman who finds that the jack has slipped while her husband was working under the car and the car has fallen on him. She reaches under the bumper of the car, generates a maximum muscular contraction in several muscle groups, and miraculously lifts the car off her husband's body. In so doing, however, she undoubtedly has suffered injury to some of her connective tissues because she overrode the threshold protection of the Golgi tendon organs.

A second example is the weight lifter who attempts to lift more weight than he has trained himself to lift and physiologically (or pharmacologically) pumps himself up to the point where he is able to overcome the threshold protection of the tendon organ. In attempting the lift, the weight lifter can actually tear the tendon, causing severe injury. The biceps tendon and the quadriceps tendon are two connective tissue structures often injured by overriding their associated tendon organ protection.

Strength training raises the threshold of force generation at which the Golgi tendon organ is stimulated, probably because the overload of training causes more connective tissue protein to be added to the tendon. The associated muscle can then generate greater contractile force before the tendon organ is stimulated.

In summary, the ability to exert more force after strength training is not solely the result of muscle fiber adaptations, but involves extremely important adaptations in connective tissue and the nervous system as well. Many scientists argue that the connective tissue and nervous system adaptations are probably more important to overall strength gains than the changes in the muscle fibers. Clearly, many successful strength athletes follow significantly different training protocols. Without a doubt, it will take continued research in the area of strength adaptations to elucidate the specific details of the current theories.

GUIDELINES FOR STRENGTH TRAINING

With an idea about how the body adapts to the progressive overload of a strength-training program, you need an understanding of general concepts to develop a strength-training program. (Please refer to Chapter 8 for a detailed discussion of the variables to be considered when developing and supervising such programs.) Strength training is a highly individualized procedure. Well-trained and highly successful power and endurance athletes have all established their own most effective training regimens. And frequently, two equally

successful strength athletes will have very different training routines. However, as with any aspect of fitness development, you must assist your clients in challenging the factors responsible for strength with an appropriate and specific overload.

Types of Strength Overloads

For many years, strength-training programs have been described as being isometric, isotonic, or isokinetic, based on the type of muscle contraction involved during the exercise. (The prefix "iso" means "same.")

Isometric (same length) refers to exercises that develop high-intensity contractions in the muscle with no change in muscle length. Generally, isometric exercises call for a maximal effort against an immovable object, like a wall or desk. Isometric training clearly increases muscle strength, but only at the joint angle where the contraction occurs.

Isotonic (same tone or tension) refers to exercises that use a given amount of external resistance that is challenged through the entire range of motion. The tension in the muscle is not constant throughout the range of motion. The actual amount of force generated by a muscle will change throughout the movement because of the biomechanics at the joint or joints involved. For example, even though a 10-pound dumbbell is obviously a constant weight throughout a biceps curl, the biceps does not generate a constant 10 pounds of force throughout its entire contraction. (The biomechanics of this concept are presented in Chapter 3.)

It has been suggested that strength exercises using a fixed amount of external resistance be referred to as **dynamic constant external resistance** training, not isotonic training. Exercises that use machines with a shaped cam can be called **dynamic variable external resistance.** These descriptions accurately suggest that even though the weight is constant throughout the movement, the amount of force generated by the overloaded muscles changes throughout the movement.

Isokinetic (same speed) refers to a type of resistance exercise that causes the exercising muscles to generate a maximum amount of force throughout the entire range of movement, while keeping the speed of movement constant. Isokinetic and dynamic resistance exercises are performed with either concentric or eccentric muscle contractions, or both. Concentric (shortening) movements are often referred to as the positive phase of a lift. Eccentric (lengthening) movements, on the other hand, are referred to as the negative phase. The type of contractions involved during strength training appears to have an impact on the degree of muscle soreness that occurs one to three days after training.

Muscle Soreness and Fatigue

Muscle Soreness. There are two general types of exercise-related muscle soreness. One is the immediate soreness felt while, or immediately after, exercising. The other type of soreness is that which persists for one to three days following a session.

Immediate soreness appears to be most directly related to the build-up of lactic acid (and other by-products) in the muscle that have leaked out of the muscle cells and stimulated sensitive nerve endings near them. This excess lactic acid is removed quite rapidly when the exercise session is completed, generally within 30 to 60 minutes. Much of the excess lactic acid is metabolized in the muscle cell in which it was produced during exercise. The lactic acid not used is carried to the liver as lactate where it is metabolized. Immediate soreness may involve minor muscle or connective tissue tears, so do not ignore it. Refer to Chapter 16 for a discussion of a wide range of exercise-related injuries and sources of soreness during exercise.

The explanation of latent soreness, the soreness unnoticed during exercise, but present from one to three days following exercise, is the subject of much research and some controversy. Available research indicates that delayed soreness (delayed onset muscle soreness, or DOMS) is most likely the result of very small tears in the connective tissues that hold individual muscle fibers together within the belly of the muscle, as well as some tearing of the membrane of the muscle cells.

Furthermore, research suggests that this latent soreness is closely associated with the eccentric, or negative, phase of muscular effort. During negative work, the muscle fibers are contracting and attempting to cause a shortening of the muscle. But the resistance is greater than the force developed, so the muscle and associated connective tissue is actually lengthening. This lends credibility to theories that implicate microscopic tears within the muscle cell membrane and/or connective tissues during aggressive negative effort. Available evidence indicates that concentric overloads produce little or no delayed soreness, compared with the significant soreness usually reported with heavy eccentric work.

Muscle Fatigue. The reasons for fatigue also are varied, but they relate primarily to the intensity and duration of the exercise bout. For instance, the fatigue felt when performing a power event or other maximum effort that lasts from 0 to 30 seconds to exhaustion occurs because the active muscle cells run out of ATP at the site of the actin-myosin crossbridge, which is part of the mechanism of muscle fiber contraction. Without ATP present, the fibers can no longer contract.

Muscle fatigue that results during heavy exercise, lasting anywhere from about 30 seconds up to about 40 to 60 minutes to exhaustion, is generally thought to be related to lactic acid accumulation. Clearly this is a broad range, and several other factors may be involved in varying degrees, but lactic acid accumulating from intense effort ultimately inhibits the ability of the muscle cell to contract.

Guidelines for Strength Training

Finally, the fatigue felt in prolonged endurance activities lasting 60 to 180 minutes or longer occurs primarily because **glycogen**—the storage form of glucose—becomes depleted in the exercising muscles. Without a source of glucose, muscle cells cannot contract even with an adequate supply of oxygen and fat. In other words, when glycogen is depleted (a marathoner calls this "hitting the wall"), the muscles being used are unable to maintain the required intensity. Other factors also implicated in fatigue during prolonged activities include **dehydration,** increased body temperature, by-products other than lactic acid, and boredom with the activity.

FLEXIBILITY TRAINING

Flexibility is defined as the range of motion about a joint. Therefore, flexibility training is designed to increase the range of motion in a specific area, such as the low back, the hamstrings, or the shoulder girdle. Flexibility is primarily limited by four factors: (1) the elastic limits of the ligaments and tendons crossing the joint, (2) the **elasticity** of the muscle tissue itself, (3) the bone and joint structure, and (4) the skin.

Many types of exercises can increase flexibility. As every system must be overloaded to generate specific gains, so must the connective and skeletal muscle be overloaded to generate increased flexibility. It appears that one of the safest overloads for flexibility training is a slow, sustained stretch. Bobbing and bouncing activities are not generally recommended. They can lead to injury in the muscle fibers and connective tissues, since there is an increased likelihood of the connective tissues being overstretched.

Only general guidelines for stretching are presented here. A detailed discussion of specific guidelines for increasing flexi-

bility is presented in Chapter 10. Slowly stretch to the point where tension (tightness) is felt in the muscles being stretched. Do not stretch to the point of pain. Hold the stretch for about 15 seconds, being sure not to hold your breath. Some research suggests that four sets of approximately 15-second stretches can lead to significant improvements in flexibility.

Just as the Golgi tendon organ serves as a protection against generating too much contractile force, fibers in the muscle tissue protect against too much stretch. These fibers are called **muscle spindles.** In ballistic (rapid, bouncing) stretching, the muscle spindle is likely stimulated, causing the muscle to contract as a protection against the excessive stretch. On the next rapid bob or bounce, when we stretch against a contracted muscle, there is a high risk of tearing in the muscle or connective tissues. Slow, sustained stretching that does not cause pain apparently does not stimulate the muscle spindles as quickly.

SUMMARY

This chapter gives you a basic introduction to the principles of exercise physiology. First, you must develop a sound understanding of the relationships between exercise intensity and energy production in exercising muscles. Then you can apply the principles of specificity and overload to design the most appropriate program for any client.

The amount of information on exercise physiology continues to grow at a rapid pace. This chapter is, by necessity, geared to present the basics of many areas of the science of exercise. All fitness professionals must recognize the responsibility of becoming students of the literature in this field to keep abreast of the constant flow of information.

REFERENCES

American College of Sports Medicine (2006). *ACSM's Guidelines for Exercise Testing and Prescription* (7th ed.). Philadelphia: Lippincott Williams & Wilkins.

American Heart Association (2002). *Scientific Position: Risk Factors and Coronary Heart Disease.* Dallas, Tex.: American Heart Association.

Berger, M. (1995). Adjustments of insulin therapy, In: *The Health Professional's Guide to Diabetes and Exercise.* Alexandria, Va.: American Diabetes Association.

Bergstrom, J. et al. (1971). Energy-rich phosphagens in dynamic and static work, In B. Pernow & B. Saltin (Eds.) *Muscle Metabolism During Exercise* (p. 341). New York: Plenum Press.

Franklin, B.A. (1999). Exercise adds up like loose change. ACSM's Health and Fitness Journal, 3, 4, 38–39.

Jakicic, J.M. et al. (1995). Prescribing exercise in multiple short bouts versus one continuous bout: effect on adherence, cardiorespiratory fitness, and weight loss in overweight women. International Journal of Obesity, 19, 12, 893–901.

Murphy, M.H. & Hardman, A.E. (1998). Training effects of short and long bouts of brisk walking in sedentary women. *Medicine and Science in Sports and Exercise,* 30, 1, 152–157.

Pollock, M.L. et al. (1998). The recommended quantity and quality of exercise for developing and maintaining cardiorespiratory and muscular fitness, and flexibility in healthy adults. *Medicine and Science in Sports and Exercise,* 30, 6, 975–991.

SUGGESTED READING

Alter, M.J. (1996). *The Science of Flexibility* (2nd ed.). Champaign, Ill.: Human Kinetics.

Katch, F.L. & McArdle, W.D. (1988). *Nutrition, Weight Control and Exercise* (3rd ed.). Philadelphia: Lea & Febiger.

McArdle, W.D., Katch, F.I., & Katch, V.L. (2007). *Exercise Physiology: Energy, Nutrition and Human Performance* (6th ed.). Philadelphia: Lippincott Williams & Wilkins.

Richmond, M. (2000). *The Physiology Storybook.* Northbrook, Ill.: Joie Publications.

Sharkey, B.J. (1990). *Physiology of Fitness* (3rd ed.). Champaign, Ill.: Human Kinetics.

Costill, D.L. & Wilmore, J.H. (2007). *Physiology of Sport & Exercise* (4th ed.). Champaign, Ill.: Human Kinetics.

References and Suggested Reading

CHAPTER 2

Human
Anatomy

Rod A. Harter, Ph.D., A.T.C./R., is an associate professor and program director of athletic training education in the Department of Exercise and Sport Science at **Rod A. Harter** *Oregon State University in Corvallis. Dr. Harter specializes in sports medicine and biomechanics and is a fellow of the American College of Sports Medicine.*

Anatomy is a broad science concerned with the study of the structure of the body and the relationships of the body parts to one another. A fundamental understanding of human anatomy is essential for you to be able to meet your responsibilities as a personal trainer and identify appropriate activities and exercises to help clients achieve their personal fitness goals. This chapter provides a brief description of the functional anatomy of five major systems operating within the human body: the cardiovascular system, the respiratory system, the nervous system, the skeletal system, and the muscular system.

ANATOMICAL TERMINOLOGY

When studying anatomy for the first time, you may encounter descriptive terms that are unfamiliar. Use of the correct anatomical terms for position, location, and direction is essential when describing a particular movement, exercise, or activity to a client or fitness professional.

Most anatomical terms have their roots in the Latin and Greek languages and are usually quite descriptive. For example, many muscle names tell of the muscle's location, shape, or action. To illustrate, consider the posterior tibialis muscle. For our purposes, **posterior** means "toward the rear." Tibialis refers to the tibia, the larger of the two bones that connect the knee to the ankle. In this case, by knowing the meanings of the root words, you can understand both the anatomical term and the location of the muscle—the posterior tibialis muscle is found on the back of the tibia. Other important terms that describe anatomical positions are defined in Table 2.1. To help you avoid having to refer continually to a medical dictionary to define the terms used throughout this chapter, a summary of commonly used anatomical and medical terms is presented in Table 2.2. A representation of anatomical position is given in Figure 2.1, along with the anatomical planes of motion.

CARDIOVASCULAR SYSTEM

Oxygen is required for energy production and, thus, sustains cellular activity (cellular metabolism) in the human body. A by-product of this activity is carbon dioxide. Since high levels of carbon dioxide in the cells produce acidic conditions that are poisonous to cells, excess carbon dioxide must be eliminated rapidly. The cardiovascular and respiratory systems are primarily responsible for this function. The cardiovascular sys-

Table 2.1
Anatomical, Directional, and Regional Terms

Anterior (ventral)	Toward the front
Posterior (dorsal)	Toward the back
Superior	Toward the head
Inferior	Away from the head
Medial	Toward the midline of the body
Lateral	Away from the midline of the body
Proximal	Toward the attached end of the limb, origin of the structure, or midline of the body
Distal	Away from the attached end of the limb, origin of the structure, or midline of the body
Superficial	External; located close to or on the body surface
Deep	Internal; located further beneath the body surface than the superficial structures
Cervical	Regional term referring to the neck
Thoracic	Regional term referring to the portion of body between the neck and the abdomen; also known as the chest (thorax)
Lumbar	Regional term referring to the portion of the back between the abdomen and the pelvis
Plantar	The sole or bottom of the foot
Dorsal	The top surface of the foot and hands
Palmar	The anterior or ventral surface of the hands
Sagittal Plane	A longitudinal (imaginary) line that divides the body or any of its parts into right and left sections
Frontal Plane	A longitudinal (imaginary) section that divides the body into anterior and posterior parts; lies at a right angle to the sagittal plane
Transverse Plane	Also known as the horizontal plane; an imaginary line that divides the body or any of its parts into superior and inferior sections

Table 2.2
Common Anatomical (Medical) Terminology

Root	Meaning	Term	Definition
arthro	joint	arthritis	inflammation in a joint
bi	two	biceps	two-headed muscle
brachium	arm	brachialis	muscle of the arm
cardio	heart	cardiology	the study of the heart
cephalo	head	cephalic	pertaining to the head
chondro	cartilage	chondro-ectomy	excision of a cartilage
costo	rib	costo-chondral	pertaining to a rib and its cartilage
dermo	skin	dermatitis	inflammation of the skin
hemo, hemat	blood	hemorrhage	internal or external bleeding
ilio	ilium	ilium	the wide, upper part of the pelvic bone
myo	muscle	myocitis	inflammation of a muscle
os, osteo	bone	osteomalacia	softening of the bone
pulmo	lung	pulmonary artery	vessel that brings blood to the lungs
thoraco	chest	thorax	chest
tri	three	triceps brachii	three-headed muscle on arm

Cardiovascular System

FIGURE 2.1
Anatomical reference position and planes of motion.

tem is composed of blood, the blood vessels, and the heart. The cardiovascular system distributes oxygen and nutrients to the cells, carries carbon dioxide and metabolic wastes from the cells, protects against disease, helps regulate body temperature, and prevents serious blood loss after injury through the formation of clots.

Blood is the only fluid tissue in the body and is composed of two parts: formed elements, which include different types of living blood cells (white blood cells, red blood cells, platelets) and plasma, the nonliving liquid portion of blood. Plasma is about 92% water and 8% dissolved solutes. There are more than 100 different types of dissolved solutes in plasma; the most abundant of these are plasma proteins. In adults, blood accounts for about 8% of body weight; an average-sized healthy woman has about 4 to 5 liters, while an average-sized healthy man has about 5 to 6 liters of blood.

There are two types of blood vessels: **arteries,** which carry blood away from the heart (Figure 2.2a); and **veins,** which transport

FIGURE 2.2a
Major arteries
of the body
(anterior view).

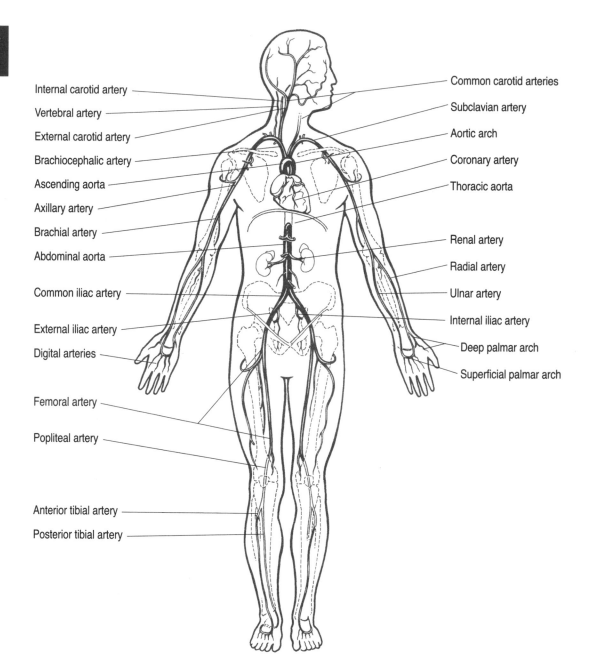

Internal carotid artery
Vertebral artery
External carotid artery
Brachiocephalic artery
Ascending aorta
Axillary artery
Brachial artery
Abdominal aorta
Common iliac artery
External iliac artery
Digital arteries
Femoral artery
Popliteal artery
Anterior tibial artery
Posterior tibial artery

Common carotid arteries
Subclavian artery
Aortic arch
Coronary artery
Thoracic aorta
Renal artery
Radial artery
Ulnar artery
Internal iliac artery
Deep palmar arch
Superficial palmar arch

blood toward the heart (Figure 2.2b). Arteries are stronger and thicker than veins, and their muscular walls help propel blood. Unlike arteries, veins contain valves to prevent the blood from flowing backward. The largest arteries are those nearest the heart; as blood flows farther away from the heart, the arteries branch into smaller vessels called **arterioles** that deliver the blood to the even smaller **capillaries.** These are microscopic blood vessels that branch to form an extensive network throughout the distal tissues. It is in the capillary beds that the critical exchange of nutrients and metabolic waste products takes place. Depleted of its oxygen and nutrients on the way from the heart to the periphery, capillary blood now begins the journey back to the heart via small vessels called **venules.** The venules are a continuation of the capillaries and join together to form veins. As the blood is transported back to the heart, the veins become larger, carrying a greater volume of blood.

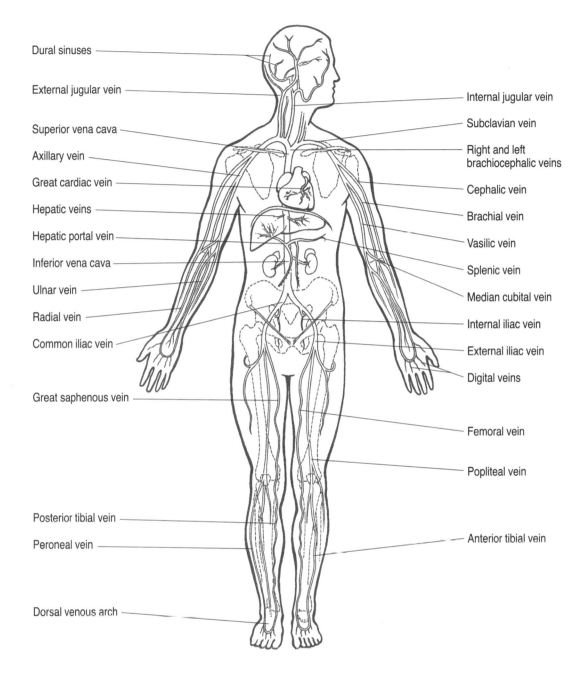

Dural sinuses

External jugular vein

Superior vena cava

Axillary vein

Great cardiac vein

Hepatic veins

Hepatic portal vein

Inferior vena cava

Ulnar vein

Radial vein

Common iliac vein

Great saphenous vein

Posterior tibial vein

Peroneal vein

Dorsal venous arch

Internal jugular vein

Subclavian vein

Right and left brachiocephalic veins

Cephalic vein

Brachial vein

Vasilic vein

Splenic vein

Median cubital vein

Internal iliac vein

External iliac vein

Digital veins

Femoral vein

Popliteal vein

Anterior tibial vein

FIGURE 2.2b
Major veins of the body (anterior view).

The human heart, a hollow, muscular organ that pumps blood throughout the blood vessels, is at the center of the cardiovascular system. In the adult, the heart is about the same size as a closed fist, and lies to the left of center, behind the sternum and between the lungs. The heart itself is divided into four chambers that receive circulating blood. The two upper chambers are called the right **atrium** and left atrium; the two lower chambers of the heart are known as the right and left **ventricles** (Figure 2.3).

The heart is a series of four separate pumps: the two primer pumps, the atria, and the two power pumps, the ventricles. Knowledge of the sequence of blood flow through the heart is fundamental to understanding the cardiovascular system. The right atrium receives blood from all parts of the body except the lungs. The superior vena cava, a large vein that drains blood from body parts above, or superior to, the heart (head, neck, arms), and the inferior vena cava, which brings blood from the

FIGURE 2.3
Structure of the
heart and flow of
blood within it.

Superior vena cava

Pulmonary veins

Right atrium

Pulmonary valve

Tricuspid valve

Right ventricle

Inferior vena cava

Aorta

Right and left
pulmonary arteries

Pulmonary trunk

Left atrium

Aortic valve

Mitral (bicuspid) valve

Left ventricle

Interventricular
septum

parts of the body below, or inferior to, the heart (legs, abdominal region), transport blood to the right atrium. During contraction of the heart, blood accumulates in the right atrium. When the heart relaxes, blood from the right atrium flows into the right ventricle, which during contraction pumps it into the pulmonary trunk. The pulmonary trunk then divides into right and left pulmonary arteries, which transport blood to the lungs, where carbon dioxide is released and oxygen is acquired. This newly oxygenated blood returns to the heart via four pulmonary veins that empty into the left atrium. The blood then passes into the left ventricle, which during contraction pumps the blood into the ascending aorta. From this point the blood is distributed to all body parts (except the lungs) by several large arteries.

RESPIRATORY SYSTEM

The respiratory system supplies oxygen, eliminates carbon dioxide, and helps regulate the acid-base balance (pH) of the body. The respiratory system

consists of the lungs and a series of passageways leading to and from them (mouth, throat, trachea, bronchi). Respiration is the overall exchange of gases (oxygen, carbon dioxide, nitrogen) between the atmosphere, the blood, and the cells. There are three general phases of respiration: external, internal, and cellular. External respiration is the exchange of oxygen and carbon dioxide between the atmosphere and the blood within the large capillaries in the lungs. Internal respiration involves the exchange of those gases between the blood and the cells of the body. Cellular respiration involves the utilization of oxygen and the production of carbon dioxide by the metabolic activity within cells. When the body is at rest, air enters the respiratory system via the nostrils and is warmed as it passes through a series of nasal cavities lined by the mucous membrane. This membrane is covered with cilia (small hairs) that filter out small particles. From the nasal cavity, inspired air next enters the pharynx (throat), which lies just posterior to the nasal and oral (mouth) cavities (Figure 2.4). The pharynx serves as a passageway for air and food and also provides a resonating chamber for

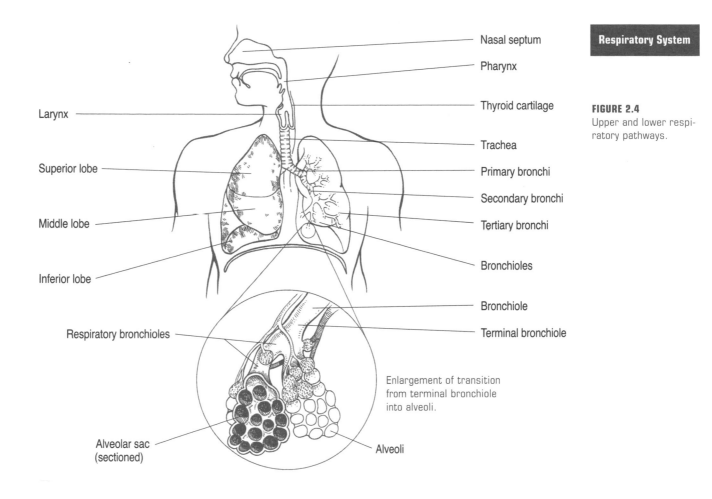

FIGURE 2.4
Upper and lower respiratory pathways.

Nasal septum

Pharynx

Thyroid cartilage

Trachea

Primary bronchi

Secondary bronchi

Tertiary bronchi

Bronchioles

Bronchiole

Terminal bronchiole

Larynx

Superior lobe

Middle lobe

Inferior lobe

Respiratory bronchioles

Enlargement of transition from terminal bronchiole into alveoli.

Alveolar sac (sectioned)

Alveoli

speech sounds. During vigorous physical activity, mouth breathing tends to predominate, and air taken in via the mouth is not filtered to the same extent as air taken in through the nostrils.

The larynx (the organ of voice) is the enlarged upper (proximal) end of the trachea (windpipe). The larynx conducts air to and from the lungs via the pharynx. An easy landmark for locating the larynx is the thyroid cartilage, or Adam's apple. The trachea is a tubular airway approximately 4½ inches (12 cm) long kept open by a series of C-shaped cartilages that function in a manner similar to the wire rings in the hose of a vacuum cleaner. The trachea extends from the larynx to approximately the level of the fifth thoracic vertebra, where it divides into the right and left primary bronchi. After the trachea divides into the right and left primary bronchi, each primary bronchus then

enters a lung and divides into smaller secondary bronchi, one for each lobe of the lung (five in total). The secondary bronchi branch into many tertiary bronchi, and these branch several times further, eventually forming tiny terminal **bronchioles.** The terminal bronchioles have microscopic branches called respiratory bronchioles that, in turn, subdivide into several alveolar ducts (plural = alveoli). The actual exchange of respiratory gases, such as oxygen and carbon dioxide, between the lungs and the blood occurs at this anatomic level. The lungs contain an estimated 300 million alveoli that provide an extremely large surface area [approximately 750 square feet (70 square meters)] for the exchange of gases. The continuous branching of the trachea resembles a tree trunk and its branches and is commonly referred to as the bronchial tree.

The final components of the respiratory system are the lungs—paired, cone-shaped

FIGURE 2.5
Spinal cord and
spinal nerves
(posterior view).

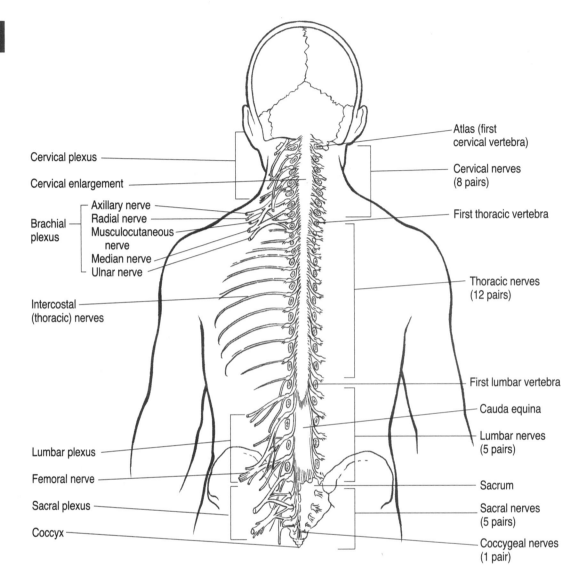

Cervical plexus

Cervical enlargement

Brachial plexus — Axillary nerve
Radial nerve
Musculocutaneous nerve
Median nerve
Ulnar nerve

Intercostal (thoracic) nerves

Lumbar plexus

Femoral nerve

Sacral plexus

Coccyx

Atlas (first cervical vertebra)

Cervical nerves (8 pairs)

First thoracic vertebra

Thoracic nerves (12 pairs)

First lumbar vertebra

Cauda equina

Lumbar nerves (5 pairs)

Sacrum

Sacral nerves (5 pairs)

Coccygeal nerves (1 pair)

organs lying in the thoracic cavity. The right lung has three lobes; the left lung has only two. The diaphragm, the muscle that forms the floor of the thoracic cavity, contracts during inspiration and relaxes to allow expiration. The lungs are separated by a space known as the mediastinum, which contains, most notably, the heart, the esophagus (the tube that connects the throat with the stomach), and a portion of the trachea.

NERVOUS SYSTEM

The nervous system is the body's control center and network for internal communication. As a personal trainer, you must understand the nervous system's

role in stimulating and controlling movement. A skeletal muscle cannot contract until it is stimulated by a nerve impulse. Without central control, coordinated human movements are impossible.

The nervous system is divided into two parts according to location: the central nervous system and the peripheral nervous system. The central nervous system (CNS), consists of the brain and the spinal cord, is completely enclosed within bony structures. The brain is protected by the skull, while the spinal cord is protected by the vertebral canal of the spinal column. The CNS is the control center of the nervous system, since it receives and integrates information from the peripheral nervous system (PNS) and formulates appropriate responses to the information. The peripheral nervous system is made up of nerves that connect the outlying parts of the body (the extremities) and their receptors within the CNS. The peripheral nervous system includes: 12 pairs of cranial nerves, 2 of which arise from the brain, while the remaining 10 pairs originate in the brain stem; and 31 pairs of spinal nerves that arise from the spinal cord. The spinal nerves include 8 cervical pairs, 12 thoracic pairs, 5 lumbar pairs, 5 sacral pairs and 1 coccygeal pair (Figure 2.5). These nerves are named and numbered according to region and the vertebral level at which they emerge from the spinal cord. For example, the first lumbar nerve (written L1) exits the spinal cord at the level of the first lumbar vertebra.

The anterior branches of the 2nd through 12th thoracic spinal nerves (written T2 through T12) innervate muscles and other structures, such as the internal organs, individually. In all other cases, the anterior branches of the spinal nerves join with adjacent nerves to form a plexus, or a network of nerve branches. There are four main plexuses in the human body: the cervical plexus (spinal nerves C1 through C4), whose nerves supply the head, neck, upper chest, and shoulders; the brachial plexus (spinal nerves C5 through T1), supplying from the shoulder down to the fingers of the hand; the lumbar plexus (spinal nerves L1 through L4), innervating the abdomen, groin, genitalia, and antero-lateral aspect of the thigh; and the sacral plexus (spinal nerves L4 through S4), which supplies the large muscles of the posterior thigh and the entire lower leg, ankle, and foot. Table 2.3 provides a summary of the primary spinal nerve roots that supply the major muscles innervated by each of these plexuses.

The nerve cells that make up the nervous system carry messages called nerve impulses that originate in either the central nervous system (brain or spinal cord) or in specialized nerve cells called receptors. Receptors are located throughout the body. Different types of receptors are sensitive to pain,

Table 2.3
Selected Spinal Nerve Roots and Major Muscles Innervated

Nerve Root	Muscles Innervated
C5	Biceps brachii, deltoid, supraspinatus, infraspinatus
C6	Brachioradialis, supinator, extensor carpi radialis longus and brevis, extensor carpi ulnaris
C7	Triceps brachii, flexor carpi radialis, flexor carpi ulnaris
C8	Extensor pollicis longus and brevis, adductor pollicis longus
T1	Intrinsic muscles of the hand (lumbricals, interossei)
L2	Psoas major and minor, adductor magnus, adductor longus, adductor brevis
L3	Rectus femoris, vastus lateralis, vastus medialis, vastus intermedius, psoas major and minor
L4	Tibialis anterior, tibialis posterior
L5	Extensor hallucis longus, extensor digitorum longus, peroneus longus and brevis, gluteus maximus, gluteus medius
S1	Gastrocnemius, soleus, biceps femoris, semitendinosus, semimembranosus, gluteus maximus
S2	Gluteus maximus, flexor hallucis longus, flexor digitorum longus
S4	Bladder, rectum

temperature, pressure, and changes in body position. Sensory nerve cells carry the impulses from the peripheral receptors to the spinal cord and brain. Motor nerve cells carry impulses away from the CNS to respond to the perceived changes in the body's internal or external environment.

An example of how this system works is the withdrawal reflex. If the hand encounters a very hot stimulus, such as an open flame, receptors in the skin of the hand send impulses to the spinal cord that communicate extreme heat and pain. In a matter of

Nervous System

milliseconds, the appropriate muscles are activated to withdraw the hand from the fire. Similarly, when performing a complex physical activity, such as an inclined bench press, the central and peripheral nervous systems work in unison to initiate, guide, and monitor all aspects of the specific activity. In this example, the nerve receptors in the periphery, located in the arm and shoulder region, provide continuous information (feedback) to the CNS regarding the amount of resistance

encountered, limb position, pressure sensed on the palms of the hands, and so on. This communication between the central and peripheral nervous systems utilizing the motor and sensory nerves is essential for us to learn, modify, and successfully perform both simple and complex physical activities.

Feeling the "burn" of fatigue in a muscle or group of muscles being heavily exercised is another example of how the feedback provided by our nervous system functions to

FIGURE 2.6
Skeletal system.

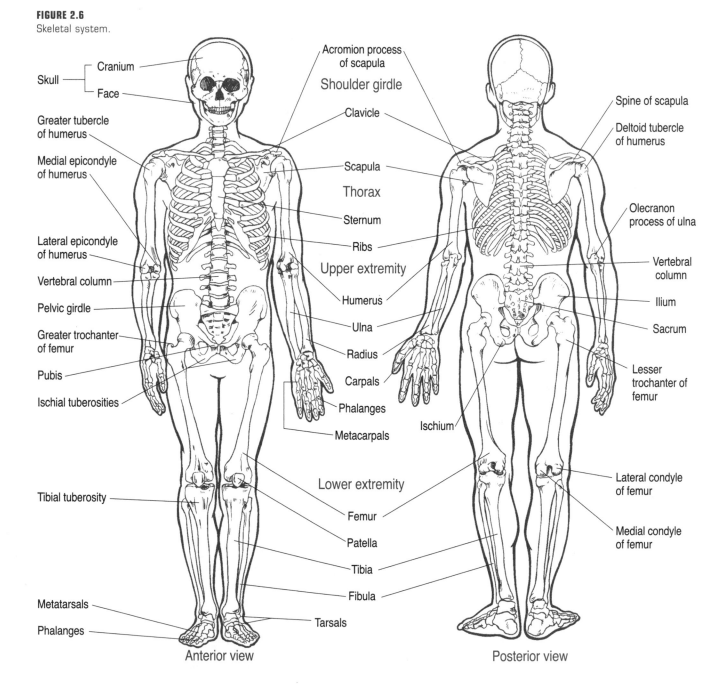

Anterior view   Posterior view

protect us. While many individuals judge the quality or quantity of a workout by the "burn" they feel in their muscles, the intense burning sensation that often accompanies muscle fatigue should be taken as a warning of an increased risk of muscle or tendon injury through overexertion, as well as a clear signal to lower the intensity level of the particular activity or workout.

SKELETAL SYSTEM

The human skeletal system consists of 206 bones (Figure 2.6) that can be divided into two sections: the axial skeleton, the 80 bones that make up the head, neck, and trunk; and the appendicular skeleton, the 126 bones that form the extremities (Table 2.4). The bones that form the skeleton combine to provide five basic yet important functions. First, the skeletal system provides protection for many of the vital organs, such as the heart, brain, and spinal cord. Second, the skeleton provides support for the soft tissues so that erect posture and the form of the body can be maintained. Third, the bones provide a framework of levers to which muscles are attached. When particular muscles contract, long bones typically act as levers to produce movement. Fourth, the red marrow of bone is responsible for the production of certain blood cells, namely red blood cells, some types of white blood cells, and platelets. Fifth, bones serve as storage areas for calcium, phosphorus, potassium, sodium, and other minerals. It is because of this high mineral content that bones remain intact for many years after death. Fat also is stored within the middle section of long bones in the medullary cavity (Figure 2.7).

Bones may also be classified according to their shape: long, short, flat, or irregular. Long bones are those in which the length exceeds the width and the thickness. Most of the bones in the lower and upper extremities are long bones, including the femur, tibia, fibula, and metatarsals in the lower limbs, and

Table 2.4
Bones in the Axial and Appendicular Skeletons

Axial Skeleton	Number of Bones
Skull	
Cranium	8
Face	14
Hyoid	1
Vertebral Column	26
Thorax	
Sternum	1
Ribs	24
(Auditory ossicles)*	6
	80

Appendicular Skeleton	Number of Bones
Lower Extremity	
Phalanges	28
Metatarsals	10
Tarsals	14
Patella	2
Tibia	2
Fibula	2
Femur	2
Pelvic Girdle	
Hip or pelvis (os coxae = ilium, ischium, pubis)	2
Shoulder Girdle	
Clavicle	2
Scapula	2
Upper Extremity	
Phalanges	28
Metacarpals	10
Carpals	16
Radius	2
Ulna	2
Humerus	2
	126

*NOTE: The auditory ossicles, three per ear, are not considered part of the axial or appendicular skeletons, but rather a separate group of bones. They were placed in the axial skeleton group for convenience.

the humerus, radius, ulna, and metacarpals in the upper extremity. Each long bone has a shaft called a diaphysis and two ends, known

FIGURE 2.7
Long bone gross
anatomy.

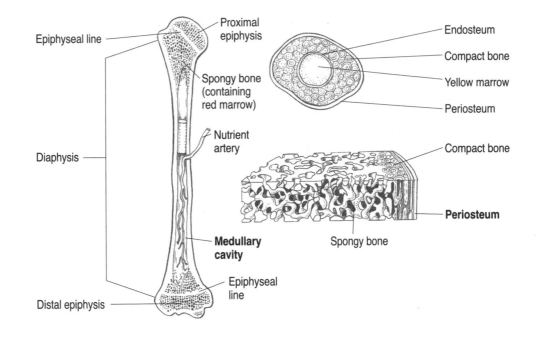

as epiphyses, that are usually wider than the shaft (singular = epiphysis). The diaphysis of a long bone is surrounded by a connective tissue sheath called the periosteum (see Figure 2.7). The periosteum has two layers: an outer layer that serves as an attachment site for muscles and tendons, and an inner layer that, when disrupted by fracture, signals the release of osteoblasts (bone-forming cells) to repair the fracture.

Short bones have no long axis but are approximately equal in length and width. They are found in the hands (carpals) and the feet (tarsals). Flat bones are partially described by their name; they are thin, but usually bent or curved rather than flat. Examples include some of the bones of the skull, the ribs, the sternum, and the scapulae (shoulder blades). Irregular bones are bones of various shapes that do not fall into the other three categories. The hip bones (os coxae), the vertebrae, and many of the bones of the skull are examples of irregular bones.

Bone is composed of an organic component made of **collagen,** a complex protein that is found in various forms within bone and other **connective tissues,** and an inorganic component composed of mineral salts, primarily calcium and potassium. According to **Wolff's Law,** bone is capable of adjusting its strength in proportion to the amount of stress placed on it. When healthy people participate in resistance-training programs for extended periods, their bones will become more dense through increases in collagen fibers and mineral salts. On the other hand, if bones are not subjected to stress, as in individuals with **sedentary** lifestyles or in the absence of gravity (as in space flight), bones will become less dense over time as mineral salts are withdrawn. An easy way to remember this important law is with the saying "Form follows function." Simply stated, the form that bone will take (strong or weak) is in direct response to the recent function of that bone.

It is important to keep this in mind when developing specific conditioning and resistance-exercise programs for your clients. Since the low levels of the hormone estrogen that accompany **amenorrhea** (two or less menstrual periods per year) and **menopause** in women lead to substantial bone mineral loss, it is important that you assist your clients in developing strength-building programs.

Axial Skeleton

As previously stated, the axial skeleton consists of the 80 bones that form the skull, the vertebral column, and the thorax (chest). This portion of the skeletal system provides the main structural support for the body and also protects the central nervous system and vital organs in the thorax (heart, lungs, etc.). Of primary importance is the adult vertebral column, consisting of 33 vertebrae divided into five groups according to the region of the body in which they are located. The upper 7 are cervical vertebrae, followed in descending order by 12 thoracic vertebrae, 5 lumbar vertebrae, 5 sacral vertebrae fused into one bone as the sacrum, and 4 coccygeal vertebrae fused together into one bone called the coccyx. The sacral vertebrae and coccygeal vertebrae become fused in the adult, so there are only 26 movable vertebrae (Figure 2.8).

Appendicular Skeleton

The appendicular skeleton consists of the bones of the lower and upper limbs and the bones that attach the legs and arms to the axial skeleton—the pelvic (hip) and pectoral (chest) girdles. The pelvic girdle consists of two large hip bones known collectively as the os coxae, with each side consisting of an ilium, an ischium, and a pubis (see Figure 2.6). Much of the weight supported by the os coxae is transferred to the bones of the lower limbs. The two pectoral girdles, each consisting of a clavicle (collarbone) and scapula (shoulder blade), attach the bones of the upper extremities to the axial skeleton at the sternum. Since this is the only attachment to or link between the upper extremities and the axial skeleton, several tradeoffs result from this configuration. Most importantly, the pectoral girdle does not provide very strong support for the upper extremity; however, the girdle does permit a wide range of movements at the shoulder, making it the most mobile joint in the body.

Articulations (Joints)

An **articulation,** or joint, is the point of contact or connection between bones, or between bones and cartilage. The stability and integrity of all joints are maintained by **ligaments,** the dense, fibrous strands of connective tissue that link together the bony segments.

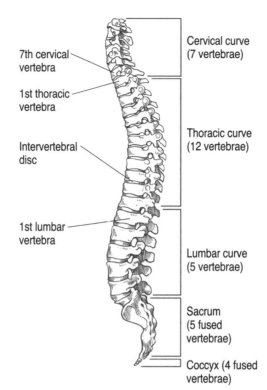

7th cervical vertebra

1st thoracic vertebra

Intervertebral disc

1st lumbar vertebra

Cervical curve (7 vertebrae)

Thoracic curve (12 vertebrae)

Lumbar curve (5 vertebrae)

Sacrum (5 fused vertebrae)

Coccyx (4 fused vertebrae)

FIGURE 2.8
Vertebral column (lateral view).

Some joints permit a large range of motion in several directions, whereas other joints permit virtually no motion at all. The various joints in the body can be classified into two general categories according to: (1) the structure of the joints; and (2) the type of movement allowed by the joints.

Structural Classification of Joints. When classifying joints according to their structure, two main characteristics differentiate the types of joints: (1) the type of connective tissue that holds the bones of the joint together, and (2) the presence or absence of a joint cavity. There are three major structural categories of joints: fibrous, cartilaginous, and synovial. Fibrous joints (syndesmoses) have no joint cavity and include all joints in which bones are held tightly together by fibrous connective tissue. Very little space separates the ends of the bones of these joints; as a result, little or no movement occurs. Examples include the joints, or sutures, between the bones of the skull, the joint between the distal tibia and fibula (Figure 2.9), and the joint between the radius and ulna.

In cartilaginous joints (synchondroses), the bones are united by cartilage. No joint cavity

Skeletal System

FIGURE 2.9
Example of a fibrous (syndesmotic) joint.

Tibia

Fibula

Fibrous connective tissue

exists and, as with fibrous joints, little or no motion occurs. Familiar examples include the joints formed by the hyaline cartilages that connect the ribs to the sternum (breastbone) and fibrocartilages that separate the bodies of vertebrae in the spinal column (Figure 2.10).

Most of the joints in the body are synovial joints (diarthroses). These joints all have a space, or joint cavity, between the bones that form them. The movement of synovial joints is limited only by the shapes of the bones of the joint and the soft tissues (ligaments, joint capsules, tendons, muscles) that surround the joint. Synovial joints have four distinguishing features that set them apart structurally from the other types of joints. First, the ends of the bones in synovial joints are covered with a thin layer of articular cartilage. The articular cartilage of synovial joints is hyaline cartilage, and although it covers the surfaces of the articulating bones, the hyaline cartilage does not attach the bones together. Second, all syn-

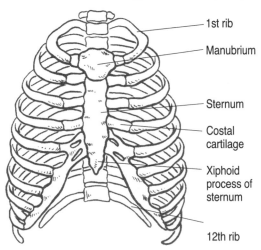

FIGURE 2.10
Example of a cartilaginous (synchrondrotic) joint.

1st rib

Manubrium

Sternum

Costal cartilage

Xiphoid process of sternum

12th rib

ovial joints are surrounded by an articular or joint capsule made of dense, fibrous connective tissue. Third, the inner surface of the joint capsule is lined with a thin synovial membrane. The primary function of the synovial membrane is the secretion of synovial fluid—the fourth unique characteristic of synovial joints. Synovial fluid acts as a lubricant for the joint and provides nutrition to the articular cartilage. Normally, only a very small amount of synovial fluid is present in even the largest joints, such as the knee and shoulder. However, acute injury to, or overuse of, a synovial joint can stimulate the synovial membrane to secrete excessive fluid, typically producing swelling and decreasing the pain-free range of motion.

In addition to these four features, some synovial joints have articular disks called menisci (singular = meniscus) that are made of fibrocartilage. In a weightbearing joint such as the knee, these cartilages help to absorb shock, increase joint stability, aid in joint nutrition by directing the flow of synovial fluid, and increase the joint contact area, thereby decreasing the pressure (load per unit area) on the weightbearing structures. A torn cartilage or meniscus, one of the most common knee injuries in sports, is simply a tearing of one of the articular disks in the joint.

Functional Classification of Joints. The functional classification of joints is based on the degree and type of movement they allow. Fibrous joints are classified as synarthroses (syn = together, arthro = joint; "an immovable joint)" (see Figure 2.9). Cartilaginous joints, which fall into the category of amphiarthroses (amphi = both sides, arthroses = joints; "cartilage on both sides of the joint"), are slightly movable (see Figure 2.10). Finally, the largest functional category of joints, diarthrodial (di = apart, arthro = joint; "apart joint"), is that of the synovial joints. Diarthroses are freely movable joints; typically, many different movements are possible at these joints.

Unlike joints classified according to the material that connects the bones together, synovial joints are classified by the movements they allow. Typically, the shapes of the bony structures forming a synovial joint are the primary factors limiting the movement of a joint. Other factors that limit motion in synovial joints are as follows: (1) ligament and/or joint capsular tension; (2) poor muscle/tendon flexibility; and (3) apposition (touching) of the soft tissues, such as the calf against the hamstrings. A summary of the major joints in the body, classified by type and movements, is presented in Table 2.5.

Movement of Synovial Joints. Recall the earlier discussion of the anatomical planes of motion used to describe the actions of the body (see Figure 2.1). For a joint to move in a given plane, there must be an axis of rotation. An **axis of rotation** is an imaginary line perpendicular to (at a right angle to) the plane of movement about which a joint rotates. Due to their configuration, many joints have several axes of rotation, enabling bones to move in the various planes.

Joints with one axis of rotation can only move in one plane and are known as uniplanar joints. Uniplanar joints also are known as "hinge" joints, since hinges only work in one plane. The ankle (talocrural) and the elbow (ulnohumeral) joints are examples of uniplanar joints. Some joints have two axes of rotation, permitting motion in two planes that are at right angles to one another. These biplanar joints, common throughout the body, include

Table 2.5
Major Joints in the Body

Region/Joint	Type	Number of Axes of Rotation	Movement(s) Possible
Lower Extremity			
Foot (metatarsophalangeal)	Synovial (condyloid)	2	Flexion & extension; abduction & adduction; circumduction
Ankle (talocrural)	Synovial (hinge)	1	Plantarflexion & dorsiflexion
Between distal tibia & fibula	Fibrous	0	Slight movement possible
Knee (tibia & femur)	Synovial (modified hinge)	2	Flexion & extension; internal & external rotation
Hip	Synovial (ball & socket)	3	Flexion & extension; abduction & adduction; circumduction; internal & external rotation
Upper Extremity			
Hand (metacarpophalangeal)	Synovial (condyloid)	2	Flexion & extension; abduction & adduction; circumduction
Thumb	Synovial (saddle)	3	Flexion & extension; abduction & adduction; circumduction; opposition
Wrist (radiocarpal)	Synovial	2	Flexion & extension; abduction & adduction; circumduction
Proximal radioulnar	Synovial (pivot)	1	Pronation & supination
Elbow (ulna & humerus)	Synovial (hinge)	1	Flexion & extension
Shoulder	Synovial (ball & socket)	3	Flexion & extension; abduction & adduction; circumduction; internal & external rotation
Ribs and sternum	Cartilaginous	0	Slight movement possible

Skeletal System

FIGURE 2.11
Movement of synovial (diarthrodial) joints.

the knee (tibiofemoral) joint, a modified hinge joint; the joints of the hand and fingers (metacarpal/phalangeal), condyloid joints; and the joints of the feet and toes (metatarsal/phalangeal joints), also condyloid joints. Multiplanar joints have three axes of motion and permit movement in three planes. Examples include the hip joint and the shoulder (glenohumeral), both of which are ball-and-socket joints, and the thumb (the first metacarpal/phalangeal joint), which is a saddle joint (Figure 2.11).

There are two basic types of movements in the various synovial joints: angular and circular. Angular movements increase or decrease

the angle between bones, and include primarily **flexion, extension, abduction,** and **adduction.** Flexion and extension occur in the **sagittal** (anterior/posterior) **plane.** Flexion usually involves a decrease in the angle between the **anterior** surfaces of articulating bones, whereas extension most often describes an increase in this angle (Figure 2.12). Exceptions are the knee and toe joints, where the reference points for flexion and extension are the **posterior** articulating surfaces of the joints.

Abduction and adduction movements always occur in the **frontal** (medial/lateral) **plane** and are defined with respect to the

Vertebral column

Shoulder joint

Elbow joint

Mediolateral axis (wrist)

Wrist joint

Extension

Flexion

Hip joint

Extension

Flexion

Mediolateral axis (hip joint)

Mediolateral axis (knee joint)

Knee joint

Flexion

Extension

Mediolateral axis (ankle)

Dorsiflexion

Plantar flexion

Ankle joint

FIGURE 2.12
Segmental movements in the sagittal plane. (Redrawn from *Biomechanics*, 3rd ed., Kreighbaum, E. & Barthels, K. Copyright 1990 by Macmillan Publishing Company. Reprinted by permission of Pearson Education, Inc.)

midline of the body. When an arm or leg is moved away from the midline of the body, abduction occurs. Adduction is the return motion from abduction and involves movement of the body part toward the midline of the body to regain **anatomical position.** Abduction and adduction movements are possible at many joints, some of which are presented in Figure 2.13.

In addition to the four primary angular movements, there are four circular movements possible at some of the synovial joints. Rotation is the motion of a bone around a central axis and is described as being either internal or external rotation of the anterior surface of the bone involved. The femur at the hip joint and the humerus at the shoulder

(glenohumeral) joint are among the most frequently rotated bones (Figure 2.14).

From the anatomical position, forearm supination and pronation are motions in the transverse or horizontal plane. Supination is a term that specifically describes the external rotation of the forearm, which causes the palm to face anteriorly. The radius and the ulna are parallel in this position, which is the anatomical position for the forearms (see Figure 2.1). Pronation describes the internal rotation of the forearm, which causes the radius to cross diagonally over the ulna and the palms to face posteriorly. The fourth circular movement, circumduction, is a sequential combination of flexion, abduction,

FIGURE 2.13
Segmental movements in the frontal plane. (Redrawn from *Biomechanics,* 3rd ed., Kreighbaum, E. & Barthels, K. Copyright 1990 by Macmillan Publishing Company. Reprinted by permission of Pearson Education, Inc.)

extension, and adduction. Similar to rotation, circumduction commonly occurs at the hip and shoulder joints. At some synovial joints, the fundamental movements are given specialized names to clarify their action. These, together with the primary angular and circular movements, are summarized in Table 2.6.

MUSCULAR SYSTEM

The anatomical system most directly affected by exercise is the muscular system. While bones and joints provide the framework for the body, it is the contraction (and relaxation) of specific

FIGURE 2.14
Segmental movements in the transverse plane. (Redrawn from *Biomechanics,* 3rd ed., Kreighbaum, E. & Barthels, K. Copyright 1990 by Macmillan Publishing Company. Reprinted by permission of Pearson Education, Inc.)

Table 2.6
Fundamental Movements (from Anatomical Position)

Plane	Action	Definition
Sagittal	Flexion	Decreasing the angle between two bones
	Extension	Increasing the angle between two bones
	Dorsiflexion	Moving the top of the foot toward the shin (only at the ankle joint)
	Plantarflexion	Moving the sole of the foot downward; "pointing the toes" (only at the ankle)
Frontal	Abduction	Motion away from the midline of the body (or part)
	Adduction	Motion toward the midline of the body (or part)
	Elevation	Moving to a superior position (only at the scapula)
	Depression	Moving to an inferior position (only at the scapula)
	Inversion	Lifting the medial border of the foot (only at the subtalar joint)
	Eversion	Lifting the lateral border of the foot (only at the subtalar joint)
Transverse	Rotation	Internal (inward) or external (outward) turning about the vertical axis of bone
	Pronation	Rotating the hand and wrist medially from the elbow
	Supination	Rotating the hand and wrist laterally from the elbow
	Horizontal flexion	From a 90-degree abducted arm position, the humerus is flexed in, toward the midline of the body in the transverse plane
	Horizontal extension	The return of the humerus from horizontal flexion
Multiplanar	Circumduction	Motion that describes a "cone"; combines flexion, abduction, extension, and adduction in sequence
	Opposition	Thumb movement unique to humans and primates

muscles that enables us to move. There are three types of muscle tissue: skeletal, cardiac, and visceral. Skeletal muscle tissue is attached to bones by **tendons** and is typically named according to its location. Skeletal muscle is voluntary muscle; that is, it can be made to contract by conscious effort. Cardiac muscle tissue forms the walls of the heart and is involuntary by nature. The third type of muscle, visceral muscle, is found in the walls of internal organs such as the stomach and intestines and in blood vessels. The contraction of visceral muscle also is involuntary and, thus, is not under conscious control. While all three types of muscle have vital functions, the structure and function of skeletal muscles warrant further discussion. Both ends of a skeletal muscle are attached to bone via tendons (a cord of connective tissue). In some cases, skeletal muscles are attached to bone by an **aponeurosis,** a broad, flat type of tendon. The wide, flat insertion of the rectus abdominis is an excellent example of an aponeurosis.

While there are more than 600 muscles in the human body, only the major muscles will be discussed in this chapter. Muscles are named according to:

- ✔ location (posterior tibialis, rectus abdominis)
- ✔ shape (deltoid, trapezius, serratus anterior, rhomboid)
- ✔ action (various muscle names include the terms extensor, flexor, abductor, adductor)
- ✔ number of divisions (biceps brachii, triceps brachii, quadriceps femoris)
- ✔ bony attachments (coracobrachialis, iliocostalis)
- ✔ size relationships (pectoralis major, pectoralis minor)

In addition, several muscles include the terms "longus" (long) and "brevis" (short) in their names.

Muscle tissue has the ability to receive and respond to input from the nervous system that may cause the muscle to contract (shorten and thicken) or relax. Muscle tissue also has elasticity so that, with proper techniques, muscles may be safely stretched. From a functional perspective, it is important to understand that most muscles of the trunk and extremities are arranged in opposing pairs. That is, when one muscle (the **agonist** muscle) is contracting to achieve a desired movement, its opposite muscle (the **antagonist** muscle) is being stretched. For example, when the abdominal muscles are contracted during a bent-knee sit-up, the erector spinae muscles are being stretched. At most joints, several muscles help (combine) to perform the same anatomical function; these muscles are functionally known as **synergists.** For example, the synergistic contractions of the gastrocnemius, soleus, and six other muscles of the leg produce plantarflexion at the ankle joint.

Muscular contraction results in motion, the maintenance of posture, and heat production. Locomotion (walking, running) is the result of the complex, combined functioning of the bones, joints, and muscles. Muscle contraction also enables the maintenance of posture in stationary positions, such as sitting and standing. Through regular contraction, muscles produce heat, which plays an important role in maintaining normal body temperature.

Muscles of the Lower Extremity

The major links of the lower extremity are the: (1) ankle joint formed by the distal tibia, distal fibula, and talus; (2) knee joint composed of the tibiofemoral and patellofemoral joints; and (3) hip joint linking the femur with the hip (coxal) bone. When compared to the muscles of the upper extremity, the muscles of the lower extremity tend to be larger and more powerful. Many of the muscles of the lower extremity cross two joints (either the hip and the knee, or the knee and the ankle). The major muscles of the lower extremity that act at more than one joint are listed in Table 2.7.

Muscles That Act at the Ankle and the Foot. The muscles of the leg are grouped into four compartments that are divided by interosseous membranes (inter = between, os = bone) between the tibia and fibula. The anterior tibial compartment muscles contract to extend the toes and dorsiflex (flex) the ankle. These muscles include the anterior tibialis, extensor digitorum longus, and extensor hallucis longus (Figure 2.15a). The muscles of the lateral tibial compartment are known as the peroneals (peroneus longus and peroneus brevis) and act to cause **eversion** (abduction) of the foot and **plantarflexion** of the ankle (Figure 2.15b). The posterior muscles of the leg are contained in two separate spaces—the **superficial** and **deep** posterior tibial compartments. The largest muscles of the calf (soleus and gastrocnemius), along with the smaller plantaris, are located in the superficial posterior tibial compartment. The deep posterior tibial compartment contains the popliteus, posterior tibialis, flexor hallucis longus, and flexor digitorum longus, (Figure 2.16). The primary functions of these posterior muscles

Table 2.7
Actions of Major Lower-extremity Multijoint Muscles

Muscle	Hip	Knee	Ankle
Rectus femoris	Flexion	Extension	—————
Biceps femoris	Extension (long head) External rotation	Flexion External rotation	—————
Semitendinosus	Extension Internal rotation	Flexion Internal rotation	—————
Semimembranosus	Extension Internal rotation	Flexion Internal rotation	—————
Gracilis	Adduction Internal rotation	Flexion Internal rotation	—————
Sartorius	Flexion External rotation	Flexion Internal rotation	—————
Gastrocnemius	————	Flexion	Plantarflexion

include plantarflexion (extension) of the ankle, flexion of the toes, and **inversion** (adduction) of the foot. The largest tendon in the body, the Achilles tendon, is found in the posterior compartment and attaches the gastrocnemius and soleus via one common tendon to the calcaneus (heel bone). The origins, insertions, primary functions, and examples of exercises to develop the muscles that act at the ankle and the foot are presented in Table 2.8.

Muscles That Act at the Knee Joint. The muscles that cross the knee joint to act on the leg (tibia and fibula) can be divided into three separate groups. The four major muscles on the front of the thigh are located in the anterior, or extensor, compartment. The primary function of these muscles is to extend the leg. They are typically grouped together and referred to as the quadriceps femoris, although each muscle has its own individual name: rectus femoris, vastus medialis, vastus intermedius, and vastus lateralis (Figure 2.17). The quadriceps insert via a common tendon known as the patellar tendon, which attaches to the tibial tuberosity (see Figure 2.6).

The muscles in the posterior, or flexor, compartment of the thigh are the biceps femoris, semitendinosus, and semimembranosus. These muscles, collectively known as the hamstrings, cross the knee joint and cause flexion of the leg. This large group of muscles has a common origin at the ischial tuberosity (see Figure 2.6). Below the knee, the biceps femoris attaches **laterally,** while the semitendinosus and semimembranosus attach on the **medial** aspect of the tibia. Between these tendons lies the popliteal space, a triangular area on the posterior aspect of the knee joint (Figure 2.18).

The third major group of muscles that act on the leg is the pes anserine group, which includes the previously mentioned semitendinosus as well as the sartorius and the gracilis (see Figures 2.17 and 2.18). These muscles are grouped together because of their common site of insertion on the medial tibia, just below the knee. The sartorius, the longest muscle in the body, originates on the ilium and courses diagonally across the anterior aspect of the thigh to its insertion on the **proximal** tibia.

FIGURE 2.15
Lower leg musculature.

a. Anterior tibial compartment muscles,
prime movers for dorsiflexion and inversion

b. Lateral tibial compartment muscles,
prime movers for eversion

Gastrocnemius   Soleus   Posterior tibialis, flexor digitorum
longus, and flexor hallucis longus

FIGURE 2.16
Posterior tibial compartment muscles primarily responsible for plantarflexion of the ankle.

Even though the sartorius is an anterior muscle, its contraction causes flexion of the leg. As a group, the three pes anserine muscles internally rotate the leg (tibia) when the knee is flexed. The origins, insertions, primary functions, and examples of exercises to develop the major muscles that act on the knee joint are presented in Table 2.9.

Muscles That Act at the Hip Joint. Most of the muscles that cross the hip joint and act on the thigh (femur) have their origins on the pelvis. Located on the anterior aspect of the hip, the psoas major and the psoas minor muscles arise from the five lumbar vertebrae. These two muscles, along with the iliacus, have a common attachment on the lesser trochanter of the femur and work together as powerful flexors of the thigh. This group of three muscles is commonly referred to as the iliopsoas muscle. The rectus femoris is the only muscle of the quadriceps femoris group that crosses the hip joint. This muscle also causes flexion of the thigh (see Figure 2.17).

Posteriorly, three large muscles combine to give shape to the buttocks and serve as

Table 2.8
Major Muscles That Act at the Ankle and Foot

Muscle	Origin	Insertion	Primary Function(s)	Selected Exercises
Anterior tibialis	Proximal ⅔ of lateral tibia	Medial aspect of 1st cuneiform and 1st metatarsal	Dorsiflexion at ankle; inversion at foot	Cycling with toe clips; resisted inversion (with dorsiflexion)
Peroneus longus	Head of fibula and proximal ⅔ of lateral fibula	Inferior aspects of medial tarsal (1st cuneiform) and 1st metatarsal	Plantarflexion at ankle; eversion at foot	Resisted eversion of foot; walking on inside of foot
Peroneus brevis	Distal ⅔ of lateral fibula	Base of the 5th metatarsal	Plantarflexion at ankle; eversion at foot	Resisted eversion of foot with rubber tubing; walking on inside of foot
Gastrocnemius	Posterior surfaces of femoral condyles	Posterior surface of calcaneus via Achilles tendon	Plantarflexion at ankle	Hill running, jumping rope, calf raises with barbell on shoulder, cycling, stair-climber machine, in-line skating
Soleus	Proximal ⅔ of posterior surfaces of tibia and fibula	Posterior surface of calcaneus via Achilles tendon	Plantarflexion at ankle	Virtually the same as for gastrocnemius; bent-knee toe raises with resistance
Posterior tibialis	Posterior surface of tibia-fibular interosseous membrane	Lower medial surfaces of medial tarsals and metatarsals	Plantarflexion at ankle; inversion at foot	Resisted inversion of foot with surgical tubing, with plantarflexion

Table 2.9
Major Muscles That Act at the Knee Joint

Muscle	Origin	Insertion	Primary Function(s)	Selected Exercises
Rectus femoris	Anterior-inferior spine of ilium	Superior aspect of patella and patellar tendon	Extension (most effective when the hip is extended)	Cycling, leg press machine, squat, vertical jumping, stair climbing, jumping rope, plyometrics
Vastus lateralis, intermedius, and medialis	Proximal ⅔ of anterior femur at midline	Patella and tibial tuberosity via the patellar tendon	Extension (particularly when the hip is flexed)	Same as for rectus femoris, resisted knee extension, in-line skating, cross-country skiing
Biceps femoris	Ischial tuberosity	Lateral condyle of tibia and head of fibula	Flexion and external rotation	Jumping rope, hamstring curls with knee in external rotation
Semitendinosus	Ischial tuberosity	Proximal anterior medial aspect of tibia	Flexion and internal rotation	Essentially the same as for biceps femoris; hamstring curls with knee in internal rotation
Semimembranosus	Ischial tuberosity	Posterior aspect of medial tibial condyle	Flexion and internal rotation	Same as semitendinosus

FIGURE 2.17
Anterior musculature of the hip and knee, prime movers for hip flexion (iliacus, psoas major and minor) and knee extension.

FIGURE 2.18
Posterior musculature of the hip and knee, prime movers for hip extension (gluteus maximus and hamstrings) and knee flexion (hamstrings and gastrocnemius).

powerful mobilizers of the hip joint. The gluteus maximus, the largest and most superficial of the three, extends and externally rotates the thigh. Underlying the gluteus maximus are the gluteus medius and the gluteus minimus, which combine to abduct and internally rotate the femur. Also on the posterior aspect of the thigh are the hamstring muscles (biceps femoris, semitendinosus, semimembranosus), whose action at the hip joint is to extend the thigh (see Figure 2.18).

The muscles located on the medial aspect of the thigh are named for both their function and their size. The adductor magnus, adductor longus, and adductor brevis work in concert to adduct the femur (Figure 2.19). The origins, insertions, primary actions, and examples of exercises to develop the major muscles that act at the hip joint are presented in Table 2.10.

Muscles That Act at the Trunk. For our discussion, the muscles of the trunk will include only the major muscles associated with the spinal column and the wall of the abdomen. Contraction of these muscles, in their agonist/antagonist relationships, results primarily in sagittal plane motion (i.e., flexion and extension of the trunk.) There are three major muscles responsible for movement of the vertebral column: the iliocostalis, the longissimus, and the spinalis, better known by their functional group name, the erector spinae. Each of the three muscles in this group has a subdivision name based on the particular portion of the spinal column to which it attaches. For example, there are three divisions of the iliocostalis muscle: the iliocostalis lumborum, iliocostalis thoracis, and iliocostalis cervicis. In addition to extending the vertebral column, unilateral contraction of the iliocostalis muscle will produce lateral flexion to that side (Figure 2.20).

Table 2.10
Major Muscles That Act at the Hip Joint

Muscle	Origin	Insertion	Primary Function(s)	Selected Exercises
Iliacus	Inner surface of the ilium and base of sacrum	Lesser trochanter of femur	Flexion and external rotation	Straight-leg sit-ups, running with knees lifted up high, leg raises
Psoas major and minor	Transverse processes of all 5 lumbar vertebrae	Lesser trochanter of femur	Flexion and external rotation	Essentially same as iliacus
Rectus femoris	Anterior-inferior spine of ilium	Superior aspect of patella and patellar tendon	Flexion	Running, leg press, squat, jumping rope
Gluteus maximus	Posterior ¼ of iliac crest and sacrum	Gluteal line of femur and iliotibial band	Extension and external rotation	Cycling, plyometrics, jumping rope, squat, stair-climbing machine
Biceps femoris	Ischial tuberosity	Lateral condyle of tibia and head of fibula	Extension	Cycling, hamstring curls with knee in external rotation
Semitendinosus	Ischial tuberosity	Proximal anterior-medial aspect of tibia	Extension	Essentially the same as for biceps femoris; hamstring curls with knee in internal rotation
Semimembranosus	Ischial tuberosity	Posterior aspect of medial tibial condyle	Extension	Same as semitendinosus
Gluteus medius and minimus	Lateral surface of ilium	Greater trochanter of femur	Abduction	Side-lying leg raises, walking, running
Adductor magnus	Pubic ramus and ischial tuberosity	Medial aspects of femur	Adduction	Side-lying bottom leg raises; manual resistance adduction exercises
Adductor brevis and longus	Pubic ramus and ischial tuberosity	Medial aspects of femur	Adduction	Side-lying bottom leg raises, resisted adduction

The walls of the abdominal cavity are supported entirely by the strength of surrounding muscles since there are no bones that provide support for this region. To make up for the lack of skeletal support, the three layers of muscles in the abdominal wall run in different directions (Figure 2.21). In the outermost (superficial) layer is the external oblique muscle, with fibers running anteriorly downward and toward the midline. In the second layer, the fibers of the internal oblique muscle run posteriorly and downward. An easy way to remember the orientations of these two muscles is to picture the fibers of the external obliques running into the front pockets of your slacks and the fibers of the internal obliques running diagonal-

ly into the rear pockets. Unilateral (one side) contraction of the lateral fibers of the obliques (external and internal) produces lateral flexion of the spinal column on that side. Trunk rotation is produced by contraction of an external oblique and an internal oblique muscle on opposite sides. Bilateral (both sides) contraction of the external and internal obliques compresses the abdominal cavity; these muscles are commonly activated during forced exhalation, defecation, and urination.

In the deepest muscular layer in the abdominal wall lies the transverse abdominis muscle. The fibers of this thin muscle run horizontally, encircling the abdominal cavity. Contraction of this muscle also compresses the abdomen (see Figure 2.21).

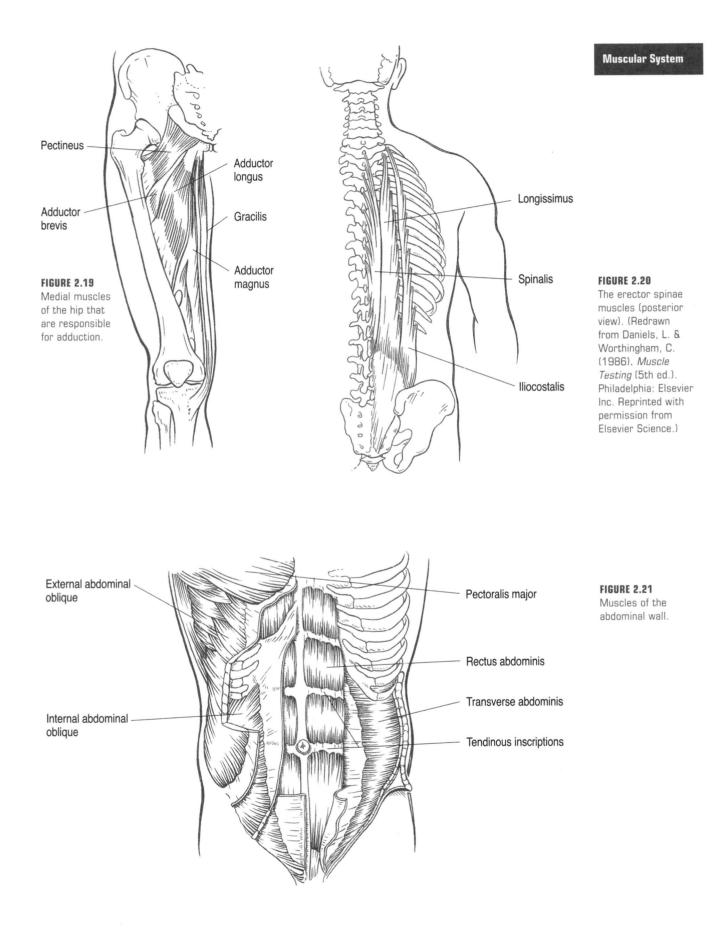

FIGURE 2.19
Medial muscles of the hip that are responsible for adduction.

Pectineus

Adductor brevis

Adductor longus

Gracilis

Adductor magnus

FIGURE 2.20
The erector spinae muscles (posterior view). (Redrawn from Daniels, L. & Worthingham, C. (1986). *Muscle Testing* (5th ed.). Philadelphia: Elsevier Inc. Reprinted with permission from Elsevier Science.)

Longissimus

Spinalis

Iliocostalis

FIGURE 2.21
Muscles of the abdominal wall.

External abdominal oblique

Internal abdominal oblique

Pectoralis major

Rectus abdominis

Transverse abdominis

Tendinous inscriptions

Muscular System

The rectus abdominis is a narrow, flat muscle on the anterior aspect of the abdominal wall that flexes the vertebral column; its fibers run vertically from the pubis to the rib cage. The rectus abdominis is crossed by three transverse fibrous bands called tendinous inscriptions (see Figure 2.21). The origins, insertions, primary functions, and examples of exercises to develop the muscles that act at the trunk are presented in Table 2.11.

Muscles of the Upper Extremity

In studying the musculature of the upper extremity, you should concentrate on understanding the motions (and muscles responsible for producing motion) at the four major links: the wrist joint, composed of the **distal** radius, ulna, and proximal carpal bones; the elbow joint, formed by the union of the olecranon process of the ulna and the distal humerus; the shoulder joint, consisting of the proximal humerus and the glenoid fossa of the scapula; and the scapulothoracic articulation. The connection between the scapula and the thorax is not a bony joint, per se, but more an important functional, soft tissue (muscle

and fascia) link between the scapula and the trunk. Similar to the lower extremity, there are many muscles in the upper extremity that act at two joints. These muscles are identified in Table 2.12.

Muscles That Act at the Wrist. The muscles that act at the wrist joint can be grouped according to their origin and function. The flexor-pronator muscles originate on the medial epicondyle of the humerus, and cause flexion of the wrist and pronation of the forearm (radius and ulna). The major wrist flexors include the flexor carpi radialis, palmaris longus, and flexor carpi ulnaris (Figure 2.22a). The major pronators of the forearm are the pronator teres at the elbow and the pronator quadratus at the wrist (Figure 2.22b). The antagonist muscles to the flexor-pronators are the extensor-supinators that arise from a common tendon on the lateral humeral epicondyle and, as their names indicate, cause extension of the wrist and supination of the forearm. The major wrist extensors are the extensor carpi radialis longus and the extensor carpi ulnaris (Figure 2.22c). Simply enough, the supinator muscle (with help from the biceps

Table 2.11
Major Muscles That Act at the Trunk

Muscle	Origin	Insertion	Primary Function(s)	Selected Exercises
Rectus abdominis	Pubic crest	Cartilage of 5th through 7th ribs and xiphoid process	Flexion and lateral flexion of the trunk	Bent-knee sit-ups, partial curl-ups, good posture, pelvic tilts
External oblique	Anteriolateral borders of lower 8 ribs	Anterior half of ilium, pubic crest, and anterior fascia	Lateral flexion of the trunk	Twisting bent-knee sit-ups (rotation opposite), and curl ups
Internal oblique	Iliac crest	Cartilage of last 3 to 4 ribs	Lateral flexion of the trunk	Twisting bent-knee sit-ups (rotation same side), and curl ups
Transverse abdominis	Iliac crest, lumbar fascia, and cartilages of last 6 ribs	Xiphoid process of sternum, anterior fascia, and pubis	Compresses abdomen	No motor function
Erector spinae	Posterior iliac crest and sacrum	Angles of ribs, transverse processes of all ribs	Extension of trunk	Squat, dead lift, prone back extension exercises, good standing posture

Muscular System

Table 2.12
Actions of Major Upper-extremity Multijoint Muscles

Muscle	Shoulder	Elbow	Forearm	Wrist
Biceps brachii	Flexion	Flexion	Supination	— —
Brachioradialis	— —	Flexion	Pronation & supination	— —
Triceps brachii	Extension (long head)	Extension	— —	— —
Flexor carpi radialis	— —	Flexion	— —	Flexion, abduction
Flexor carpi ulnaris	— —	Flexion	— —	Flexion, adduction
Extensor carpi radialis (longus and brevis)	— —	Extension	— —	Extension
Extensor carpi ulnaris	— —	Extension	— —	Extension, adduction

brachii) is responsible for supination of the forearm (see Figure 2.14). The origins, insertions, primary functions, and examples of exercises to develop the muscles that act at the wrist and forearm are presented in Table 2.13.

Muscles That Act at the Elbow Joint. The muscles that act at the elbow joint produce motion of the forearm (radius and ulna),

and are easily remembered by the motions that their contractions produce. As you recall, the elbow (ulnohumeral) joint is a hinge joint and permits motion in only one plane. In the case of the elbow, that one plane is the sagittal plane, and the only motions in the sagittal plane are flexion and extension. The flexors of the elbow, the biceps brachii, brachialis, and brachioradialis,

Medial epicondle of the humerus
Palmaris longus
Flexor carpi radialis
Flexor carpi ulnaris
Pronator teres
Pronator quadratus
Extensor carpi ulnaris
Extensor carpi radialis longus
Extensor carpi radialis brevis

a. Flexors b. Pronators c. Extensors

FIGURE 2.22
Muscles of the wrist.

Table 2.13
Major Muscles That Act at the Wrist

Muscle	Origin	Insertion	Primary Function(s)	Selected Exercises
Flexor carpi radialis	Medial epicondyle of humerus	2nd and 3rd metacarpals	Flexion	Wrist curls against resistance; grip strengthening exercises for humerus; baseball and softball; racquet sports, particularly racquetball and badminton
Flexor carpi ulnaris	Medial epicondyle of humerus	5th metacarpal	Flexion	Same as flexor carpi radialis
Extensor carpi radialis longus	Lateral epicondyle of humerus	2nd metacarpal	Extension	"Reverse" wrist curls; racquet sports, particularly tennis
Extensor carpi ulnaris	Lateral epicondyle of humerus	5th metacarpal	Extension	Same as extensor carpi radialis longus

are located on the anterior aspect of the arm (humerus) (Figure 2.23). The triceps brachii is the major extensor of the elbow joint and is located on the posterior aspect of the arm. As its name suggests, the triceps has three heads, or origins: one on the scapula and two on the proximal humerus. All three heads converge and insert, via a common tendon, into the olecranon process of the ulna (Figure 2.24). The origins, insertions, primary functions, and examples of exercises to develop muscles that act at the elbow joint and forearm are listed in Table 2.14.

Muscles That Act at the Shoulder Joint. As mentioned, the shoulder (glenohumeral) joint is the most mobile joint in the body. We will concern ourselves here with only the nine major muscles that cross the shoulder joint and act on the arm (humerus). The two largest muscles, the pectoralis major and the

Table 2.14
Major Muscles That Act at the Elbow and Forearm

Muscle	Origin	Insertion	Primary Function(s)	Selected Exercises
Biceps brachii	Long head from tubercle above glenoid cavity; short head from coracoid process of scapula	Radial tuberosity and bicipital aponeurosis	Flexion at elbow; supination at forearm	"Curling" with barbell, chin-ups, rock climbing, upright "rowing" with barbell
Brachialis	Anterior humerus	Ulnar tuberosity and coronoid process of ulna	Flexion at elbow	Same as for biceps brachii
Brachioradialis	Distal ⅔ of lateral condyloid ridge of humerus	Radial styloid process	Flexion at elbow	Same as for biceps brachii
Triceps brachii	Long head from lower edge of glenoid cavity of scapula; lateral head from posterior humerus; short head from distal ⅔ of posterior humerus	Olecranon process of ulna	Extension at elbow	Push-ups, dips on parallel bars, bench press, military press
Pronator teres	Distal end of medial humerus and medial aspect of ulna	Middle ⅓ of lateral radius	Flexion at elbow; pronation at forearm	Pronation of forearm with dumbbell

latissimus dorsi have their origins on the thorax. The pectoralis major has several important functions at the shoulder: flexion in the sagittal plane, adduction in the frontal plane, and internal rotation in the transverse plane (see Figure 2.23). The latissimus dorsi arises posteriorly from the pelvis and the lumbar and lower thoracic vertebrae. Interestingly, due to its medial insertion on the arm, the latissimus shares two functions with the pectoralis major. While the latissimus dorsi is a prime extensor of the shoulder joint, it complements the pectoralis as an adductor and internal rotator of the arm (Figure 2.25).

The remaining muscles that act at the shoulder joint have their origins on the scapula itself. The deltoid muscles, superficial muscles located on the superior aspect of the shoulder joint, resemble their name in several ways. The deltoid is shaped like a triangle (Greek letter delta = Δ) and is divided into three functional sections. The anterior deltoid fibers flex and internally (inwardly) rotate the arm. The middle portion of the deltoid is a primary abductor of the arm. The posterior deltoid fibers extend the arm as well as produce

Muscular System

FIGURE 2.23
Superficial musculature of the anterior chest, shoulder, and arm (humerus).

external rotation when activated (see Figures 2.23 and 2.24).

The rotator cuff muscles, a group of four small muscles, are functionally very important. These muscles act against the pull of gravity to hold the arm in the transverse plane. These muscles are frequently injured due to errors in training, such as general overuse, improper or insufficient

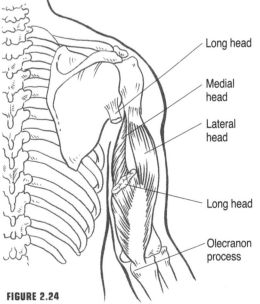

FIGURE 2.24
Triceps brachii muscle, responsible for elbow extension.

FIGURE 2.25
Superficial musculature of the superior and inferior shoulder joint, prime movers for shoulder abduction (deltoid) and adduction (latissimus dorsi and teres major). (Redrawn from Luttgens, K., Deustch, H., & Hamilton, N. (1992). *Kinesiology* (8th ed.). Madison, Wis.: Brown & Benchmark. Reprinted with permission from The McGraw-Hill Companies.)

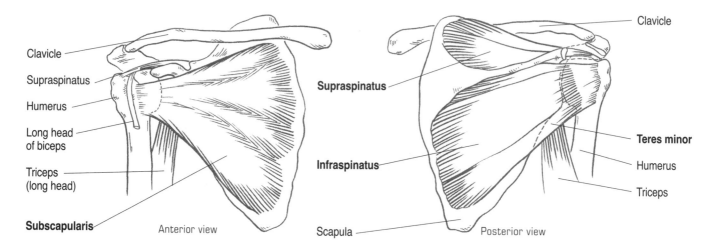

Clavicle
Supraspinatus
Humerus
Long head of biceps
Triceps (long head)
Subscapularis
Anterior view

Supraspinatus
Infraspinatus
Scapula

Clavicle
Teres minor
Humerus
Triceps
Posterior view

FIGURE 2.26
Rotator cuff muscles. (Redrawn from Luttgens, K., Deustch, H., & Hamilton, N. (1992). *Kinesiology* (8th ed.). Madison, Wis.: Brown & Benchmark. Reprinted with permission from The McGraw-Hill Companies.)

warm-up, or excessive repetitions of shoulder abduction with internal rotation. Inflammation of the rotator cuff muscles commonly results in a painful condition known as impingement syndrome in which the swollen rotator cuff muscles and the bursa are "pinched" by the scapula when the arm is abducted. If you recommend exercise regimens that include repeated overhead arm motions, such as swimming, weight training, racquet sports, and gymnastics, you should closely monitor your client's performance to avoid inducing shoulder impingement syndrome. The rotator cuff muscles are easily remembered as the SITS muscles: the supraspinatus, which abducts the arm; the infraspinatus and teres minor, which externally rotate the arm; and the subscapularis, which, as its name implies, is located on the inferior surface of the scapula, and internally rotates the arm (Figure 2.26). The origins, insertions, primary functions, and examples of exercises designed to develop the muscles that act at the shoulder joint are presented in Table 2.15.

Muscles That Act at the Scapulothoracic Articulation. The primary function of the muscles and fascia that make up the soft tissue "joint" between the scapula and the trunk is to stabilize the scapula during movement of the arm (humerus). The four major muscles that anchor the scapula are named according to their shape (trapezius, rhom-

boid major, and rhomboid minor) and function (levator scapulae) (Figure 2.27). Due to its shape and the varied directions of its fibers, the superficial trapezius has several different functions. The upper portion of the trapezius is responsible for elevation of the scapula (example: shrugging the shoulders). The middle section of the trapezius has horizontally directed fibers, resulting in adduction of the scapula when stimulated. The fibers of the lower portion of the trapezius angle downward toward their attachment on the thoracic vertebrae. Contraction of the lower trapezius primarily results in depression and adduction of the scapula.

Deep to the trapezius are the rhomboids (major and minor), which work in unison to produce adduction and slight elevation of the scapula (see Figure 2.27). Good muscle tone in the rhomboids will help maintain good upper-back posture and, thereby, avoid the "rounded shoulders" posture. The levator scapulae muscle runs from the upper cervical vertebrae to the medial border of the scapula and, together with the upper part of the trapezius, elevates the scapula. The origins, insertions, primary functions, and examples of exercises to develop the muscles of the scapulothoracic "articulation," or shoulder girdle, are presented in Table 2.16.

Table 2.15
Major Muscles That Act at the Shoulder

Muscle	Origin	Insertion	Primary Function(s)	Selected Exercises
Pectoralis major	Clavicle, sternum, and first six costal cartilages	Greater tubercle of humerus	Flexion; adduction; internal rotation	Push-ups, pull-ups, incline bench press, regular bench press, climbing a rope, all types of throwing, tennis serve
Deltoid	Anterolateral clavicle, border of the acromion, and lower edge of spine of the scapula	Deltoid tubercle of humerus on mid-lateral surface	Entire muscle: abduction; anterior fibers: flexion, internal rotation; posterior fibers: extension, external rotation	Lateral "butterfly" (abduction) exercises with dumbbells; anterior deltoid has similar functions to the pectoralis major
Latissimus dorsi	Lower six thoracic vertebrae, all lumbar vertebrae, crests of ilium and sacrum, lower four ribs	Medial side of intertubercular groove of humerus	Extension; adduction; internal rotation	Chin-ups, rope climbing, dips on parallel bars, rowing, any exercise that involves pulling the arms downward against resistance, (e.g., "lat" pulls on exercise machine)
Rotator cuff	Various aspects of scapula	All insert on greater tubercle of humerus except for the subscapularis, which inserts on the lesser tubercle of humerus	Infraspinatus and teres minor: external rotation; subscapularis: internal rotation; supraspinatus: abduction	Exercises that involve internal and external rotation, (e.g., tennis serve, throwing a baseball), internal and external rotation exercises from prone position with dumbbells

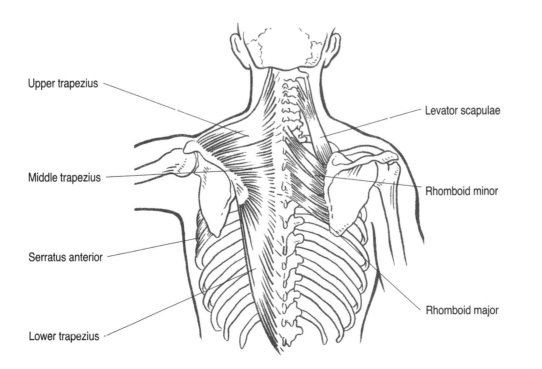

Upper trapezius

Middle trapezius

Serratus anterior

Lower trapezius

Levator scapulae

Rhomboid minor

Rhomboid major

FIGURE 2.27
Superficial and deep muscles that act at the scapulothoracic articulation.

Table 2.16
Major Muscles That Act at the Shoulder Girdle

Muscle	Origin	Insertion	Primary Function(s)	Selected Exercises
Trapezius	Occipital bone, spines of cervical and thoracic vertebrae	Acromion process and spine of scapula	Upper: elevation of scapula Middle: adduction of scapula Lower: depression of scapula	Upright rowing, shoulder shrugs with resistance
Levator scapulae	Upper four or five cervical vertebrae	Vertebral border of scapula	Elevation of scapula	Shoulder shrugs with resistance
Rhomboid major and minor	Spines of 7th cervical through 5th thoracic vertebrae	Vertebral border of scapula	Adduction and elevation of scapula	Chin-ups, supported dumbbell bent-over rows

SUMMARY

As a personal trainer, you are required to design programs that are safe and effective and that accomplish the desired fitness and/or personal goals of your clients. Without a fundamental understanding of human anatomy, this task is nearly impossible. Anatomical terminology and the five major anatomical systems—cardiovascular, respiratory, nervous, skeletal, and muscular—were presented. You now have sufficient information to identify specific exercises and physical activities that will efficiently accomplish the fitness goals of your clients.

SUGGESTED READING

Bowden, B. & Bowden, J. (2002). *An Illustrated Atlas of the Skeletal Muscles.* Englewood, Colo.: Morton.

Calais-Germain, B. (1993). *Anatomy of Movement.* Seattle: Eastland Press.

Calais-Germain, B. (1996). *Anatomy of Movement: Exercises.* Seattle: Eastland Press.

Clemente, C. (1997). *A Regional Atlas of the Human Body* (4th ed.). Philadelphia: Lippincott Williams & Wilkins.

Golding, L.A. & Golding, S.M. (2003). *Musculoskeletal Anatomy and Human Movement.* Monterey, Calif.: Healthy Learning.

Guyton, A. (2005). *Textbook of Medical Physiology* (11th ed.). Philadelphia: WB Saunders.

Hamill, J. & Knutzen, K.M. (2003). *Biomechanical Basis of Human Movement* (2nd ed.). Philadelphia: Lippincott Williams & Wilkins.

Hamilton, N. & Luttgens, K. (2002). *Kinesiology: Scientific Basis of Human Motion* (10th ed.). Boston: McGraw-Hill.

Marieb, E. (2006). *Human Anatomy and Physiology* (6th ed.). Redwood City, Calif.: Benjamin-Cummings.

Neumann, D.A. (2002). *Kinesiology of the Musculoskeletal System: Foundations for Physical Rehabilitation.* St. Louis: Mosby.

Smith, L., Weiss, E., & Lehmkuhl, L. (1996). *Brunnstrom's Clinical Kinesiology* (5th ed.). Philadelphia: F. A. Davis.

Strete, D. & Creek, C.H. (2000). *An Atlas to Human Anatomy.* Boston: McGraw-Hill.

Thompson, C. & Floyd, R. (2000). *Manual of Structural Kinesiology* (14th ed.). St. Louis: WCB/McGraw-Hill.

Tortora, G. (1999). *Principles of Human Anatomy* (8th ed.). New York: John Wiley & Sons.

Watkins, J. (1999). *Structure and Function of the Musculoskeletal System.* Champaign, Ill.: Human Kinetics.

Biomechanics and Applied Kinesiology

*Deborah Ellison, P.T., is a
registered physical therapist,
yoga instructor, and personal trainer. She has worked
with the American Council
on Exercise as director of
education, an
item-writer for
certification
exams, chair of the
Accreditation Commission,
and designer of the personal
trainer practical training
course. She has taught at
San Diego State University,
authored articles for
SHAPE and SELF
magazines, and published
several books on strength,
aerobic, flexibility, and
yoga-based training.*

**Deborah
Ellison**

The human body is a magnificent, extremely sophisticated machine. Its many parts (bones, joints, muscles, connective tissue, nerves, vessels, and organs) can produce an infinite number of movements, positions, and postures. Kinesiology is the study of those movements and postures and is grounded in the principles of two sciences: anatomy and mechanics. To understand human movement, you must know the physical struc-tures of the component parts (bones, joints, muscles) and how the physical laws of motion govern these structures (mechanics). The goal is to understand how the component parts work together to provide the stability and mobility needed for effective human performance in sports and the activities of daily living. Applying the principles of biomechanics (mechanics

Biomechanics

applied to living things) and **kinesiology** will enable you to design exercise programs that are safe, effective, and compatible with the body's function and design.

BIOMECHANICS

Motion is a change in an object's position in relation to another object. It is necessary to choose a reference point to determine whether an object is moving or at rest. For example, a sleeping baby in a car traveling 30 mph is at rest if the car seat is the reference point. If the road is the reference point, however, the baby is in motion.

To avoid confusion it also is necessary to choose a reference point to analyze the motion of the body and its parts. We use two primary reference points in the body: the joints and segments, which are body parts between two joints. For example, the upper-arm segment is between the shoulder and elbow, while the lower-leg segment is between the knee and ankle joints.

Four Types of Motion

There are four basic types of motion: rotary (Figure 3.1), translatory (Figure 3.2), curvilinear, and general plane motion.

If an object is tied down at a fixed point, it turns around that fixed point in rotary (angular) motion, much like a tetherball. Body segments generally move in rotary motion as they rotate around the joint at one end (the fixed point). When an object

in motion is not tied down anywhere and moves in a straight line, it moves in translatory or linear motion; all parts move in the same direction and at the same speed.

However, many human movements combine translatory and rotary movements to accomplish such a task as reaching for an object. In this case, the forearm and hand move straight forward because of rotary motion at the shoulder and elbow. This creates a third type of motion: curvilinear motion, which is similar to the path of a ball thrown through the air. A small gliding motion within the joint (linear or translatory) combines with the more obvious rotary motion of the segment. The gliding within the joint slightly changes the axis of rotation throughout the movement, particularly at the knee and shoulder, and is an important part of normal movement patterns.

When motions at various joints are simultaneously linear and rotary, "general plane motion" occurs. The whole body is

FIGURE 3.2
Translatory motion. Each point on the forearm/hand segment moves in a parallel path through the same distance at the same time.

FIGURE 3.1
Rotary motion. Each point in the forearm/hand segment follows the same angle, at a constant distance from the axis of rotation (A), and at the same time.

Table 3.1
Fundamental Movements (from Anatomical Position)

Plane	Action	Definition
Sagittal	Flexion	Decreasing the angle between two bones
	Extension	Increasing the angle between two bones
	Hyperextension	Increasing the angle between two bones beyond anatomical position (continuing extension past neutral)
	Dorsiflexion	Moving the top of the foot toward the shin (ankle only)
	Plantarflexion	Moving the sole of the foot downward (ankle only)
Frontal	Abduction	Motion away from the midline of the body (or body part)
	Adduction	Motion toward the midline of the body (or body part)
	Elevation	Moving the scapula to a superior position
	Depression	Moving the scapula to an inferior position
	Inversion	Lifting the medial border of the foot (subtalar joint only)
	Eversion	Lifting the lateral border of the foot (subtalar joint only)
Transverse	Rotation	Medial (inward) or lateral (outward) turning about the vertical axis of bone in the transverse plane
	Pronation	Of the forearm, rotating the hand and wrist from the elbow to the palm down position (elbow flexed) or back (elbow extended)
		Of the foot, rotation so that the sole of the foot faces somewhat laterally and the weight is borne on the inside edge of the foot.
	Supination	Of the forearm, rotating the hand and wrist from the elbow to the palm up position (elbow flexed) or forward (elbow extended)
		Of the foot, rotation so that the sole of the foot faces somewhat medially and the weight is borne on the outside edge of the foot.
	Horizontal flexion (horizontal adduction)	From a 90-degree abducted arm position, the humerus moves toward the midline of the body in the transverse plane
	Horizontal extension (horizontal abduction)	The return of the humerus from horizontal flexion (adduction) to 90-degree abduction
Multiplanar	Circumduction	Motion that describes a "cone"; combines flexion, abduction, extension, and adduction in sequential order
	Opposition	Thumb movement unique to primates and humans that follows a semicircle toward the little finger

in linear motion when we ride a bicycle, some body segments also experience rotary motion around the joints (hips, knees, ankles). The body as a whole undergoes rotary motion during a somersault or a cartwheel. At the same time, we are in linear motion across the floor. Table 3.1 provides a list of the fundamental movements with respect to anatomical position.

Forces and Motion

A force is something that tends to cause motion. Simply stated, it is a push or pull exerted by one object or substance on another. A force can be external to the body, such as gravity (the pull of the earth on a body), water, air (wind), other objects or other people. Muscular forces are considered internal forces when the body as a whole is the reference point. However, when the joint or joint axis is the reference point, muscular forces are classified as "external" because they act outside the joint itself.

In describing human movement, we often refer to motive and resistive forces. A **motive force** causes an increase in speed or a change in direction. A **resistive force** resists the motion of another external force.

In weight training the contracting muscle may be the motive force (tending to cause motion) and gravity (acting on the body segment and the dumbbell) is the resistive force (resists the motion of the motive force). This occurs in the up-phase of a lifting motion such as a "biceps curl." The contraction of the elbow flexors causes upward motion of the forearm, and the force of gravity acting on the dumbbell and the arm resists the upward movement. In the return phase of the same biceps curl the opposite occurs: the motive force is gravity, which causes downward motion. The elbow flexor contraction in the return phase resists the downward motion and is the resistive force.

There are several terms used in kinesiology to describe the various muscular actions described above. When the muscle acts as the motive force, it shortens as it cre-ates muscle tension. This is called a **concentric action.** When the muscle acts as the resistive force, it lengthens as it creates muscle tension. This is called an **eccentric action.** When muscle tension is created, but no apparent change in length occurs, the muscle action is called **isometric.** These terms are explained further on pages 76–77 (see Terms for Types of Muscular Action).

We often refer to the tools we use in strength training, such as free weights, variable-resistance machines, elastic bands or tubing, manual resistance, and body weight, as "resistance." It is important to remember, though, that they are the resistive force in one phase of the movement and the motive force in the other phase.

Levers and Torque

Body segments work as a system of levers as they rotate around the joints. A **lever** is a rigid bar with a fixed point around which it rotates when an external force is applied. The fixed point is called its **fulcrum.** In general, the center of a joint acts as a fulcrum for rotary motion of the body segments.

Rotary motion occurs in one of three planes of motion (Figure 3.3). When the body is in anatomical position, **flexion** and

FIGURE 3.3
Planes of motion.

Transverse Plane   Frontal Plane   Sagittal Plane

extension occur in the sagittal plane, **abduction** and **adduction** occur in the frontal plane, and internal and external rotation occur in the transverse plane.

The **axis of rotation** is the imaginary line or point about which the lever rotates. It intersects the center of the joint (Figure 3.4) and is perpendicular to the plane of movement. The axis of rotation is in the frontal or coronal plane (side-to-side) for movements occurring in the sagittal plane. The axis of rotation is in the sagittal plane (anterior-posterior) for movements occurring in the frontal plane. The axis of rotation is called longitudinal (superior-inferior) for movements occurring in the transverse plane.

For rotation to occur, the motive force must contact the lever at some distance from the axis of rotation. If the motive force passes through the axis of rotation, no movement will occur.

The perpendicular distance from the axis of rotation to the line of applied force is called a lever arm. The lever arm length of the motive force (F) is the force arm (Fa). The lever arm length of the resistance (R) is the resistance arm (Ra). Equilibrium occurs (the lever is in balance) if the force times the force arm equals the resistance times the resistance arm (F x Fa = R x Ra).

When a force acts on a lever at some distance from the axis of rotation a turning effect occurs. This turning effect is called **torque.** The magnitude of torque is found by multiplying the amount of force by the length of the lever arm (perpendicular distance from the axis of rotation). Therefore, F x Fa is the torque of the motive force, and R x Ra is the torque of the resistance. Rotation occurs in the direction of the greater torque.

PHYSICAL LAWS AFFECTING MOTION

To understand forces and their effects on human movement, it helps to know the physical laws

formulated by Sir Isaac Newton that govern the motion of all objects. They are the law of inertia, the law of acceleration and momentum, and the law of impact and reaction forces.

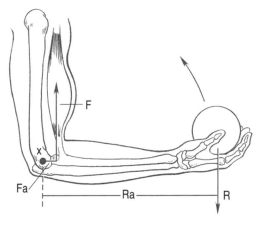

FIGURE 3.4
Example of a lever system in the human body. X = axis of rotation; F (biceps contraction) = motive force; R (weight in hand) = resistance; Fa (biceps force x distance of biceps attachment from axis) = lever arm of the motive force; Ra (weight x distance from axis) = lever arm of the resistance.

Sample Torque Calculation

A client holding a weight in his or her hand is asked to hold it steady at 90 degrees of elbow flexion. The force of the weight and the arm segment is considered to be 10 pounds. The elbow flexors are considered to act at a perpendicular distance from the elbow joint of 2 inches. The lever arm length of the weight + the arm segment is 15 inches. What is the torque of the elbow flexors in a balanced system? To calculate the torque of the elbow flexors, use the following equation:

R x Ra = F x Fa*

10 pounds x 15 inches = 150 pound-inches

In the balanced system the torque of the resistance and the torque of the elbow flexors would be equal at 150 pound-inches.

To answer the question of how much force must be created by the elbow flexors to hold the 10-pound weight steady, solve for F:

R x Ra = F x Fa

10 pounds x 15 inches = F x 2 inches

150 pound-inches = F x 2 inches

150 pound-inches / 2 inches = F

75 pounds = F

* R=resistance; Ra=resistance arm; F=motive force; Fa=force arm

**Physical Laws
Affecting Motion**

Inertia

The **law of inertia** states: A body at rest stays at rest, and a body in motion stays in motion with the same velocity and direction unless acted upon by an external force. In other words, force is required to start an object into motion and to decelerate or stop an object that is already moving.

A body's inertia is proportional to its mass. For example if you are lifting weights, a heavier weight requires more force both to set it in motion and to slow down or stop its motion than a light weight does.

Acceleration and Momentum

Newton's second law is the **law of acceleration.** It states that the force (F) acting on a body moving in a given direction is equal to the body's mass (m) multiplied by the body's acceleration (a): $F = ma$. From this we can see that the acceleration of a body is proportional to the magnitude of the force applied: $a = F/m$. So, a body's acceleration depends on how hard you push it, divided by its mass. The harder you push or pull something, the faster it will accelerate in the direction of the force.

The second law also relates to a moving body's momentum. Linear or angular momentum is the quantity of motion that a moving body possesses and is equal to its mass times its velocity. This means that a body's momentum can increase in two ways: by increasing its mass or increasing its velocity. So, when lifting a 10-pound weight and then a 20-pound weight at the same velocity, the 20-pound weight will have more momentum. Lifting a 10-pound weight at a high velocity requires more force than lifting the same weight at a lower velocity, even though the resistance is the same. As momentum increases, more force is also required to stop or change the direction of motion.

Momentum can be a positive force when playing sports like football in which players race down the field, hoping the opponents cannot match their momentum. However, in a progressive fitness-training program, your own body must be able to stop the momentum you create. Excessive momentum can cause injury, especially when working with weights, so strength training should occur at velocities that are under complete muscular control.

In other words, if you "cheat" by initiating a movement with momentum from a body part other than the one you are focusing on, the momentum of the moving weight may be greater than the muscle's ability to decelerate and stop it. The "stopping muscles" may not be strong enough to match the forces involved. Similarly, if momentum resulting from an external force, rather than muscular force (internal), is used to lift a weight that is too heavy, the opposing muscles may not be strong enough to stop the motion. This may expose the ligaments, fascia, and joints to over-stress and injury.

Impact and Reaction Forces

Newton's third law, the **law of impact and reaction forces,** states that for every force applied by one body to a second, the second applies an equal force on the first, but in the opposite direction. Thus, for every action there is an equal and opposite reaction.

This law applies to the impact forces that the body must absorb during activities such as running, jumping and high-impact aerobics, as the earth exerts a force against the body that is equal to the force applied to the earth as one runs or jumps.

Overuse and stress injuries can result from the body's inability to withstand impact and reaction forces. Impact on the feet and body mounts quickly during impact activities, especially in larger people or during activities with high acceleration. Landing impact is the body's mass (m) multiplied by its acceleration (a). The body exerts a force (m x a) on the earth; the earth exerts an equal reactive force on the body that must be dissipated through its shock-absorbing structures. Injuries often occur when the body is misaligned so that the forces are not evenly distributed, or are concentrated in the tissues that were not designed to absorb such strong forces.

This further explains why overuse and stress injuries can also occur in weight-training activities which involve momentum: the force of the tissues involved in stopping the motion must match the mass of the weight and body segment multiplied by the acceleration of the weight and body segment.

Lever Classes

As mentioned previously, the body operates as a system of levers (rigid bars rotating around fixed points). If you possess knowledge of the types and mechanics of levers, you will better understand the motion and workings of the human body.

There are three classes of levers, each determined by the relative location of its axis, force, and resistance. The first two classes are seen primarily outside the body (Figure 3.5). Levers such as the crow bar and the wheelbarrow enable us to lift or push heavy objects with relatively small forces. In these levers, the motive force acts farther away from the axis of rotation than the resistive force, allowing smaller forces to easily move large amounts of resistance. A mechanical advantage is utilized with a long lever arm. We use a relatively small amount of force at the end of a long lever arm to move a relatively large force at the end of a short lever arm.

Internally, the body operates primarily as a series of third-class levers in which the force (F) acts between the axis (X) and the resistance (R), as in the example of the biceps action at the elbow in Figure 3.4. That is, the motive force has a short lever arm and the resistance has a long lever arm. In a third-class lever system, the motive force muscles are at a mechanical disadvantage and must create a strong force to lift small amounts of resistance.

Since muscle attachments are typically close to the joint and use a short lever arm, and the bones are relatively long, with resistance

applied at the end (long lever arm), the forces necessary to lift even small weights are larger than we might imagine. For example, to abduct the arm to 80 degrees (lateral raise) with a 10-pound weight in the hand may require up to 300 pounds of tension in the deltoid. If the deltoid connected one inch farther down (longer lever arm for the motive force) and the arm were two inches shorter (shorter lever arm for the resistance), it would take much less muscular force to lift the same weight. This is why world-class weight lifters usually have relatively short arms and legs.

This is also why a lateral raise (abducting the shoulder to 80 degrees) is easier if we bend the elbow slightly or attach the weight higher on the arm. When the lever arm of the resistance is shortened, we can move it with much less tension in the deltoid. You can use the principles of levers when varying resistance for a client. To create more resistance with the same amount of weight, move the weight farther from the working joint. To lessen the resistance as fatigue occurs, move the weight closer to the working joint.

Muscles and Force Production

Although the body's lever system puts the muscles at a mechanical disadvantage in terms of force production for lifting heavy weights, it is very conducive to force production when high velocities of motion are involved. Since force equals mass times acceleration, muscular forces of the shoulders and arms can create significant striking or

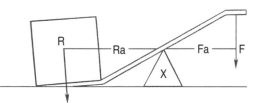

FIGURE 3.5
The first two classes of levers. X = axis of rotation (fulcrum); R = resistance load; F = effort force; Fa = lever arm distance from the force to the axis (force arm); Ra = lever arm distance from the resistance to the axis (resistance arm). The product of force and force lever arm balances the product of the resistance and resistance lever arm in this example (F x Fa = R x Ra); therefore, the resulting torques (turning effects) are equal.

FIGURE 3.6
Muscle fiber
arrangements.

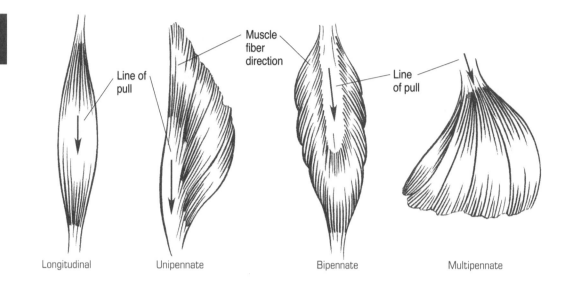

Longitudinal　　Unipennate　　Bipennate　　Multipennate

throwing forces but relatively small lifting forces. A strong contraction of upper-body muscles can provide considerable acceleration of the hand. With tools that extend the lever arm beyond the hand, such as an ax, significant forces can be achieved to accomplish a task such as splitting wood.

There also are anatomical and physiological factors that influence a muscle's ability to create force, such as the number and size of muscle fibers, fiber type and arrangement, as well as neurological training and recruitment.

There are several kinds of muscle fiber arrangements, including penniform (unipennate, bipennate, multipennate) and longitudinal (Figure 3.6). Penniform muscles are designed for higher force production than longitudinal muscles. Most muscles in the body are penniform muscles, in which the fibers lie diagonal to the line of pull. (The line of pull is generally thought of as a straight line between the muscle's two points of attachment.) A penniform muscle allows a greater number of fibers to be packaged into a given cross-sectional area, making it possible for more fibers to contribute to force production. The quadriceps is an example of a penniform muscle that can produce significant amounts of force. (Its attachments also are relatively far from the moving joints.)

Longitudinal muscles are long and thin and have parallel fibers that run in the same direction as the length of the muscle. This type of fiber arrangement allows for speed of contraction. However, since the cross section of a longitudinal muscle is small, its force of contraction is small. The sartorius and the rectus abdominis are examples of longitudinal muscles.

Anatomical, physiological, and biomechanical factors play an important role in determining the appropriate resistance for a client and in designing their conditioning program. A muscle's structure will tell you much about its primary function and how it should be trained.

BALANCE AND ALIGNMENT

To understand human motion and design appropriate exercises, you must understand several other mechanical principles that relate to the body's balance and alignment: center of gravity, the line of gravity, and base of support.

Center of Gravity

To track an object's motion we look at its center of gravity. In a rigid object of uniform density, like a baseball, this point is at its geometric center. The location of the cen-

The center of gravity (COG) lies approximately at the second sacral vertebra, point S2, anterior to the sacrum (see inset).

COG
S2
COG
Sacrum

Location of the center of gravity in the upper-trunk and lower-limb segments.

The added weight of the suitcase to the shoulder girdle causes the center of gravity to shift up and to the right. The man leans laterally to the left to bring the line of gravity back to the middle of his base of support.

FIGURE 3.7
Center of gravity.

ter of gravity in the ever-changing human body is more difficult to find. The body's center of gravity is the point at which its mass is considered to concentrate and where it is balanced on either side in all planes (frontal, sagittal, transverse). We also consider gravity as enacting its constant downward pull through this point. Thus, a body's center of mass is considered to be its center of gravity.

In an average person this point is generally located at the level of the second sacral vertebra, but it changes from person to person, depending on their build. It also changes with a person's position in space and depends on whether they are supporting external weight. See Figure 3.7 for various locations of a person's center of gravity.

Line of Gravity and Base of Support

Gravity acts on a body in a straight line through its center of gravity toward the center of the earth. This line of gravitational pull is called the line of gravity. To maintain balance without moving, a person's line of gravity must fall within the base of support, the area beneath the body that is encompassed when you connect, via one continuous line, all points of the body

that are in contact with the ground (e.g., the space between the feet if a person is standing). A large, wide base of support is more stable than a small, narrow one (Figure 3.8). Thus, standing with one's feet apart and toes turned out is more stable than placing them parallel and close together. This is why a person with balance

LOG

FIGURE 3.8
A wide base of support allows a wide excursion of the line of gravity (LOG) without permitting it to fall outside the base of support.

problems will automatically stand and walk with their feet apart. If you want to work on balance with a client, make their base of support more narrow to stimulate adaptation to the imposed demand.

To stand without excessive muscular effort or strain, the body parts must be equally distributed about the line of gravity (within the base of support). Such balanced, neutral alignment prevents excessive stress on muscles and ligaments. An important goal of exercise and training is to stimulate and reinforce neutral, symmetrical alignment about the line of gravity (static balance).

Linear and rotary motion of the whole body (walking, running, doing a flip or a dive) involve shifting the line of gravity beyond the base of support, then moving to reestablish a new base of support beneath it. The muscles exert forces to rotate and move, then reestablish equilibrium (dynamic balance).

POSTURE AND MUSCLE IMBALANCE

Neutral alignment occurs when the parts of the body are balanced and symmetrical around the line of gravity: the right and left halves of the body are mirror images of each other and the body is balanced from the front to the back allowing the spine to display its natural curves. The ankles, knees, hips, and shoulders are even and parallel to the floor, and there is a slight inward curve of the spine at the lumbar level, a slight outward curve of the spine at the thoracic level, and a slight inward curve at the cervical level (Figure 3.9). In neutral alignment the line of gravity is considered to pass just anterior to the ankle, through the center of the knee, hip, and shoulder joints and through the external meatus of the ear. A client's alignment may be assessed by comparing it to the straight vertical line of a plumb line. A plumb line follows the line of gravity and is made by

tying a weight to a string that is suspended from the ceiling.

Neutral alignment is an important consideration when working as a personal trainer. It is the position in which the spine is best equipped to deal with external stress and strain, so it is the safest position for lifting heavy objects, including weights and other tools used in strength training.

The ability to assume and maintain neutral alignment is an important neuromuscular skill that comes with repeated practice. Most acute and chronic injuries are caused by a person's inability to maintain neutral alignment during various activities. Therefore, building the strength, endurance, and flexibility necessary to attain and hold neutral in all activities is the cornerstone to an effective and functional training program. It requires static and dynamic balance and coordination as well as muscular balance in all aspects of fitness: flexi-

FIGURE 3.9
Ideal (neutral) alignment.

bility, strength, and endurance, especially when adding resistance in various body positions and in various sports maneuvers.

Muscular imbalances manifest themselves in a person's posture and alignment and are frequently influenced by work and standing, sitting, and moving habits. For example, if a person sits most of the day (working, eating, driving, watching TV) they spend many hours with their back and shoulder blades in an unbalanced, (stretched) position, and their chest, hips, and shoulders in an unbalanced, shortened position. Figure 3.10 illustrates proper sitting posture.

Habitual postures also influence a person's kinesthetic awareness, or their ability to know where their body is in space without looking. For example, many people sit with their head forward and chest collapsed. This position "feels right" to them, but the low back is in a lordosis, causing the muscles to fatigue. Their awareness of their own body alignment is inaccurate.

Allowing clients to observe their movements in a mirror or on video will help increase their awareness of correct and incorrect postures, and going through the full range of motion of the exercise several times, ending in the neutral position, can sharpen **kinesthetic awareness.**

There are several classic postural deviations that you should be able to recognize and describe: kyphosis-lordosis, flat-back posture, sway-back posture, forward-head posture, and scoliosis. **Kyphosis-lordosis** (Figure 3.11) is an increase in the normal inward curve of the low back, often accompanied by a protruding abdomen and buttocks (lordosis), increased flexion (outward curve) of the thoracic spine, rounded shoulders, and a forward-tilted head (kyphosis). **Flat-back posture** (Figure 3.12) is a decrease in the normal inward curve of the lower back, with the pelvis in posterior tilt. **Sway-back posture** (Figure 3.13) is a long outward curve of the thoracic spine with an accentuated lumbar curve and a backward shift of the upper

trunk. It is often accompanied by rounded shoulders, a sunken chest, and a forward-tilted head. **Scoliosis** (Figure 3.14) is a lateral curve of the spine. There are usually two curves on opposite sides of the spine that compensate for each other.

Table 3.2 lists several common muscle imbalances that accompany postural misalignment.

Postural deviations may be temporary or permanent. If they are temporary and caused by muscle or **connective tissue** imbalances, they can be changed with exercise. However, if the deviations are due to abnormalities of the bones, exercise will not have a primary impact. Attention to postural deviations is important because over time, the tissues, including the bones, adapt to these postures and cause the deviations to become irreversible. Clients with any of these conditions should be referred to a physician or therapist.

HUMAN MOTION TERMINOLOGY

As discussed in Chapter 2, several terms are important to know when discussing human motion. They are usually one-word descriptions of movements,

FIGURE 3.10
Good alignment of the body in the sitting position can reduce or prevent pain associated with posture-related problems and requires the least amount of muscle energy.

directions, relationships, and positions, so that discussions can be concise.

There also are terms for muscle functions and the roles muscles play during movement. An **agonist,** also called a prime mover, is a muscle that causes a desired motion. **Antagonists** are muscles that have the potential to oppose the action of the agonist. For example, if shoulder flexion is the desired action (without gravity as a factor), the shoulder flexors are the agonists and the shoulder extensors are the antagonists.

Synergist muscles assist the agonist in causing a desired action. They may act as joint stabilizers or may neutralize rotation or be activated when the external resistance increases or the agonist becomes fatigued. The term **co-contraction** describes when the agonist and antagonists contract together and a joint must be stabilized. It is an important component of functional or

usable strength because the torso muscles must be able to stabilize the spine to safely move external resistance. The muscles that co-contract to protect a joint and maintain alignment are called **stabilizers.** Stimulating strength and endurance of the stabilizers is a vital component of effective fitness training.

Terms for Types of Muscular Action

When a muscle contracts it develops tension or force as cross-bridges within muscle fibers are formed and broken. There are several types of muscle actions, named after the muscle's apparent length during the action. A muscle may actually shorten (come together), lengthen (away from the middle), or remain the same.

Static (Isometric) Action. In an **isometric action** no visible movement occurs and the resistance matches the muscular ten-

FIGURE 3.11
Kyphosis-lordosis posture.

FIGURE 3.12
Flat-back posture.

FIGURE 3.13
Sway-back posture.

FIGURE 3.14
Scoliosis.

Table 3.2
Postural Deviations and Associated Muscle Imbalances

Malalignment	Possible Tight Muscles	Possible Weak Muscles
Lordosis	Lower back (erectors), hip flexors	Abdominals (especially obliques), hip extensors
Flat-back	Upper abdominals, hip extensors	Lower back (erectors), hip flexors
Sway-back	Upper abdominals, hip flexors	Oblique abdominals, hip extensors
Kyphosis	Internal oblique, shoulder adductors (pectorals and latissimus), intercostals	Erector spinae of the thoracic spine, scapular adductors (mid and lower trapezius)
Forward-head	Cervical extensors, upper trapezius	Neck flexors

sion. The resistance may come from the opposing muscle group (co-contraction) or from another force such as gravity, an immovable object, or weight-training equipment. Bodybuilders use isometric action when striking a pose to show their muscle development, and physical therapists use isometrics in rehabilitation following an injury when a joint must not move. Isometric action also is used in PNF stretching techniques (see pages 311–312). Isometric muscle action can be used in balance and stabilization training and may be included in strength-training programs. Holding the torso upright in neutral position during a V-sit exercise (sitting on the floor with straight legs extended to form a V), or a brief hold at the top of a push-up are good examples. If isometric methods are used, the client must be able to take deep, fluid breaths throughout the individual muscle action. (See Chapter 8 for further discussion on isometric action.)

Concentric (Shortening) Action. In a **concentric action** the muscle shortens and overcomes the resistive force. For example, the biceps brachii act concentrically in the up-phase of a biceps curl with a dumbbell.

Eccentric (Lengthening) Action. In an **eccentric action** the muscle is producing force and is "lengthening," or returning to its resting length from a shortened position. The muscle "gives in" to, or is overwhelmed by, the external force and can be thought of as "putting on the brakes," or slowing the descent of a weight.

An eccentric action occurs when an external force exceeds the contractile force generated by a muscle. For example, the biceps brachii act eccentrically in the return phase of a biceps curl performed with a dumbbell.

An understanding of muscle actions is crucial to exercise analysis. Joint motion alone does not accurately reveal the muscle causing that motion.

MUSCLES AND MOVEMENTS OF THE PELVIS AND LOWER EXTREMITY

Movements of the lower body include motion of the lumbar spine, pelvis, hip, knee, and ankle joints. Figure 3.15 represents the movements of the lower body and the "normal" range of motion at each joint. The range of motion required for specific sports or activities such as dance, martial arts, or gymnastics may vary greatly and go beyond what is considered the "normal" range of motion.

The ranges of motion pictured in Figure 3.15 serve as the functional range of motion for most people, but when working with clients you will find that the range of possible movement varies from person to person. It is determined by their individual bone and joint

FIGURE 3.15
Movements of the lower body and the normal range of motion at each joint.

Hip flexion
120°
Extension
0° Neutral

Range of motion of hip flexion and extension.

Range of motion of hip abduction.
90°
50° Abduction
0° Neutral

Hip extension and hyperextension (<20°).

Hyperextension <20°
0° Neutral
Extension to neutral

Range of motion of the knee: flexion-extension, hyperextension.

Hyperextension 10°
0° Neutral
Flexion
90°
135°

Range of motion for rotation at the hip.

Neutral
35° Internal rotation
50° External rotation

Ankle range of motion with knee flexed.

0° Neutral
20° Dorsiflexion
50° Plantarflexion
90°
90°

structure, muscle mass, and soft tissue flexibility. If an individual's range is less than average, they probably need to work on flexibility.

Table 3.3 summarizes the muscles and movements of the lower body along with selected exercises for each.

Pelvis and Lumbar Spine

To teach a client to maintain neutral alignment you must understand pelvis and lower-back movements and how the two relate. Neutral position of the lumbar spine and pelvis is the central position, not flexed, extended, tilted, or rotated.

Pelvic motion is called tilt and can be anterior, posterior, or lateral (Figure 3.16). If we think of the pelvis as a bucket, then the anterior tilt is like tipping the bucket forward and spilling the water in front. It is associated with increased hip flexion and low-back **hyperextension.** The posterior tilt is tipping the bucket backward and spilling the water behind. It is associated with hip hyperextension and flexion of the low back at the lumbosacral joint. A lateral tilt is like lifting the hip to walk with a stiff knee; the pelvis would be tipped to the side. In neutral, the bucket would be straight up, not tipped in any direction. The pelvis can also rotate, which is important to normal walking. Pelvic rotation is like grasping the rim of the bucket and twisting back and forth.

Motion of the lumbar spine includes flexion, extension, hyperextension, lateral flexion, and rotation. Flexion is bending forward; extension is the return to neutral; hyperextension is further extension backward past the neutral position; lateral flexion is bending toward the side, away from the midline; and rotation is a twist, clockwise or counterclockwise, around the axis of the spine. Motion of the pelvis and the lumbar spine occur together. Therefore, the muscles responsible for lumbar motion also will cause pelvic motion. For example, the abdominals flex the spine and posteriorly tilt the pelvis. It is important to include all these lumbar spine and pelvis motions in a training program, but progressive loads must be carefully integrated.

There is nothing inherently wrong or unsafe about any spinal motion under normal circumstances. It is when static positions are maintained for long periods of time, such as sitting forward flexed at your desk all day, week after week, that problems occur. For example, constant spinal flexion loads the discs unevenly, overstretches the posterior ligaments of the back, and causes poor alignment of the upper body as well (upper spine, head, neck, and shoulders). The likelihood of problems increases if the spine is overloaded (lifting weights) when it is out of the neutral position. The spine is designed to bear loads and stresses in neutral; if it is not aligned properly those loads and stresses are transmitted unevenly and transferred to structures that were not designed for load-bearing.

Pelvic and lower-back movement can also be caused by hip muscles that attach to the pelvis. If the hamstrings (hip extensors) are tight, they can cause the pelvis to tilt posteriorly and the lumbar spine to flex. Likewise, if the hip flexors are tight, they can cause the pelvis to tilt anteriorly and the lumbar spine to hyperextend (see Figures 3.11 and 3.12). Therefore, an effective training program for the lower back and pelvis must also include strength and flexibility training for the hip muscles: flexors, extensors, abductors, adductors, and rotators. Weak or tight hip/pelvic muscles can have a significant impact on the spine.

Lumbar Extensors: Erector Spinae

The erector spinae group has three main divisions (lateral, medial, and intermediate) and extends from the sacrum to the occiput. These muscles attach to the transverse and spinous processes of all vertebrae. The muscle is large in the lumbosacral region, but divides into several segments (iliocostalis, longissimus, and spinalis) as it continues upward toward the head. The erector spinae muscles extend, hyperextend, and laterally flex the spine. When standing in neutral alignment, the activity of this muscle is very slight, but it is

Muscles and Movements of the Pelvis and Lower Extremity

Muscles and Movements of the Pelvis and Lower Extremity

Table 3.3
Lower-body Muscles—Functions and Selected Exercises

Muscle	Primary Function	Selected Exercises
Erector spinae	Trunk extension, hyperextension, lateral flexion	S/E: Active spinal extension (Figure 3.17), squats, return to good sitting posture from flexion
		F: Erector spinae stretch (Figure 3.18)
Rectus abdominis	Flexion and lateral flexion of the spine	S/E: Standing and supine pelvic tilts with resistance, supine abdominal curl-ups, straight reverse abdominal curls, abdominal crunches
External oblique	Lateral flexion of the spine	S/E: Holding neutral "press and reach," oblique abdominal curls, straight and oblique reverse abdominal curls, resisted pelvic tilts, straight abdominal curls with feet away from buttocks
Internal oblique	Lateral trunk flexion	S/E: Holding neutral "press and reach," side-lying torso raises, supine pelvic tilts, oblique abdominal curls, reverse abdominal curls
Transverse abdominis	Compresses abdominal viscera	S/E: Forceful expiration while lifting
Iliopsoas	Hip flexion and lateral rotation	S/E: Straight-leg raises, bench-stepping, knee lifts
		F: Hip flexor stretch (Figure 3.24)
Rectus femoris	Hip flexion and knee extension	S/E: Squats, bench-stepping, lunges, lunge walk, standing straight-leg raise
		F: Standing, passive knee flexion holding to ankle, posterior pelvic tilt
Sartorius	Hip flexion, abduction, and lateral rotation; knee flexion and medial rotation	S/E: Knee lift with hip external rotation, wide stance onto bench
Tensor fasciae latae	Hip flexion, medial rotation, abduction	S/E: Side-lying leg lifts with the hip slightly flexed and internally rotated
		F: Side-lying, hips extended; let top leg drop behind
Gluteus maximus	Hip extension and lateral rotation	S/E: Bench-stepping, squats, lunges, resisted hip extension in standing, jumping
Biceps femoris (hamstring)	Hip extension and knee flexion	S/E: Squat, lunge, dead lift
		F: Standing hamstring stretch (Figure 3.26)
Semitendinosus	Hip extension and knee flexion	S/E: Squat, lunge, dead lift
Semimembranosus	Hip extension and knee flexion	S/E: Same as for semitendinosus
Hip external rotators	Hip lateral rotation	S/E: Maintain hips in neutral with arches of feet lifted
		F: Rotator stretch (Figure 3.28)
Adductor magnus, brevis, and longus	Hip adduction and rotation	S/E: Walking lunges

S/E (Strength/Endurance): Exercises to improve strength and/or endurance of the muscle, depending upon the resistance and repetitions. Each exercise is not isolated to that particular muscle because muscles work in groups to cause movement; however, the exercises listed would include the designated muscle as a prime mover.

F (Flexibility): Exercises to improve the flexibility of the designated muscle. Flexibility exercises do not stretch the muscle fiber itself but are designed to lengthen the connective tissue associated with each particular muscle group. For maximum effectiveness, these exercises should be performed after the muscle group is thoroughly warmed.

Table 3.3 continued

Muscle	Primary Function	Selected Exercises
Gracilis	Hip adduction, knee flexion, and medial rotation	S/E: Same as for adductors
Pectineus	Hip flexion and hip adduction	S/E: Sitting, lift flexed knee toward opposite shoulder
Gluteus medius and minimus	Hip abduction and medial rotation	S/E: Standing leg raises to the side with elastic resistance
Quadriceps: vastus medialis, intermedius, and lateralis	Knee extension	S/E: Resisted knee extension, straight leg raises, squats, one-legged squats, lunges, bench-stepping F: Same as rectus femoris
Gastrocnemius	Ankle plantarflexion and assists with knee flexion	S/E: Bilateral heel raises, unilateral heel raises F: Sitting hamstring stretch position + active dorsiflexion
Soleus	Ankle plantarflexion	S/E: Same as for gastrocnemius, bent-knee resisted heel raises, bi- and unilateral F: Same as for gastrocnemius with knee flexed
Posterior tibialis	Foot inversion, assists with ankle plantarflexion	S/E: Resisted inversion with plantarflexion using elastic resistance
Anterior tibialis	Ankle dorsiflexion, foot inversion	S/E: Resisted dorsiflexion with inversion, toe-tapping side to side
Peroneus longus	Plantarflexion and eversion	S/E: Resisted eversion, alternate toe-and-heel lifts moving right and left
Peroneus brevis	Plantarflexion and eversion	Same as for peroneus longus

S/E (Strength/Endurance): Exercises to improve strength and/or endurance of the muscle, depending upon the resistance and repetitions. Each exercise is not isolated to that particular muscle because muscles work in groups to cause movement; however, the exercises listed would include the designated muscle as a prime mover.

F (Flexibility): Exercises to improve the flexibility of the designated muscle. Flexibility exercises do not stretch the muscle fiber itself but are designed to lengthen the connective tissue associated with each particular muscle group. For maximum effectiveness, these exercises should be performed after the muscle group is thoroughly warmed.

active in the upright position as the spine flexes forward (eccentric contraction) and when it extends again to neutral (concentric contraction).

To strengthen the erector spinae muscles, use an extension machine or have the client flex forward over the edge of a bench, table, or stability ball for full range of motion (Figure 3.17); you will have to help them stabilize their legs in the prone position. Begin with the client's arms at the side (short lever arm) and progress to crossing them on the chest or overhead, which increases lever arm length. Slowly hyperextend the spine from the prone position.

To stretch the erector spinae, have the client lie supine with the hips and knees flexed toward the shoulders (Figure 3.18). You may gently assist them by pressing upward from beneath the hips.

An important part of training the lumbar muscles is holding the lower back in neutral when lifting heavy objects and when performing squats and lunges, particularly when using resistance. When the lower back is in neutral during a lift, the spinal muscles co-contract with other torso

FIGURE 3.16
Pelvic tilt can be anterior, posterior, or lateral. The bucket of water serves as a visual aid to better illustrate the direction of the pelvic tilt.

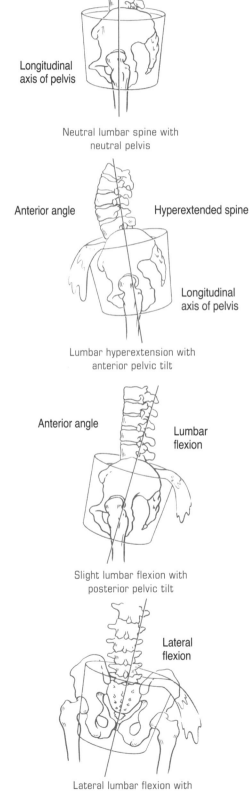

Anterior angle — Neutral spine

Longitudinal axis of pelvis

Neutral lumbar spine with neutral pelvis

Anterior angle — Hyperextended spine

Longitudinal axis of pelvis

Lumbar hyperextension with anterior pelvic tilt

Anterior angle — Lumbar flexion

Slight lumbar flexion with posterior pelvic tilt

Lateral flexion

Lateral lumbar flexion with lateral pelvic tilt

muscles to stabilize the back, keeping the load evenly distributed over the spinal structures. The actual lifting is performed by the larger, more powerful hip and knee extensors (Figure 3.19).

If the spine is flexed while lifting a heavy object, the erector spinae muscles must generate tremendous force. Consider the biomechanics of lifting with the spine in flexion: the weight held by the arms is relatively far from the fulcrum of motion, the lumbar spine (long lever arm). The spinal extensors are very close to the fulcrum of motion (short lever arm). The spinal extensors are small muscles with relatively small cross-sections and are not designed for high force production. For example, a person must lift a large box and the combined weight of the box and the upper body is 100 pounds. If the box is held where the total lever arm length is 10 inches long, the torque of the resistance is 1,000. If the spinal extensors act with a lever arm of 2 inches, their force production must be more than 500 pounds in order to lift the box by themselves. These muscles are easily strained in such a lift. The discs and posterior ligaments also are at high risk. For safety, keep the spine neutral and use the larger thigh muscles to lift heavy loads.

Lumbar Flexors: Posterior Tilters of the Pelvis

Various abdominal muscles are responsible for trunk flexion and stabilization. Consider the structure and location of the various abdominal muscles, which relate to their purpose and effective training.

The most **superficial** of the abdominal muscles are the external obliques. They arise from the outer surfaces of ribs 5 through 12, extend toward the midline of the abdomen, and insert into a broad, flat **aponeurosis.** This aponeurosis forms the outer layer of the connective-tissue sheath that covers the rectus abdominus muscle. The attachments to the ribs reach around the torso toward the back. The uppermost fibers **interdigitate** with the serratus anterior. The direction of the anterior fibers is diagonal, like putting your hands in your pockets, forward and downward toward the center, but ending several centimeters from it. This muscle also has **lateral** fibers that are more vertically aligned, between the ribs and the iliac crests (Figure 3.20).

The internal obliques are beneath the external obliques. Their fibers also run diagonally, but in the opposite direction, like an inverted V. The muscles arise from various parts of the pelvis: the inguinal ligaments, iliac crests, and lumbar aponeurosis. The fibers attach to the lower ribs and into the aponeurosis.

The obliques are thin muscles, not designed for high force production. The right and left sides of the internal and external obliques connect into the same aponeurosis, and with their other connections to the back and pelvis they essentially form a continual wrap around the torso, enclosing the internal structures, including the vertebrae, in a protective support.

The fibers of the rectus abdominus run vertically from the sternum and upper ribs

Muscles and Movements of the Pelvis and Lower Extremity

FIGURE 3.18
Erector spinae stretch. To increase the range of motion of this stretch, clients can separate the knees so that they fall on either side of the upper torso.

to the pubic bone. The rectus abdominis is a longitudinal, or "strap-like" muscle, designed for long, smooth movements.

The deepest abdominal muscle is the transversus abdominis. Its fiber direction is essentially horizontal, extending from the inner surfaces of the lower six ribs, the thoracolumbar fascia, internal surfaces of the iliac crest, and the inguinal ligaments to the linea alba by means of an aponeurosis. Its primary function is forced expiration such as coughing or sneezing, and it acts as a girdle to flatten the abdominal wall and compress the abdominal viscera.

We usually think of the abdominals as serving two functions: flexing the spine and providing support for the lower back. The rectus abdominis is the primary spinal flexor; however, it only flexes the spine in the **supine** position or in returning the torso to the upright position from hyperextension. In the upright posture, flexion is controlled by eccentric contraction of

FIGURE 3.17
Active spinal extension. The trainer should spot this exercise movement above the knees to avoid placing stress on the knee joints.

**Muscles and
Movements of
the Pelvis and
Lower Extremity**

the back extensors as they lower the weight of the torso in the same direction as gravity. The rectus is seldom used in the upright position. According to electromyograph (EMG) studies, it is not active when straining or lifting. What seems to be a rectus abdominis contraction during these activities (except coughing) is just a passive bulging of the muscles and their sheaths.

EMG studies show that the active muscles in such lifting and straining actions are the obliques. The pattern is the same with forced expiration and singing: the obliques are active, the rectus is quiet. The obliques also have a function in upright movement because as you lean or twist sideways the obliques on the opposite side contract to control the motion.

It is the obliques and the sheath of the rectus (formed by the aponeuroses of the external and internal obliques and the transversus) that protect the abdominal area during the functions of straining, lifting, bearing down, sneezing, and forced expiration. It seems logical, then, to focus training time on the obliques as well as the rectus abdominis.

Injuries occur when we fail to stabilize the torso as we push, pull, or lift or move large objects. We need "torso-stabilizing strength," not "torso-moving strength," to keep gravity from constantly pulling us out of neutral while sitting or standing.

One way to train the abdominals to stabilize the pelvis against the changing resistance of moving arms and legs is the press-and-reach exercise (Figure 3.21). Have the client lie supine with a neutral spine and shoulders and hips flexed to 90 degrees. Straighten one leg toward the floor; the movement should be slow and smooth. Return to the starting position and repeat, straightening the opposite leg. To overload, use enough resistance to fatigue the abdominals in one to two minutes.

FIGURE 3.19
Correct lifting
technique.

Stand close to the object with a wide stance. Bend knees to lower yourself to the object and keep the curve in the low back.

Stand by straightening the knees and hips, keeping the abdominal stabilizers (transverse and obliques) lifted and firm. Do not jerk up.

When upright, pivot your feet; do not simply twist your torso.

FIGURE 3.20
External and internal obliques.

Anterior fibers

Lateral fibers

Lateral fibers

Anterior fibers

External obliques

Internal obliques

Muscles Acting to Tilt the Pelvis

Active anterior pelvic tilt is achieved by contraction of the iliopsoas muscle and/or the lower-back muscles, depending on the body's position relative to gravity. The fact that the iliopsoas originates on the lumbar vertebrae tells us that it exerts a force on the pelvis as well as on the hip joint. When the hips are extended, as when standing, this muscle is too short if it passively pulls the pelvis into an anterior tilt.

The antagonists to the iliopsoas at the pelvis are those muscles that tilt the pelvis posteriorly, primarily the abdominals.

If tightness exists in the hip flexors, clients may wish to flex the hips slightly during abdominal strengthening exercises such as trunk curls (the hips should be flexed only enough to accommodate the existing muscle shortness). With their hips slightly bent and feet on the floor, the shortened iliopsoas will not pull the pelvis forward. It will be stabilized in a position of posterior tilt by an active abdominal contraction. Meanwhile, work on flexibility training for the iliopsoas. Perform torso curls at the limit of hip flexor length, so that the back is actively stabilized on the floor by abdominal action. Avoid doing this exercise when the hips are fully flexed with the feet near the buttocks, since the

FIGURE 3.21
Abdominal training for stabilization.

Lie supine with the shoulders and hips flexed.

Raise both arms overhead and straighten one leg toward the floor. Repeat, alternating legs.

Muscles Acting at the Hip Joint

back is stabilized passively with no abdominal action required. Use the tilt-and-curl to train the abdominals to actively flex the spine through the full range of motion (Figure 3.22). It should be noted that emerging evidence suggests that posteriorly tilting the pelvis when performing abdominal exercises may increase spine tissue loading (McGill, 2002). Some leading experts recommend that individuals with a history of low-back pain maintain a normal or natural lumbar curve when training their abdominal muscles (see Curl-up, page 299).

MUSCLES ACTING AT THE HIP JOINT

The hip joint is a triaxial joint that allows motion to occur in several planes. The hip has inherent stability in its bone and ligament structure and its movements include flexion and extension, hyperextension, abduction and adduction, **circumduction,** internal and external rotation,

and the hybrid horizontal abduction and adduction. All the hip muscles connect the lower extremity with the pelvis, except the psoas minor and major, which attach the femur to the lumbar spine (Figure 3.23). The psoas do, however, have action at the pelvis since they cross it.

Anterior Hip Muscles: Hip Flexors

The anterior hip muscles cause the hip to flex. They include the iliopsoas, rectus femoris, sartorius, tensor fasciae latae, and the pectineus. Hip flexion can occur by lifting the thigh toward the torso as in a knee lift or straight-leg raise, or by lifting the torso toward the thigh as in a full sit-up. The flexors also contract eccentrically to control hip extension, as in the return phase of a straight-leg raise.

Iliopsoas. The iliopsoas is actually three muscle—the psoas major, the psoas minor, and the iliacus—that function as one. It flexes the hip when the lumbar spine is sta-

FIGURE 3.22
Abdominal curl.

1. Starting position.

2. Tilt the pelvis to flatten the lower back.

3. Curl the upper torso, lifting the scapula from the floor.

5. Allow the spine to return to its natural curve.

4. Lower the upper torso.

bilized, such as in a straight-leg raise performed while lying face-up on the floor. It moves the trunk toward the thighs if the femur is stabilized, as in a sit-up done with the legs held down.

There is another condition that must be met for the iliopsoas to move the trunk toward the thighs: the movement must occur against gravity or another external resistance. Thus, bending forward from the standing position does not involve the hip flexors, but is controlled by an eccentric contraction of the hip and/or lower-back extensors.

Rectus Femoris. The rectus femoris is one of four parts of the quadriceps muscle. It attaches to the anterior inferior iliac spine and to the tibia via the patellar tendon (ligament). The concentric action of the muscle against resistance is to flex the hip and/or extend the knee. It also works eccentrically to control knee flexion in a weightbearing position, such as a squat or lunge.

Sartorius. The sartorius also originates on the anterior superior iliac spine and inserts on the medial side of the tibia below

the knee. It is a **synergist** to flex, abduct, and externally rotate the hip and to flex and inwardly rotate the knee.

Tensor Fasciae Latae. The origin of this muscle is on the outer surface of the anterior superior iliac spine and the front part of the iliac crest. It inserts into the iliotibial band about one-third of the way down the femur. It acts to flex, internally rotate, and abduct the hip, and it may also contribute to the stability of the extended knee.

Pectineus. This muscle originates on the pubic bone and inserts along the pectineal line which is found on the posterior surface of the femur. It is a synergist to hip flexion and adduction.

As a group the hip flexors are often short and tight. (See Chapter 6 for specific flexibility tests.) Tight hip flexors are not identified by hip flexion in a standing position. The tightness is seen as a forward tilt of the pelvis and lordosis of the lower back and results from the hip extension that occurs while standing. The short iliopsoas pulls the lumbar spine forward as a result of being put in a stretched position.

Muscles Acting at the Hip Joint

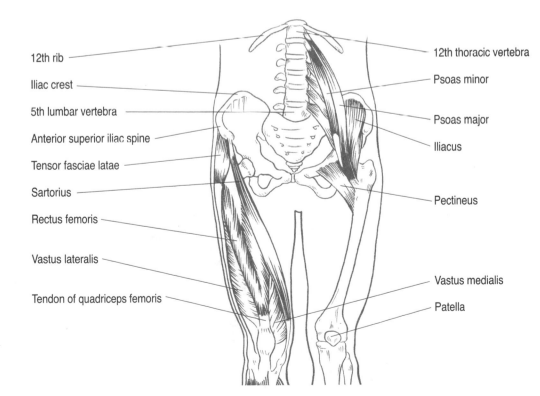

12th rib

Iliac crest

5th lumbar vertebra

Anterior superior iliac spine

Tensor fasciae latae

Sartorius

Rectus femoris

Vastus lateralis

Tendon of quadriceps femoris

12th thoracic vertebra

Psoas minor

Psoas major

Iliacus

Pectineus

Vastus medialis

Patella

FIGURE 3.23
Anterior muscles of the hip and knee.

Muscles Acting at the Hip Joint

Stretching the hip flexors is a priority in an exercise program. Figure 3.24 demonstrates an effective hip flexor stretch that will be safe for most clients. Assume a forward lunge position with the back knee bent and back heel off the floor. Use the abdominals to tilt the pelvis backward, stretching the iliopsoas. Add a stretch of the rectus femoris by dipping into a deep lunge position and adding increased flexion of the back knee.

Posterior Hip Muscles: Hip Extensors

The hip extensor muscles include the gluteus maximus and hamstrings (biceps femoris, semimembranosus, and semitendinosus). They extend the hip against gravity, as when lifting your leg behind you, and they also control hip flexion by contracting eccentrically, as in the down phase of a squat or lunge. In weightbearing positions, they work with the knee extensors (quadriceps) to move the torso up and down.

Gluteus Maximus. The largest and most superficial of the **posterior** hip muscles is the gluteus maximus. It attaches to the pelvic rim at one end and broadly along the iliotibial tract (IT band) at the other (Figure 3.25).

This muscle is a good example of why we can seldom assign a single purpose to a muscle. Its function depends on how the fibers cross the joint. Most of the fibers in the gluteus maximus cross behind the joint, so its primary role is to extend the hip. There are other fibers, though, that synergistically contribute to abduction and adduction and external rotation, depending on the position of the hip joint at the time.

The gluteus maximus plays its greatest role during walking up an inclined plane, stair climbing, jumping, and hyperextending the hip against resistance from the erect standing position.

Hamstrings. The hamstrings cross the hip and the knee and originate (except the short head of the biceps femoris) on the ischial tuberosity (see Figure 3.25). The semimembranosus and semitendinosus attach medially to the tibia, and the biceps femoris attaches laterally to the fibular head. The hamstrings extend the hip and

FIGURE 3.24
Hip flexor stretch.

Begin in a forward lunge position.

Use the abdominals to tilt the pelvis posteriorly and push the hip bone of the back leg forward.

flex the knee against resistance and are important knee stabilizers. They also help to control hip flexion in a weightbearing position by contracting eccentrically when the flexion occurs in the same direction as gravity, such as in a "dead-lift," or hip-hinge position as you bend to sit down.

Many clients have tight hamstrings. As with hip flexor tightness, you will observe it as a pelvic tilt rather than as hyperextended hips or flexed knees. Very tight hamstrings can cause the pelvis to tilt posteriorly, which shows up as a "flat-back" posture.

To effectively stretch the hamstrings combine an anterior tilt of the pelvis with hip flexion and knee extension (Figure 3.26). Place one foot on a step with a relatively straight knee and bend forward from the hip keeping the back straight and sternum lifted. Turn the tailbone toward the ceiling, as if sliding the buttocks up a wall. This tilts the pelvis forward and gives the hamstrings a better stretch. To increase the stretch, rotate the leg slightly in then out. This isolates the medial and lateral hamstrings.

The hamstrings may be weak as well, particularly in relation to quadriceps strength. It is important to include strengthening exercises in weightbearing positions that use the muscle in the same way it is used in sports or in everyday life. Squats and lunges are good examples of hamstring strengthening exercises in weightbearing positions. Isolated hamstring curls can also be used in cases of imbalance.

Deep External Rotators

The six primary hip rotators are located beneath the gluteus maximus (Figure 3.27). Their order, from top to bottom, is: piriformis, gemelli superior, obturator internus, gemelli inferior, obturator externus, and quadratus femoris. They have horizontal fibers that cross behind the joint. Their attachment to the femur is very close and behind the joint, meaning they rotate the hip externally and help the femoral head to stay in its socket. Because of their small

Iliac crest
Gluteus medius
Gluteus maximus
Gracilis
Adductor magnus
Iliotibial band
Long head ⎱ Biceps femoris
Short head ⎰
Semi-tendinosus
Medial head ⎱ Gastrocnemius
Lateral head ⎰
Semi-membranosus
Popliteal space

FIGURE 3.25
Posterior muscles of the hip and knee.

FIGURE 3.26
Standing hamstring stretch, starting position. Instruct your client to initiate the stretch by curling the buttocks upward to create more lordosis, not by bending at the waist (see arrow). Also, there should be isometric contraction of the quadriceps.

Muscles Acting at the Hip Joint

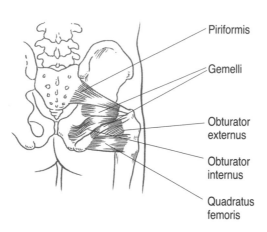

Piriformis

Gemelli

Obturator externus

Obturator internus

Quadratus femoris

FIGURE 3.27
Deep rotators of the hip. Avoid overloading these muscles with long lever arm exercises.

FIGURE 3.28
Hip rotator stretch. As a trainer, you can provide a passive over-stretch.

size and short lever arm, they are not designed to resist large forces. Their primary function seems to be stabilization and alignment of the hip.

Tightness or spasm in these muscles, particularly the piriformis, can lead to hip and leg pain, since the sciatic nerve passes through the piriformis and can become irritated. These muscles frequently become tight in runners. To stretch and relax the rotators, have the client position the hip in internal rotation (opposite to the muscles' concentric function). Greater range of motion can be achieved if the client flexes the hip (Figure 3.28).

Medial Hip Muscles: Hip Adductors

The muscles located **medial** to the hip joint adduct the hip. They include the pectineus (see Anterior Hip Muscles: Hip Flexors, page 86), and the adductor magnus, minimus, longus, and brevis (Figure 3.29). The last adductor, the gracilis, crosses the knee joint as well as the hip joint.

These muscles seem to function primarily as thigh stabilizers, especially during movements such as lunges (Figure 3.30). Their stabilizing function can also be trained by doing squats with the knees held together or by placing a ball between the knees. Figure 3.31 shows an effective stretch for these muscles.

Many female clients may want to eliminate the fat deposits and "tone" the inner thigh. You will have to explain to them that spot-reducing does not work and that they must exercise aerobically to decrease body fat stores. Muscles will become "toned" if they are functioning correctly.

Lateral Hip Muscles: Hip Abductors

The muscles that abduct the hip include the gluteus medius and minimus (Figure 3.32) and the tensor fasciae latae (see Figure 2.17, page 53).

Gluteus Medius and Minimus. These muscles are located high on the hip, not the outer thigh, and their origin is the external surface of the ilium. They insert laterally (medius) and anteriorly (minimus) on the greater trochanter of the femur. In addition to abduction, these muscles internally rotate the hip. This can occur as movement of the leg around the hip joint, but more often occurs as movement or stabilization of the pelvis (ilium) around the hip joint.

FIGURE 3.29
Adductor muscles of the hip.

— Pectineus

— Adductor brevis

— Adductor longus

— Gracilis

— Adductor magnus

Muscles Acting at the Knee and Ankle Joints

FIGURE 3.30
Hip adductor muscles help to stabilize the body in a variety of weightbearing movements. During a lunge, emphasize medial and lateral knee stabilization.

Like the hip adductors, the primary function of the abductors is that of stabilizing the hip and pelvis. Abduction occurs when the muscles contract but is not evidenced as a side leg lift. Instead it prevents adduction and keeps the pelvis even during locomotion. To clarify this function, look at Figure 3.33. As the left leg is lifted during walking, the left side of the pelvis is unsupported and would drop toward the ground if nothing stabilized it. The right hip abductors contract and pull down on the upper right rim of the pelvis to hold it even and keep the left side from dropping. So, the right hip abductors function to prevent right hip adduction and lateral tilt of the pelvis during walking.

Again, many clients are concerned about reducing the fat deposits in the upper thigh. Specific exercises for the hip abductors will not diminish body fat; only systematic aerobic exercise and proper nutrition will accomplish that goal.

MUSCLES ACTING AT THE KNEE AND ANKLE JOINTS

The knee is a hinge joint, so for general training purposes, primary motions are flexion and extension. The knee is supported medially and laterally

FIGURE 3.31
Hip adductor stretch. The objective is to move the knees as close to the floor as possible. Clients can move the feet further from the body if needed, but should not sacrifice upper-body form and alignment.

FIGURE 3.32
Abductors of the posterior hip.

Gluteus medius

Gluteus minimus (deep to gluteus medius)

Muscles Acting at the Knee and Ankle Joints

Abductors

FIGURE 3.33
Action of the abductors during walking.

Rectus femoris

Vastus lateralis

Vastus intermedius

Vastus medialis

FIGURE 3.34
Quadriceps muscles.

by ligaments. The muscles controlling knee motion are located anteriorly (the extensors) and posteriorly (the flexors).

Anterior Muscles: Knee Extensors

The knee extensors are the four quadriceps muscles: rectus femoris, vastus medialis, vastus intermedius, and vastus lateralis (Figure 3.34). As penniform muscles, they have large cross sections and are capable of producing significant force. The fibers converge at the patella, wrap around it, and attach to the tibia by way of the patellar ligament, sometimes called the patellar tendon. The patella acts like a pulley, enabling the muscle to have a favorable angle of pull even when the knee is flexed past 90 degrees.

Strong knee extensors are needed to lift heavy objects, climb stairs, and walk downhill. Therefore, weightbearing exercises such as squats, lunges, lifting, or stair climbing will probably be the most effective means of preparing them for optimum function. It is important to maintain an appropriate progression of resistance and proper alignment in these activities. Knee and lower back safety is important when

performing a squat or deep knee bend. During a squat the hip and knee extensors contract eccentrically to control hip and knee flexion in the down-phase of the movement (Figure 3.35). The motive forces are the weight of the torso and upper body; the resistive forces are the eccentric contractions of the hip and knee extensors. Although the muscles are able to sustain large forces, problems can occur with muscle imbalance and poor alignment of the knee joint. There also is potential for the patella to slip out of its track if the quadriceps' line of pull is not balanced, resulting in damage to the cartilage on the underside.

Some experts suggest that the best way to avoid knee injury in squats and lunges is to limit the degree of knee flexion to no more than 90 degrees. It may, however, be necessary to flex more than 90 degrees to lift objects from the floor.

Posterior Muscles: Knee Flexors

The primary knee flexors are the hamstrings, which were previously discussed with the hip extensors. Secondary knee flexors include the gastrocnemius, sartorius, gracilis, and popliteus (see Figures 3.23, 3.25, 3.29, and 3.36). The popliteus is a stabilizer that prevents knee dislocation when a squatting position is maintained. It also unlocks the knee by inwardly rotating from the anatomical position. The gastrocnemius, though primarily an ankle muscle, acts in certain instances to stabilize or flex the knee.

Posterior Muscles Acting at the Ankle: Plantarflexors

The gastrocnemius and soleus group make up the bulk of the muscles on the **posterior** calf (see Figure 3.36). They both cross posterior to the ankle joint so they plantarflex the ankle. Their primary function is to rotate the leg (and everything above it) around the ankle. This is a massive muscle group, designed to lift and propel the full body weight forward, not just rotate the foot at the ankle.

Gastrocnemius. This is a two-joint muscle, with a penniform fiber arrangement and a large angle of pull. It is capable of creating very large forces. Overload is achieved by performing multiple sets of heel raises on both feet, progressing to one foot. Vary the speed of contraction to train the muscle for power.

Soleus. The soleus acts with the gastrocnemius to plantarflex the ankle. It does not cross the knee. It is designed to plantarflex with the knee flexed or straight. To isolate

Muscles Acting at the Knee and Ankle Joints

FIGURE 3.35
Squat. Aim to flex knees 90° so thighs are parallel to the floor. Make sure the knees stay aligned over the ankles (do not extend the knees beyond the toes).

the soleus from the gastrocnemius, flex the knee to strengthen or stretch it.

Posterior Tibialis. This muscle is located between the tibia and fibula and connects to several bones of the foot. It is deep below the gastrocnemius and soleus muscles. It inverts the foot and participates in plantarflexion, and it also is important in maintaining the longitudinal arch of the foot.

These calf muscles are often shortened and tight. You can help your clients stretch them effectively by utilizing the stretch pictured in Figure 3.37.

Plantaris

Popliteus

Gastrocnemius

Soleus

Achilles tendon

Popliteus

Posterior tibialis

FIGURE 3.36
Posterior calf muscles.

Upper-body
Muscles:
Movements,
Functions, and
Exercise
Implications

Anterior Muscles Acting at the Ankle: Dorsiflexors

Figure 3.38 shows the **anterior** muscles of the lower leg, primarily the tibialis anterior, which functions to **dorsiflex** the foot around the ankle. These muscles located along the shin are the first line of defense in high-impact activities with regard to shock absorption. They also control the foot movements important to balance during walking and running, particularly on uneven ground. Toe tapping will provide a thorough warm-up of these muscles prior to impact activities.

When you compare the mass of the gastrocnemius and soleus group with that of the anterior muscles, their respective functions become more apparent. The small anterior muscle is designed to move the foot (small load); the large posterior muscles are designed to move the body (large load). It is easy to see how the anterior muscles become injured with the impact and momentum of running when they are not adequately conditioned.

Lateral Muscles Acting at the Ankle and Foot

The peroneus longus and brevis are the muscles that compose the lateral compartment of the lower leg (Figure 3.39). Their tendons curve around the lateral malleolus of the ankle and attach to the first and fifth metatarsal, respectively. They are designed for plantarflexion and **eversion,** so they are active in walking and also are important in maneuvering on uneven ground. For strengthening exercises for these muscles, see Ellison's *Advanced Exercise Design for Lower Body.*

UPPER-BODY MUSCLES: MOVEMENTS, FUNCTIONS, AND EXERCISE IMPLICATIONS

Upper-body motion includes movement of the head and neck, scapulae, shoulders, elbows, wrists, and hands, as well as of the cervical and thoracic spine. Table 3.4 summarizes the muscles, movements, and selected exercises for the upper body. For the purposes of this text, we

FIGURE 3.37
Stretches for the calf.

Gastrocnemius stretch. Using the wall or a chair as support, place one foot behind the other. With front knee slightly bent, back knee straight, and heel down, lean hips forward. Repeat on the opposite side.

Soleus stretch. Using a wall or chair as support, place one foot behind the other. With both knees bent and heels down, lean forward from the hips. Repeat on the opposite side.

Anterior tibialis

Extensor
digitorum longus

Extensor
hallucis
longus

FIGURE 3.38
Anterior muscles
of the lower leg.

Peroneus longus

Peroneus brevis

FIGURE 3.39
Lateral muscles
of the lower leg.

**Upper-body
Muscles:
Movements,
Functions, and
Exercise
Implications**

will not discuss the intricate, complex muscles and functions of the hand and wrist.

Shoulder and upper-arm movements are the result of a combination of movements of several joints, primarily the scapulae and the glenohumeral joint. For example, shoulder abduction to 90 degrees is a combination of 30 degrees of upward rotation of the scapula and 60 degrees of abduction at the shoulder joint. This synchronization of movement is known as scapulohumeral rhythm (Figure 3.40).

Scapular movements controlled by the shoulder girdle muscles are pictured in Figure 3.41. They include **retraction** and **protraction** (also known as scapular adduction and abduction), elevation and depression, and upward and downward rotation. These movements describe scapulae motion alone; do not confuse them with shoulder joint motion.

Scapular muscles are classified into two groups according to their location: posterior shoulder girdle and anterior shoulder girdle muscles. In activities of daily living the scapular muscles move and stabilize. They hold the upper body in position so that we can reach, flex, push, or pull with our arms and hands. Some also stabilize the humerus in its socket. Proper training

techniques can add power to arm and shoulder motions by strengthening the scapulohumeral rhythm.

Posterior Shoulder Girdle Muscles

Posterior shoulder girdle muscles earned their name because of their stabilizing function. They connect the scapula to the back of the head and torso, particularly to the spine, and they include the trapezius, rhomboids major and minor, and the levator scapulae (Figure 3.42).

Trapezius. The largest and most superficial of the posterior shoulder girdle muscles is the trapezius. It attaches along the base of the skull, at all the cervical and thoracic vertebrae, and to the scapular spine.

Because the muscle's origin is very broad, the fibers actually travel in three very different directions; as such, they almost function as three different muscles. But it is very important to seek balance among the three parts for proper upper-body function and injury prevention.

If contracting alone, the upper trapezius will elevate and retract the scapula (the scapula would move up and toward the spine). When the middle trapezius contracts alone, the scapula retracts, or moves toward the spine. The lower trapezius,

**Upper-body
Muscles:
Movements,
Functions, and
Exercise
Implications**

**Table 3.4
Upper-body muscles—Functions and Selected Exercises**

Muscle	Primary Function	Selected Exercises
Trapezius: upper	Scapular elevation; stabilizer for scapular adduction; upward rotation of the scapula, with insertion fixed, acting bilaterally; head and neck extension, unilaterally; head extension, lateral flexion, rotation to the opposite side	S/E: Lateral raises, overhead presses. Emphasize scapular rotation function to balance with lower and middle. Decrease emphasis on isolated function F: Upper trapezius stretch: depress shoulder, tilt head diagonally to opposite side (Figure 3.43)
Trapezius: middle	Scapular adduction, stabilizer for upward rotation	S/E: Middle trapezius strengthener: prone or simulated prone for antigravity position; bilateral or unilateral scapular adduction (double- or single-arm row) (Figure 3.44); Standing scapular adduction against elastic resistance pull-up F: Often already overstretched
Trapezius: lower	Scapular depression, stabilizer for scapular adduction, upward rotation	S/E: Lower trapezius strengthener: pull scapulae down and toward the middle (Figure 3.45). Prone overhead lifts, pull-up (Figure 3.46)
Rhomboids (major and minor)	Scapular adduction and elevation, downward rotation of scapula	S/E: Prone or simulated prone for antigravity position: arms extended and adducted; pull scapulae up and together upright, same motion with elastic resistance under feet
Levator scapulae	Scapular elevation, downward rotation; with insertion fixed, rotates and laterally flexes the cervical vertebrae to the same side	S/E: Prone: rotate head to the side and extend neck while lifting head off the ground F: In supine position depress scapulae, tuck chin, and flex head forward
Serratus anterior	Upward rotation of scapula, holds scapula flat on thorax, scapular abduction	S/E: Scapular push-ups (Figure 3.48), scapular abduction at end of supine pectoral fly or press; upright anterior shoulder press against elastic resistance around midback
Pectoralis minor	Tilts scapulae anteriorly; with scapulae stabilized in adduction may lift chest and assist with forced inspiration	S/E: Squeeze scapulae together, then lift chest F: Manual stretch with trainer assistance
Deltoid (anterior)	Shoulder flexion and internal rotation, stabilizer for shoulder abduction	S/E: Diagonal raise: abduct arm halfway between front and side
Deltoid (middle)	Shoulder abduction	S/E: Lateral shoulder raises with weights or elastic resistance under feet; avoid abduction with internal rotation to protect the rotator cuff from impingement
Deltoid (posterior)	Shoulder extension and external rotation, stabilizer for shoulder abduction	S/E: Forward lunge position: arms down toward the floor; abduct, extend, and externally rotate the arm; seated manual resistance
Supraspinatus (rotator cuff)	Shoulder abduction, stabilizes humeral head in glenoid fossa	S/E: Lateral shoulder raises in neutral rotation

Table 3.4 continued

Muscle	Primary Function	Selected Exercises
Infraspinatus (rotator cuff)	Shoulder external rotation, stabilizes humerus in glenoid fossa during shoulder motion	S/E: Holding elastic resistance in front at waist level, arms adducted, pull hands apart, rotating back
Teres minor (rotator cuff)	Shoulder external rotation, stabilizes humeral head in glenoid fossa during shoulder motion	S/E: Same as for infraspinatus
Subscapularis (rotator cuff)	Shoulder internal rotation, stabilizes humeral head in glenoid fossa during shoulder motion	S/E: Holding elastic resistance in back at waist level, arms adducted and elbows flexed, cross hands in front, rotating inwardly at the shoulder
Latissimus dorsi	Shoulder adduction, extension, and internal rotation	S/E: Pulling the arms downward against elastic resistance held overhead, "dips" on bench with arms abducted, lat "pull-down" to chest with neutral head, neck, and spine
Teres major	Shoulder adduction, extension, and internal rotation	S/E: Same as for latissimus dorsi
Pectoralis major	Shoulder adduction and internal rotation; upper fibers: shoulder flexion and horizontal adduction to opposite shoulder; lower fibers: horizontal adduction toward opposite iliac crest	S/E: Push-ups, (Figure 3.51) standing horizontal adduction against elastic resistance around midback, supine "bench press" or "fly"; incline bench press or fly on stability ball F: Pole stretch
Coracobrachialis	Shoulder flexion and adduction	S/E: Shoulder flexion and adduction with elbow flexed and forearm supinated
Biceps brachii	Shoulder flexion; long head assists with shoulder abduction if the humerus is externally rotated; elbow flexion and forearm supination	S/E: Biceps curls adding supination, with weights or elastic resistance under feet; use in conjunction with scapular retraction
Brachialis	Elbow flexion	S/E: Biceps curls without supination, with weights or elastic resistance under feet
Brachioradialis	Elbow flexion; assists with supination to midposition; assists with pronation to midposition	S/E: "Hammer curls": curls with forearm in neutral position (not pronated or supinated)
Triceps brachii	Elbow extension; long head may assist in shoulder adduction and extension	S/E: Push-ups; dips from bench; bench press; triceps kickback with scapular stabilization
Pronator teres	Forearm pronation; assists with elbow flexion	Curls with pronation and supination

S/E (Strength/Endurance): Exercises to improve strength and/or endurance of the muscle, depending upon the resistance and repetitions. Each exercise is not isolated to that particular muscle because muscles work in groups to cause movement; however, the exercises listed would include the designated muscle as a prime mover.

F (Flexibility): Exercises to improve the flexibility of the designated muscle. Flexibility exercises do not stretch the muscle fiber itself, but are designed to lengthen the connective tissue associated with each particular muscle group. For maximum effectiveness, these exercises should be performed after the muscle group is thoroughly warmed.

Upper-body Muscles: Movements, Functions, and Exercise Implications

Shoulder joint abduction to 90° is 30° scapular rotation and 60° abduction of the glenohumeral joint.

180°

90°

0°

As the arm is abducted over-head, the scapula outwardly (upwardly) rotates to 60°.

180°

90°

60°

0°

FIGURE 3.40
Scapulohumeral rhythm.

Elevation

Depression

Adduction (retraction)

FIGURE 3.41
Scapular movements.

Abduction (protraction)

Upward rotation

Downward rotation (return to neutral position)

acting alone, will depress and retract the scapula (the scapula moves down and in).

The trapezius, however, is designed to function not in isolated segments, but together with the other scapular muscles and muscles of the shoulder (scapulohumeral rhythm). The upper and lower trapezius, along with the serratus anterior, upwardly rotate the scapula, which occurs each time the arm is raised to the front or to the side. Downward rotation of the scapula occurs with action of the middle trapezius and rhomboids.

Imbalance of the scapular muscles can produce problems such as impingement at the shoulder joint and has also been implicated in some cases of headache and carpal tunnel syndrome. It is important to correct any imbalance that exists among the scapular muscles and to prevent its progression. Imbalances typically exist in clients before they begin a training program.

The upper trapezius is often imbalanced with the middle and lower regions of the muscle. To help create balance, concentrate more training time on the middle and lower portions of the muscle (low rows), and less time on isolated upper trapezius work (shrugs, upright rows). Design and cue exercises so that the stronger upper trapezius cannot take over for the weaker areas and reinforce the existing imbalance.

The upper trapezius may also be short and tight because of habitual postures and everyday stress. It needs stretching. Habit-ual forward-head posture with hyperextended cervical vertebrae causes the upper trapezius muscles to adapt over time to the restricted range of motion. This is especially true if work is done with the arms in front and unsupported.

To effectively stretch the upper trapezius, the muscle should be positioned with the shoulder depressed and the head tilted slightly forward and to the other side (opposite of a shoulder shrug) (Figure 3.43).

If working with free weights, strengthen the middle trapezius in antigravity positions. Have the client lie face down on a stability ball with arms out to the sides and elbows bent. Squeeze the shoulder blades together and lift the arms, keeping them parallel to the floor (Figure 3.44). Start with a short lever arm (elbows bent), progress to a long lever arm (elbows straight), and then progress to holding weights, first with elbows bent, then straight.

To perform a seated row without a machine, wrap elastic tubing around your feet and hold the ends or handles at chest level while sitting upright. Watch carefully for fatigue—it shows as the upper trapezius takes over and the shoulders begin to elevate.

A latissimus pull-down machine can be used to strengthen the lower trapezius: grip the bar and pull only the shoulder blades down and together (the elbows remain extended and the shoulders flexed) (Figure 3.45).

FIGURE 3.42
Posterior shoulder girdle muscles.

Upper trapezius

Middle trapezius

Serratus anterior

Lower trapezius

Levator scapulae

Rhomboid minor

Rhomboid major

Upper-body Muscles: Movements, Functions, and Exercise Implications

FIGURE 3.43
Upper trapezius stretch. Have your client apply passive pressure on the back of the head.

An advanced exercise for the lower and middle fibers is a pull-up (Figure 3.46). In the starting position, the scapulae are abducted and upwardly rotated due to the arm position. To perform a pull-up, the lower and middle fibers of the trapezius must strongly contract to stabilize the scapulae (retract, depress, and downwardly rotate) so that the arms can adduct and lift the body to clear the chin over the bar. The muscles are having to lift the body weight against gravity.

FIGURE 3.44
Middle trapezius and posterior deltoid strengthener. You can stimulate contraction of the middle trapezius by placing a hand between the shoulder blades.

Rhomboids. The major and minor rhomboids are located beneath the middle and upper trapezius (see Figure 3.42). They connect the entire medial border of the scapula to the spine and retract and elevate the scapula. They also participate in downward scapula rotation. The fibers are diagonal.

Levator Scapulae. This muscle connects the scapula to the transverse processes of the cervical vertebrae with a vertical line of pull (see Figure 3.42). Its function is scapular elevation and downward scapular rotation.

Anterior Shoulder Girdle. The anterior shoulder girdle muscles attach the scapulae to the front of the chest. They include the serratus anterior and the pectoralis minor (Figure 3.47).

Serratus Anterior. The serratus anterior connects the medial border of the scapulae on its underside to the front of the rib cage (ribs one through nine). The muscle interdigitates with the external oblique. Its function is protraction and upward rotation of the scapula and it also participates in reaching motions, such as a punch.

If this muscle is weak, the shoulder blade may protrude from the surface of the back, particularly along the medial border and will be clearly visible during a push-up. This muscle will become relatively weaker as others substitute for its weakened function. To strengthen the serratus, have the client do wall push-ups or scapular push-ups (Figure 3.48). Spot carefully to make sure the shoulder blades stay flat.

People whose shoulder blades are protracted (pulled forward, away from the spine), may also have a tight serratus. At rest, the medial border of the scapula should be about 2 inches (5 cm) from the spine.

Pectoralis Minor. This muscle connects the coracoid process of the scapula to the third, fourth, and fifth ribs. It can have a positive or negative effect on posture, depending on the condition of the scapular retractors. If the middle and lower trapezius are weak or overstretched, the pectoralis minor can become shortened and tilt the scapulae forward and down. If the scapular retractors are properly stabilizing the scapulae, the pectoralis minor assists with respiration by pulling the ribs upward.

Muscles of the Shoulder and Elbow

The shoulder is called the glenohumeral joint. It is the **articulation** between the glenoid fossa of the scapula and the humerus, and it is a multiaxial joint.

The movements and normal ranges of motion of the shoulder are pictured in Figure 3.49. They include: flexion and extension in the sagittal plane, abduction and adduction in the frontal plane, external and internal rotation and horizontal flexion and extension in the transverse plane, and circumduction in a combination of planes.

The muscles acting at the glenohumeral joint attach the humerus to the scapula and cause movement of the upper arm. Remember that the shoulder girdle muscles act as stabilizers during all arm movements, so scapular motion and stabilization occurs simultaneously with shoulder movements. If there is a problem with arm movement, it

may stem from weakness or tightness either of the arm or shoulder girdle or both.

Each muscle acting at the shoulder has many functions depending on the shoulder's current angle. The muscles include the deltoid, coracobrachialis, latissimus dorsi, and teres major, as well as the group called the rotator cuff (supraspinatus, infraspinatus, teres minor, and subscapularis).

Deltoid. The deltoid is identified by three names, relative to fiber location around the joint (Figure 3.50). The muscle is

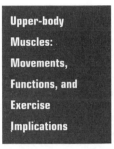

Upper-body Muscles: Movements, Functions, and Exercise Implications

FIGURE 3.45
Lower trapezius strengthener, pull only the shoulder blades down and together.

FIGURE 3.46
Pull-up, an advanced exercise for the middle and lower trapezius fibers.

Upper-body Muscles: Movements, Functions, and Exercise Implications

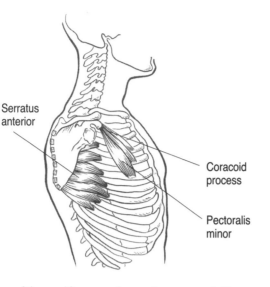

FIGURE 3.47
Anterior shoulder girdle muscles.

Serratus anterior

Coracoid process

Pectoralis minor

multipenniform and attaches a good distance from the joint, making it a powerful mover of the shoulder joint.

The anterior deltoid originates along the lateral third of the clavicle and inserts on the deltoid tuberosity of the humerus. It acts with the posterior deltoid as a stabilizer and synergist during shoulder abduction and also flexes, horizontally adducts, and internally rotates the arm at the shoulder. Front raises and many traditional pectoral exercises work the anterior deltoid.

The middle deltoid originates on the acromion and inserts on the deltoid tuberosity (see Figure 3.50). With shoulder girdle muscles acting as synergists, the middle deltoid abducts the arm at the shoulder, as in a lateral raise. It also controls the down-phase of a lateral raise (shoulder adduction in the same direction as gravity).

Perform a lateral raise with the shoulder in neutral rotation to prevent injury. Forcing a lateral raise with internal rotation at the shoulder can impinge and damage the rotator cuff. Impingement also can occur if the raise is performed in poor alignment, such as with rounded shoulders or protracted scapulae.

The posterior deltoid originates on the posterior border of the scapular spine, and passes behind the shoulder joint to insert on the deltoid **tuberosity.** It functions as a shoulder extensor and horizontal abductor. If using free weights when exercising the posterior deltoid, position the client prone on an incline bench. Use dumbbells or apply manual resistance to the rear of the upper arm (see Figure 3.44).

Latissimus Dorsi and Teres Major. The position and fiber direction of these two muscles are very similar (see Figure 3.50). The teres major attaches to the lower corner of the scapula. The latissimus dorsi is much larger with a broad attachment along the lower thoracic and lumbar spine, sacrum, and pelvis. They both insert on the anterior surface of the upper humerus, and their function is to extend, adduct, and internally rotate the arm on the torso at the shoulder. They also act to propel the torso forward and upward on the arms such as in swimming, rowing, cross-country skiing, performing pull-ups or pulling the body along the ground as one might do on a military obstacle course.

The most common strengthening exercise for these muscles is the "lat pull-down" (see page 289). To achieve the maximum

FIGURE 3.48
Scapular push-up.

Starting position, with the torso sagging and the scapula adducted (retracted).

Push the hands "through the floor," moving into scapular abduction (protracted) and lifting the torso.

Upper-body Muscles: Movements, Functions, and Exercise Implications

Elbow range of motion: flexion 150°; extension (to 0°); hyperextension (<10°).

Forearm range of motion: pronation 90°; supination 90°.

Wrist range of motion: flexion 80°; extension (to 0°); hyperextension 70°.

Range of motion of the wrist: radial deviation 20°; ulnar deviation 30°.

FIGURE 3.49
Upper extremity movements and ranges of motion.
continued on next page

effectiveness of this exercise, pull the bar down to the chest rather than the back of the shoulders. Pulling to, and lifting the chest toward, the bar also engages the lower trapezius and does not compromise the shoulder or head and neck positions. Keep the chest lifted and the back in neutral throughout the exercise.

In the absence of variable-resistance equipment, a good way to provide progressive resistance to these muscles is to have clients perform a lat pull-down against elastic bands or tubing that is held in a door jamb. Swimming, rowing, and lifting the body up on parallel bars also will strengthen these muscles.

Pectoralis Major. The origin of the pectoralis major is broad and ranges from the medial half of the clavicle, anterior surface of the sternum, cartilages of the first six or seven ribs, and the aponeurosis of the external oblique (see Figure 3.50). It inserts near the latissimus dorsi on the anterior surface of the upper humerus and functions as a shoulder adductor and internal rotator. It also participates in shoulder flexion and horizontal adduction.

The push-up is an important exercise to strengthen the pectorals. The pectoralis major, serratus anterior, and triceps contract eccentrically to lower the weight of the body toward the floor. The same muscles contract concentrically to lift the body up from the floor. For maximum effectiveness, use the torso stabilizers to maintain neutral alignment of the head, neck, spine, and hip joints as shown in Figure 3.51.

To stretch the pectoralis major effectively, the client should lie supine on a bench with the back pressed against it. The hands touch the head just behind the ears with the elbows flexed. You may assist with the stretch by applying slow, mild, downward pressure just above the elbows.

There are several common training errors related to the latissimus dorsi and pectoralis

Upper-body Muscles: Movements, Functions, and Exercise Implications

FIGURE 3.49 continued

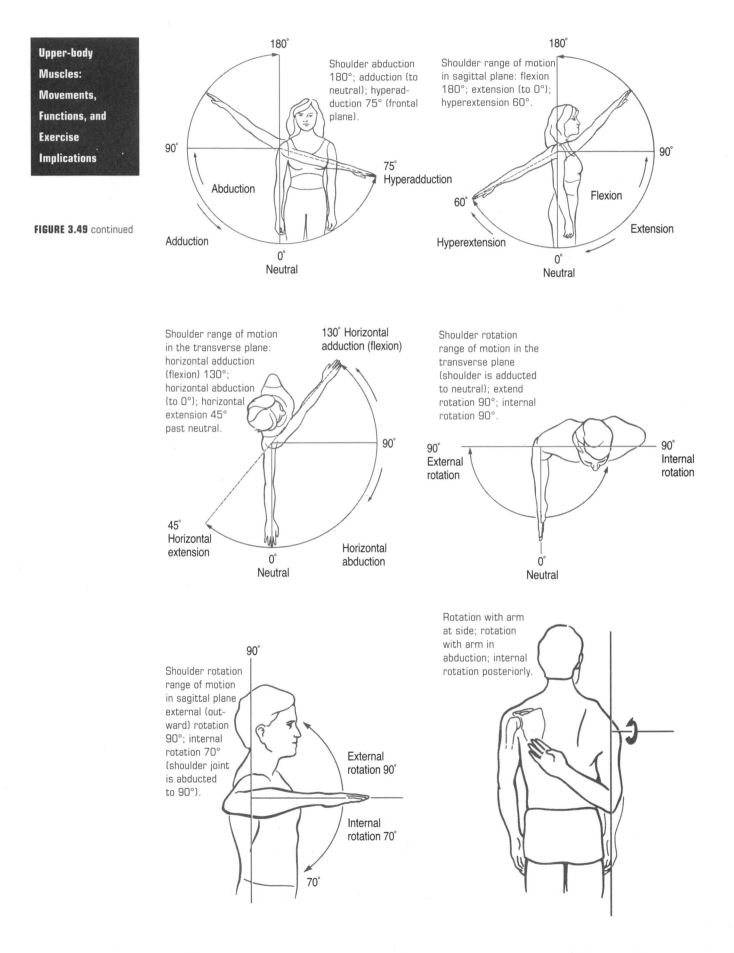

Shoulder abduction 180°; adduction (to neutral); hyperadduction 75° (frontal plane).

Shoulder range of motion in sagittal plane: flexion 180°; extension (to 0°); hyperextension 60°.

Shoulder range of motion in the transverse plane: horizontal adduction (flexion) 130°; horizontal abduction (to 0°); horizontal extension 45° past neutral.

Shoulder rotation range of motion in the transverse plane (shoulder is adducted to neutral); extend rotation 90°; internal rotation 90°.

Shoulder rotation range of motion in sagittal plane external (outward) rotation 90°; internal rotation 70° (shoulder joint is abducted to 90°).

Rotation with arm at side; rotation with arm in abduction; internal rotation posteriorly.

Anterior deltoid and
pectoralis major

Latissimus dorsi, pectoralis,
and deltoid, lateral view

Posterior muscles of the
shoulder (glenohumeral) joint

FIGURE 3.50
Superficial shoulder
muscles.

major. One occurs when swimmers and body-builders work hard to build up their pectorals and latissimus but fail to stretch those muscles. Their shoulders are always internally rotated, possibly because the pecs and lats are too short. A less severe version of this standing posture is evidenced by shoulders that are rounded forward and hands that face backward instead of toward each other during relaxed standing. In an undeveloped individual, this may be due to weak, overstretched scapular retractors and shoulder external rotators that passively allow the shoulder to fall forward into internal rotation. The scapular retractors become overstretched because,

in a habitually poor sitting and standing posture, the scapulae passively slide away from the spine, keeping the muscles that connect the scapulae to the spine in a state of perpetual stretch. This may be accompanied and accentuated by a tight pectoralis minor that exerts a downward pull on the upper front part of the scapula.

Training time is often spent strengthening the pectoralis major and latissimus dorsi without stretching. Trainers must be sure to consider muscular balance when planning time with a client.

For a pectoral stretch, the arm should be in a combined position of abduction, external rotation, and some hyperextension as in Figure 3.52. Varying the angle of abduction would stretch different parts (sternal and clavicular) of the muscle. The

FIGURE 3.51
Correct push-up
alignment (mid-
range position).

**Upper-body
Muscles:
Movements,
Functions, and
Exercise
Implications**

posterior scapular muscles should actively contract to stabilize the scapulae in a depressed, retracted position.

Coracobrachialis and Biceps Brachii. The coracobrachialis and biceps brachii originate on the top front of the scapula and insert on the humerus (coracobrachialis) and radius (biceps) (Figure 3.53). They are **anterior** to the joint, so they flex the shoulder. The biceps brachii has two heads that attach to the scapula; if the shoulder is externally rotated, the long head moves laterally and will assist with shoulder abduction.

In addition to shoulder motion, the biceps flexes the elbow and **supinates** the forearm. The biceps curl is commonly used to strengthen this muscle. Incorporating supination with the curl will utilize both functions at the elbow.

However, the biceps is not the prime mover when the forearm is **pronated** (palms face down). The brachialis is the "pure flexor of the elbow." It is the prime mover for all positions of the forearm. This is demonstrated by feeling the biceps

muscle as we first flex the elbow with the palm up, then down. Feeling it once more as we pull up against the bottom of a table with the back of the hand (resisted elbow flexion with pronation), we see that the biceps is a synergist when there is resistance. Because the biceps brachii is wrapped around the radius when the forearm is pronated, it cannot provide as much force for elbow flexion as it can when the forearm is supinated.

Triceps. The triceps also is a two-joint muscle, crossing posterior to the shoulder and elbow, attaching to the scapula proximally and the forearm distally (Figure 3.54). It therefore extends the shoulder and elbow joints. If using free weights as resistance, place the client's arm into an antigravity position. For example, the client could stand in a slight forward lunge and hold the shoulder in hyperextension, then extend the elbow. Or they could lie supine, pointing their elbow toward the ceiling, and then lift the hand toward the ceiling.

Rotator Cuff Muscles. The muscles that rotate the shoulder joint are located on the scapula. They are stabilizers as well as movers. Their tendons form a cuff around the upper and posterior part of the joint. You may remember them better as SITS muscles: supraspinatus, infraspinatus, teres minor, and subscapularis. They attach to the humerus in that order, starting at the top and moving toward the back and then around and underneath to the front (Figure 3.55). The supraspinatus is above (supra) the scapular spine (spinatus). It does not rotate the shoulder in neutral, but helps abduct and stabilize the head of the humerus in the socket. The infraspinatus is below (infra) the scapular spine and the teres minor is located inferior to the infraspinatus. These muscles externally rotate the shoulder. The subscapularis is located on the anterior side, or beneath (sub) the scapula (scapularis), and attaches to the front of the humerus. It internally rotates the shoulder.

FIGURE 3.52
Effective, trainer-assisted pectoral stretch.

FIGURE 3.53
Biceps and coracobrachialis.

FIGURE 3.54
Triceps: long, medial, and lateral heads.

Impingement of these muscle attachments can occur when the shoulder is abducted and internally rotated simultaneously. In this position, the humerus contacts the acromion, pinching the tendons, and they may fray and become inflamed. To prevent injury, abduct the shoulder when it is neutral or externally rotated.

Forearm and Wrist

The muscles located along the forearm act to control wrist and finger motion. The forearm muscles are usually exercised in all movements of the shoulder and elbow when using a machine or gripping a weight. They may also benefit from individual strengthening since restricted grip strength is sometimes the limiting factor for other exercises such as pull-ups or lunges performed while holding heavy dumbbells.

APPLIED KINESIOLOGY

The purpose of learning the location and functions of various muscles, as well as the mechanical principles of movement, is to enhance your ability to analyze movement and design effective exercises.

The body's position and the direction of gravity's pull often are clues to which muscle is contracting and how. If the movement occurs against the pull of gravity, the agonist that normally performs that joint action is contracting concentrically. If the movement is slow and controlled and occurs in the same direction as the pull of gravity, the agonist muscle is contracting eccentrically. (The motion must be slower than the segment during free fall with no muscle action. An eccentric contraction then

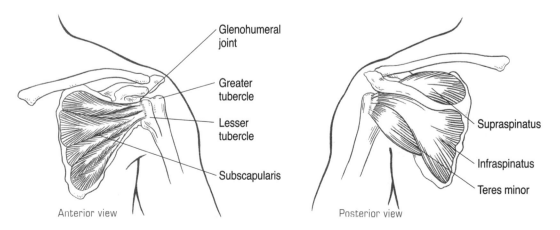

FIGURE 3.55
Rotator cuff muscles. Avoid shoulder abduction with internal rotation to prevent impingement.

provides a "braking" action on the movement.) If the motion occurs in the direction of gravity, but is faster than the acceleration of gravity or occurs against external resistance, the cause is a concentric contraction of the antagonist. When the movement occurs perpendicular to the pull of gravity, it is usually due to alternating concentric contractions of the expected muscle groups.

As an illustration, analyze hip abduction and adduction in different body positions. In Figure 3.56a (side-lying leg raise), the joint action is hip abduction, against gravity. The hip abductors (agonists) are contracting concentrically. In the return phase, the joint action is hip adduction. However, since the motion occurs slowly in the same direction as gravity, the hip abductors contract eccentrically. In Figure 3.56b (lying supine, legs extended on the floor), the joint actions are hip abduction and adduction (same movement as before). However, in this case, gravity is not a factor; the muscular action is what one would expect: the hip abductors, contract concentrically as the hip abducts (legs apart), and the hip adductors contract concentrically as the hip adducts (legs together).

FIGURE 3.56
Hip abduction and adduction.

a. Side-lying leg raise, hip abduction against gravity.

b. Supine with legs extended on the floor. The muscular action is the same, but the effect of gravity has been eliminated.

Exercise Analysis

The following questions may guide you in analyzing and designing effective exercises:

1. What movements occur at each joint?
2. Is the movement slow or fast, against resistance or not?
3. Is the motion occurring against gravity or in its same direction? Is it against some other resistance (pulleys, elastic)?
4. What muscles are causing the joint movement?
5. Is the contraction concentric, eccentric, or isometric?
6. Which muscles are movers and which are stabilizers?
7. Does the movement achieve the stated goal of the exercise?
8. Does the exercise train the primary function of the muscle?
9. Does the movement compromise the safety of other body parts? Are non-moving joints stabilized adequately in neutral?
10. How can the exercise be adapted to meet the specific needs of the client (made more or less difficult)?

EXAMPLES OF EXERCISE ANALYSIS

Having reviewed the locations and functions of most of the major muscles of the trunk and extremities, and having applied biomechanical principles pertinent to each muscle group and analyzed the type of muscle contractions involved in many joint movements, you can now put it all together to analyze two exercises commonly employed by personal trainers: the push-up and the seated lat pull-down.

Push-up

Up-phase. To press the torso away from the floor, the body is raised by extending the elbows and horizontally flexing the shoulders. (Horizontal flexion occurs if the elbows are wide but not if the elbows are held close to the sides.) Motion occurs at the shoulders, shoulder girdle, elbows, and wrists. And though no movement occurs, critical stabilization happens at the neck, torso, hips, and knees.

Shoulders: The joint movement is horizontal flexion and internal rotation. The movement occurs against gravity, so it is controlled by concentric contraction of the shoulder flexors and internal rotators: pectoralis major, anterior deltoid, coracobrachialis, and subscapularis.

Shoulder girdle: The motion is scapular abduction and upward rotation controlled by concentric contraction of the agonists: pectoralis minor, serratus anterior, upper and middle trapezius, and rhomboids.

Elbows: The movement is extension against gravity, so muscular action is concentric contraction of the extensors: triceps.

Wrists: Hyperextension occurs here by concentric contraction of the wrist extensors.

Head and neck: Cervical vertebrae are maintained in neutral alignment by isometric contraction of the cervical extensors. (When there is no movement, imagine what would happen if all muscles relaxed, then decide which muscles are contracting to prevent that motion.)

Lumbar spine: A neutral spine is maintained by isometric contraction of the abdominals.

Hips: No movement occurs, but the joint is stabilized by isometric contraction of the flexors since gravity would tend to cause hip extension.

Down-phase. In the down-phase of the movement, the opposite movements occur at the shoulder, shoulder girdle, elbows, and wrists. Since the down-phase movements occur in the same direction as gravity, they are controlled by eccentric contractions of the muscles just listed. The head, spine, and hips are maintained in a neutral position by the same muscles contracting isometrically.

Lat Pull-down

Next, analyze the "lat pull-down" pictured in Chapter 9 (see page 289).

Down-phase. In the down-phase the resistance of the machine is lifted by adducting and extending the shoulders. The prime motion occurs at the shoulders, shoulder girdle, and elbows. Stabilization occurs at the wrist, neck, lumbar spine, and hips. In the analysis of an exercise performed against an external resistance other than gravity, the direction of the movement in relation to gravity is a lesser consideration.

Shoulders: The primary joint movements are adduction and extension. The movement occurs against the external resistance of the machine, so it is controlled by concentric contractions of the agonists: shoulder adductors (pectoralis major, latissimus dorsi, and teres major), and extensors (latissimus, teres major, posterior deltoid, and triceps). Also, some internal rotation may occur depending on the exact start and end positions, so the subscapularis also contracts concentrically.

Shoulder girdle: The motion is scapular adduction, depression, and downward rotation occurring against the external resistance of the machine (the resistance is being lifted against gravity). Therefore, it is controlled by concentric contraction of the agonists: primarily the lower and middle trapezius muscles and the rhomboids.

Elbows: The movement is flexion against the resistance of the machine. (It occurs in the same direction as gravity, but we must remember that the resistance is being lifted against gravity.) The muscular action is concentric contraction of the biceps, and because the forearm is pronated, the brachialis also contracts concentrically.

Wrists: Ideally, the wrists should be stabilized in neutral by isometric co-contraction of the flexors and extensors.

Head and neck: Cervical vertebrae are maintained in neutral, with minimal muscle contraction if they are properly aligned.

Lumbar spine: In a seated position, gravity tends to pull the pelvis into a posterior tilt (spinal tilt). Neutral position is achieved by isometric contraction of the spinal extensors.

Hips: No movement occurs ordinarily, though a slight forward lean at the hips may occur, controlled by eccentric contraction of the hip extensors.

Return Phase. In the return phase of the exercise, the opposite motions occur at the shoulder, shoulder girdle, and elbows. They are controlled by eccentric contractions of the muscles just listed for those three joints. They are applying "braking" action to the weight moving with gravity.

EXERCISE DESIGN, INSTRUCTION, AND CORRECTION

The effective personal trainer applies the principles of biomechanics and kinesiology to analyze and design exercises appropriate for each individual client. It is important for you to begin the exercise program at the proper level and to progress slowly to prevent risk of injury.

To progressively overload muscles, use the principles of biomechanics presented earlier in this chapter. First, the body position can be changed from one in which gravity is not a factor to an antigravity position. Second, the trainer can utilize a series of concentric, eccentric, and (when appropriate) isometric contractions of the same muscle group. Third, the lever arm of the resistance can be increased, as in a lateral raise with the elbow extended instead of flexed. External resistance can be added in the form of either your own manual resistance, elastic bands or tubing, or free weights applied with various lever arm lengths.

Injury prevention should be a major consideration when designing exercise programs. Body parts such as the neck and low back should not be put at risk for injury to gain advantage for another muscle group. Progressive resistance should be added gradually. Decrease the resistance if form is not perfect. Thorough instruction and continual reminders also are important.

Spotting is particularly crucial when working with large amounts of resistance. You should be able to recognize muscle substitution patterns that occur as muscles fatigue and approach failure. This will show as subtle variations in body position that allow other muscles to substitute. The client may be focused on more reps and often will not even realize that their form has changed. You must take responsibility for recognizing these substitutions and signs of fatigue so that the spine and surrounding structures are not injured.

There are two effective methods for correcting a client's position. First, place your hand in the desired position and ask the client to touch it. For example, if the client has a forward head posture, put your hand where their head would be with good alignment and instruct them to glide their head back to touch your hand. An alternative is to place your hand in the undesired position and instruct them to avoid contact with your hand. For example, if the client is allowing their knees to go forward past the toes in a squat, place your hand even with the toes and instruct the client to keep the knees behind your hand. These techniques encourage the person to actively assume the correct position. They set up the desired neurological pathways and recruitment patterns, improving kinesthetic awareness of the correct position.

Pushing or pulling a person's body into a desired position will usually produce a reflex response in the opposite direction and may actually interfere with the ability to actively return to the desired position.

SUMMARY

The body is an incredible machine. Its function actually improves with use if its movement is compatible with its design and the physical laws of motion. However, if repetitive movement occurs that is incompatible with the body's design, a breakdown results, either as an acute injury or degeneration over time. It is vital that the exercises and activities you employ as a personal trainer not only enhance the body's performance, but also prevent its injury in the gym and in real life.

Use the tools and knowledge base of kinesiology to prepare your clients for an active lifestyle. Consider the body's daily activities, postures, and the physical stresses it undergoes in those positions. Next, identify possible areas of weakness or tightness caused by those habitual positions and activities. Then design activities to improve the body's function under those performance conditions. The result will be a balanced fitness program, which not only includes cardiovascular endurance, but also muscular balance, neutral alignment, and good body mechanics.

Summary

Suggested Reading

SUGGESTED READING

Basmajian, J.V. & Deluca, C.J. (1985). *Muscles Alive* (5th ed.). Baltimore: Williams & Wilkins.

Ellison, D. (1993). *Advanced Exercise Design for Lower Body.* San Diego: E & C Productions.

Ellison, D. (1995). *Advanced Exercise Design for Upper Body.* San Diego: E & C Productions.

Enoka, R. (2002). *Neuromechanical Basis of Human Movement.* (3rd ed.). Champaign, Ill.: Human Kinetics.

Golding, L.A. & Golding, S.M. (2003). *Musculoskeletal Anatomy and Human Movement.* Monterey, Calif.: Healthy Learning.

Kapit, W. & Elson, L. (2001). *The Anatomy Coloring Book.* (3rd ed.). New York: Benjamin/Cummings.

Kendall, F.P., McCreary, E.K., & Provance, P. (2005). *Muscles: Testing and Function.* (4th ed.). Baltimore: Williams & Wilkins.

Kreighbaum, E. & Barthels, K. (1995). *Biomechanics.* (4th ed.). Minneapolis: Burgess.

Levangie, P.K. & Norkin, C.C. (2000). *Joint Structure and Function.* (3rd ed.). Philadelphia: F.A. Davis.

Luttgens, K., Deutsch, H. & Hamilton, N. (2001). *Kinesiology: Scientific Basis of Human Motion.* New York: WCB/McGraw-Hill.

Rasch, P. (1993). *Kinesiology and Applied Anatomy.* (7th ed.). Philadelphia: Lea & Febiger.

CHAPTER 4

Nutrition

Jacqueline R. Berning, Ph.D., R.D., holds a master's degree in exercise science from the University of Colorado-Boulder and a doctorate in nutrition from Colorado State University.

Jacqueline R. Berning *She is an associate professor in the department of biology at the University of Colorado in Colorado Springs, and is the co-author of TRAINING NUTRITION: The Diet and Nutrition Guide for Peak Performance with Ed Burke, Ph.D. She is the nutrition consultant for the University of Colorado Athletic Department in Boulder, the Denver Broncos, and the Cleveland Indians.*

A lack of nutrition knowledge and poor eating habits can contribute to poor fitness, low energy stores, and the development of such lifestyle-related diseases as heart disease, diabetes, some types of cancer, and obesity. The time is right to start making wise food choices and commit to an exercise program. Eating well is not difficult in principle. All that is needed is to eat a selection of foods that supplies appropriate amounts of the essential nutrients and energy. Yet to put this into practice may be extremely difficult for some. As a personal trainer, you will help your clients commit to fitness programs and make appropriate food selections for good health. You should become knowledgeable about nutrition so you can provide sound, credible nutrition information to your clients in terms they can understand and follow, as well as know when to refer them to a registered dietitian or physician. Find a local resource in nutrition, possibly a registered dietitian capable of giving sensible responses to your questions, or a group of dietitians who practice in sports and cardiovascular nutrition (SCAN). To locate local SCAN dietitians, contact the American Dietetic Association and ask for the SCAN referral list. And most important, be a role model and practice healthful eating habits to show a commitment to good nutrition.

WHY IS IT SO HARD TO MAKE WISE FOOD CHOICES?

Why are we so tempted to eat foods that we know we should avoid? What triggers our eating habits? Why do we like high-fat, high-calorie foods?

Many factors influence our eating patterns, including hunger, habits, economics, marketing, availability, convenience, and nutritional value. Probably the strongest reason we choose to eat certain foods is for taste. We like the taste of sweet and salty foods and, as a result, we tend to eat too many of them. We also like foods that have happy associations, such as those we eat at family gatherings or on holidays.

Social pressure has a very powerful influence on food choices and it is at work in every culture and social circle. Many of us have been programmed to feel that it is rude not to accept food in certain social situations and we have all felt the pressure of being forced to eat at office celebrations even though we are not hungry or are trying to watch caloric intake. Availability, convenience, and economics also play a role in choosing the foods we do. You cannot eat foods that are unavailable or unaffordable. In addition, because we are all so busy, we tend to pick foods based on convenience. We are more likely to choose foods that we can pop in the microwave and eat in five minutes than take the time to prepare a

meal from scratch. Both physical and emotional stress affect our eating habits. Some people respond to stress, whether positive or negative, by eating; others may use food to ward off loneliness, boredom, or anxiety.

As you can see, there are a variety of reasons for choosing the foods we do. So how do you get your clients, and perhaps yourself, to select foods with good nutritional value? To do so successfully, you need to educate your clients about the nutrients that the body needs and, specifically, what foods supply them in adequate amounts for optimal health and fitness.

NUTRIENTS

Nutrients are life-sustaining substances found in food. They work together to supply the body with energy and structural materials, and to regulate growth, maintenance, and repair of the body's tissues.

Protein, carbohydrate, fat, vitamins, minerals, and water are the six major classes of nutrients. Table 4.1 lists the nutrient classes and their major functions. While the amount of each nutrient a body needs varies widely, there are guidelines for making sure that the body receives enough nutrients to sustain a healthy and active lifestyle.

The Caloric Nutrients

Protein, carbohydrate, and fat are the three nutrients that provide calories. These calories are used by the body to sustain life by helping to maintain body temperature and facilitating the growth and repair of all organs and tissues. Many people believe carbohydrate calories are "good" calories and fat calories are "bad" calories. In reality, they both serve a vital purpose in our diet. One reason fat calories are considered bad is that Americans eat too many of them, which can result in excess body fat and weight. Fat is a very concentrated source of energy and contains more than twice the calories of protein and carbohydrate. Alcohol also provides calories, but is not considered a nutrient since it does not contribute to the growth, maintenance, or repair of body tissue. Furthermore, alcohol can be converted to fat when total caloric intake exceeds caloric output.

- 1 gram protein = 4 calories
- 1 gram carbohydrate = 4 calories
- 1 gram fat = 9 calories
- 1 gram alcohol = 7 calories

Essential Nutrients

The body can make certain nutrients from other nutrients. For example, it can convert some amino acids into carbohydrates, and it can manufacture some vitamins from amino acids as well. However, certain compounds that the body cannot make for itself, called **essential amino acids,** are absolutely indispensable to bodily functions. There are about 40 essential nutrients to be concerned about, so it may be a relief to discover that diet planning can be reduced to a few simple principles to ensure that we take in all the nutrients in the appropriate amounts without having to count and weigh each one.

Recommended Nutrient Intakes

Normal, healthy adults of average size who engage in physical activity should consume the following amounts of nutrients daily to remain in optimal health.

- ✔ Protein—approximately 50 to 70 grams, depending on body size, or 12 to 20% of caloric intake as protein
- ✔ Carbohydrate—a minimum of 125 grams, optimal 350 to 400 grams, or 55 to 65% of caloric intake as carbohydrate
- ✔ Fat—approximately 30 to 65 grams, depending on caloric consumption, or 25 to 30% of caloric intake from fat
- ✔ Vitamins—specific amounts are listed in the Recommended Dietary Allowances (RDA)
- ✔ Minerals—specific amounts are listed in the RDA
- ✔ Water—2 to 3 quarts per day

Table 4.1
The Six Classes of Nutrients and Their Major Functions

Nutrient	Function
Protein	✔ Builds and repairs body tissue ✔ Major component of enzymes, hormones, and antibodies
Carbohydrate	✔ Provides a major source of fuel to the body ✔ Provides dietary fibers
Lipids	✔ Chief storage form of energy in the body ✔ Insulate and protect vital organs ✔ Provide fat-soluble vitamins
Vitamins	✔ Help promote and regulate various chemical reactions and bodily processes ✔ Do not yield energy themselves, but participate in releasing energy from food
Minerals	✔ Enable enzymes to function ✔ A component of hormones ✔ A part of bone and nerve impulses
Water	✔ Enables chemical reactions to occur ✔ About 60% of the body is composed of water ✔ Essential for life as we cannot store it, nor conserve it

Recommended Dietary Allowance

RECOMMENDED DIETARY ALLOWANCE

The **Recommended Dietary Allowances (RDAs)** are nutrient recommendations designed to meet the needs of essentially all people of similar age and gender. Established by the Food and Nutrition Board of the National Academy of Science, they are a general guide for estimating your nutritional needs. RDAs are expressed as an optimal amount with upper and lower limits—meaning too little is not good and too much also may present problems. Many people mistakenly believe that if a little is good, more has to be better. In nutrition, however, that kind of thinking may lead to toxicities, especially with some **fat-soluble** vitamins.

Dietary Guidelines

The RDA is to be used as a guide—a ballpark figure. It does not mean that if you do not consume the RDA for a certain vitamin or mineral that you will come down with a deficiency disease. On the contrary, symptoms of nutritional deficiencies may be subtle and develop over a long period of time. The opposite also is true. Taking large amounts of specific vitamins or minerals also may lead to toxicity problems. The RDAs are not minimums. Be careful when assessing a client's diet using the RDA. Use it to see if your clients are getting the nutrients they need. If a client is consistently three quarters below the RDA for a particular nutrient for a long period, they may be at risk for certain nutritional deficiencies. You should consult with the client's physician and/or a registered dietitian rather than diagnose dietary deficiencies. You can make dietary suggestions by using the MyPyramid Food Guidance System approach, emphasizing variety and moderation.

DIETARY GUIDELINES

The Dietary Guidelines issued by the U.S. Department of Agriculture and the Department of Health and Human Services were revised in 2005. They provide science-based recommendations to promote health and reduce risk for major chronic diseases (e.g., cardiovascular disease, type 2 diabetes, hypertension, osteoporosis, certain cancers) through proper diet and physical activity. Revised every five years, the Dietary Guidelines summarize current scientific knowledge of individual nutrients and food components into recommendations for a pattern of eating that can be adopted by the public. Implemented as a whole, the Dietary Guidelines encourage most Americans to eat fewer calories, become more physically active, and make wiser food choices.

The 2005 edition of the Dietary Guidelines are as follows:

1. *Consume adequate nutrients within calorie needs.* Balanced eating patterns such as those described in the USDA MyPyramid Food Guidance System and the Dietary Approaches to Stop Hypertension (DASH) Eating Plan help individuals consume a variety of nutrient-dense foods that limit the intake of saturated and trans fats, cholesterol, added sugars, salt, and alcohol. Both eating patterns provide energy intake recommendations across a range of calorie levels to meet the needs of various age and gender groups (Tables 4.2–4.5). These eating patterns are not promoted as weight-loss diets, rather they are examples of how to eat in accordance with the Dietary Guidelines.

2. *Promote weight management.* Adults should strive to maintain a healthy body

---

A New Standard on the Way?

The Food Nutrition Board and the National Academy of Science, working with Health Canada and Canadian scientists and hoping for future involvement from their Mexican counterparts, are in the midst of an ongoing project to standardize nutrition norms across North America. By combining four distinct ways of measuring nutritional needs into one universally accepted guideline—Dietary Reference Intakes (DRI)—they are hoping to increase consumers' abilities to plan and assess their own diets. The Dietary Reference Intakes are based on the following:

Recommended Dietary Allowances (RDA) represent the average daily dietary intake levels sufficient to meet the nutritional needs of nearly all healthy individuals.

Adequate Intake (AI) is only used when an RDA cannot be determined. AIs provide the recommended daily intake value based on observed or experimentally determined approximations of nutrient intake by a group of healthy people that are assumed to be adequate.

Tolerable Upper Intake Level (UL) is the highest level of daily nutrient intake that will likely pose no health risks to almost all individuals. As intake increases above the UL, risk of adverse effects also increases.

Estimated Average Requirement (EAR) is a daily nutrient intake value that is estimated to meet the requirements of half of the healthy individuals in a group.

Visit www.nap.edu to learn more about DRIs and to see the published *Dietary Reference Intake Reports.*

Anatomy of MyPyramid

One size doesn't fit all

USDA's new MyPyramid symbolizes a personalized approach to healthy eating and physical activity. The symbol has been designed to be simple. It has been developed to remind consumers to make healthy food choices and to be active every day. The different parts of the symbol are described below.

Activity
Activity is represented by the steps and the person climbing them, as a reminder of the importance of daily physical activity.

Moderation
Moderation is represented by the narrowing of each food group from bottom to top. The wider base stands for foods with little or no solid fats or added sugars. These should be selected more often. The narrower top area stands for foods containing more added sugars and solid fats. The more active you are, the more of these foods can fit into your diet.

Personalization
Personalization is shown by the person on the steps, the slogan, and the URL. Find the kinds and amounts of food to eat each day at MyPyramid.gov.

Proportionality
Proportionality is shown by the different widths of the food group bands. The widths suggest how much food a person should choose from each group. The widths are just a general guide, not exact proportions. Check the Web site for how much is right for you.

Variety
Variety is symbolized by the 6 color bands representing the 5 food groups of the Pyramid and oils. This illustrates that foods from all groups are needed each day for good health.

Gradual Improvement
Gradual improvement is encouraged by the slogan. It suggests that individuals can benefit from taking small steps to improve their diet and lifestyle each day.

USDA U.S. Department of Agriculture Center for Nutrition Policy and Promotion April 2005 CNPP-16

USDA is an equal opportunity provider and employer.

GRAINS | VEGETABLES | FRUITS | OILS | MILK | MEAT & BEANS

Source: U.S. Department of Agriculture, 2005

FIGURE 4.1
The MyPyramid Food Guidance System.

weight by balancing calories consumed with calories expended. Those who need to lose weight should aim for slow, steady weight loss by decreasing calorie intake and increasing physical activity.

3. *Incorporate physical activity.* New to the Dietary Guidelines in 2005 is the addition of specific physical activity recommendations for different population groups. Adults who desire to lower their risk of chronic disease should engage in at least 30 minutes of moderate-intensity physical activity most days of the week. Although

regular participation in 30 minutes of moderate-intensity exercise promotes health and psychological well-being, most people will receive greater health benefits by engaging in activities of more vigorous intensity for longer durations. Engaging in approximately 60 minutes of moderate- to vigorous-intensity physical activity on most days of the week while not exceeding caloric requirements will help adults manage body weight and help prevent gradual weight gain. For adults who have lost weight, 60 to 90 minutes of daily moderate-intensity exercise while not exceeding caloric intake requirements may help to sustain previous weight-loss achievements. Other recommendations include guidelines for children and adolescents (engage in at least 60 minutes of physical activity on most days of the week) and older adults (participate in regular exercise to reduce functional declines associated with aging).

4. *Emphasize the consumption of certain food groups.* Daily consumption of a variety of fruits and vegetables, whole grains, and non-fat or low-fat dairy products within caloric intake requirements is recommended. For example, individuals at the 2,000 calorie per day level are advised to consume 2 cups of fruit, 2.5 cups of vegetables, 3 or more ounce-equivalents of whole-grain products, and 3 cups of fat-free or low-fat milk products daily.

5. *Select the appropriate fats.* Total fat intake should range between 20–35% of daily calories, with most fats coming from polyunsaturated and monounsaturated sources (e.g., fish, nuts, vegetable oils). Consuming lean meats and poultry, dry beans, and low-fat or fat-free dairy products is recommended for ensuring adequate protein intake without increasing unhealthy (saturated) fat intake. In addition, no more than 10% of calories should come from saturated fats and consuming less than 300 mg per day of cholesterol is advised. Products containing trans fatty acids should be limited or avoided.

6. *Select the appropriate carbohydrates.* Fiber-rich fruits, vegetables, and whole grains represent the majority of carbohydrate consumption in a healthy diet. Foods and beverages that contain little added sugars or caloric sweeteners should be chosen and prepared. Limiting sugar- and starch-containing foods and beverages along with good oral hygiene will help to reduce the incidence of dental caries.

7. *Balance sodium and potassium consumption.* Americans are advised to choose and prepare foods with little salt and to limit consumption to less than 2,300 mg of sodium (approximately 1 teaspoon of salt) per day. Potassium-rich foods, such as fruits and vegetables, should be consumed daily in the amounts recommended by the USDA MyPyramid Food Guidance System and the DASH Eating Plan.

8. *Limit alcoholic beverage intake.* Sensible and moderate consumption of alcoholic beverages—defined as no more than one drink per day for women and no more than two drinks per day for men—is recommended. Certain individuals, such as women of childbearing age who may become pregnant, pregnant and lactating women, children and adolescents, individuals taking medication that may interact with alcohol, and those with specific medical conditions should avoid alcoholic beverages. Furthermore, individuals planning to drive or operate machinery should avoid consuming alcohol.

9. *Enhance food safety.* The incidence of microbial food-borne illness may be limited or prevented by practicing the following key recommendations for handling food. Hands, food contact surfaces, and fruits and vegetables should be cleaned prior to food preparation. Raw, cooked, and ready-to-eat foods should be separated from each other while shopping, preparing, or storing them. Foods should be cooked to a safe temperature and perishable foods should be refrigerated and/or defrosted properly. Unpasteurized milk products and juices, raw eggs and sprouts, or undercooked or raw meats and poultry should be avoided.

THE MYPYRAMID FOOD GUIDANCE SYSTEM

The MyPyramid Food Guidance System (Figure 4.1) provides food-based guidance to help implement the recommendations of the 2005 Dietary Guidelines for Americans. MyPyramid provides specific recommendations for making food choices that will improve the quality of an average

Table 4.2
Sample USDA Food Guide and the DASH Eating Plan at the 2,000-Calorie Level[1]

Food Groups & Subgroups	USDA Food Guide Amount[2]	DASH Eating Plan Amount
Fruit Group	2 cups (4 servings)	2 to 2.5 cups (4 to 5 servings)
Vegetable Group	2.5 cups (5 servings)	2 to 2.5 cups (4 to 5 servings)
• Dark green vegetables	• 3 cups/week	
• Orange vegetables	• 2 cups/week	
• Legumes (dry beans)	• 3 cups/week	
• Starchy vegetables	• 3 cups/week	
• Other vegetables	• 6.5 cups/week	
Grain Group	6 ounce-equivalents	7 to 8 ounce-equivalents
• Whole grains	• 3 ounce-equivalents	(7 to 8 servings)
• Other grains	• 3 ounce-equivalents	
Meat & Beans Group	5.5 ounce-equivalents	• 6 ounces or less: meat, poultry and fish
		• 4 to 5 servings per week: nuts, seeds and dry beans[3]
Milk Group	3 cups	2 to 3 cups
Oils	24 grams (6 tsp)	8 to 12 grams (2 to 3 tsp)
Discretionary Calorie Allowance	267 calories	
• Example of distribution: Solid fat[4]	18 grams	~ 2 tsp (5 Tbsp per week)
Added sugars	8 tsp	

[1] All servings are per day unless otherwise noted. USDA vegetable subgroup amounts and amounts of DASH nuts, seeds, and dry beans are per week.

[2] The 2,000-calorie USDA Food Guide is appropriate for many sedentary males 51 to 70 years of age, sedentary females 19 to 30 years of age, and for some other gender/age groups who are more physically active.

[3] In the DASH Eating Plan, nuts, seeds and dry beans are a separate food group from meat, poultry and fish.

[4] The oils listed in this table are not considered to be part of discretionary calories because they are a major source of the vitamin E and polyunsaturated fatty acids, including the essential fatty acids, in the food pattern. In contrast, solid fats (i.e., saturated and trans fats) are listed separately as a source of discretionary calories.

SOURCE: United States Department of Agriculture, 2005

American diet as it translates the Dietary Guidelines into a total diet that meets nutrient needs from food sources. If followed properly, MyPyramid results in the following changes to a typical diet:

- Increased intake of vitamins, minerals, dietary fiber, and other essential nutrients through increased consumption of fruits, vegetables, and whole-grains
- Lowered intake of saturated fats, trans fats, and cholesterol
- Calorie intake balanced with energy needs to prevent weight gain and/or promote a healthy weight

There are six general topic areas presented in the MyPyramid Food Guidance System. The topics represent a personalized approach to eating and physical activity and are meant to remind consumers to make healthy food choices and be active every day. First, MyPyramid emphasizes daily physical activity which is represented by the person climbing the steps on the left side of the pyramid. The second topic is moderation and is symbolized by the narrowing of each food group from the bottom of the pyramid to the top. The wider base stands for food selections with little or no saturated and trans fats or added sugars.

MyPyramid Food Guidance System

The narrower top portion of the pyramid stands for foods containing more added sugars and solid fats that should be limited in the typical diet. Personalization is the third topic and can be applied by understanding the kinds and amounts of food to eat each day based on an individual's age, gender, and activity level. Proportionality, the fourth topic is shown by the different widths of the food groups displayed in the pyramid. The widths suggest the relative amount of food one should select from each group. For example, the food groups represented by larger widths (i.e., grains, vegetables, fruits, milk) should be consumed in relatively larger amounts than the food groups represented by smaller widths (i.e., meat and beans, oils). The fifth topic, variety, suggests that individuals eat foods from all food groups daily. Variety is symbolized by the six different colored stripes that make up the pyramid. Finally, the sixth topic, gradual improvement, implies that improvements in diet and lifestyle are best achieved by taking small steps daily. For the average person, preventing gradual weight gain over time or improving current health status involves making small decreases in calorie intake and moderate increases in physical activity.

Table 4.3

Daily Amount of Food from Each Group

Calorie Level[1]	1,600	1,800	2,000	2,200
Fruits[2]	1.5 cups	1.5 cups	2 cups	2 cups
Vegetables	2 cups	2.5 cups	2.5 cups	3 cups
Grains	5 oz-eq	6 oz-eq	6 oz-eq	7 oz-eq
Meat and Beans	5 oz-eq	5 oz-eq	5.5 oz-eq	6 oz-eq
Milk	3 cups	3 cups	3 cups	3 cups
Oils	5 tsp	5 tsp	6 tsp	6 tsp
Discretionary Calorie Allowance	132	195	267	290

[1] A wider range of calorie levels (1,000–3,200) is available on www.mypyramid.gov. See Table 8.7 for help in assigning individuals to the food intake patterns at particular calorie levels.

[2] See www.mypyramid.gov for information on each of the food groups and tips for reaching these amounts for each calorie level.

SOURCE: United States Department of Agriculture, 2005

Table 4.4

Vegetable Subgroup Amounts Per Week

Calorie Level[1]	1,600	1,800	2,000	2,200
Dark green vegetables	2 cups	3 cups	3 cups	3 cups
Orange vegetables	1.5 cups	2 cups	2 cups	2 cups
Legumes	2.5 cups	3 cups	3 cups	3 cups
Starchy vegetables	2.5 cups	3 cups	3 cups	6 cups
Other vegetables	5.5 cups	6.5 cups	6.5 cups	7 cups

[1] A wider range of calorie levels (1,000–3,200) is available on www.mypyramid.gov.

SOURCE: United States Department of Agriculture, 2005

Table 4.5
Estimated Daily Calorie Needs

	Calorie Range
Children	**Sedentary →Active[1]**
2–3 years	1,000 → 1,400
Females	
4–8 years	1,200 → 1,800
9–13 years	1,600 → 2,200
14–18 years	1,800 → 2,400
19–30 years	2,000 → 2,400
31–50 years	1,800 → 2,200
51+	1,600 → 2,200
Males	
4–8 years	1,400 → 2,000
9–13 years	1,800 → 2,600
14–18 years	2,200 → 3,200
19–30 years	2,400 → 3,000
31–50 years	2,200 → 3,000
51+	2,000 → 2,800

[1] Sedentary = a lifestyle that includes only the light physical activity associated with typical day-to-day life; Active = a lifestyle that includes physical activity equivalent to walking more than 3 miles per day at 3 to 4 miles per hour, in addition to the light physical activity associated with typical day-to-day life.

SOURCE: United States Department of Agriculture, 2005

VEGETARIANS

The vegetarian faces a special challenge in diet planning—obtaining the needed nutrients from fewer food groups. There are two major classes of vegetarians (with many variations): the **lacto-ovo vegetarian** eats milk and eggs but excludes meat, fish, and poultry from the diet, whereas a pure vegetarian, or **vegan,** eats only foods from plant sources.

For both types, it is necessary to know how to combine foods to obtain the nutrients for health, as well as performance. Foods derived from animal sources such as chicken, fish, beef, milk, and eggs contain all the essential amino acids and are called **complete proteins.** Plant sources of food contain **incomplete proteins** because they are missing one or more amino acids. Incomplete proteins can be made complete by combining them either with other foods that are complete proteins, such as cereal with milk, and rice with cheese, or with other incomplete proteins, such as beans with rice, and peanut butter with bread. Many cultures have dishes or food combinations that meet the requisite amino acid combinations. In most cases, these dishes have been served for many generations. For example, Mexicans serve beans and tortillas and/or rice; Indians eat lentils and rice; Lebanese prepare humus tahini (garbanzo beans and sesame seed paste) with pita bread; and cornbread and beans are served in the southern United States. Figure 4.2 gives examples of how to combine incomplete proteins to make a complete protein. Eating extra servings of grains, nuts, and seeds will supply the necessary quantities of riboflavin, iron, and zinc.

A Vegetarian MyPyramid Food Guidance System is available through the American Dietetic Association (2005). For the lacto-ovo vegetarian, the MyPyramid Food Guidance System can be adapted by making a change in the meat group and by using non-meat proteins such as eggs, dairy products, legumes, and nuts. The strict vegetari-

Vegetarians

FIGURE 4.2
Protein complementarity chart. Adapted, with permission, from: Lappé, F.M. (1992). *Diet for a Small Planet.* New York: Ballantine Books.

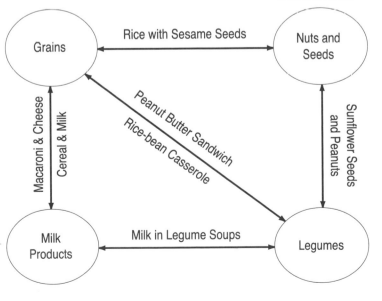

an who does not eat dairy products or animal protein should take a vitamin B_{12} supplement, or use soy or rice milk fortified with vitamin B_{12} and calcium.

NUTRIENT NEEDS FOR THE PHYSICALLY ACTIVE ADULT

Carbohydrates

Carbohydrates are the most important nutrient for exercising muscles. Adequate amounts of carbohydrates are essential not only for muscular performance but for the brain and central nervous system. The principal functions of carbohydrates are to

✔ serve as the primary energy source for working muscles
✔ ensure that the brain and nervous system function properly
✔ help the body use fat more efficiently

Stored carbohydrates, in the form of **glycogen,** are the primary fuel for exercise. If your clients are having a hard time maintaining normal workout intensities, they may have inadequate muscle carbohydrate or glycogen stores. Unless adequate glycogen levels are restored, exercise performance will continue to deteriorate to the point where even a low-intensity workout causes fatigue.

Carbohydrate Recommendations

Clients should consume at least 55 to 65% of their total calories from carbohydrates. Those who exercise more than one hour every day should consume close to 65% of their calories as carbohydrates. Those who work out every other day should consume around 55 to 60% of their calories from carbohydrates. Current consumption of carbohydrates for Americans is about 45%, and much of this is in the form of simple carbohydrates or sugars rather than complex carbohydrates such as whole grain breads, cereal, rice, and pasta. Complex carbohydrates also contain ample amounts of B vitamins and fiber and some trace minerals. While telling a client to consume 65% of their total calories

from carbohydrates is excellent advice, most individuals have no idea how much carbohydrate that is or what foods they should be eating to reach that goal. It appears that most consumers find it easier to count grams of carbohydrate or number of servings from the MyPyramid Food Guidance System than calculate percentages. The recommended carbohydrate intake in gram weight is 4 to 6 grams of carbohydrate per kilogram (1.8 to 2.7 grams per pound) of body weight, depending on activity level. Give your clients a list of carbohydrate foods so that they can determine how many servings and what carbohydrate foods they should consider eating in greater quantities (Table 4.6).

Carbohydrate Loading

Muscle glycogen depletion is a well-recognized limitation to endurance exercise that exceeds 90 minutes (Figure 4.3). **Carbohydrate loading** can nearly double an individual's muscle glycogen stores. Obviously, the greater the pre-exercise glycogen content, the greater the endurance potential.

The classic study on carbohydrate loading compared exercise time to exhaustion. Subjects exercised at 75% of $\dot{V}O_2$ max after consuming diets with varying amounts of carbohydrate—a low-carbohydrate diet, a normal diet, and a high-carbohydrate diet. The low-carbohydrate diet sustained only

FIGURE 4.3
After three days of training, individuals can use most of their muscle glycogen. A low-carbohydrate diet does not replace the glycogen quickly enough.

Table 4.6
Foods Listed by Groups with Carbohydrate and Fat Content

	Calories	Carbohydrate (gm)	Fat (gm)		Calories	Carbohydrate (gm)	Fat (gm)
Milk Group				**Fruits**			
2% milk, 1 cup	121	12	5	Apple, medium	80	20	0
Skim milk, 1 cup	86	12	0	Applesauce, ½ cup	53	14	0
Lowfat yogurt, 1 cup	225	42	3	Apricots, dried, 4 halves	33	9	0
Cottage cheese, 1 cup	164	7	2	Banana, medium	105	27	0
Lowfat cheddar cheese	80	8	5	Cantaloupe, 1 cup pieces	57	13	0
Lowfat American cheese	72	6	4	Cherries, sweet, 10	49	11	0
Lowfat mozzarella cheese	79	8	5	Dates, dried, 10	228	61	0
				Grapefruit, 1 half	39	10	0
Meat Group				Grapes, 1 cup	58	16	0
Lean ground beef, 3 oz.	214	0	14	Orange	65	16	0
Flank steak, 3 oz.	209	0	12	Peach	37	10	0
Chicken, light meat w/o skin, roasted, 3 oz.	148	0	4	Pear	98	25	0
Chicken, dark meat, w/o skin, roasted, 3 oz.	176	0	8	Pineapple, 1 cup pieces	77	19	0
Turkey, light meat, w/o skin, roasted, 3 oz.	135	0	3	Raisins, ⅔ cup	300	79	0
				Strawberries, 1 cup	45	11	0
Turkey, dark meat, w/o skin, roasted, 3 oz.	160	0	6	Watermelon, 1 cup	50	12	0
Turkey sandwich slices, 1 oz.	44	0	1	**Vegetables**			
Tuna, spring water, 1 oz.	60	0	1	Asparagus, 6 spears	22	4	0
Rainbow trout, broiled, 3 oz	129	0	4	Green beans, ½ cup	22	5	0
Salmon, 3 oz.	99	0	3	Broccoli, ½ cup	23	4	0
Beans, refried, 1 cup	270	47	3	Carrots, 1 medium	31	7	0
Kidney beans, 1 cup	216	40	1	Cauliflower, ½ cup	15	3	0
Ham, lean, 3 oz.	124	1	5	Celery, 1 stalk	6	2	0
Peas, black-eyed, 1 cup	198	36	1	Corn, ½ cup	89	21	0
Peanut butter, 1 Tbsp.	95	2	8	Green peas, ½ cup	67	13	0
				Baked potato	220	51	0
				Mushrooms, ½ cup	9	2	0
				Spinach, ½ cup	6	1	0
				Tomato	24	5	0

continued on next page

Table 4.6 continued

	Calories	Carbohydrate (gm)	Fat (gm)
Grain Group			
Bagel	163	31	1
Whole wheat bread, 1 slice	61	11	1
White bread, 1 slice	64	12	1
French bread, 1 slice	81	15	1
Bread sticks, 2	77	15	1
Graham crackers, 2 squares	60	11	1
Saltines, 10	125	20	4
Oatmeal, Quaker, ¾ cup	105	18	2
English muffin	135	26	1
Life Cereal, Quaker, ⅔ cup	111	19	2
Pancake, 4-inch dia.	61	9	2
Pasta, ½ cup	100	19	1
Rice, ½ cup	112	25	0
Flour tortilla, 8-inch dia.	105	18	3

an hour of exercise; the mixed diet sustained 115 minutes of exercise; and the high-carbohydrate diet sustained 170 minutes of the high-intensity exercise (Bergstrom, 1967).

Following additional research, the carbohydrate-loading sequence developed into a week-long regimen, beginning with an exhaustive training session one week before competition. For the next three days, the athlete consumed a low-carbohydrate diet, yet continued exercising to lower muscle glycogen stores even further. Then, for three days prior to competition, the athlete rested and consumed a high-carbohydrate diet to promote glycogen supercompensation. For many years, this week-long sequence was considered the optimal way to achieve maximum glycogen storage. However, it has many drawbacks. The three days of reduced carbohydrate intake can cause **hypoglycemia** (low blood sugar) and **ketosis** (increased blood acids),

which is associated with nausea, fatigue, dizziness, and irritability. These dietary manipulations prove to be too cumbersome for many athletes, and an exhaustive training session the week before competition may predispose the athlete to injury.

A revised method of carbohydrate loading eliminates many of the problems associated with the old regimen. Six days before the competition, the athlete exercises hard (70 to 75% of aerobic capacity for 90 minutes) and consumes a diet of 60% carbohydrates. On the second and third days, training is decreased to 40 minutes at 70 to 75% of aerobic capacity and, again, the athlete consumes the same diet. On the next two days, the athlete consumes a high-carbohydrate diet providing 70% carbohydrate (about 550 grams, or 10 grams per kilogram) and reduces training to 20 minutes at 70 to 75% of aerobic capacity. On the last day, the athlete rests while maintaining the high-carbohydrate diet. The modified regimen results in muscle glycogen stores equal to those provided by the classic low-carbohydrate regimen (Table 4.7).

Today, most athletes no longer practice the full technique of carbohydrate loading simply because they train and need to have glycogen stores maximized every day. It appears that most exercising individuals are now concerned about reloading muscle glycogen stores following heavy training to minimize fatigue associated with repeated days of it. This means that most

Table 4.7
Modified Carbohydrate Loading Technique

Day	Exercise Duration	Dietary Carbohydrate %
1	90 minutes	60
2	40 minutes	60
3	40 minutes	60
4	20 minutes	70
5	20 minutes	70
6	rest	70
7	competition	70

individuals need to consume adequate amounts of carbohydrates every day.

Glycogen Resynthesis

It takes about 24 hours before muscle glycogen is fully restored (Figure 4.4). However, some individuals may exercise again in 12 hours or less. It appears that *when* carbohydrate is consumed, relative to exercise, is important for refilling muscle glycogen. Studies have shown that when carbohydrate consumption is delayed after exercise, muscle glycogen storage is reduced and recovery is impaired. Ivy and associates found that individuals who consume about 1.5 grams of carbohydrate per kilogram (0.68 grams per pound) of body weight (about 100 grams) within 30 minutes after a moderate- to high-intensity exercise session, followed by an additional 1.5 grams of carbohydrate per kilogram of body weight every two hours, maximizes muscle glycogen levels (Ivy et al., 1988). Keep in mind that these guidelines are for highly fit exercisers; glycogen resynthesis is less of a concern for moderate exercisers.

Zawadzki and colleagues found that combining protein with carbohydrates induced a faster rate of glycogen resynthesis in four hours than either the carbohydrates or protein alone. They found significantly higher blood glucose and insulin levels, factors that stimulate glucose uptake by the muscles and activation of the enzyme that converts glucose to glycogen (Zawadski et al., 1992). Table 4.8 lists foods that contain 100 grams of carbohydrates as well as some protein.

Research shows that when a specific amount of carbohydrates (measured in calories) is compared to an equal amount of combined carbohydrates and protein, they reload muscle glycogen at the same rate (Jentjens & Jeukendrup, 2003; Jentjens et al., 2001; Van Hall, Shirreffs, & Calbet, 2000; van Loon et al., 2000). Therefore, while protein may not be necessary for glycogen recovery, it might assist with muscle synthesis.

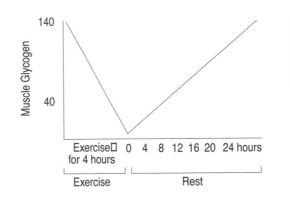

FIGURE 4.4
It takes 24 hours to replenish muscle glycogen after strenuous exercise.

Glycemic Index

A number of different types of carbohydrates have been studied, using white bread as the standard, to determine which might be optimal for glycogen resynthesis. White bread is assigned a glycemic index (GI) of 100. Carbohydrates that quickly empty into the blood stream (high glycemic) are recommended immediately after exercise. High-glycemic foods such as simple carbohydrates raise blood glucose and insulin levels and facilitate glycogen synthesis. The remaining carbohydrates should be derived from other natural resources, such as the complex and simple carbohydrates found in fruits, vegetables, breads, cereals, pasta, and rice. Table 4.9 lists foods with different glycemic indices. It should be noted that when these carbohydrates are combined with other nutrients,

---

Table 4.8
Postexercise Meals/Snacks for Glycogen Resynthesis

✔ One bagel with peanut butter and ⅔ cup of raisins

✔ One cup lowfat yogurt, one banana, and a cup of orange juice

✔ One turkey sandwich on whole wheat bread with one cup of applesauce

✔ Spaghetti with meat sauce and garlic bread

✔ 8 ounces of skim milk, one apple, one orange, two slices of bread, and three pancakes

✔ 12 ounces of a carbohydrate-loading drink and a bagel

Protein

Table 4.9
Glycemic Index of Various Foods

High Glycemic Foods (greater than 85)

Honey, corn syrup

Bagel, white bread

Cornflakes

Raisins

Potato (baked, boiled, or mashed)

Sweet corn

Moderate Glycemic Foods (60–85)

Spaghetti, macaroni

Oatmeal

Banana, grapes, oranges

Rice

Yams

Baked beans

Low Glycemic Foods (less than 60)

Apple, applesauce

Cherries, dates, figs, peaches, pears, plums

Kidney beans, chick peas, green peas, navy beans,
    red lentils

Whole milk, skim milk, plain yogurt

such as protein or fat, it changes the glycemic index. For this reason, some experts consider the glycemic load (i.e., how the combination of nutrients affects blood glucose) as a more realistic approach.

PROTEIN

The principal role of protein in the body is to build and repair body tissues, including muscles, ligaments, and tendons. Protein also is important for the synthesis of hormones, enzymes, and antibodies, as well as for fluid transport and energy. Contrary to popular belief, protein is not a primary source of energy, except when you do not consume enough calories or carbohy-

drates. If your clients fail to eat enough calories or put themselves on restricted-energy diets, then protein is stripped from the muscle and used as an energy source instead of being used for its intended job of building tissue, enzymes, hormones, etc.

Proteins are structural and regulatory molecules made up of specific combinations of 20 different amino acids. Eight of these amino acids cannot be synthesized in the body and therefore must be supplied by the diet. Generally, the dietary intake of most individuals exceeds even the highest recommendation. If you consume more protein than the body can use, the excess amino acids may be stored as fat in the body. Available research suggests that an active adult needs about 0.8 to 1.0 grams of protein per kilogram of body weight. This would mean that a 45-year-old male who weighs 155 pounds (70.45 kilograms) needs 56 to 70 grams of protein per day. Use the following equation to determine protein requirements:

Your weight in lbs. _____
÷ 2.2 = _____ weight in kilograms
Your weight in kilograms _____
x 0.8 = _____ protein requirement
per day

To determine the amount of protein in food, use the following as a guide:

✔ 8 grams of protein are found in 1 cup of milk or yogurt

✔ 8 grams of protein are found in 1 ounce of cheese

✔ 8 grams of protein are found in ¾ cup of cottage cheese

✔ 7 grams of protein are found in 1 ounce of meat (chicken, fish, pork, beef) and in one egg

✔ 3 grams of protein are found in ½ cup of pasta, rice, corn, beans, or one slice of bread

Table 4.10 lists the specific amounts of protein in some common protein-rich foods.

Table 4.10
Protein in Common Foods

Food	Portion Size	Protein (grams)
Milk (skim, 2%, whole)	1 cup	8
Yogurt (nonfat, lowfat)	1 cup	8
Cheese (any variety)	1 ounce	8
Lean hamburger patty	3 ounces	26
Egg/egg white	1	7
Lean steak	3 ounces	21
Chicken breast	3.5 ounces	30
Taco	1	11
Pizza	2 slices	32
Tuna	3 ounces	24
Peanut butter	1 tablespoon	4
Whole wheat bread	1 slice	2
Pasta	1 cup	6

Protein Requirements for Exercising Individuals

Because protein can be used as a metabolic fuel during exercise, much controversy surrounds the need for protein in exercising individuals. There are now sufficient data in the literature to suggest that protein requirements do vary with the type and intensity of exercise performed and the total energy consumed.

In general, protein recommendations for athletes are about 1.2 to 1.8 grams of protein per kilogram of body weight. When active individuals fail to consume enough protein, their available stores are used for fuel, leaving little left for muscle repair and general body maintenance. Reports of food intake in athletes consistently indicate that protein represents from 12 to 20% of total energy intake, or 1.2 to 2 grams of protein per kilogram of body weight per day. The exception to the rule will be the small, active woman who may consume a low energy intake in conjunction with an exercise or training program. While these women may consume close to the RDA for protein, it may be inadequate to maintain lean mass (Lemon, 1995).

Consuming more protein than the body can use should be avoided. When athletes consume diets that are high in protein, they compromise their carbohydrate status, possibly affecting their ability to train and compete at peak performance. The National Research Council also points out that because protein-rich foods are often high in fat, eating too much protein makes it difficult to maintain a low-fat diet. In addition, the **hypercalciuric effect** of high-protein diets is still considered by some a significant factor in calcium balance and is often cited as a potentially adverse side effect, especially for women.

Amino Acid Supplementation

Protein or amino acid supplementation in the form of powders or pills is not necessary and should be discouraged. Taking large amounts of these supplements can lead to dehydration, loss of urinary calcium, weight gain, and kidney and liver stress. Taking single amino acids or combinations, such as arginine and lysine, may interfere with the absorption of certain essential amino acids (Slavin, 1991). An additional concern is that substituting amino acid supplements for food may cause deficiencies of other nutrients found in protein-rich foods such as iron, niacin, and thiamin. Amino acid imbalances and toxicities are possible if single amino acid supplements, such as arginine and ornithine, are consumed in large quantities to achieve growth hormone release and muscle development. Because single amino acid supplements have not been routinely consumed by humans in the past, little scientific data is available. You need to realize that amino acid supplements taken in large doses have not been tested in human subjects, and no margin of safety is available. They are essentially drugs with unknown physiological effects. It is important for you to develop a strategy to effectively approach and discuss supplement use with clients.

Fat

FAT

Fat is the primary fuel for light- to moderate-intensity exercise. It is the most concentrated source of food energy and supplies more than twice as many calories by weight (9 kcal/gram) as protein (4 kcal/gram) or carbohydrate (4 kcal/gram). Fat provides **essential fatty acids** and is necessary for the proper functioning of **cell membranes,** skin, and hormones, and for transporting fat-soluble vitamins. The body has total glycogen stores (both muscle and liver) equaling about 2,500 calories, whereas each pound of body fat supplies 3,500 calories. This means that an athlete weighing 163 pounds (74 kg) with 10% body fat has 16.3 pounds (7.4 kg) of fat, which equals 57,000 calories.

Although fat performs many important functions in the body and is a valuable metabolic fuel for muscle activity during long-term aerobic exercise, no attempt should be made to consume more fat, especially since individuals consuming a high-fat diet typically consume fewer carbohydrate calories. Simonsen and colleagues had elite rowers consume either 40% or 20% of their calories from fat and then compared the two diets for power output and speed. After taking a biopsy of the rowers' muscles, they found that those who consumed the low-fat, high-carbohydrate diet had more muscle glycogen. Rowers on the high-fat, low-carbohydrate diet had moderate levels of muscle glycogen and actually were able to complete the workout sets. However, when it came to power output and faster speeds, those athletes who consumed the lower-fat, higher-carbohydrate diets had significantly higher power and speed (Simonsen et al., 1991). This has implications for individuals who participate in muscular endurance sports that require bursts of power, such as rowing, swimming, gymnastics, figure skating, judo, boxing, or any other sport that needs energy generated by the anaerobic pathway (see pages 6–8). Following a low-fat, high-carbohydrate diet is important for

health reasons as well, since a high-fat diet has been associated with cardiovascular disease, obesity, **diabetes,** and some types of cancers (Krause & Mahan, 2003).

You need to recognize the many sources of hidden fat in foods. Fat is present, but not visible, in dairy products such as cheese, ice cream, and whole milk, and in bakery items, granola bars, french fries, avocados, chips, nuts, and many processed foods. Fat is more clearly visible in margarine, butter, mayonnaise, salad dressing, oil, and highly-marbled meats.

Most athletes should consume 20 to 30% of their calories from fat. Aside from decreasing overall calories, limiting consumption of dietary fat is the first step toward losing excess body fat. Doing so eliminates excess calories, but not nutrients as long as the client consumes nutritious, low-fat foods. Suggestions for reducing fat intake are listed in Table 4.11.

HEART DISEASE

There are nearly two million deaths in this country each year and almost 30% of them are the result of **coronary heart disease.** Most coronary heart disease is due to blockages in the arteries that supply blood to the heart muscle. Fat, saturated fat, and **cholesterol** that circulate in the blood are deposited on the inner walls of the arteries. Over time, scar tissue builds up as more fat and cholesterol are deposited, and the arteries become progressively narrower. This process is known as **atherosclerosis.**

Cholesterol

Human and animal studies have shown that elevated levels of blood cholesterol lead to early development of coronary heart disease. Available research also shows that individuals with high blood cholesterol have a greater chance of developing heart disease than do people with lower levels of cholesterol, and that the chances of developing coronary heart disease increase in proportion to the amount the cholesterol is elevated. The National

Table 4.11
Fat Substitutions

Instead of	Try
Whole milk	Skim milk
Cheddar, jack, or swiss cheese	Part-skim mozzarella, string or lowfat cottage cheese, other cheeses that contain less than 5 grams of fat per ounce
Ice cream	Ice milk or lowfat/nonfat frozen yogurt
Butter or margarine	Jam, yogurt, ricotta cheese, light or nonfat cream cheese, lowfat yogurt, light sour cream, blender-whipped cottage cheese dressing
Bacon	Lowfat turkey bacon, Canadian bacon, bacon bits
Ground beef	Extra lean ground beef or ground turkey
Fried chicken	Baked chicken without the skin
Doughnuts and pastries	Bagels, whole-grain breads, homemade breads, muffins, quick breads
Apple pie	Baked or raw apples
Chocolate candy or bars	Jelly beans, hard candy, licorice
Cookies, cakes, brownies	Vanilla wafers, gingersnaps, graham crackers, fig bars

Cholesterol Education Program (NCEP) has set standards to determine an individual's risk for cardiovascular disease (Expert Panel on Detection, Evaluation, and Treatment of High Blood Cholesterol in Adults, 2001). The NCEP suggests that blood cholesterol levels should be classified as follows (in mg/dL):

Desirable	< 200
Borderline high	200–239
High	≥240

These categories apply to all adults over age 20, regardless of age or sex.

A physician can assess a person's risk for heart disease, offer advice on how to make dietary changes, monitor progress toward cholesterol reduction, or refer your client to an R.D. for comprehensive dietary planning. Persons with very high cholesterol levels might need a prescribed cholesterol-lowering drug.

Clients with desirable blood cholesterol levels (less than 200 mg/dL) are advised to have a serum cholesterol test again within three years. Clients with cholesterol levels of 200 mg/dL or greater should repeat the test to confirm the value and use the average as a guide.

Those who have high blood cholesterol (240 mg/dL or greater) should undergo **lipoprotein** analysis. Clients with borderline high blood cholesterol (200–239 mg/dL) who are considered high risk because they have coronary heart disease or two other risk factors should also have their lipoprotein levels analyzed. See Table 4.12 and Chapter 5 for a discussion of risk factors.

Table 4.12
Risk Factors for Heart Disease

Hypertension (high blood pressure)*

Cigarette smoking*

Elevated total cholesterol (>200 mg/dL) and/or low HDL cholesterol (<40 mg/dL)*

Sedentary lifestyle*

Obesity

Diabetes or impaired fasting glucose

Family history of heart disease before the age of 55 in father or 65 in mother

* Classified as a primary risk factor for heart disease by the American Heart Association.

Lipoproteins

Low-density lipoproteins (LDLs) and **high-density lipoproteins (HDLs)** are made by the body to transport fat and cholesterol through the blood. LDLs contain the greatest amounts of cholesterol and may be responsible for depositing it on the artery walls. For this reason, they are sometimes called "bad" cholesterol. The NCEP also has set standards for LDLs (in mg/dL):

Optimal	<100
Near or above optimal	100–129
Borderline high	130–159
High	160–189
Very high	≥190

LDL cholesterol can be lowered by exercising, losing weight, incorporating more monounsaturated and polyunsaturated fats into the diet, and decreasing the overall percentage of fat calories consumed. Clients with extremely high LDL levels may need medication to control LDL cholesterol.

HDLs contain more protein than cholesterol. They remove cholesterol from the cells in the arteries and transport it back to the liver for repackaging and removal from the body. Studies have shown that individuals with higher levels of HDL have a lower incidence of heart disease. Thus, HDLs have become known as the "good" cholesterol. HDL cholesterol levels below 40 mg/dL are considered a significant risk factor for coronary heart disease. Several factors, including regular consistent exercise, have been found to raise HDLs. Regular moderate-to-vigorous aerobic exercise has been shown to cause an increase in HDL levels. Moderate alcohol consumption also appears to raise HDL levels, but most health professionals recommend exercise as a better method.

With the technology available today, you can easily provide initial cholesterol screening for your clients. However, if lipoprotein analysis is desired, which involves a 12-hour fast and a venipuncture blood draw, a referral to a medical professional is necessary. All clients with an LDL cholesterol level greater than 160 mg/dL, or a level of 130–159 mg/dL combined with high-risk status, should be clinically evaluated by a physician.

Triglycerides

The bulk of dietary fat is ingested in the form of **triglycerides,** which are made up of a glycerol backbone with three **fatty acids** attached (Figure 4.5). The fatty acids attached to the glycerol may differ from one another in either chain length and degree of saturation, or in chemical structure. A **saturated fatty acid** is one that carries the maximum number of hydrogen atoms, leaving no points unsaturated, whereas an unsaturated fatty acid has one or more double bonds, and therefore less hydrogen. There are two types of unsaturated fatty acids: **monounsaturated** and **polyunsaturated.** Food fats contain a mixture of the three kinds of fatty acids.

When a fat contains predominantly saturated fatty acids, it is said to be a saturated fat. Similarly, when a fat or oil contains a large proportion of monounsaturated or polyunsaturated fatty acids, it is called a monounsaturated fat or a polyunsaturated fat, respectively. The more saturated fat an individual eats, the higher the blood cholesterol will be. The major sources of saturated fatty acids in the diet come from animal products such as meats and whole milk dairy products that are solid at room temperature. Lowfat dairy products are lower in saturated fats and are recommended for adults who need to lower their levels of saturated fats and cholesterol. The exceptions to this rule are coconut,

FIGURE 4.5
Structure of a triglyceride.

palm, and palm kernel oils, which are unsaturated but act like saturated fats and raise blood levels of cholesterol. (Mono- and polyunsaturated fatty acids come from plants and are liquid at room temperature.) While these oils are not available for consumer purchase, they are often used in commercial baked goods and other processed foods.

Since saturated fats raise blood cholesterol, eating less of them is recommended. Remember:

✔ Reducing total fat can reduce saturated fat as well.

✔ Most animal fats contain high proportions of saturated fat, whereas vegetable foods provide a higher proportion of polyunsaturated fatty acids.

✔ Vegetable oils from palm kernel, coconut, palm, and cocoa fat will raise blood cholesterol.

✔ Some margarines are lower in saturated fat and higher in unsaturated fats than butter.

Hydrogenation

Hydrogenation is the process of breaking the double bonds in unsaturated fats (liquid at room temperature), thereby turning them solid. This reduces the number of double bonds and makes them more saturated and more resistant to spoilage.

When fatty acids are hydrogenated, their shapes change (Figure 4.6). A cis-fatty acid

Cis-fatty Acid

Trans-fatty Acid

FIGURE 4.6
Transformation of a fatty acid as a result of hydrogenation.

has its hydrogen atoms on the same side, whereas a trans-fatty acid has them on opposite sides. The cis- configuration is typical of the fatty acids found in natural foods, but during hydrogenation, some hydrogen atoms shift and form trans-fatty acids. Trans-fatty acids are more stable, but their safety is questionable. Trans-fatty acids raise blood cholesterol even higher than saturated fats. Clients need to be educated about finding hydrogenated fats in their foods and margarines, and they should know that food processors can control the extent of hydrogenation—they do not have to automatically convert all unsaturated fatty acids to saturated ones. Any margarine that lists hydrogenated fats first on the label is going to have more trans-fatty acids than cis-fatty acids. It seems desirable to take advantage of all opportunities to select foods and design meals that are low in both fat and hydrogenated fat.

VITAMINS AND MINERALS

Vitamins and minerals are food components that serve as coenzymes in the metabolic reactions that release energy, transport and consume oxygen, and maintain cell integrity. Because of these important functions, their use as **ergogenic aids** has been highly touted, even though there is little scientific evidence to document their effect. The need for vitamins and minerals for exercise has been reviewed by Haymes and Clarkson, and resulted in the consensus that unless an individual is deficient in a given nutrient, supplementation of that nutrient does not have a major effect on performance (Haymes, 1991; Clarkson, 1991).

Nutrient Deficiencies

Nutrient deficiencies for the exercising population are similar to those of the general population. In other words, just because you exercise does not mean that you need special amounts of any vitamin or mineral. The nutrients that people often do not get enough of include folate, vitamin B$_6$, **antioxidants,** calcium, and zinc. Because many women exercisers also are vegetarians, iron, vitamin B$_{12}$, and zinc may be of specific concern to this subgroup.

Vitamin/Mineral Supplementation

Because consumers experience a lot of confusion over what makes up a nutritionally balanced diet, and because most individuals do not understand the RDA, many Americans turn to vitamin and mineral supplementation as nutritional insurance. But should most people be taking a supplement? Generally, no, although the consumer who takes a simple one-a-day type of vitamin or mineral supplement that does not exceed the nutrient levels of the RDA is probably not doing any harm. It may even be appropriate to suggest a multiple one-a-day to clients who limit their food selection and calories, since they may have a difficult time getting the recommended levels of nutrients. Of greater concern is the client who has a whole medicine cabinet full of supplements. These individuals take a handful of supplements for breakfast, perhaps several tablespoons of nutritional yeast, assorted pills containing trace minerals, powdered protein, and herbs. They are asking the pills and supplements to play a role that is better delegated to food.

Many athletes, in search of a competitive edge, also turn to supplements in the form of pills, powders, or magical elixirs in an effort to make the body perform at its best. They listen to self-proclaimed "experts" who try to convince the athletes that their product will elevate their performance by improving muscle contractions, preventing fat gain, enhancing strength, or supplying energy. These "experts" may insist that fatigue and muscle soreness is due to a vitamin or mineral deficiency when, in fact, if there is a nutritional reason for fatigue, it is usually a lack of calories, fluids, and/or carbohydrates.

Takers of self-prescribed supplements need a warning about the risks of overdosing. There are two types of vitamins: **water-soluble** and **fat-soluble.** Concern should be expressed if individuals are taking high doses of fat-soluble vitamins (A, D, E, and K). These particular vitamins are stored in body fat, principally in the liver, and toxic levels have been found in people who take megadoses of these nutrients.

The water-soluble vitamins (B complex and C) are not stored by the body, and any excesses are excreted in the urine. It was once thought that a toxic level of water-soluble vitamins was impossible. Consumption of **megadoses** of water-soluble vitamins can, however, reach toxic levels. Table 4.13 lists all of the vitamins, their physiologic function, and major food sources.

Vitamin toxicity usually affects the nervous system. Both vitamins A and B$_6$ are known to produce adverse neurologic reactions (such as nerve transmission) when ingested in megadoses rather than the Recommended Dietary Allowances (RDAs). The RDA is the daily amount of a nutrient recommended for practically all healthy individuals to promote optimal health. It is not a minimal amount needed to prevent disease symptoms—a large margin of safety is included. The symptoms of vitamin or mineral toxicity are vague at best; diarrhea, vomiting, skin rashes, and overall "just not feeling right" have been reported. Because these symptoms could describe any disease or illness, it is best for you not to make recommendations about vitamin toxicity to clients. You should, however, suggest that such clients seek professional medical advice about the symptoms. Encourage them to take their supplements to the physician and/or dietitian for assessment.

Because consumers may have strong beliefs in their vitamin supplement program, several strategies can be used to avoid upsetting them. Acknowledge their feelings and the values that underlie their

Table 4.13
Vitamin Facts

Vitamin	RDA/AI* Men†	Women†	Best Sources	Functions
A (carotene)	**900 μg**	**700 μg**	Yellow or orange fruits and vegetables, green leafy vegetables, fortified oatmeal, liver, dairy products	Formation and maintenance of skin, hair and mucous membranes; helps you see in dim light; bone and tooth growth
B₁ (thiamine)	**1.2 mg**	**1.1 mg**	Fortified cereals and oatmeals meats, rice and pasta, whole grains, liver	Helps body release energy from carbohydrates during metabolism; growth and muscle tone
B₂ (riboflavin)	**1.3 mg**	**1.1 mg**	Whole grains, green leafy vegetables, organ meats, milk, eggs	Helps body release energy from protein, fat, and carbohydrates during metabolism
B₆ (pyridoxine)	**1.3 mg**	**1.3 mg**	Fish, poultry, lean meats, bananas, prunes, dried beans, whole grains, avocados	Helps build body tissue and aids in metabolism of protein
B₁₂ (cobalamin)	**2.4 μg**	**2.4 μg**	Meats, milk products, seafood	Aids cell development, functioning of the nervous system and the metabolism of protein and fat
Biotin	30 μg	30 μg	Cereal/grain products, yeast, legumes, liver	Involved in metabolism of protein, fats, and carbohydrates
Choline	550 mg	425 mg	Milk, liver, eggs, peanuts	A precursor of acetylcholine; essential for liver function
Folate (folacin, folic acid)	**400 μg**	**400 μg**	Green leafy vegetables, organ meats, dried peas, beans, lentils	Aids in genetic material development; involved in red blood cell production
Niacin	**16 mg**	**14 mg**	Meat, poultry, fish, enriched cereals, peanuts, potatoes, dairy products, eggs	Involved in carbohydrate, protein, and fat metabolism
Pantothenic Acid	5 mg	5 mg	Lean meats, whole grains, legumes, vegetables, fruits	Helps release energy from fats and carbohydrates
C (absorbic acid)	**90 mg**	**75 mg**	Citrus fruits, berries and vegetables— especially peppers	Essential for structure of bones, cartilage, muscle and blood vessels; helps maintain capillaries and gums and aids in absorption of iron
D	5 μg	5 μg	Fortified milk, sunlight, fish, eggs, butter, fortified margarine	Aids in bone and tooth formation; helps maintain heart action and nervous system
E	**15 mg**	**15 mg**	Fortified and multigrain cereals, nuts, wheat germ, vegetable oils, green leafy vegetables	Protects blood cells, body tissue, and essential fatty acids from harmful destruction in the body
K	120 μg	90 μg	Green leafy vegetables, fruit, dairy and grain products	Essential for blood clotting functions

* Recommended Dietary Allowances are presented in bold type; Adequate Intakes are presented in ordinary type
† RDAs and AIs given are for men aged 31–50 and non-pregnant, non-breastfeeding women aged 31–50; mg = milligrams; μg = micrograms

Reprinted with permission from *Dietary Reference Intakes* (various volumes). Copyright 1997, 1998, and 2000 by the National Academy of Science. Courtesy of the National Academies Press, Washington, D.C.

Minerals

practice, and then distinguish between practices that are dangerous and those that are not. For example, clients using supplements at pharmacological doses (greater than 100 times the RDA) are headed for toxic levels, unlike those who are just taking a multivitamin/mineral supplement once a day. Confront only the dangerous practices; ignore the harmless ones. Try to wean such clients off of their supplements gradually instead of asking them to quit all at once, and encourage them to get their nutrients from foods. Let your clients know that there is a lot of information that scientists have not yet discovered about nutrients and the effects of their combinations in foods, and teach them to attain nutritional adequacy and balance by adopting the principles of the MyPyramid Food Guidance System.

While it has been shown that a severely inadequate intake of certain vitamins can impair performance, it is unusual for individuals who exercise to have such deficiencies. Even marginal deficiencies do not appear to markedly affect the ability to exercise efficiently. Most individuals can meet the RDA by making wise food selections from the MyPyramid Food Guidance System.

The Antioxidant Vitamins

Antioxidants are compounds that preserve and protect other compounds in the body from free radical damage. Five nutrients have been identified as having antioxidant properties: beta carotene, vitamin C, vitamin E, and the minerals sulfur and selenium.

Free radicals are oxygen molecules with a single electron. Oxygen is composed of two atoms that are bound together, but occasionally these oxygen atoms split and create two individual or singlet oxygen atoms. It is these molecules that cause damage to tissues and create health problems. Sometimes these singlet oxygen molecules will attach to other compounds in the

body, particularly polyunsaturated fats, and start chain reactions that create even more free radicals and further health problems. Free radicals have been linked to the development of cancer, atherosclerosis, and cataracts, as well as to the aging process.

Out of all the antioxidant nutrients, vitamin E appears to be the most promising. It appears that vitamin E helps prevent LDL cholesterol from becoming oxidized, thus inhibiting the formation of plaque in veins and arteries.

Clients may ask about adding vitamin E to their diets. A typical low-fat diet may provide as much as 25 mg of vitamin E per day, roughly three times the RDA, and by adding a bowl of fortified cereal to their diet, clients could more than double that level. If they do decide to take a vitamin E supplement, it is wise to stay within a modest range [65 to 260 mg, or 100 to 400 International Units (IU)].

Phytochemicals

Some **phytochemicals,** which are plant chemicals found in fruits, vegetables, many spices and herbs, as well as beans, grains, and seeds, may reduce the risk of cancer and cardiovascular disease if consumed regularly. Phytochemicals, of which more than 900 have been identified, are not absolutely required elements of the diet, but many of these substances probably provide significant health benefits. Because most vitamin and mineral supplements contain few, if any, phytochemicals, they must be consumed through food sources.

MINERALS

Minerals perform a variety of functions in the body. While some are used to build tissue, such as calcium and phosphorus for bones and teeth, others are important components of hormones, such as iodine in thyroxine. Iron is critical for the formation of hemoglobin, which carries oxygen within the red blood cells. Minerals also are important for regulating muscle contractions and body fluids, conducting nerve impulses, and regulating normal heart rhythm.

Minerals are divided into two groups. The first are referred to as macro minerals and are needed in amounts from 100 mg to 1 gram. These include calcium, phosphorus, magnesium, sodium, potassium, chloride, and sulfur. The others fall under the category of trace minerals and include copper, iodine, zinc, cobalt, fluoride, and selenium. Food sources

Minerals

Table 4.14
Mineral Facts

Vitamin	RDA/AI*		Best Sources	Functions
	Men†	Women†		
Calcium	1,000 mg	1,000 mg	Milk and milk products	Strong bones, teeth, muscle tissue; regulates heart beat, muscle action and nerve function; blood clotting
Chromium	35 µg	25 µg	Corn oil, clams, whole grain cereals, brewer's yeast	Glucose metabolism (energy); increases effectiveness of insulin
Copper	900 µg	900 µg	Oysters, nuts, organ meats, legumes	Formation of red blood cells, bone growth and health, works with vitamin C to form elastin
Fluoride	4 mg	3 mg	Fluorinated water, teas, marine fish	Stimulates bone formation; inhibits or even reverses dental caries
Iodine	150 µg	150 µg	Seafood, iodized salt	Component of hormone thyroxine, which controls metabolism
Iron	8 mg	18 mg	Meats and organ meats, legumes	Hemoglobin formation, improves blood quality, increases resistance to stress and disease
Magnesium	420 mg	320 mg	Nuts, green vegetables, whole grains	Acid/alkaline balance; important in metabolism of carbohydrates, minerals and sugar
Manganese	2.3 mg	1.8 mg	Nuts, whole grains, vegetables, fruits	Enzyme activation; carbohydrate and fat production; sex hormone production; skeletal development
Molybdenum	45 µg	45 µg	Legumes, grain products, nuts	Functions as a cofactor for a limited number of enzymes in humans
Phosphorus	700 mg	700 mg	Fish, meat, poultry, eggs, grains	Bone development; important in protein, fat and carbohydrate utilization
Potassium	No RDA		Lean meat, vegetables, fruits	Fluid balance; controls activity of heart muscle, nervous system, kidneys
Selenium	55 µg	55 µg	Seafood, organ meats, lean meats, grains	Protects body tissues against oxidative damage from radiation, pollution, and normal metabolic processing
Zinc	11 mg	8 mg	Lean meats, liver, eggs, seafood, whole grains	Involved in digestion and metabolism; important in development of reproductive system; aids in healing

*, † See Table 4.10, page 135 for notes and sources.

and the physiologic functions for each mineral are listed in Table 4.14.

Iron

Iron is present in all cells of the body and plays a key role in numerous reactions. It is vital to the transport and activation of oxygen and is present in several pathways that create energy. The diets of many women are deficient in iron, a result of dieting and limiting calories. Due to the fact that women face a potentially greater chance of lacking iron because of increased physiological need, low-calorie intakes, and increased iron loss through menstruation, it has been suggested that they consider routine use of iron supplements, particularly during periods of heavy training. In one report, 42% of the female distance runners studied were modified vegetarians and consumed fewer than 200 grams of meat per week (Brooks et al., 1984). Iron supplementation in non-anemic women, however, has not been shown to be useful and may even be potentially harmful. Clearly, there is some hazard from prolonged administration of large doses of iron to persons who are not iron deficient. They are needlessly exposed to **hemosiderosis,** a disorder of iron metabolism in which large deposits of iron are made in the liver. Routine screening tests for women should be performed by medical professionals to detect early stages of iron depletion. Those women found to be iron-deficient, or **anemic,** should receive professional dietary counseling from a physician or dietitian. Supplemental iron may be indicated in individual cases; however, routine use of iron supplements by all females is not warranted.

While dietary intake of iron is tied to caloric intake, iron absorption depends upon the bioavailability, or rate of absorption, of the iron. Meats contain heme-iron, which is a highly bioavailable source of iron. Heme-iron also enhances the absorption of the non-heme-iron found in plant foods like leafy greens, legumes, cereals, whole grains,

and enriched breads. Combining these foods with a source of vitamin C can significantly enhance the absorption of iron (for example, combine orange juice with an iron-enriched cereal, pasta with broccoli, or tomatoes and green peppers).

Regular monitoring of iron levels in physically active individuals, including biochemical evaluations and dietary assessments, is recommended to ensure optimal health and performance.

To ensure an adequate iron intake you should encourage the following for your clients:

✔ Eat foods high in vitamin C at each meal to help the body absorb iron. For example, eat salsa and/or chili peppers with a bean burrito.

✔ Include meat, preferably lean red meat and the dark meat of chicken and turkey, as part of the training diet. These foods provide the body with heme-iron.

✔ To enhance the absorption of non-heme-iron (vegetable and grain sources of iron), combine vegetable proteins with meat. For example, split pea soup with ham, tuna noodle casserole, turkey vegetable soup, chicken soup with lentils, or chili beans with lean ground turkey or hamburger.

✔ To increase iron and carbohydrate intake, eat cereals, breads, and pastas labeled "enriched" or "fortified."

Calcium

Osteoporosis is a major health concern, especially for women. Although the disease has been regarded as an elderly women's problem, young females, especially those who have had interrupted menstrual function, may be at risk for decreased bone mass. Three major risk factors for osteoporosis have been identified: hormonal status (particularly estrogen deficiency), calcium consumption, and physical activity.

Bone mass is developed until the ages of 35 to 40 years. Peak bone mass, however, is obtained between the ages of 14 to 24. The amount of bone mass a woman has by age 35 will strongly influence her susceptibility to fractures in later years. Therefore, it is important that young women consume calcium throughout early life, through the peak bone mass years, and into early adulthood.

The National Institutes of Health (NIH) recommends that **premenopausal** adult women consume 1,000 mg of calcium per day. **Postmenopausal** women who are not taking estrogen should consume 1,500 mg of calcium per day. Unfortunately, though specific calcium levels have been recommended for women, the National Health and Nutrition Examination Survey (NHANES) found that 50% of all females age 15 and older consume less than 75% of the RDA of 1,200 mg, and that 75% of women over 35 consume less than the RDA of 800 mg.

Lowfat and nonfat dairy products, such as milk, buttermilk, yogurt, cheese, and cottage cheese, are excellent sources of dietary calcium.

You can recommend that your clients try the following to incorporate more calcium into their diet:

✔ Prepare canned soup with skim milk instead of water.

✔ Add nonfat dry milk to soups, stews, casseroles, and even cookie recipes.

✔ Add grated lowfat cheese to salads, tacos, and pasta dishes.

✔ Eat yogurt as a snack, or use it to make low-calorie dressings.

✔ Choose calcium-rich desserts, such as lowfat cheese and fruit, frozen nonfat or lowfat yogurt, and puddings made with skim milk.

✔ Drink hot chocolate made with skim milk.

Athletic Amenorrhea

Some women who exercise strenuously stop menstruating due to a condition known as athletic **amenorrhea.** It is associated with many factors, such as nutritional inadequacy, physical stress, energy drain, and acute and chronic hormonal alterations (Sanborn, Albrech, & Wagner, 1987). Amenorrhea can also lead to infertility, unfavorable changes in blood lipoprotein profiles, and an increased risk of fractures, particularly stress fractures.

Young women, driven to excel in their chosen sports and pressured to fit a specific body image (e.g., leanness, low percent body fat, or lower weight) to attain their performance goals, place themselves at risk for developing disordered eating patterns. Such eating behavior may lead to menstrual dysfunction and, subsequently, premature osteoporosis (Bryant, Franklin, & Conviser, 2002).

Spinal bone mass has been found to be lower in amenorrheic women runners compared to **eumenorrheic** women runners (Drinkwater, Nilson, & Chestnut, 1984). What is especially disturbing about this is that further follow-up with these women indicated that bone mineral density remained well below the average for their age group four years after the resumption of normal menses (Drinkwater et al., 1986).

Women with athletic amenorrhea should consult a physician to rule out any serious medical problems, and all amenorrheic women should be consuming 1,500 mg of calcium per day. A physician may suggest several strategies to promote the resumption of menses, including estrogen replacement therapy, weight gain, diet modification, and reduced training.

Regardless of menstrual history, most female athletes need to increase their calcium intake to meet the RDA for calcium.

Lactose Intolerance

One of the more common problems of the gastrointestinal tract is lactose intolerance. Lactase is the enzyme responsible for breaking down lactose, a carbohydrate commonly found in dairy products. Without lactase, lactose cannot be digested and absorbed. As individuals get older, lactase activity appears to decrease and can cause bloating, gas, diarrhea, and sometimes nausea.

It seems that lactose intolerance is not an "all or nothing phenomenon." A person with lactose intolerance does not need to give up

Fluid and Hydration

all dairy products. Some individuals with lactose intolerance may be able to handle small amounts of lactose throughout the day, and others can tolerate fermented dairy products because the bacteria in the products provide their own lactase activity. Have clients try yogurt, buttermilk, some cheeses, and frozen yogurt. For those who are very sensitive to lactose in dairy products, products such as Lactaid can be added to milk and will, in most cases, reduce symptoms.

Probiotics

Probiotics are bacterial cultures that promote the metabolic activity of "good" bacteria, while inhibiting the growth of "bad," or illness-causing, bacteria. Some forms of probiotics have become available in the United States as dietary supplements and are effective in the treatment of several types of diarrhea. They also have been found to inhibit the growth of heliocobacter pylori, the bacteria that is the cause of most cases of peptic ulcers and gastritis. The most well-known source of probiotics is yogurt.

FLUID AND HYDRATION

Maintaining hydration is by far the greatest concern for regular exercisers. Clients who are **dehydrated** will fatigue earlier and lose coordination skills. Their performance can suffer when they lose as little as 2% of body weight due to dehydration. To prevent this from happening, exercising individuals must drink plenty of fluids before, during, and after a workout. Relying on thirst as an indicator of how much fluid is lost is not an accurate method. If your clients relied on thirst, they would only put back 50 to 75% of the fluid they have lost and would start their next workout already in a state of dehydration. Do not wait until you are thirsty to drink, and do not stop drinking once your thirst has been quenched. Most peo-

ple have no idea how much fluid they need, let alone how much they have lost during the day or during exercise. The Adequate Intake for fluids from beverages and food is 3.7 L/day for adult males and 2.7 for adult females. Physically active individuals, however, need more and should take care to follow the recommendations of the National Athletic Trainers' Association (Table 4.15). It should be noted that while the recommendations provided in Table 4.15 provide good general guidelines, the best practice is to replace fluids lost in sweat. To gain insight into fluid losses, have your clients self-monitor their fluid levels by one of two methods:

✔ Weigh in before and after a workout. Consume two to three cups of fluid for each pound of body weight lost.

✔ Check urine color. A dark gold color means the client is dehydrated. A pale yellow color, or no color at all, means the client is headed toward a state of hydration. Clients who consume a lot of caffeine, which is a **diuretic,** will have pale or clear urine even though they are, in fact, dehydrated. Alcohol also is a very powerful diuretic.

Table 4.15

Fluid-intake Recommendations During Exercise

2 hours prior to exercise, drink 500–600 mL (17–20 oz)
Every 10–20 minutes during exercise, drink 200–300 mL (7–10 oz)
Following exercise, drink 450–675 mL for every 0.5 kg body weight lost (or 16–24 oz for every pound)

Adapted with permission from Casa, D.J. et al. (2000). National Athletic Trainers' Association:
Position statement: Fluid replacement for athletes. *Journal of Athletic Training*, 35, 212–224

Sports Drinks

Most experts will now recommend sports drinks to exercising individuals, especially if their workout lasts longer than 60 minutes. The fear that sports drinks impair fluid absorption is unfounded, and it has been shown that sports drinks formulated with 6 to 8% carbohydrates plus at least 100 mg sodium per 8 oz replace fluids just as fast as water, improve performance, and help ensure optimal rehydration (Table 4.16). They also maintain physiological function as well as, if not better than, water.

Remind your clients to pay attention to the percentage of carbohydrates in each drink. Those containing less than 5% carbohydrate do not provide enough energy to enhance performance, and beverages containing 10% carbohydrate or more (fruit juices and soda) are associated with intestinal cramping, nausea, diarrhea, and impaired absorption.

**Table 4.16
Comparison of Sport Drinks and Other Beverages**

Beverage	Carbohydrate Concentration (%)	Sodium Concentration Per 8 oz (mg)
Gatorade	6.0	110
AllSport	9.0	55
Met-RX	8.0	125
Powerade	8.0	55
Cytomax	8.0	50
Endurox	15.0	153
Revenge	4.2	48
Ultima	1.7	8
Cola	11.0	34
Orange Juice	11.0	7
Red Bull*	11.0	207
Water	0.0	0

*Also contains caffeine

Reprinted with permission from the Gatorade Sports Science Institute.

DISPELLING SPORT NUTRITION MYTHS

M*yth:* Large amounts of protein will increase muscle strength and size.

Reality: There is no evidence to show that consuming excess amounts of protein will increase muscle strength or size. In fact, protein consumed in excess of what the body needs will be converted to fat. Also of concern is that excessive protein consumption can cause dehydration and place added stress on the kidneys and liver.

It is true that athletes in heavy training (muscular endurance training lasting 60 to 90 minutes) may need to allocate a slightly greater percentage of their calories from protein, while nonathletes require only 12 to 15%. This is because the body may have reduced protein stores during heavy training periods. People do not, however, necessarily need to consume excess amounts of protein to meet this increased requirement since it can be met by eating a well-balanced diet with protein-rich foods during periods of heavy training.

Myth: Eating honey, candy bars, soft drinks, or sugar before competing will provide a quick burst of energy.

Reality: Such foods have a high sugar content and eating them within an hour of competition causes the amount of insulin in the blood to rise and, consequently, the sugar in the blood is removed too quickly (i.e., rebound hypoglycemia). The exerciser may feel tired and weak as a result of low blood sugar. High-carbohydrate foods consumed two to three hours prior to competition may, however, improve performance since the exerciser is no longer compensating for low blood sugar, and the food can serve as a source of fuel. Does this mean that endurance athletes should load up on soft drinks and candy bars a few hours before they exercise? It appears that individuals differ in their susceptibility to a lowering of blood glucose during exercise. The physiological basis for this difference has not been determined, so at this time, advise your clients that consuming sugar-containing foods less than one hour prior to exercise could harm their performance if they are sensitive to a lowering of their blood glucose level.

Myth: Drinking water prior to and during exercise causes upset stomach and cramps.

Reality: Water is the most important nutrient to an exercising individual. Restricting fluids during exercise, especially in hot weather, can cause severe dehydration and limit performance. Remind your clients to drink 7 to 10 ounces of water every 10 to 20 minutes during exercise to help replace body fluids lost through perspiration. They should monitor water losses and rehydrate with the appropriate amount (Table 4.15).

Myth: Carbohydrates encourage weight gain, while protein promotes weight and fat loss.

Reality: Sugar Busters!, The Zone, Dr. Atkins' New Diet Revolution, Protein Power, and The Carbohydrate Addict's Diet are some of the latest fad diets that have become popular—and controversial. The basic claim of these diets is that carbohydrates make you fat and that insulin causes obesity. These diets focus on blood-sugar levels and blame carbohydrates for causing a sudden rise in blood-sugar levels. As blood-sugar levels rise, insulin is released and sends sugar to the brain and to the muscles to be burned for energy, while the excess gets stored as fat. The theory is that if you eat more protein and fat and limit your intake of carbohydrate, the rapid rise in blood sugar is avoided and less sugar will be stored for fat. These diets also claim that by eating a high-fat/high-protein diet, the body will metabolize fat instead of carbohydrates for energy. However, there is no scientific evidence to back up the authors' claims. The rapid weight loss that people may experience while on these diets is primarily from water and protein losses from muscle, not fat.

According to Bryant, Franklin, and Conviser (2002), low-calorie diets that limit carbohydrate intake can have serious nutrition and health consequences. They eliminate many food groups that provide essential nutrients, energy, and fiber to the diet (e.g., breads, grains, cereals, fruits, and vegetables). They also do not teach or promote good nutritional habits. The dieter learns very little regarding wise food choices or about making lifestyle changes that will help to

maintain weight loss. In addition, these diets can cause dehydration that persists until the diet is over. Finally, low-calorie diets provide limited carbohydrates for glycogen replacement. As a result, the dieter quickly becomes glycogen depleted, making exercising difficult, especially when combined with dehydration. These factors help set any exercising dieter up for ultimate failure.

Myth: Muscle cramps are caused by inadequate salt intake.

Reality: Cramps are caused by excess water loss through perspiration. Ingesting salt tablets can aggravate existing dehydration by drawing water out of body tissues and into the stomach. Water should be consumed before, during, and after exercise to prevent dehydration.

Myth: Taking vitamin and mineral supplements will provide more energy.

Reality: Not one of the 14 vitamins has been shown to supply energy; their role is to release the energy from food. Some vitamins are involved in energy production, but taking excess amounts, or megadoses, of them will not result in increased energy. Part of the confusion may be due to nutrition terminology. Most laypersons equate energy with subjective mental and physical feelings, while nutrition experts define energy as calories. Vitamins and minerals provide no calories. You should stress to your clients that all 14 vitamins can be supplied by a well-balanced diet.

Myth: Tea and coffee are the best precompetition beverages.

Reality: Tea and coffee contain caffeine, which is a stimulant. Some research suggests that caffeine can improve endurance performance by increasing the use of fat as an energy source, thus sparing muscle glycogen, but not all individuals will experience this effect (MacIntosh & Wright, 1995; Pasman et al., 1995; Costill et al., 1978). In fact, a hypersensitive response resulting in increased heart rate and anxiety is a more likely occurrence. There also is evidence of increased urine production, which can lead to dehydration.

Myth: Crash diets are the fastest, most effective way to lose weight.

Reality: Though crash dieting can result in large amounts of weight loss, it is muscle mass, glycogen stores, and water, not excess body fat, that is lost. This can impair an individual's endurance and cause poor performance. Other problems associated with crash diets include electrolyte imbalances, calcium deficiency, iron deficiency anemia, and vitamin and mineral deficiencies. It is important to be sensible about modifying a diet to lose weight. A person should lose no more than 2 pounds per week. If they reduce their caloric intake by 500 calories per day and increase their activity to burn an additional 500 calories per day, they will likely lose two pounds by the end of one week. (See pages 362–363 for more information on weight control.)

Myth: Most low-fat foods are also low in calories.

Reality: Foods naturally low in fat (e.g., fruits, vegetables, grains) tend to be low in calories. However, foods that are manufactured to be low in fat (e.g., reduced fat snacks and desserts) can be relatively high in calories. During the process of removing fat, some of the taste and texture of the food items is lost. In an effort to add taste and texture, food manufacturers often add carbohydrates and protein, thus adding calories. Inform your clients that just because a food item is "low-fat" it does not give them a license to overeat.

Myth: All-natural or herbal supplements are safe and effective in enhancing weight loss and improving overall performance.

Reality: Many nutritional supplements are marketed using deceptive, misleading, or fraudulent advertising. Although many claims are unsubstantiated, such substances can be marketed without the FDA review of safety and effectiveness. Since the passage of the Dietary Supplement Health and Education Act of 1994 (DSHEA),

dietary ingredients used in dietary supplements are no longer subject to the premarket safety evaluations required of other new food ingredients or for new uses of old food ingredients, thereby allowing companies to sell supplements without first testing and proving their safety and efficacy. A major problem with these "magic pills, powders, and potions" is that the concentration of active ingredients can greatly differ from product to product due to the lack of regulatory control. Although some supplements may confer beneficial effects, most are associated with varied adverse side effects. When a supplement label refers to "research" that has proved a supplement's powers, it may actually be referring to animal studies, not research involving humans. As a fitness professional (unless you hold the proper credentials), it is beyond your scope of practice to recommend nutritional supplement use to your clients—from both a professional and legal liability standpoint.

SUMMARY

Fortunately, the same diet that enhances good health also will maximize performance for most people. A basic knowledge of nutrition should aid you in helping your clients make wise food choices that will contribute to their health. Clients should be aware of the nutrients they are consuming and the effect those nutrients are having on their body. Because carbohydrates are the main fuel for exercising muscles, it is extremely important that at least 55 to 65% of total daily calories come from carbohydrates. Consuming excess protein may result in a gain in fat weight. Being aware of fat in the diet and recognizing heart-healthy foods will help reduce the risk of cardiovascular disease.

Help your clients integrate the dietary guidelines into their nutrition plans to reduce their risk for diet-related diseases. The MyPyramid Food Guidance System

Summary

will enable clients to visualize contemporary ways they can combine foods to meet the guidelines and recommended dietary allowances.

Probably one of the most important nutritional concerns for exercising individuals is fluids and hydration. A 2% decrease in body weight due to perspiration will decrease performance, so exercisers must monitor their water losses. It also is important to closely monitor calcium and iron intake, especially for female and adolescent male athletes, since performance can be impaired with even a mild iron deficiency. Though most people are not aware of it, they can consume the RDAs of most nutrients by eating a balanced diet (except iron and calcium for women). Instead, many choose to supplement their diets with vitamins and minerals and often believe that the more they take the better. Make clients aware that megadoses of vitamins and minerals will not boost their performance. If they still feel the need to take a supplement, a multiple-type vitamin is recommended.

REFERENCES

American Dietetic Association (1997). Vegetarian diets—Position of the American Dietetic Association. *Journal of the American Dietetic Association,* 97, 1317–1321.

Bergstrom, J. et al. (1967). Diet, muscle glycogen and physical performance. *Acta Physiology Scandinavia,* 71, 140–150.

Brooks, S.M. et al. (1984). Diet in athletic amenorrhea. *Lancet,* 1, 559.

Bryant, C.X., Franklin, B.A., & Conviser, J.M. (2002). *Exercise Testing and Program Design.* Monterey, Calif.: Healthy Learning.

Clarkson, P.M. (1991). Vitamins and trace minerals, In: *Perspectives in exercise science and sports medicine, Vol 4: Ergogenic enhancement of performance in exercise and sport,* 123–182. Lamb, D.R. & Williams, M.H. (Eds.) Ann Arbor: Brown and Benchmark.

Costill, D.L. et al. (1978). Effects of caffeine ingestion on metabolism and exercise performance. *Medicine and Science in Sports and Exercise,* 10, 155.

Drinkwater, B.L., Nilson, K., & Chestnut, C.H. (1984). Bone mineral content of amenorrheic and eumenorrheic athletes. *New England Journal of Medicine,* 311, 277–281.

Drinkwater, B.L. et al. (1986). Bone mineral density after resumption of menses in amenorrheic athletes. *Journal of the American Medical Association,* 256, 380–382.

Expert Panel on Detection, Evaluation, and Treatment of High Blood Cholesterol in Adults (2001). Executive Summary of the Third Report of the National Cholesterol Education Program (NCEP) Expert Panel on Detection, Evaluation, and Treatment of High Blood Cholesterol in Adults (Adult Treatment Panel II). *Journal of the American Medical Association,* 285, 19, 2486–2497.

Haymes, E.M. (1991). Vitamin and mineral supplementation to athletes. *International Journal of Sport Medicine,* 1, 146–169.

Ivy J.L. et al. (1988). Muscle glycogen synthesis after exercise effect of time of carbohydrate ingestion. *Journal of Applied Physiology,* 64, 4, 1480–1485.

Jentjens, R.L. & Jeukendrup, A. (2003). Determinants of post-exercise glycogen synthesis during short-term recovery. *Sports Medicine,* 33, 2, 117–144.

Jentjens, R.L. et al. (2001). Addition of protein and amino acids to carbohydrates does not enhance postexercise muscle glycogen synthesis. *Journal of Applied Physiology,* 91, 839–846.

Krause, M.E & Mahan, C.K. (2003). *Food Nutrition and Diet Therapy* (11th ed.). Philadelphia: Saunders.

Lemon, P. (1995). Do athletes need more protein and amino acids? *International Journal of Sports Nutrition,* 1, 2, 127–145.

MacIntosh, B.R. & Wright, B.M. (1995). Caffeine ingestion and performance of a 1500-metre swim. *Canadian Journal of Applied Physiology,* 20, 168.

Pasman, W.J. et al. (1995). The effect of different dosages of caffeine on endurance performance time. *International Journal of Sports Medicine,* 16, 225.

Sanborn, C.F., Albrech, B.H., & Wagner, W.W. (1987). Athletic amenorrhea, lack of association with body fat. *Medicine and Science in Sports and Exercise,* 19, 207–212.

Simonsen, J.C. et al. (1991). Dietary carbohydrate, muscle glycogen, and power output during rowing training. *Journal of Applied Physiology,* 70, 4, 1500–1505.

Slavin, J. (1991). Protein needs for athletes, In: Berning, J.R. and Steen, S.N. (Eds.). *Sports Nutrition for the Nineties: The Health Professionals Handbook.* Gaithersburg, Md.: Aspen Publishers.

Van Hall, G., Shirreffs, S.M., & Calbet, J.A.L. (2000). Muscle glycogen resynthesis during recovery from cycle exercise: No effect of additional protein ingestion. *Journal of Applied Physiology,* 88, 1631–1636.

Van Loon, L. et al. (2000). Maximizing postexercise muscle glycogen synthesis: Carbohydrate supplementation and the application of amino acid or protein hydrolysate mixtures. *American Journal of Clinical Nutrition,* 72, 106–111.

Zawadski, K.M., Yaspelkis, B.B., & Ivy J.L. (1992). Carbohydrate-protein complex increases the rate of muscle glycogen storage after exercise. *Journal of Applied Physiology,* 72, 5, 1854–1859.

SUGGESTED READING

Benardot, D. (2000). *Nutrition for Serious Athletes.* Champaign, Ill.: Human Kinetics.

Berning, J.R. (2002). *Sports Nutrition Patient Education Resource Manual.* Gaithersburg, Md.: Aspen Publishers.

Berning, J.R. & Steen, S.N. (1998). *Nutrition for Sport and Exercise.* Gaithersburg, Md.: Aspen Publishers.

Brouns, F. (2002). *Essentials of Sport Nutrition.* New York: John Wiley & Sons.

Burke, E.R. & Berning, J.R. (1995). *Training Nutrition: The Diet and Nutrition Guide for Peak Performance.* Carmel, Ind.: Cooper Publishing.

Burke, L. & Deakin, V. (Eds.) (2000). *Clinical Sports Nutrition.* (2nd ed.). New York: McGraw-Hill.

Clark, N. (2003). *Sports Nutrition Guidebook.* (3rd ed.). Champaign, Ill.: Human Kinetics.

Coleman, E. (2003). *Eating for Endurance.* (4th ed.). Palo Alto, Calif.: Bull Publishing.

Coleman, E. & Steen, S.N. (2000). *Ultimate Sports Nutrition.* (2nd ed.). Boulder, Colo.: Bull Publishing.

Houtkooper, L. (1994). *Winning Sports Nutrition: Training Manual.* Tucson, Ariz.: University of Arizona.

Kies, C.V. & Driskell, J. (Eds.) (1995). *Sports Nutrition: Minerals and Electrolytes.* Boca Raton, Fla.: CRC Press.

Manone, M. & Thompson, J. (2000). *Sport Nutrition for Health and Performance.* Champaign, Ill.: Human Kinetics.

McArdle, W.D., Katch, F.I., & Katch, V.L. (2005). *Sports and Exercise Nutrition.* (2nd ed.). Philadelphia: Lippincott Williams & Wilkins.

Ryan, M. (1999). *Complete Guide to Sports Nutrition.* Boulder, Colo.: Velo Press.

Williams, M.H. (2001). *Nutrition for Fitness and Sport.* (6th ed.) Dubuque, Iowa: William C. Brown.

Wolinsky, I. & Hickson, J.F. (1997). *Nutrition in Exercise and Sport.* (3rd ed.). Boca Raton, Fla.: CRC Press.

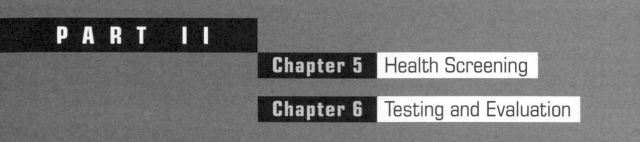

PART II

Screening
and Evaluation

CHAPTER 5

Health
Screening

Jeff Anthony, D.O., is a team physician at San Diego State University and for the San Diego SOCKERS professional soccer team. He is a senior partner at the San Diego Sports Medicine and Family Health Center and frequently lectures on sports medicine topics at medical conferences. He is a past member of the IDEA Advisory Board.

Jeff Anthony

Health screening is a vital first step in the personal trainer/client relationship. Not only does it give you essential information that will assure safety and effectiveness in exercise programming, but it also raises the quality and professionalism of your services. Health screening allows you to (1) identify health conditions and risk factors that may necessitate referral or place the client at risk when participating in certain activities; (2) identify possible contraindicated activities; (3) assist in designing an exercise program that includes safe activities and/or appropriate modifications; (4) fulfill legal and insurance requirements for you or the health club; and (5) open lines of communication between you and physicians that will help you to gain a reputation as a concerned professional and ally in health promotion. This chapter outlines the components of an effective health screening and identifies some conditions that may require modifications to an exercise program and/or healthcare professional participation.

Because the primary purpose of a physical activity program is to improve one's quality of life, aggravating an existing medical condition is counterproductive. To set up the most effective program, you need to evaluate your clients' health conditions and their goals. If a significant health condition or risk factor for injury exists, a client may need medical clearance or specific recommendations from a physician. This should not deter you from working with a client if you possess the appropriate training and experience. With proper modifications to the exercise program, almost everyone can, and should, engage in physical activity. Your client and his or her physician should work with you to coordinate the most effective program, giving careful consideration to the risks, benefits, and goals of exercise.

It is only in the last two decades that exercise has truly been appreciated as a medical necessity. In the early 1900s, the average life expectancy was 50 years; most people died of infections or **acute** diseases. With the advent of antibiotics, immunizations, and better health care, people are now living much longer. The average life expectancy today approaches 80 years and statistics tell us that 80% of the deaths in the United States are from **chronic diseases** that are largely a result of lifestyle (Rosenstein, 1987). This is exciting because by taking responsibility for how we live, we can gain some control over our health and mortality.

For the human body, the key components to a healthy life are

✔ Physical activity
✔ Good nutrition
✔ Stress alleviation/management
✔ Psychological balance
✔ Routine check-ups

As a personal trainer, you focus on the importance of physical activity, which positively influences the other components. A **sedentary** lifestyle is now recognized as a health hazard (Paffenbarger et al., 1993; American College of Sports Medicine, 2000; Blair, 1993) and everyone can benefit from some form of physical activity. However, before beginning to work with a client, you must take a health and exercise history to assess client goals, commitment to an active lifestyle, and fitness level. Refer to Figure 5.1 for a flowchart of specific health screening procedures, results, and decisions based on these results.

HEALTH SCREENING FORMS

A client's health history is your primary tool for setting up a safe and effective training program. The necessary components of a health his-

---

Intensity Defined

The American College of Sports Medicine (ACSM) has defined what is considered moderate and vigorous exercise to assist in determining the need for referral and/or physician clearance for certain individuals.

Moderate exercise is defined as an intensity of 40 to 59% $\dot{V}O_2R$. Note: the $\dot{V}O_2R$ is the difference between $\dot{V}O_2max$ and resting $\dot{V}O_2$ and correlates well with the Karvonen heart rate reserve method of establishing and monitoring exercise intensity. If you are not able to accurately determine the intensity of an activity, moderate exercise also can be defined as "an intensity well within the individual's current capacity that can be sustained for a prolonged period of time, that is, approximately 45 minutes, which has a gradual initiation and progression, and is generally noncompetitive."

Vigorous exercise is defined as activities of >6 **METs**. Vigorous exercise may alternatively be defined as exercise intense enough to represent a substantial cardiorespiratory challenge. If an individual's exercise capacity is known, vigorous exercise may be defined as an intensity of >60% maximal oxygen uptake (American College of Sports Medicine, 2000). Keep in mind your client and the activity he or she wants to pursue when deciding on the need for referral or physician clearance.

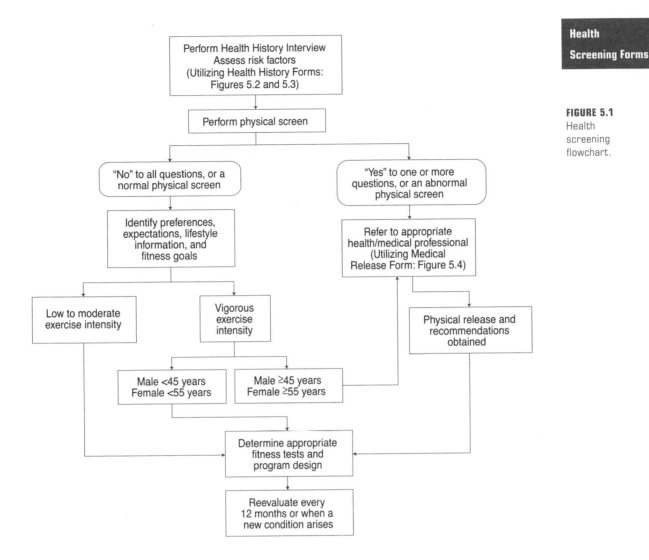

FIGURE 5.1
Health
screening
flowchart.

tory form include: (1) demographic information, such as age, sex, and occupation; (2) past and present exercise history; (3) health risk factors; (4) medications; (5) recent or current illness and injuries; (6) surgery and injury history; and (7) family medical history. Demographic information is important because gender, age, and occupation all bring risks, needs, expectations, and referral differences to programming. Information on activity patterns will help to identify the client's current fitness level and the most appropriate type and progression of the exercise program. It also will help you to identify the risks of activity for that individual. Cardiovascular **risk factors,** medications,

and illness/injury information all have a tremendous impact on both referral and programming issues. And family medical history is important for determining risk as well. The Physical Activity Readiness Questionnaire (PAR-Q) has been recommended as a minimal prerequisite for beginning a low- to moderate-intensity exercise program (Figure 5.2). A sample of a more comprehensive health history form is shown in Figure 5.3 and serves as a model that you can modify as needed. Listing common conditions that affect the ability to exercise enables you to identify the major health risks for clients beginning a program. Update the information on the form every year or any time a new condition arises.

The Physical Activity Readiness Questionnaire — PAR-Q
(revised 2002)
PAR-Q & YOU (A Questionnaire for People Aged 15 to 69)

Regular physical activity is fun and healthy, and increasingly more people are starting to become more active every day. Being more active is very safe for most people. However, some people should check with their doctor before they start becoming much more physically active.

If you are planning to become much more physically active than you are now, start by answering the seven questions below. If you are between the ages of 15 and 69, the PAR-Q will tell you if you should check with your doctor before you start. If you are over 69 years of age, and you are not used to being very active, check with your doctor.

Common sense is your best guide when you answer these questions. Please read the questions carefully and answer each one honestly: check YES or NO.

YES	NO	
☐	☐	1. Has your doctor ever said that you have a heart condition *and* that you should only do physical activity recommended by a doctor?
☐	☐	2. Do you feel pain in your chest when you do physical activity?
☐	☐	3. In the past month, have you had chest pain when you were not doing physical activity?
☐	☐	4. Do you lose your balance because of dizziness or do you ever lose consciousness?
☐	☐	5. Do you have a bone or joint problem (for example, back, knee, or hip) that could be made worse by a change in your physical activity?
☐	☐	6. Is your doctor currently prescribing drugs (for example, water pills) for your blood pressure or heart condition?
☐	☐	7. Do you know of *any other reason* why you should not do physical activity?

If you answered YES to one or more questions:

✔ Talk with your doctor by phone or in person BEFORE you start becoming much more physically active or BEFORE you have a fitness appraisal. Tell your doctor about the PAR-Q and which questions you answered YES.

✔ You may be able to do any activity you want—as long as you start slowly and build up gradually. Or, you may need to restrict your activities to those that are safe for you. Talk with your doctor about the kinds of activities you wish to participate in and follow his/her advice.

✔ Find out which community programs are safe and helpful for you.

If you answered NO honestly to all PAR-Q questions, you can be reasonably sure that you can:

✔ Start becoming much more physically active—begin slowly and build up gradually. This is the safest and easiest way to go.

✔ Take part in a fitness appraisal—this is an excellent way to determine your basic fitness so that you can plan the best way for you to live actively. It is also highly recommended that you have your blood pressure evaluated. If your reading is over 144/94, talk with your doctor before you start becoming much more physically active.

FIGURE 5.2
The Physical Activity
Readiness Questionnaire.

Delay becoming much more active:

✔ If you are not feeling well because of a temporary illness such as a cold or a fever—wait until you feel better; or

✔ If you are or may be pregnant—talk to your doctor before you start becoming more active.

Please note: If your health changes so that you then answer YES to any of the above questions, tell your fitness or health professional. Ask whether you should change your physical activity plan.

Informed Use of the PAR-Q: The Canadian Society for Exercise Physiology, Health Canada, and their agents assume no liability for persons who undertake physical activity, and if in doubt after completing this questionnaire, consult your doctor prior to physical activity.

> **No changes permitted. You are encouraged to copy the PAR-Q but only if you use the entire form.**

Note: If the PAR-Q is being given to a person before he or she participates in a physical activity program or a fitness appraisal, this section may be used for legal or administrative purposes.

I have read, understood, and completed this questionnaire. Any questions I had were answered to my full satisfaction.

_____

Name

_____

Signature   Date

_____

Signature of Parent   Witness
or Guardian (for participants under the age of majority)

> Note: This physical activity clearance is valid for a maximum of 12 months from the date it is completed and becomes invalid if your condition changes so that you would answer YES to any of the seven questions.

© Canadian Society for Exercise Physiology   Supported by: Health   Santé
Societe canadienne de physiologie de l'exercice   Canada   Canada

FIGURE 5.2 continued

Sample Health History Form

Name_____ Date_____

Age _____ Sex ☐ M ☐ F

Physician's Name _____

Physician's Phone (_____)_____

Person to contact in case of Emergency:

Name _____ Phone_____

Are you taking any medications or drugs? If so, please list medication, dose, and reason.

_____
_____

Does your physician know you are participating in this exercise program?

_____
_____

Describe any physical activity you do somewhat regularly.

_____
_____

Do you now, or have you had in the past:	Yes	No
1. History of heart problems, chest pain, or stroke	☐	☐
2. Increased blood pressure	☐	☐
3. Any chronic illness or condition	☐	☐
4. Difficulty with physical exercise	☐	☐
5. Advice from physician not to exercise	☐	☐
6. Recent surgery (last 12 months)	☐	☐
7. Pregnancy (now or within last 3 months)	☐	☐
8. History of breathing or lung problems	☐	☐
9. Muscle, joint, or back disorder, or any previous injury still affecting you	☐	☐
10. Diabetes or thyroid condition	☐	☐
11. Cigarette smoking habit	☐	☐
12. Obesity (more than 20% over ideal body weight)	☐	☐
13. Increased blood cholesterol	☐	☐
14. History of heart problems in immediate family	☐	☐
15. Hernia, or any condition that may be aggravated by lifting weights	☐	☐

Please explain any "yes" answers on the back.

Comments:

_____
_____
_____
_____

FIGURE 5.3
Sample Health
History Form.

Clients who answer "yes" to one or more of the questions on either form may be at increased risk for injury during exercise and may benefit from further screening before becoming more physically active or having a fitness assessment. Also, if a client has a medical condition you are not thoroughly equipped to handle, you should obtain recommendations from their physician or, preferably, refer the client to a more qualified professional.

The physician's release provides you with clarification of a client's status and explains any limitations to physical activity. It also enables the physician to direct modifications to the exercise program. Figure 5.4 is an example of a physician release form, which outlines the planned exercise program for the physician and enables him or her to return their consent and recommendations, if any.

Once the health history has been obtained, the information should be used, not just filed away. This information is crucial to designing a safe and effective exercise program and can provide support and guidance for the client's overall health and fitness program.

It is your responsibility to be familiar with appropriate local healthcare professionals for referral. These professionals may include psychotherapists, registered dietitians, physical therapists, athletic trainers, and clinical exercise physiologists, among others. When making referrals, it is imperative that the professionals you recommend be degreed, licensed, boarded, and/or otherwise qualified in their area of expertise. It also is important that you recommend at least two professionals to avoid bias and allow your clients a choice in their care.

HEALTH CONDITIONS THAT AFFECT PHYSICAL ACTIVITY

The benefits of regular physical activity are well established (American College of Sports Medicine, 2000). But there also are risks inherent in physical activity. Identifying these risks is the first step in preventing them. Regular physical activity increases the risk of both musculoskeletal injury and cardiovascular problems, such as cardiac arrest. While your clients need to be informed of these risks (see pages 476–482 for more information on informed consent), they also should know that the overall absolute risk in the general population is low, especially when weighed against the health benefits of regular exercise (American College of Sports Medicine, 2000). Injuries related to physical activity usually come from:

✔ aggravating an existing condition (either known or unknown by the client); or

✔ precipitating a new condition.

The primary systems of the body that experience stress during physical activity are the cardiovascular, respiratory, and musculoskeletal systems. Certain metabolic and other medical conditions also will be affected by regular physical activity. Obtaining a complete health history provides you with essential information in these areas that will ensure your client gets the most benefit from an exercise program with the lowest degree of risk. The following material covers health conditions that may affect your client's benefit-to-risk ratio and should be considered when developing a physical activity program.

Cardiovascular Disease

Atherosclerosis is a process in which fatty deposits of **cholesterol** and calcium accumulate on the walls of the arteries, causing them to harden, thicken, and lose elasticity. When this process affects the arteries that supply the heart, it is called **coronary artery disease (CAD).** As with other muscles, the heart contracts when we exercise. The increased contraction of the heart muscle occurs because of an increased supply of oxygen-rich blood that provides necessary nutrients. The greater the exercise intensity, the larger the demand for blood and

Health Conditions That Affect Physical Activity

Sample Medical Release Form

Date _____

Dear Doctor:

Your patient, _____, wishes to start a personalized training program. The activity will involve the following:

(type, frequency, duration, and intensity of activities)

If your patient is taking medications that will affect his or her heart rate response to exercise, please indicate the manner of the effect (raises, lowers, or has no effect on heart-rate response):

Type of medication _____

Effect _____

Please identify any recommendations or restrictions that are appropriate for your patient in this exercise program:

_____

_____

_____

Thank you.
Sincerely,

Fred Fitness
Personalized Gym
Address
Phone

_____ has my approval to begin an exercise program with the recommendations or restrictions stated above.

Signed Date   Phone

FIGURE 5.4
Sample Medical Release Form.

Table 5.1
Coronary Artery Disease Risk-factor Thresholds

Instructions:

Determine the total number of risk factors using the following risk-factor criteria, scoring a point for each risk factor identified. If high-density lipoprotein (HDL) levels exceed 60 mg/dL, subtract one point from the sum of positive risk factors, as high HDL levels lower the risk for coronary artery disease.

Positive Risk Factors

Family History +1
- Myocardial infarction, coronary revascularization, or sudden death before 55 years of age in father or other first-degree male relative
- Myocardial infarction, coronary revascularization, or sudden death before 65 years of age in mother or other first-degree female relative

Cigarette Smoking +1
- Current cigarette smokers or those who quit within the previous six months

Hypertension +1
- Systolic blood pressure ≥140 mmHg or diastolic blood pressure ≥90 mmHg, confirmed by measurements on at least two separate occasions, or on anti-hypertensive medications

Dyslipidemia +1
- Low-density lipoprotein (LDL) cholesterol ≥130 mg/dL or HDL cholesterol <40 mg/dL, or on lipid-lowering medication
- If serum cholesterol is all that is available, use serum cholesterol ≥200 mg/dL

Impaired Glucose Fasting +1
- Fasting blood sugar ≥100 mg/dL confirmed by measurements on at least two separate occasions

Obesity +1
- Body mass index of ≥30 kg/m^2
  or
- Waist girth >102 cm (40 inches) for men and ≥89 cm (35 inches) for women
  or
- Waist/hip ratio ≥0.95 for men and ≥0.86 for women

As professional opinions vary regarding the most appropriate markers and thresholds for obesity, use additional valid markers to evaluate obesity as a risk factor (this may include a valid measure of percent body fat).

Sedentary Lifestyle +1
- Persons not participating in a regular exercise program or not meeting the minimal recommendations from the Surgeon General's Report/USDA Guidelines

Negative Risk Factor

High serum HDL Cholesterol - 1
- Score >60 mg/dL   **TOTAL SCORE** _____

American College of Sports Medicine (2006). *ACSM's Guidelines for Exercise Testing and Prescription* (7th ed.). Philadelphia: Lippincott Williams & Wilkins.

---

oxygen to the heart muscle. If the vessels that supply this blood to the heart are narrowed from atherosclerosis, the blood supply is limited, and the increased oxygen demand by the heart cannot be met. This can result in chest discomfort, called **angina,** and possibly a **myocardial infarction,** or heart attack.

Angina is usually described as a pressure or tightness in the chest, but can also be experienced in the arm, shoulder, or jaw.

This pain may be accompanied by shortness of breath, sweating, nausea, and palpitations (pounding or racing of the heart).

Although regular exercise may be an important part of the treatment and rehabilitation for CAD, limitations may be necessary. Anyone with a history of CAD or chest pain should have a physician's release, along with a description of any specific limitations, before beginning an exercise program.

Risk Factors. Unfortunately, many people with CAD have no known symptoms and are unaware of their potential risk for a heart attack. Long-term studies have helped researchers identify several factors that correlate with an increased risk for CAD. ACSM has identified several positive (increased risk) coronary artery disease risk factors (Table 5.1).

ACSM also has defined the following negative (decreased risk) risk factor: High serum **high-density lipoprotein (HDL) cholesterol** greater than 60 mg/dL.

Note: It is common to add up, or sum, risk factors in determining increased risk. If HDL is high, subtract one risk factor from the sum of positive risk factors, since high HDL reduces CAD risk.

The more risk factors a person has, the greater their chance of having or developing CAD. An important goal of any exercise program should be to minimize these risk factors as much as possible to reduce the risk of heart disease. Any client with two or more risk factors should be referred to a physician before beginning a vigorous exercise program (see, Intensity Defined on page 150). In addition, ACSM recommends that males over age 45 and females over age 55 have a medical evaluation, including a maximal exercise test, before beginning vigorous exercise programs. You and the physician can then work together to develop an ideal program. If low-to-moderate exercise is the goal, only those persons diagnosed with cardiopulmonary disease, or those with one or more major signs or symptoms suggestive of cardiopulmonary disease, need to have a medical examination and clinical exercise test prior to beginning an exercise program (Tables 5.2 and 5.3).

**Table 5.2
Physician Supervision During Exercise Test**

	Low Risk	Moderate Risk	High Risk
Submaximal	Not necessary	Not necessary	Recommended
Maximal	Not necessary	Recommended	Recommended

**Table 5.3
Medical Exam (Within Past Year) and
Exercise Test Recommendation**

	Low Risk*	Moderate Risk[†]	High Risk[‡]
Moderate Exercise Intensity[¨]	Not necessary	Not necessary	Recommended
Vigorous Exercise Intensity[††]	Not necessary	Recommended	Recommended

* Younger individuals (men <45, women <55), asymptomatic and have no more than one risk factor

[†] Older individuals who have two or more risk factors and are asymptomatic

[‡] Individuals with one or more signs/symptoms or known cardiac (CVD, PVD, or CVA), pulmonary (COPD, asthma, cystic fibrosis, or interstitial lung disease) or metabolic (DM, thyroid disorders, liver or kidney) disease

[¨] Moderate exercise implies 40–59% $\dot{V}O_2$max or heart-rate reserve, or 11–12 on the rating of perceived exertion on the Borg 6–20 RPE for at least 45 minutes

[††] Vigorous implies ≥60% $\dot{V}O_2$max or heart-rate reserve, or an RPE ≥13 sustained for 20 minutes

Note: CVD = Cardiovascular disease; PVD = Peripheral vascular disease; CVA = Cerebral vascular accident; COPD = Chronic obstructive pulmonary disease; DM = Diabetes mellitus.

American College of Sports Medicine (2006). *ACSM's Guidelines for Exercise Testing and Prescription* (7th ed.). Philadelphia: Lippincott Williams & Wilkins.

Hypertension. Hypertension, or high blood pressure, is more prevalent among the elderly and the African-American population but is becoming more common in the general population. An individual's risk of CAD, **stroke,** and kidney disease increases progressively with higher levels of **systolic** and **diastolic blood pressure** (Young, 1995). This is important information for you as a personal trainer because blood pressure increases with exercise, especially in activities involving heavy resistance, such as weight lifting, or isometric exercises. If a person's resting blood pressure is already high, it may elevate to dangerous levels during exercise, increasing the likelihood of a stroke.

Respiratory

The lungs (respiratory system) extract oxygen from the air we breathe and deliver it to the body's tissues via the cardiovascular system. Oxygen is essential to all body tissues for survival. A problem in the respiratory system will interfere with the body's ability to provide enough oxygen for the increasing demand that occurs during aerobic exercise. Bronchitis, **asthma,** and **chronic obstructive pulmonary disease** are some of the more common respiratory problems. Each of these conditions may result in **dyspnea** (difficult breathing), making exercise difficult. Regular exercise may aggravate the condition for some people, and may improve it for others. Anyone with a disorder of the respiratory system should have a physician's clearance and recommendations before beginning or continuing an exercise program. More information on respiratory conditions and programming concerns can be found in Chapter 12.

Musculoskeletal

The musculoskeletal system consists of the muscles, bones, **tendons,** and **ligaments** that support and move the body. This is the system most commonly injured during exercise. Aside from the pain and discouragement of an injury, there are other factors to contend with. Client motivation and your **scope of practice** create concerns when working with a client with previous or current musculoskeletal injuries. Changes or modifications in the exercise program are necessary to accommodate the injury. For these reasons, it is important to be cognizant of potentially hazardous situations before they occur. Most minor sprains and strains are easily managed, but a persistent problem or a more serious injury requires physician referral for appropriate treatment.

The health screening evaluation is crucial to identifying both old injuries and risk factors for potential new injuries. Asking the client about current conditions, previous injuries, and pain that comes and goes is critical in detecting potential problems. The most common type of injury sustained by persons participating in physical activity is the **overuse injury.** These injuries are usually the

result of poor training techniques, poor body mechanics, or both. Examples of overuse injuries include runner's knee, swimmer's shoulder, tennis elbow (epicondylitis), shin splints (pain in the anterior lower leg), and iliotibial (IT) band syndrome (pain along the outside of the thigh and knee). To avoid aggravating an existing injury, and to allow for healing to occur, modify the client's exercise program using a **cross-training** strategy.

Other common conditions to screen for in the health history interview are **sprains** (ligament) or **strains** (muscle or its tendon), **herniated disc, bursitis, tendinitis,** and **arthritis.** Information on arthritis and low-back disorders can be found in Chapter 12. These conditions must be recognized before implementing an exercise program to avoid worsening the condition. Guidelines for recognizing and preventing injuries can be found in Chapter 16. Any musculoskeletal disorder that you are not qualified to deal with should be referred to an appropriate health professional, and a client with an injury more severe than a simple sprain or strain must have a physician's approval before beginning an exercise program. If a specific muscle weakness or joint looseness exists, medical referral is recommended, and appropriate accommodations to the program are necessary.

A client who has recently undergone orthopedic surgery may not be ready for a standard exercise program. Depending on the type of surgery performed, it may take up to one year (in the case of knee reconstruction, for example) for the tissues to heal completely. Also, disuse **atrophy** of the muscles surrounding an injury may begin after just two days of inactivity. Properly rehabilitating the weakened area requires knowledge of the type of surgery as well as the indicated rehabilitation program. This information can be obtained from the client's surgeon and physical therapist. Beginning an exercise program before complete rehabilitation may lead to biomechanical imbalances that could predispose the client to other injuries. Commun-

> **Health Conditions That Affect Physical Activity**

ication with the physician is paramount, particularly for clients who have had surgery within the last year.

Metabolic

There are many metabolic diseases that may interfere with metabolism, or the utilization of energy. Two of the more common types are **diabetes** and thyroid disorders. A client with either condition requires physician approval before initiating an exercise program. Exercise, both as a means to regulate blood glucose and to facilitate fat loss, is an important component of the lifestyle of an individual with diabetes. Your clients with diabetes should discuss their situations and exercise programs with their physicians before working with you. Physician referral is especially important if a client is receiving insulin. Diabetes types and exercise programming concerns are discussed further in Chapter 12.

The thyroid is a small gland in the neck that secretes a hormone that regulates the rate of metabolism. Hyperthyroid persons have an increased level of this hormone and a higher metabolic rate. Hypothyroid persons have a reduced level of this hormone and require thyroid medication to increase their metabolism to a normal rate. Because exercise also increases the metabolism, it could be dangerous in a person with uncontrolled thyroid disease.

Other Conditions

Hernia. Another condition that needs consideration, especially when incorporating weight lifting into a program, is a history of an inguinal or abdominal **hernia.** This is a protrusion of the abdominal contents into the groin or through the abdominal wall, respectively. Pain is usually present, but may not be in some cases. During an activity involving increased abdominal pressure, such as the **Valsalva maneuver,** the hernia may be further aggravated. A hernia is a relative contraindication for weight lifting unless cleared by a physician. If

there is a history of a hernia, it is very important to instruct and educate the client on proper breathing and lifting techniques.

Pregnancy. Optimum fitness levels during pregnancy are beneficial to both the mother's and the unborn infant's health. This is not a good time to pursue maximum fitness goals, but rather to focus on maintaining a good fitness level. A client should have a physician's approval for exercise during pregnancy and until three months after delivery. Please refer to Chapter 12 for more information on modifying an exercise program during pregnancy.

Illness or Infection. A recent history of illness or infection may impair a client's ability to exercise. Moderate exercise may be acceptable during a mild illness such as a cold. A more serious condition, however, requires more of the body's energy reserves, and exercise would be contraindicated until the client improves. Our bodies have a given amount of available energy that must be balanced between the body's physiological requirements, which include fighting infections, and the energy used during exercise. This balance varies from person to person, but it is generally not advisable to start a new exercise program during an illness. To distinguish between a minor and a major illness, you may need to consult with the client's physician.

MEDICATIONS

Medication or drug use is another important topic to cover when taking a health history. These substances alter the biochemistry of the body and may affect a client's ability to perform or respond to exercise. The properties of these drugs must be understood and discussed with your client. In designing and supervising an exercise program, it is important to realize that many over-the-counter medications and prescription or illicit drugs affect the heart's response to exercise. There are hundreds of thousands of different drugs on the market and each may be referred to by the manufacturer's brand name (e.g., Inderal) or by the scientific generic name (e.g., propranolol). Table 5.4 lists many medication categories that may affect a person's response to exercise. To use the table, consult the client, the client's physician, or a medical reference to find the correct category for the medication. *Note: Appendix D provides a list of generic and brand names of common medications by category.* Then refer to the general category under which each drug is grouped, such as **beta blockers,** antihistamines, or **bronchodilators.** The drugs in each group are thought to have a similar effect on most people, although individual responses will vary.

A particular response is usually dose dependent; the larger the dose, the greater the response. An important factor to consider in this dose-related response is the time when the medication is taken. As medications are metabolized, their effects diminish. If you have any questions concerning a client's medications, discuss them with the client and his or her physician. Any client taking a prescription medication that could potentially have an effect on exercise should have a physician's clearance for physical activity. The following are some of the most common categories of medications of which you should be aware.

Antihypertensives

High blood pressure, or hypertension, is common in our society, and there are many medications used for its treatment. Most antihypertensives primarily affect one of four different sites: the heart, to reduce its force of contraction; the peripheral blood vessels, to open or dilate them to allow more room for the blood; the brain, to reduce the sympathetic nerve outflow; or the kidneys, to deplete body water and decrease blood volume. The site that the medication acts on helps to determine its effect on the individual as well as any potential side effects. The following are common antihypertensives:

Beta blockers. Beta-adrenergic blocking agents, or beta blockers, are commonly prescribed for a variety of cardiovascular and other disorders. These medications block beta-adrenergic receptors and limit sympathetic nervous system stimulation. In other words, they block the effects of catecholamines (epinephrine and norepinephrine) throughout the body, and reduce resting, exercise, and maximal heart rates. This reduction in heart rate requires modifying the method used for determining exercise intensity. Using the Borg Scale of Perceived Exertion, for example, would be appropriate for a safe and effective aerobic exercise program for someone on beta blockers (see page 348).

Calcium channel blockers. Calcium channel blockers prevent calcium-dependent contraction of the smooth muscles in the arteries, causing them to dilate, which lowers blood pressure. These agents also are used for angina and heart dysrhythmias (rapid or irregular heart rate). There are several types of calcium blockers on the market, and their effect on blood pressure and heart rate depends on the specific agent. Notice in Table 5.4 that calcium channel-blocking drugs may increase, decrease, or have no effect on the heart rate. Therefore, while it is important to know the general effects of a category of medication, remember that individual responses can vary.

Angiotensin-converting enzyme (ACE) inhibitors. ACE inhibitors block an enzyme secreted by the kidneys, preventing the formation of a potent hormone that constricts blood vessels. If this enzyme is blocked, the vessels dilate, and blood pressure decreases. ACE inhibitors should not have an effect on heart rate, but will cause a decrease in blood pressure at rest and during exercise.

Angiotensin-II receptor antagonists. Angiotensin-II receptor antagonists (or block-

Medications

Table 5.4
Effects of Medication on Heart-rate (HR) Response

Medications	Resting HR	Exercising HR	Maximal Exercise HR	Comments
Beta-adrenergic Blocking Agents	↓	↓	↓	Dose-related response
Diuretics	↔	↔	↔	
Other Antihypertensives	↑, ↔, or ↓	↑, ↔, or ↓	Usually ↔	Many antihypertensive medications are used. Some may decrease, a few may increase, and others do not affect heart rates. Some exhibit dose-related response.
Calcium Channel Blockers	↑, ↔, or ↓	↑, ↔, or ↓	Usually ↔	Variable and dose-related responses
Antihistamines	↔	↔	↔	
Cold medications: without sympathomimetic activity (SA)	↔	↔	↔	
with SA	↔ or ↑	↔ or ↑	↔	
Tranquilizers	↔, or if anxiety reducing may ↓	↔	↔	
Antidepressants and some Antipsychotic Medications	↔ or ↑	↔	↔	
Alcohol	↔ or ↑	↔ or ↑	↔	Exercise prohibited while under the influence; effects of alcohol on coordination increase possibility of injuries
Diet Pills: with SA	↑ or ↔	↑ or ↔	↔	Discourage as a poor approach to weight loss; acceptable only with physician's written approval
Containing Amphetamines	↑	↑	↔	
without SA or Amphetamines	↔	↔	↔	
Caffeine	↔ or ↑	↔ or ↑	↔	
Nicotine	↔ or ↑	↔ or ↑	↔	Discourage smoking; suggest lower target heart rate and exercise intensity for smokers

↑ = increase   ↔ = no significant change   ↓ = decrease

Note: Many medications are prescribed for conditions that do not require clearance. Do not forget other indicators of exercise intensity (e.g., client's appearance, rating of perceived exertion).

ers) are a newer class of antihypertensive agents. These drugs are selective for angiotensin II (type 1 receptor). Angiotensin-II receptor antagonists are well tolerated, and cough occurs much less often with these agents than with ACE inhibitors. In addition, they do not adversely affect blood lipid profiles or cause "rebound hypertension" after discontinuation. Clinical trials indicate that angiotensin-II receptor antagonists are effective and safe in the treatment of hypertension.

Diuretics. **Diuretics** are medications that increase the excretion of water and electrolytes through the kidneys. They are usually prescribed for high blood pressure, or when a person is accumulating too much fluid, as occurs with congestive heart failure. They have no primary effect on the heart rate, but they can cause water and **electrolyte** imbalances, which may lead to dangerous cardiac **arrhythmias.** Since diuretics can decrease blood volume, they may predispose an exerciser to dehydration. A client taking diuretics needs to maintain adequate fluid intake before, after, and during exercise, especially in a warm, humid environment. Diuretics are sometimes used by athletes to try to lose weight for sport. This is a dangerous practice and should not be condoned by a responsible trainer.

Bronchodilators

Asthma medications, also known as **bronchodilators,** relax or open the air passages in the lungs, allowing better air exchange. There are many different types, but the primary action of each is to stimulate the **sympathetic nervous system.** Bronchodilators increase exercise capacity in persons limited by bronchospasm.

Cold Medications

Decongestants act directly on the smooth muscles of the blood vessels to stimulate **vasoconstriction.** In the upper airways, this constriction reduces the volume of the swollen tissues and results in more air space. Vasoconstriction in the peripheral vessels may raise blood pressure and increase heart rate both at rest and possibly during exercise.

Antihistamines block the histamine receptor, which is involved with the mast cells and the allergic response. These medications do not have a direct effect on the heart rate or blood pressure, but they do produce a drying effect in the upper airways and may cause drowsiness.

Most cold medications are a combination of decongestants and antihistamines and may have combined effects. However, they are normally taken in low doses and have minimal effects on exercise.

CLIENTS' PREFERENCES, EXPECTATIONS, AND LIFESTYLE INFORMATION

A simple questionnaire that you can use with your clients in an interview format will give you invaluable information about what they want and need from you. Figure 5.5 is an example of a Lifestyle Information Questionnaire that can be quickly administered in an orientation session. This information not only serves as an important adjunct to the health history (past musculoskeletal injuries resulting from activity), but allows you to personalize the physical activity program to the highest degree and avoid potential errors. This interview also serves as a stepping stone for assisting the client in establishing realistic goals. The important components of a lifestyle information form are (1) physical activity feelings, barriers, preferences, and history; (2) family and social support; (3) occupation; (4) stressors; (5) dietary patterns; and (6) hobbies and leisure activities. Information on the client's expectations of you and/or physical activity will aid in developing a sound program.

Clients'
Preferences,
Expectations, and
Lifestyle
Information

Lifestyle Information Form

Name_____ Date _____

Physical Activity

1. In the past year, how often have you been engaged in physical activity?
   - ☐ Regularly (3 to 4 times/week)
   - ☐ Semiregular (1 to 2 times/week)
   - ☐ Sporadic (1 to 2 times/month)
   - ☐ None
2. What types of physical activity do you consider "fun"?_____
3. What are your personal barriers to exercise (i.e., your reasons for not exercising)? _____
   _____
4. What physical activity have you been successful with in the past (liked and participated in regularly)?
   _____
5. How do you think your weight affects your daily activities?_____
   _____

Support

6. Do you feel any family, friends, or co-workers have negative feelings (i.e., disapproval, resentment) toward your efforts at physical activity? _____
7. Is your significant other or a close friend involved in any regular physical activity? _____
   _____

Occupation/Leisure

8. What is your present occupation? _____
9. Does your occupation require much activity (i.e., walking, getting up and down, carrying things)?
   _____
10. What are your usual leisure activities? _____

Stressors

11. What types of things make you feel stressed?_____
12. How do you deal with your stress normally? _____

Dietary Patterns

13. How many meals and/or snacks do you have per day? _____
14. What would you estimate your caloric intake to be per day? _____
15. Do you feel you eat healthy "most of the time"? _____

Expectations

16. Specifically describe what you would like to accomplish through your fitness program during the next:
   1 month_____
   4 months_____
   1 year _____

FIGURE 5.5
Lifestyle Information Form.

PHYSICAL SCREEN

The medical history is very important, but it has the limitation of defining only the conditions that a client is aware of and remembers to report. A client may be completely unaware of a significant risk factor. The purpose of a physical evaluation is to identify these unknown conditions and to further delineate a known condition. The physical screen also establishes an initial baseline and can uncover specific areas that need work. Finally, it commun- icates to clients that you are interested in them and are designing an individualized program to meet their needs.

Two important components of the screening are resting blood pressure and resting heart rate. Optimal blood pressure with respect to cardiovascular risk is <120/80 mmHg. However, as stated earlier, a blood pressure reading below 130/85 is considered normal. There are many factors that can elevate blood pressure, including atherosclerosis, medications, obesity, and stress. Exercise training can be a form of treatment if performed correctly. However, exercise in a person with uncontrolled hypertension can be dangerous and should be postponed until the condition is treated. A blood pressure greater than 140/90 in an adult is classified as hypertension and needs the attention of a physician (see Table 5.1). Normal blood pressure for children varies depending on age and body mass (Kaplan, 1986).

Resting heart rate in adults is usually 60 to 100 beats per minute and is regular in rhythm. Well-trained endurance athletes have developed an efficient cardiovascular system and often have resting heart rates in the low 40s. If an untrained client's resting heart rate is greater than 100, or less than 60, or if the heart rate is irregular, medical referral is recommended.

Observation is the next part of the physical screen and should begin as soon as you meet a client. You should look for shortness of breath at rest, perform a simple postural analysis, check for muscle tightness imbalances, and observe their **gait.** Be aware of any physical characteristics or limitations that may influence the design of the program.

After observation comes the more specific evaluation, beginning with range of motion. It is easiest to do this in a systematic fashion (e.g., starting from the head and moving downward). It is important to assess the quality as well as the quantity of motion. Look for a limited range of motion or asymmetry (Kendall, McCreary, & Provance, 1993).

Evaluation of strength is an important, albeit possibly risky, ordeal. Your goal is to establish a baseline from which to safely start a program, as well as to further delineate any potential asymmetries or weaknesses. You need to consider your client's health history and gathered information before determining which strength testing, if any, is appropriate. The type of strength evaluation should relate to the type of program you will design for them, in consideration both of their goals and your recommendations. For example, if you intend to design a program using elastic resistance, you could evaluate their strength using that type of equipment. See Chapter 6 for more information on testing and evaluation.

SUMMARY

Exercise is a vital component of good health. An effective exercise program improves a client's quality of life without aggravating or precipitating an injury or illness. Health screening is a crucial first step in working with a client and requires recognizing any significant medical conditions or risk factors for injury so a program can be modified accordingly.

The medical history is an important component of the health screening and you should pay particular attention to the cardiovascular and musculoskeletal systems. It also is important to address risk factors for different diseases, as the client may not be aware of a potential or underlying problem. Finally,

Summary

medications should be evaluated because they can alter exercise performance and increase risk factors.

Comprehensive health screening for the personal trainer involves the following steps and tools:

- ✔ Health history form and interview
- ✔ Assessment of risk factors and need for referral and/or physician clearance
- ✔ Assessment of any medications and their effect on exercise response
- ✔ Identification of lifestyle factors that may affect program design
- ✔ Physical screening

In many cases, a safe and appropriate exercise program requires a coordinated effort by you, your client, and his or her physician to safely achieve the desired goals.

REFERENCES

American College of Sports Medicine (2006). *ACSM's Guidelines for Exercise Testing and Prescription* (7th ed.). Philadelphia: Lippincott Williams & Wilkins.

Blair, S.N. (1993). 1993 C.H. McCloy Research Lecture: Physical Activity, Physical Fitness, and Health. *Research Quarterly for Exercise and Sport,* 64, 4, 365–378.

Kaplan, N. (1998). *Clinical Hypertension* (7th ed.). Baltimore: Williams & Wilkins.

Kendall, F.P., McCreary, E.K., & Provance, P.G. (1993). *Muscles: Testing and Function* (4th ed.). Philadelphia: Lippincott Williams & Wilkins.

Paffenbarger, R.S. et al. (1993). The association of changes in physical activity level and other lifestyle characteristics with mortality among men. *New England Journal of Medicine,* 328, 538–545.

Rosenstein, A. (1987). The benefits of health maintenance. *The Physician and Sportsmedicine,* 15, 57–69.

Young, J.M. (1995). The Fifth Report of the Joint Committee on Detection, Evaluation and Treatment of High Blood Pressure. *AAOHN Journal,* 43, 6, 301–305.

SUGGESTED READING

Expert Panel on Detection, Evaluation, and Treatment of High Blood Cholesterol in Adults (2001). Executive Summary of the Third Report of the National Cholesterol Education Program (NCEP) Expert Panel on Detection, Evaluation, and Treatment of High Blood Cholesterol in Adults (Adult Treatment Panel II). *Journal of the American Medical Association,* 285, 19, 2486–2497.

Heyward, V.H. (2006). *Advanced Fitness Assessment & Exercise Prescription.* (5th ed.). Champaign, Ill.: Human Kinetics.

Howley, E.T. & Franks, B.D. (2007). *Health Fitness Instructor's Handbook.* (5th ed.). Champaign, Ill.: Human Kinetics.

Medical Economics Staff, Eds. (2007). *Physician's Desk Reference.* (61st ed.). Montvale, N.J.: Medical Economics.

References and
Suggested Reading

CHAPTER 6

Testing and Evaluation

Richard Cotton, M.A., chief exercise physiologist at MyExercisePlan.com, has been in the health and fitness industry for nearly 30 years. Cotton is the former chief exercise physiologist of the Scripps Clinic & Research Foundation as well as the American Council on Exercise, where he also served as a spokesperson and as editor of five of ACE's fitness professional training manuals. He is certified by the American Council on Exercise, holds the American College of Sports Medicine's (ACSM) two highest-level certifications, and has served as an ACSM certification director since 1983.

Richard T. Cotton

The testing and evaluation of a client is an essential first step in the training process and provides valuable information for both you and your client. Fitness testing and evaluation offers an opportunity to gather information related to a client's current level of physical fitness. The purpose may be any or all of the following:

✔ to assess current fitness levels relative to age and sex

✔ to aid in the development of an exercise program

✔ to identify areas of health and injury risks with possible referral to the appropriate health professional

✔ to establish goals and provide motivation

✔ to evaluate progress

While the specific tests administered may vary from client to client, a comprehensive assessment measures the following four components:

✔ cardiorespiratory efficiency
(at rest and during exercise)
✔ muscular strength and endurance
✔ muscle and joint flexibility
✔ body composition

A sound fitness testing battery should assess the function of the heart, blood vessels, lungs, and muscles according to the physical demands of the individual's optimal lifestyle. Many clients desire a level of fitness that supports daily activities, an active lifestyle, and the ability to confront unforeseen emergencies. Others desire a level of physical fitness that is more athletic and will want to achieve more competitive levels of **cardiovascular endurance, muscular strength** and **endurance, flexibility,** and **body composition.**

REQUIRED VS. OPTIONAL EVALUATION COMPONENTS

Not all clients need or desire comprehensive exercise testing, but some form of evaluation is necessary to obtain the health-screening information you need to assess their cardiovascular risk and suitability for any level of testing and training.

Cardiovascular risk and the consequent necessity of physician referral are determined by applying the cardiovascular **risk factor** guidelines developed by the American College of Sports Medicine; these are explained in detail in Chapter 5. Additionally, a client's exercise history and attitudes toward exercise must be considered. Figure 6.1, the exercise history and attitude questionnaire, is an example of a preexercise assessment tool. It can be used in conjunction with comprehensive fitness testing and also as a minimum evaluation for a client who, for whatever reason, is not being tested.

While many of your clients will look forward to testing and evaluation, it is important to understand that others are very uncomfortable with the process, and that in these cases, it may actually be counterproductive to the success of an exercise program. Some may be embarrassed about their physical condition and would rather be tested at a later date or perhaps not at all. Others are extremely competitive with themselves and understand that poor test results might be too much to tolerate when attempting to make such an important lifestyle change. The minimum evaluation you should require is the assessment of health-risk factors (see Chapter 5), and the completion of an exercise history and attitude questionnaire (see Figure 6.1). The risk factor assessment must be completed to determine the necessity of physician clearance and/or physician-supervised exercise testing. The history and attitude questionnaire is necessary to help you design a unique program geared to each client's habits and motivation.

Pretest and Safety Procedures

While the **submaximal aerobic exercise test** and other tests outlined in this chapter carry a relatively low risk of cardiovascular or other medical complications, it is essential that you follow accepted procedure in the assessment of cardiovascular and other medical risks before testing or training a client. Before a client is tested, the cardiovascular risk assessment should be administered and reviewed. The American College of Sports Medicine (ACSM) (2000) recommends that men over 45 and women over 55 with two or more positive cardiovascular risk factors have a physician-supervised maximal graded exercise test before taking part in any vigorous exercise (i.e., greater than 60% of capacity). The cardiovascular risk assessment should include questions related to all the cardiovascular risk factors recognized by the ACSM and outlined in Chapter 5.

Required vs. Optional Evaluation Components

Exercise History and Attitude Questionnaire

Name _____ Date _____

General Instructions: Please fill out this form as completely as possible. If you have any questions, DO NOT GUESS; ask your trainer for assistance.

1. Please rate your exercise level on a scale of 1 to 5 (5 indicating very strenuous) for each age range through your present age:

    15–20 _____   21–30 _____   31–40 _____   41–50 _____   51+_____

2. Were you a high school and/or college athlete?

    ☐ Yes   ☐ No   If yes, please specify _____

3. Do you have any negative feelings toward, or have you had any bad experience with, physical activity programs?

    ☐ Yes   ☐ No   If yes, please explain _____

4. Do you have any negative feelings toward, or have you had any bad experience with, fitness testing and evaluation?

    ☐ Yes   ☐ No   If yes, please explain _____

5. Rate yourself on a scale of 1 to 5 (1 indicating the lowest value and 5 the highest). Circle the number that best applies.

    Characterize your present athletic ability.
    1   2   3   4   5

    When you exercise, how important is competition?
    1   2   3   4   5

    Characterize your present cardiovascular capacity.
    1   2   3   4   5

    Characterize your present muscular capacity.
    1   2   3   4   5

    Characterize your present flexibility capacity.
    1   2   3   4   5

6. Do you start exercise programs but then find yourself unable to stick with them?

    ☐ Yes   ☐ No

7. How much time are you willing to devote to an exercise program?

    _____ minutes/day   _____ days/week

8. Are you currently involved in regular endurance (cardiovascular) exercise?

    ☐ Yes   ☐ No   If yes, specify the type of exercise(s) _____
    _____ minutes/day   _____ days/week

    Rate your perception of the exertion of your exercise program (circle the number):
    (1) Light   (2) Fairly light   (3) Somewhat hard   (4) Hard

FIGURE 6.1
A sample exercise history and attitude questionnaire.

continued on next page

FIGURE 6.1 continued

9. How long have you been exercising regularly?
   _____ months   _____ years

10. What other exercise, sport, or recreational activities have you participated in?
    In the past 6 months? _____
    In the past 5 years?_____

11. Can you exercise during your work day?
    ☐ Yes   ☐ No

12. Would an exercise program interfere with your job?
    ☐ Yes   ☐ No

13. Would an exercise program benefit your job?
    ☐ Yes   ☐ No

14. What types of exercise interest you?
    ☐ Walking   ☐ Jogging   ☐ Other aerobic
    ☐ Cycling   ☐ Traditional aerobics   ☐ Strength training
    ☐ Stationary biking   ☐ Elliptical striding   ☐ Racquet sports
    ☐ Stair climbing   ☐ Swimming   ☐ Yoga/Pilates

15. Rank your goals in undertaking exercise:
    What do you want exercise to do for you? _____
    _____
    _____

    Use the following scale to rate each goal separately:

Not at all important				Somewhat important				Extremely important	
1	2	3	4	5	6	7	8	9	10

    a. Improve cardiovascular fitness   ____
    b. Body-fat weight loss   ____
    c. Reshape or tone my body   ____
    d. Improve performance for a specific sport ____
    e. Improve moods and ability to cope with stress ____
    f. Improve flexibility   ____
    g. Increase strength   ____
    h. Increase energy level   ____
    i. Feel better   ____
    j. Enjoyment   ____
    k. Other   ____

16. By how much would you like to change your current weight?
    (+) _____ lbs   (-) _____ lbs

FIGURE 6.2
Radial pulse is palpated with two fingers on the wrist at the base of the thumb.

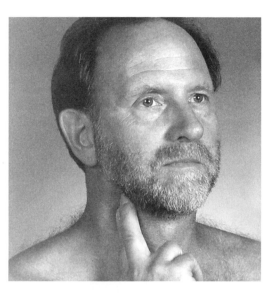

FIGURE 6.3
To palpate the carotid pulse, place the fingertips on the neck, just to the side of the larynx.

Written Consent. All clients should read and sign an **informed consent** before being tested. This consent should explain the purpose and process of the testing and include a statement of the potential for discomfort, pain, or even death associated with its implementation. While this may sound extreme, it is your legal responsibility to adequately inform your clients of even the most unlikely occurrences that could take place during a procedure. In the event of an incident, properly written emergency procedures and consents may help to protect you or the exercise facility (see Chapters 17 and 18).

Written Emergency Procedures. All trainers and exercise facilities should have written emergency procedures that include everything from how to report an emergency and what to do for minor injuries in the gym, to how to respond to an apparent cardiovascular event. All procedures should include a detailed delineation of responsibilities and documentation in the event of an incident (see Chapter 17).

CARDIORESPIRATORY TESTING AND EVALUATION

Cardiorespiratory testing can give you valuable information to aid in both the development and maintenance of your client's program. Regular

resting heart rate and **blood pressure** checks provide some basic cardiovascular health status and program progress information. Aerobic fitness testing not only helps you develop your client's exercise program, but periodic testing can also be motivating as improvements are documented.

Measuring Heart Rate

The resting heart rate may be measured indirectly by placing the fingertips on a pulse site (**palpation**), or directly by listening through a stethoscope (**auscultation**). Resting heart rate is most accurately measured just before the client gets out of bed in the morning. Accuracy is further enhanced by averaging three separate morning readings. To determine the number of beats per minute, take the resting pulse rate for a full minute, or for 30 seconds and then multiply by two. One of the points at which the resting pulse can be accurately measured by palpation is at the radial pulse on the wrist, in line with the base of the thumb (Figure 6.2). Place the tips of your index and middle fingers (not the thumb, which has a pulse of its own) over the artery and lightly apply pressure.

The resting pulse, as well as the exercise pulse, also is accurately palpated from the larger carotid artery on the side of the larynx (Figure 6.3). Heavy pressure should

Cardiorespiratory
Testing and
Evaluation

FIGURE 6.4
Correct stethoscope
position for measuring
resting and exercise
heart rates.

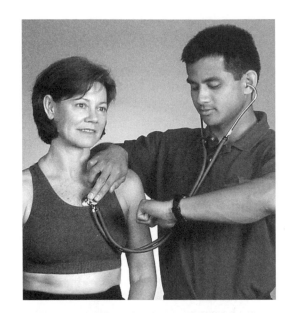

FIGURE 6.5
Chest-strap heart-rate
monitor.

FIGURE 6.6
Correct cuff position
for measuring blood
pressure.

not be applied to the carotid arteries because they contain **baroreceptors** that sense increases in pressure and respond by slowing the heart rate. Exercise pulse should be taken for 10 seconds, counting the first pulse beat as zero at the start of the 10-second period. When measuring by auscultation, place the bell of the stethoscope to the left of the sternum just above the nipple line (Figure 6.4).

Another very accurate and easy method of measuring heart rate, for both testing and training, uses one of the portable heart-rate monitors currently on the market. These consist of a chest strap that contains electrodes that pick up the actual heart rate (not pulse rate) and transmit the signal to a digital readout on a wrist receiver (Figure 6.5). These monitors currently cost between $40 and $350 and are an indispensable tool for personal trainers.

Interpreting resting heart rate as it relates to cardiovascular fitness is difficult. A normal resting heart rate can vary from as low as 40 beats per minute to as high as 100 beats per minute. Men average about 70 beats per minute and women average about 75 beats per minute. Endurance-trained persons generally have a lower resting heart rate due to the increased amount of blood that the heart pumps with each beat (**stroke volume**). Resting heart rate can vary widely for both endurance-trained athletes and deconditioned subjects. It can be used to measure improvements in cardiovascular fitness because it usually decreases as cardiovascular fitness improves. Also, an elevated resting heart rate can be an indication that a client may not quite be recovered from the previous workout. A chronically elevated resting heart rate in a vigorous exerciser is a sign of overtraining.

Measuring Blood Pressure

Blood pressure reflects the force of the heartbeat and the resistance of the arteries to the pumping action of the heart. It is measured in millimeters of mercury (mmHg). The higher number, **systolic blood pressure,** represents the pressure created by the heart as it pumps blood (via ventricular contraction) to the body; this is the maximum pressure created by the heart during a complete cardiac cycle. The lower number, **diastolic blood pressure,** represents the pressure that remains in the arteries during the filling phase of the **cardiac cycle,** when the heart relaxes. It is the minimum pressure within the arteries during a complete cardiac cycle.

Blood pressure is measured using a medical-grade **sphygmomanometer** and stethoscope after a client has been seated with both feet flat on the floor for two full minutes. The cuff should be smoothly and firmly wrapped around the arm with its lower margin about one inch above the **antecubital space** (Figure 6.6). (Use an appropriate-sized cuff as very obese clients may have falsely elevated blood pressure readings with small, standard-sized cuffs.) The arm should be comfortably supported on either an arm chair, or by you, at an angle of 10 to 45 degrees. Place the stethoscope over the brachial artery using a minimal amount of pressure so as not to distort the artery. The stethoscope should not touch the cuff or its tubing. Rapidly inflate the cuff to 20 to 30 mmHg above the point when the pulse can no longer be felt at the wrist. Release the pressure at a rate of about 2 mmHg per second, listening for sounds. The systolic pressure is determined by the first perception of sound. The diastolic pressure is determined when the sounds cease to be heard or when they become muffled. A duplicate measurement should be made using the other arm. Normative values for blood pressure readings are presented in Table 6.1.

If a blood pressure reading needs to be repeated, allow 30 to 60 seconds between trials so normal circulation can return. Record each of the results for comparison with subse-

Table 6.1
Classification of Blood Pressure for Adults Age 18 and Older*

Category	Systolic (mmHg)		Diastolic (mmHg)
Normal†	<120	and	<80
Prehypertension	120–139	or	80–89
Hypertension‡			
Stage 1	140–159	or	90–99
Stage 2	≥160	or	≥100

* Not taking antihypertensive drugs and not acutely ill. When systolic and diastolic blood pressures fall into different categories, the higher category should be selected to classify the individual's blood pressure status. For example, 140/82 mmHg should be classified as stage 1 hypertension, and 154/102 mmHg should be classified as stage 2 hypertension. In addition to classifying stages of hypertension on the basis of average blood pressure levels, clinicians should specify presence or absence of target organ disease and additional risk factors. This specificity is important for risk classification and treatment.

† Normal blood pressure with respect to cardiovascular risk is below 120/80 mmHg. However, unusually low readings should be evaluated for clinical significance.

‡ Based on the average of two or more readings taken at each of two or more visits after an initial screening.

Source: National Institutes of Health (2003). *The Seventh Report of the Joint Committee on Prevention, Detection, Evaluation, and Treatment of High Blood Pressure.* NIH Publication No. 03-5233.

quent measurements. If abnormal readings result, repeat the measurement on the opposite arm. If there is a significant discrepancy between readings from arm to arm, it could represent a circulatory problem, and the client should be referred to a physician for a medical evaluation.

Cardiorespiratory Fitness Testing

Cardiorespiratory fitness is directly assessed by measurement of oxygen uptake during a **maximal graded exercise test,** or indirectly by estimating **maximal oxygen uptake ($\dot{V}O_2$ max)** from the heart-rate response to a submaximal workload. The direct measurement of maximal oxygen uptake is by far the most accurate method, but it requires specialized equipment. Depending on the age and cardiovascular risk of the client, this method is often limited to clinical or research facilities and is usually performed in the presence of a physician trained in advanced cardiac life support. Depending on the type of submaximal test administered, the submaximal exercise test provides a reasonably accurate estimation of maximal oxygen uptake (±10 to 20%). To keep the test submaximal, the intensity should not exceed 85% of **heart-rate reserve** (Karvonen formula) or maximal oxygen uptake (see page 220 for a discussion of this formula).

While there may be some error in the estimation of maximal oxygen uptake, the heart rates measured at equivalent submaximal workloads can be very informative. Therefore, it is the comparison of the heart rates at equivalent workloads during follow-up testing that will show a relative change in aerobic fitness. Even though the maximal oxygen uptake estimated from the test may be somewhat inaccurate, if the heart rates are precise and the testing procedures are correct and consistent, a change in estimated maximal oxygen uptake will be a valid measurement of relative change in aerobic fitness.

It also is very important for you to record perceived exertions during submaximal fitness tests (Table 6.2). **Ratings of perceived exertion** give you an indication of your clients' status during a test and will be valuable in the determination of a **training heart-rate range** following the test.

Absolute vs. Relative Maximal Oxygen Uptake

Because cycling is nonweightbearing, the maximal oxygen consumption figures measured from bike tests will usually be given in liters per minute (L/min) so weight is not a factor in the measurement. Maximal oxygen uptake measurements that are taken from weightbearing activi-

**Table 6.2
Ratings of Perceived Exertion**

RPE		Category Ratio Scale	
6		0	Nothing at all
7	Very, very light	0.5	Very, very weak
8		1	Very weak
9	Very light	2	Weak
10		3	Moderate
11	Fairly light	4	Somewhat strong
12		5	Strong
13	Somewhat hard	6	
14		7	Very strong
15	Hard	8	
16		9	
17	Very hard	10	Very, very strong
18		*	Maximal
19	Very, very hard		
20			

Source: Adapted, with permission, from American College of Sports Medicine (2006). *Guidelines for Exercise Testing and Prescription* (7th ed.). Philadelphia: Lippincott Williams & Wilkins.

ties such as walking, jogging, and stepping are usually given in milliliters of oxygen per kilogram of bodyweight per minute ($mL\ O_2/kg_{BW}/min$).

You can convert absolute oxygen uptake to relative oxygen uptake using the following formula:

$$\text{Relative } O_2 \text{ uptake} = \frac{O_2 \text{ uptake (L/min)} \times 1{,}000}{\text{bodyweight (kg)}}$$

Calculate oxygen uptake in $mL\ O_2/kg_{BW}/min$ by multiplying the oxygen uptake in L/min by 1,000 to convert to mL/min. Divide this figure by the subject's weight, in kilograms, to determine relative oxygen uptake in $mL\ O_2/kg_{BW}/min$.

The calculation of relative oxygen uptake allows for comparison to others of different body weights. A heavy person may have a somewhat high absolute maximal oxygen uptake (L/min) when compared to a lighter person, but when expressed in relative terms (mL/kg/min), the lighter person may show a higher level of cardiovascular fitness. For example:

	Subject A	**Subject B**
Weight	231 lb	132 lb
	(105 kg)	(60 kg)
Absolute $\dot{V}O_2$ max	3.8 L/min	3.2 L/min
Relative $\dot{V}O_2$ max	3.8 x 1,000/ 105 = 36.1 mL/kg/min	3.2 x 1,000/ 60 = 53.3 mL/kg/min

The norms for relative maximal oxygen uptake are given in Table 6.3, which describes "aerobic fitness" of adults. Table 6.4 gives health-related minimums for maximal oxygen consumption for both men and women. To realize the health benefits of aerobic activity, your clients should aim for these levels. For those interested in optimizing both health and aerobic fitness the figures given in Table 6.3 can become the basis for goal setting.

YMCA Submaximal Bicycle Test

The YMCA adapted a submaximal bicycle ergometer test from the tests developed by Sjostrand (1947) to evaluate **physical working capacity,** and by Astrand and Rhyming (1954) to estimate maximal oxygen uptake. The YMCA uses the bicycle ergometer instead of the treadmill because it is less expensive, requires little space, is easily transported and makes it easier to take a heart rate. And, because its external work is known (treadmill workload must be calculated from rate and grade), it requires little training or practice. The ergometer used should be accurate, easily calibrated and have a range of 6 to 2,100 kilogram-meters per minute (kgm/min), or 1 to 350 watts. Two of the most com-

Cardiorespiratory Testing and Evaluation

Table 6.3
Percentile Values for Maximal Aerobic Power (mL/kg/min)

Percentile	Age				
	20–29	30–39	40–49	50–59	60–69
Men					
90	54.0	52.5	51.1	46.8	43.2
80	51.1	48.9	46.8	43.3	39.5
70	48.2	46.8	44.2	41.0	36.7
60	45.7	44.4	42.4	38.3	35.0
50	43.9	42.4	40.4	36.7	33.1
40	42.2	41.0	38.4	35.2	31.4
30	40.3	38.5	36.7	33.2	29.4
20	39.5	36.7	34.6	31.1	27.4
10	35.2	33.8	31.8	28.4	24.1
Women					
90	47.5	44.7	42.4	38.1	34.6
80	44.0	41.0	38.9	35.2	32.3
70	41.1	38.8	36.7	32.9	30.2
60	39.5	36.7	35.1	31.4	29.1
50	37.4	35.2	33.3	30.2	27.5
40	35.5	33.8	31.6	28.7	26.6
30	33.8	32.3	29.7	27.3	24.9
20	31.6	29.9	28.0	25.5	23.7
10	29.4	27.4	25.6	23.7	21.7

Source: Adapted, with permission, from the *Personal Trainer Workshop Manual,* The Cooper Institute, Dallas, Tex. (revised 2006).
Study population for the data set was predominately white and college educated. A modified Balke treadmill test was used with $\dot{V}O_2$max estimated from the last grade/speed achieved. The following may be used as descriptors for the percentile rankings: well above average (90), above average (70), average (50), below average (30), and well below average (10).

Cardiorespiratory Testing and Evaluation

Table 6.4
Suggested Health-related Minimums for
V̇O₂ max (mL O₂/kg_BW/min)

Age Group	V̇O₂ max	
	Men	Women
<45	36	32
50	34	31
55	32	29
60	31	28
>65	30	27

Source: Adapted, with permission, from Baumgartner, T.A. & Jackson, A.S. (1995). *Measurement for Evaluation.* Madison: Brown & Benchmark.

monly used ergometers are manufactured by Monark and Body-guard. The test also requires the use of a metronome to time the test duration, a stethoscope and stopwatch to measure heart rate (or a heart-rate monitor), and the proper form on which to record data. See page 233 for guidelines for using stationary cycling machines.

To estimate maximal oxygen uptake you must record two steady-state submaximal heart rates between 110 and 150 beats per minute. Heart rate is considered to be at a steady state in this test when it is measured within five beats at the end of the second and third minute of each stage. Each workload/heart-rate point is plotted on a graph and connected to form a line segment. This

line segment is then extended up and to the right to the point of intersection with the horizontal line extending from the predicted maximal heart rate (220 minus age). A vertical line perpendicular to the maximal heart-rate line is then drawn down from that point to the baseline. The point of intersection with the baseline marks the estimated maximal oxygen uptake (Figure 6.7). Maximal oxygen uptake estimates that are the result of bicycle ergometer testing are given in liters per minute (absolute measurement). To calculate the relative maximal oxygen uptake you will need to convert the liters to milliliters and divide that figure by the client's weight in kilograms. The result can then be used for comparison to established norms (see Table 6.3).

Ross Submaximal Treadmill Protocol

The Ross Submaximal Treadmill Protocol given in Table 6.5 is an easy-to-use alternative to bicycle ergometer testing. The treadmill speed is held constant at a comfortable walk of 3.4 mph, and the elevation is increased every three minutes. The change is 4% per stage for men, and 3% per stage for women. Submaximal heart rate is measured during the last 15 seconds of every minute. Since the movement produced by walking on a treadmill makes it difficult to measure heart rate by palpitation, electronic equipment is necessary to measure exercise heart rate for treadmill tests. Individual heart-rate responses to the power output will vary according to fitness levels. The submaximal heart rate at any stage should not exceed 150 to 155 beats per minute. The following guidelines are offered to ensure that submaximal exercise is achieved:

✔ Do not go to Stage II if the heart rate exceeds 140 at Stage I; this person is unfit.

✔ Stages IV and V should only be used for individuals under age 50.

✔ Never go to the next stage if the heart rate exceeds 145 beats per minute.

FIGURE 6.7
Extrapolating submaximal heart rates to age-adjusted maximal heart rate to estimate aerobic capacity. Note that in this example, a 25-year-old has heart rates plotted and extrapolated on two different occasions. This results in a 12% error.

*The validity of this equation has recently been called into question (see page 220).

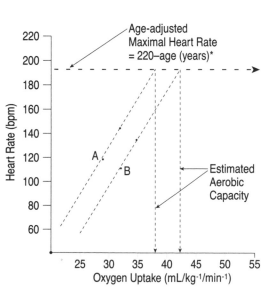

Table 6.5 lists the submaximal oxygen uptake and **MET** levels for each stage. The submaximal oxygen uptake estimations and their associated heart rates are used to estimate maximal oxygen uptake by using the formulas given below. If maximal heart rate is known, substitute it for the 220-minus-age portion of the formula.

Formulas for estimating $\dot{V}O_2$ max from Ross Submaximal Treadmill Protocol:

Women

$$\dot{V}O_2 \text{ (mL/kg/min)} = \frac{(\dot{V}O_2 \text{ from Table 6.5}) \times (220 - \text{Age} - 73)}{\text{ExHR} - 73}$$

Men

$$\dot{V}O_2 \text{ (mL/kg/min)} = \frac{(\dot{V}O_2 \text{ from Table 6.5}) \times (220 - \text{Age} - 63)}{\text{ExHR} - 63}$$

Note: ExHR = exercise heart rate; Exercise heart rates for this test must be within the range of 45 to 70% of heart-rate reserve (Karvonen formula).

YMCA Submaximal Step Test

The three-minute step test developed by Dr. Fred Kasch of San Diego State University also is used by the YMCA. The aerobic stimulus is controlled by stepping to a standardized cadence. This type of test is easier to administer than the bicycle ergometer test. It requires less equipment, costs less, and can be used in mass testing situations. A disadvantage of this test is that it does not result in an estimation of maximal oxygen consumption. The comparison to established norms are based on a one-minute recovery heart rate.

The following equipment is needed to administer the test:

✔ a 12-inch-high (30.5 cm) step bench
✔ a metronome for accurate pacing (96 bpm)
✔ a timer for timing the three-minute test and the one-minute recovery
✔ stethoscope to count recovery heart rate
✔ test forms on which to record data

Table 6.5
Ross Submaximal Treadmill Protocol

Stage	Minutes	MPH	Percent Grade	$\dot{V}O_2$ (mL/kg/min)	METs
Women					
I	1–3	3.4	0	14.9	4.25
II	4–6	3.4	3	18.4	5.27
III	7–9	3.4	6	22.0	6.29
IV	10–12	3.4	9	25.6	7.31
V	13–15	3.4	12	29.2	8.33
Men					
I	1–3	3.4	0	14.9	4.25
II	4–6	3.4	4	19.6	5.61
III	7–9	3.4	8	24.4	6.97
IV	10–12	3.4	12	29.2	8.33
V	13–15	3.4	16	33.9	9.09

Source: Adapted, with permission, from Baumgartner, T.A. & Jackson, A.S. (1995). *Measurement for Evaluation*. Madison: Brown & Benchmark.

Before beginning the test, demonstrate the stepping procedure. With the metronome set to 96 bpm (24 stepping cycles per minute), start stepping to a four-beat cycle—up, up, down, down (Figure 6.8). It does not matter which foot begins the cycle, although both feet must touch the top of the bench on the up portion of the cycle, and both feet must touch the floor during the down portion. The lead foot may change during the test.

Remind the client that they will step for three minutes and be seated immediately afterward for a one-minute pulse count. Have the client face the bench and step in place, in time with the metronome. Start timing the three minutes when the client begins stepping. Check stepping rhythm throughout the test, announcing when one minute, two minutes, and two minutes and 40 seconds have elapsed. You may want to provide additional verbal cues by clapping your hands or saying "up, up, down, down" in cadence with the metronome. At the end of the three-minute stepping period, immediately begin counting the heart rate of the seated subject for one minute. The one-minute postexercise heart rate is used to score the test and can be compared to both the norms in Tables 6.6 and 6.7 and previous test results if appropriate.

McArdle Step Test

An alternative test developed by McArdle and colleagues (1972) may be useful for more fit clients. Though this test results in an estimation of maximal oxygen uptake, the standard error of estimation of ±16% is still comparable to other submaximal tests. You will need a 16.25-inch-high step (41.28 cm). Men should step at a 24-step-per-minute rate (96 bpm), while women step at 22 steps per minute (88 bpm).

Have the client step for three minutes and remain standing. Wait 5 seconds and take a 15-second pulse. Multiply the 15-second pulse by four to convert it to beats per minute. The maximal oxygen uptake in mL/kg/min is estimated using the following equations:

Men: $\dot{V}O_2 \text{ max} = 111.33 - (0.42 \times HR)$
Women: $\dot{V}O_2 \text{ max} = 65.81 - (0.1847 \times HR)$

These results can then be compared to the norms in Tables 6.3 and 6.4.

The Rockport Fitness Walking Test (1-Mile Walk)

The Rockport Fitness Walking Test is routinely used to assess the cardiovascular fitness of those with a low-to-moderate aerobic fitness level. The test involves a timed 1-mile walk on a smooth and level surface (preferably a ¼-mile running track). The only other equipment necessary is a timing device and a form for recording results.

Whereas lab tests measure parameters (e.g., estimated $\dot{V}O_2$ workload or heart rate) that give a very good indication of how well an individual will perform during aerobic activity, the Rockport Fitness Walking Test evaluates performance directly. This test also is excellent for mass testing. It does, however, have its limits. Pacing ability and body-fat weight may adversely affect performance, and because the test requires the mile to be walked as fast as possible, lack of motivation may result in an underestimation of cardiovascular fitness.

Before beginning the test, have clients

FIGURE 6.8
Three-minute step test
—stepping cycle.

Table 6.6
Postexercise Heart Rate Norms for 3-minute Step Test (Men)

Rating	% Rating	Age (years)					
		18–25	26–35	36–45	46–55	56–65	66+
Excellent	100	50	51	49	56	60	59
	95	71	70	70	77	71	74
	90	76	76	76	82	77	81
Good	85	79	79	80	87	86	87
	80	82	83	84	89	91	91
	75	84	85	88	93	94	92
Above average	70	88	88	92	95	97	94
	65	90	91	95	99	99	97
	60	93	94	98	101	100	102
Average	55	95	96	100	103	103	104
	50	97	100	101	107	105	106
	45	100	102	105	111	109	110
Below average	40	102	104	108	113	111	114
	35	105	108	111	117	115	116
	30	107	110	113	119	117	118
Poor	25	111	114	116	121	119	121
	20	114	118	119	124	123	123
	15	119	121	124	126	128	126
Very poor	10	124	126	130	131	131	130
	5	132	134	138	139	136	136
	0	157	161	163	159	154	151

Source: *YMCA Fitness Testing and Assessment Manual,* Copyright 2000. Reprinted and adapted with permission of the YMCA of the USA, 101 N. Wacker Drive, Chicago, IL 60606.

FIGURE 6.8
continued

Table 6.7
Postexercise Heart Rate Norms for 3-minute Step Test (Women)

Rating	% Rating	Age (years)					
		18–25	26–35	36–45	46–55	56–65	66+
Excellent	100	52	58	51	63	60	70
	95	75	74	77	85	83	85
	90	81	80	84	91	92	92
Good	85	85	85	89	95	97	96
	80	89	89	92	98	100	98
	75	93	92	96	101	103	101
Above average	70	96	95	100	104	106	104
	65	98	98	102	107	109	108
	60	102	101	104	110	111	111
Average	55	104	104	107	113	113	116
	50	108	107	109	115	116	120
	45	110	110	112	118	118	121
Below average	40	113	113	115	120	119	123
	35	116	116	118	121	123	125
	30	120	119	120	124	127	126
Poor	25	122	122	124	126	129	128
	20	126	126	128	128	131	129
	15	131	129	132	132	135	133
Very poor	10	135	134	137	137	141	135
	5	143	141	142	143	147	145
	0	169	171	169	171	174	155

Source: *YMCA Fitness Testing and Assessment Manual,* Copyright 2000. Reprinted and adapted with permission of the YMCA of the USA, 101 N. Wacker Drive, Chicago, IL 60606.

warm up by walking and performing light stretching exercises. Explain that while this test requires a near maximal effort, clients should not walk to exhaustion and should stop at any time if necessary. Elapsed times should be announced with every lap. After completing the test, take a 10-second exercise pulse. This 10-second value and its corresponding per-minute pulse (the 10-second pulse times six) should be recorded along with the time it took to complete the mile walk. After test completion, all participants should walk for at least five minutes to cool down.

In addition to completion time and immediate postexercise heart rate, the highest rating of perceived exertion (see Table 6.2) should also be recorded to provide an indication of effort and a comparison to subsequent tests. Completion time and minute pulse rate are used to estimate maximal oxygen uptake using the following formulas:

Women
$\dot{V}O_2$ (mL/kg/min) = 132.85 − (0.388 x Age) − (0.077 x Weight$_{lbs}$) − (3.265 x Mile Walk Time$_{min}$) − (0.156 x Exercise HR)

Men
$\dot{V}O_2$ (mL/kg/min) = 139.168 − (0.388 x Age) − (0.077 x Weight$_{lbs}$) − (3.265 x Mile Walk Time$_{min}$) − (0.156 x Exercise HR)

The standard error of the estimate of maximal oxygen uptake from the Rockport walking test is 5.0 mL O_2/kg$_{BW}$/min. This is about 1.0 mL O_2/kg$_{BW}$/min better than most submaximal bike, treadmill, or step tests.

BYU Jog Test
Researchers at Brigham Young University (BYU) developed a test similar to the

Rockport test by replacing walking with jogging. It is a good test for more fit clients. The test requires a 1-mile jog at a steady pace, and exercise heart rate is measured immediately after the run.

Your client should first take a two- to three-minute warm-up jog. The goal is to jog the mile at a steady and suitable pace. Remind your client that this is a submaximal test and they should not run at an "all-out" rate. Set run time and exercise limits to ensure a submaximal effort. Clients' exercise heart rates should be less than 180 beats per minute, and men should not jog at a pace faster than eight minutes per mile and women should not jog faster than nine minutes per mile. Use the following equations to estimate maximal oxygen uptake:

Women

$$\dot{V}O_2 = 100.5 - (0.164 \times Weight_{kg}) - (1.438 \times Mile\ Jog\ Time_{min}) - (0.193 \times Exercise\ HR)$$

Men

$$\dot{V}O_2 = 108.44 \quad (0.164 \times Weight_{kg}) - (1.438 \times Mile\ Jog\ Time_{min}) - (0.193 \times Exercise\ HR)$$

Note: The standard error of this test (SE = 3.0 mL/kg/min) is half that of the submaximal bike, treadmill, and step tests.

BODY COMPOSITION TESTING AND EVALUATION

Excess body fat has been associated with a number of health risks, including heart disease, **diabetes, hypertension,** arthritis, gall bladder disease, cirrhosis of the liver, **hernia,** intestinal obstruction, and sleep disorders. It also is associated with reduced endurance performance and an increased risk for injury. The primary reason most adults begin exercise programs is to reduce body weight, so it is important to be able to assess body composition to determine a reasonable body-weight goal and to develop a safe and effective exercise program to reach it.

Body composition refers to the quality or makeup of total body mass, which can be divided into **fat-free mass** and fat mass. Fat-free mass is composed of bone, muscle, and organs, and fat mass is composed of **adipose tissue.** Body composition assessment determines the relative percentages of fat-free and fat mass.

Ideal body weight has historically been determined without concern for body composition and involved the use of the standardized height-weight tables. Ideal body weight is estimated only from height and frame size without consideration of the composition of the weight. Therefore, a well-muscled bodybuilder would most likely be considered overweight, while another person could fall within the accepted range and actually be over-fat by body-composition standards. It is not uncommon for an exerciser to lose fat weight and gain muscle weight without any change in total body weight. Without an assessment of body composition, this favorable change could go undetected and possibly lead to frustration on the part of the exerciser.

The four most common methods of assessing body composition are hydrostatic weighing, circumference measurements, bioelectrical impedance, and skinfold measurements.

Hydrostatic Weighing

Hydrostatic weighing, also known as underwater weighing, is considered the "gold standard" of body composition assessment. The test involves suspending a client, seated in a chair attached to a scale, in a tank of water. Body density is calculated from the relationship of normal body weight to underwater weight. Body-fat percentage is calculated from body density. This method is most accurate when combined with a measurement of **residual volume** (the amount of air left in the lungs after a complete expiration). When residual volume is estimated from a formula, the accuracy of the hydrostatic method can be significantly

Body Composition Testing and Evaluation

decreased. Though hydrostatic weighing is accurate, it is often impractical in terms of expense, time, and equipment.

Bioelectrical Impedance

Bioelectrical impedance is a popular method for determining body composition. It is based on the principle that the conductivity of an electrical impulse is greater through lean tissue than through fatty tissue. An imperceptible electrical current is passed through two pairs of electrodes, which are placed on a hand and foot. The analyzer, essentially an ohmmeter and a computer, measures the body's resistance to electrical flow and computes body density and body-fat percentage. The subject must lie still, with wrist and ankle electrodes accurately placed. The client should be well-hydrated and not

have exercised in the past 6 hours or consumed any alcohol in the past 24 hours. Some research has shown the impedance method to be as accurate as the skinfold method, depending on the quality of the analyzer, the formula used to compute body density and the adherence of the client to the aforementioned restrictions. Assessing body composition via bioelectrical impedance is both fast and easy and requires minimal technical training. The cost of the analyzers ranges from $300 to $5,000, depending on design and report-generation capabilities (from simple digital readouts to elaborate multipage reports).

Body-fat scales are now available for around $100, though they are not accurate enough to be reliable measurement tools. The problem stems from the scales' inability

---

Table 6.8
Body Mass Index

Height (inches)	19	20	21	22	23	24	25	26	27	28	29	30	35	40
							Weight (pounds)							
58	91	95	100	105	110	115	119	124	129	134	138	143	167	191
59	94	99	104	109	114	119	124	128	133	138	143	148	173	198
60	97	102	107	112	118	123	128	133	138	143	148	153	179	204
61	100	106	111	116	121	127	132	137	143	148	153	158	185	211
62	104	109	115	120	125	131	136	142	147	153	158	164	191	218
63	107	113	118	124	130	135	141	146	152	158	163	169	197	225
64	110	116	122	128	134	140	145	151	157	163	169	174	203	233
65	114	120	126	132	138	144	150	156	162	168	174	180	210	240
66	117	124	130	136	142	148	155	161	167	173	179	185	216	247
67	121	127	134	140	147	153	159	166	172	178	185	191	223	255
68	125	131	138	144	151	158	164	171	177	184	190	197	230	263
69	128	135	142	149	155	162	169	176	182	189	196	203	237	270
70	132	139	146	153	160	167	174	181	188	195	202	209	243	278
71	136	143	150	157	165	172	179	186	193	200	207	215	250	286
72	140	147	155	162	169	177	184	191	199	206	213	221	258	294
73	144	151	159	166	174	182	189	197	204	212	219	227	265	303
74	148	155	163	171	179	187	194	202	210	218	225	233	272	311
75	152	160	168	176	184	192	200	208	216	224	232	240	279	319
76	156	164	172	180	189	197	205	213	221	230	238	246	287	328

Note: Find your client's height in the far left column and move across the row to the weight that is closest to the client's weight. Their body mass index will be at the top of that column.

to differentiate between body types and to provide consistent readings.

Body Mass Index

More useful estimates of body composition can be obtained by adjusting weight for height or stature and calculating a height-normalized index. The most commonly used index is the **body mass index (BMI),** which is calculated as follows:

$$BMI = \frac{Weight\ (kg)}{Height^2(m)}$$

Example:
Convert weight from pounds to kilograms by dividing by 2.2:
Weight = 209.5 pounds

$$\frac{209}{2.2} = 95.2\ kg$$

Convert height from inches to centimeters, and then to meters, by multiplying by 2.54 and then dividing by 100:

Height = 67.7 inches

$$67.7 \times 2.54 = 172\ cm$$

$$\frac{172}{100} = 1.72\ m$$

$$BMI = \frac{95.2}{(1.72)^2} = 32.2$$

Use Table 6.8 to determine body mass index. People in a normal weight range usually have a BMI between 18.5 and 24.9. According to NHANES III data, as reported in the National Heart, Lung, and Blood Institute's obesity guidelines (1998), "54.9% of U.S. adults aged 20 years and older are either overweight or obese; 32.6% are overweight, defined as having a body mass index (BMI) of 25.0 to 29.9 kg/m²; and 22.3% are obese with a BMI of 30 kg/m²" (Table 6.9).

Since BMI uses total body weight (i.e., not estimates of fat and lean body mass separately) in the calculation, it does not discriminate between the overfat and the athletic or more muscular body type. Therefore, BMI should ideally be used in conjunction with other body composition assessments.

Anthropometry

Anthropometric assessments of body composition are perhaps the easiest and least expensive methods for assessing body composition. These include circumference and skinfold measures, which are readily used in the field. Anthropometric measures also can be used to estimate body fat and its distribution (i.e., central vs. peripheral, or upper vs. lower body).

Circumference Measures. Circumference measures can easily be used to assess body composition, even with significantly overweight clients. However, to ensure accuracy, you must use exact anatomical landmarks for taking each circumference measurement (Table 6.10 and Figures 6.9–6.12). A thorough review of anthropometric measurement sites and techniques for optimizing accuracy is presented in Lohman et al. (1988).

A cloth or fiberglass (i.e., non-elastic) metric measurement tape must be used. The tape

Table 6.9
BMI Reference Chart

Weight Category	BMI Range
Underweight	<18.5
Normal weight	18.5–24.9
Overweight	25.0–29.9
Grade I Obesity	30.0–34.9
Grade II Obesity	35.0–39.9
Grade III Obesity	>40

Table 6.10
Anatomic Locations of Circumference Measurement Sites

Circumference	Anatomic Site
Abdomen	At the level of the umbilicus
Hips	The largest circumference at the posterior extension of the gluteals
Iliac	Level with the iliac crests
Waist	The narrowest part of the torso

Body Composition Testing and Evaluation

FIGURE 6.9
Abdominal circumference.

FIGURE 6.10
Hip circumference.

FIGURE 6.11
Iliac circumference.

Table 6.11
Waist-to-Hip Ratios and Associated Level of Health Risks

Classification	Men	Women
High risk	>1.0	>0.85
Moderately high risk	0.90–1.0	0.80–0.85
Lower risk	<0.90	<0.80

Adapted, with permission, from: Van Itallie, T.B. (1988). Topography of Body Fat: Relationship to Risk of Cardiovascular and Other Diseases. In: *Anthropometric Standardization Reference Manual.* Lohman, T.G., Roche, A.F., & Martorell, R. (Eds.). Champaign, Ill.: Human Kinetics.

should be periodically calibrated against a meter stick to ensure it has not been stretched. When assessing significantly overweight clients, be sure to use a long enough tape. Pull the tape tight enough to keep it in position without causing an indentation of the skin. There are tapes available that have a gauge that indicates the correct tension.

Estimating Body Fat from Circumference Measures. Body density (BD) for women and men can be predicted from generalized equations that use girth measurements (Tran and Weltman, 1989; Tran, Weltman, & Seip, 1988):

FIGURE 6.12
Waist circumference.

BD for women = 1.168297 − (0.002824 x abdomen$_{cm}$) + (0.0000122098 x abdomen$^2_{cm}$) − (0.000733128 x hips$_{cm}$) + (0.000510477 x height$_{cm}$) − (0.000216161 x age)

BD for men = 1.21142 + (0.00085 x weight$_{kg}$) − (0.00050 x iliac$_{cm}$) − (0.00061 x hip$_{cm}$) − (0.00138 x abdomen$_{cm}$)

Body density can then be converted to percent fat by using the following formula:

$$\text{Percent fat} = \left(\frac{495}{\text{BD}}\right) - 450$$

Estimating Body-fat Distribution. Upper-body or abdominal obesity is known to increase health risk (e.g., type 2 diabetes, hypertension, hypercholesterolemia). A quick and reliable technique is the **waist-to-hip circumference ratio (WHR).** To calculate the WHR ratio, divide the waist measurement by the hip measurement. Table 6.11 illustrates the relative risk ratings for WHR ratios. It should also be noted that waist circumference is a reliable and easily measured indicator of abdominal obesity (National Heart, Lung, and Blood Institute, 1998). Waist circumferences of greater than 40 inches (102 cm) in men and 35 inches (89 cm) in women are considered strong indicators of abdominal obesity.

Skinfold Measurements. Skinfold measurements are a relatively inexpensive way to assess body composition, and, if the measurements are taken properly, the results are both valid and reliable. The standard error associated with this method is 3.5%, depending on the equation applied. This is compared to a 2.7% error for a hydrostatically determined measurement. Skinfold measurement is based on the belief that approximately 50% of total body fat lies under the skin, and involves measuring the thickness of the skinfolds at standardized sites. These measurements are summed and applied to one of many equations available.

For the most part, the equations calculate body density, with percent fat being calculated from the same formula used for hydrostatic weighing. Calculation is often simplified through the use of a table or nomogram. Calipers specifically designed for skinfold measurement are the only equipment needed for this method of body-fat assessment, and range in cost from $3 to $300.

The procedure for measuring skinfolds is as follows:

1. Identify the anatomical location of the skinfold. Take all measurements on the right side of the body. (Optional: Mark the site with a common eyebrow pencil to expedite site relocation in repeated measures.)

2. Grasp the skinfold firmly with the thumb and index finger of the left hand.

3. Holding the calipers perpendicular to the site, place the pads of the calipers approximately ¼ inch from the thumb and forefinger.

4. Approximately one or two seconds after the trigger has been released, read the dial to the nearest 0.5 millimeter.

5. A minimum of two measurements should be taken at each site, with at least 15 seconds between measurements to allow the fat to return to its normal thickness.

6. Continue to take measurements until two measurements vary by less than 1 millimeter.

Improper site determination and measurement are the two primary sources of error when using this method. The technique is best learned by locating and measuring the standard sites numerous times and comparing results with those of a well-trained associate. Skinfold measurements should not be taken after exercise because the transfer of fluid to the skin could result in overestimations.

Of the many equations for estimating body composition, two developed by Jackson and Pollock (1985) have the smallest margin of error for the general population. These equations are based on the sum of measurements taken at three sites.

Body Composition Testing and Evaluation

For men the skinfold sites are as follows:

1. Chest (Figure 6.13): a diagonal skinfold taken midway on the anterior axillary line (crease of the underarm and the nipple.)

2. Thigh (Figure 6.14): a vertical skinfold taken midway between the hip and knee joints on the front of the thigh.

3. Abdomen (Figure 6.15): a vertical skinfold taken 1 inch lateral to the umbilicus.

For women, the skinfold sites are as follows:

1. Triceps (Figure 6.16): a vertical fold on the back of the upper arm taken halfway between the acromion (shoulder) and olecranon (elbow) processes.

2. Thigh (Figure 6.17): a vertical skinfold taken midway between the hip and knee joints on the front of the thigh.

3. Suprailium (Figure 6.18): a diagonal fold taken at, or just anterior to, the crest of the ilium.

After obtaining three satisfactory measurements, add them and refer to Table 6.12 for men and Table 6.13 for women (pages 191 and 192).

For example, a 47-year-old man has the following measurements: chest, 20; abdomen, 30; and thigh, 17, for a total measurement of 67. According to Table 6.12, at the intersection of the row corresponding to the sum of the skinfolds and the column corresponding to the age, his estimated body-fat percentage is 21.3%. Table 6.14 contains various ranges of body-fat. This man is 5% above the upper limit of the 14 to 17% range for men desiring optimal fitness. In order to calculate this man's weight for the desired range, his lean body weight must first be calculated. Since 21.3% of his body weight is fat weight, subtract 21.3% from 100%, which

equals 78.7% of his weight as lean body mass. Assuming a total body weight of 212 pounds, we then use the decimal form of the percentage figure to derive a lean body weight of 166.8 pounds. To summarize:

Step 1: 100% − fat percentage
= lean body percentage
100 % − 21.3% = 78.7%

Step 2: body weight x lean body percentage = lean body weight
212 x .787 = 166.8 pounds

A body weight for a desired percent fat is then calculated by first subtracting the desired percent fat from 100% and then dividing the lean body weight by the decimal form of this percentage:

Step 3: 100 - desired percent fat =
desired lean percent
Upper limit: 100% − 17% = 83%
Lower limit: 100% − 12% = 88%

Step 4: lean body weight/desired lean percentage = desired body weight

$$\frac{167}{0.83} = 201 \text{ pounds}$$

$$\frac{167}{0.88} = 190 \text{ pounds}$$

The weight range corresponding to a desired body fat of 12 to 17% is 190 to 201 pounds. With regular aerobic activity, resistance training and dietary management, this man would need to lose a minimum 11 pounds of fat weight (212 − 201 = 11).

It is important to understand that muscle weight can increase even when exercise participation is limited to aerobic activity. Body composition should be assessed periodically throughout an exercise program. This can provide motivating information, especially when fat weight loss appears to have plateaued.

Girth Measurements

Girth measurements may be used alone or with skinfold measurements to assess

Table 6.14
General Body-fat Percentage Categories

Classification	Women (% fat)	Men (% fat)
Essential fat	10–13%	2–5%
Athletes	14–20%	6–13%
Fitness	21–24%	14–17%
Average	25–31%	18–24%
Obese	32% and higher	25% and higher

FIGURE 6.13
Chest skinfold measurement for men:

Locate the site midway between the anterior axillary line and the nipple.

Grasp a diagonal fold and pull it away from the muscle.

FIGURE 6.14
Thigh skinfold measurement for men:

Locate the hip and the knee joints and find the midpoint on the top of the thigh.

FIGURE 6.15
Abdominal skinfold measurement for men:

Grasp a vertical skinfold one inch to the right of the umbilicus.

**Body Composition
Testing and
Evaluation**

FIGURE 6.16
Triceps skinfold mea-
surement for women.

Locate the site midway
between the acromial
(shoulder) and olecra-
non (elbow) processes.

Grasp a vertical fold on
the posterior midline
and pull it away from
the muscle.

FIGURE 6.17
Thigh skinfold mea-
surement for women:

Locate the hip and the
knee joints and find the
midpoint on the top of
the thigh.

Grasp a vertical skin-
fold and pull it away
from the muscle.

FIGURE 6.18
Suprailium skinfold
measurement for
women:

Grasp a diagonal skin-
fold just above, and
slightly forward of, the
crest of the ilium.

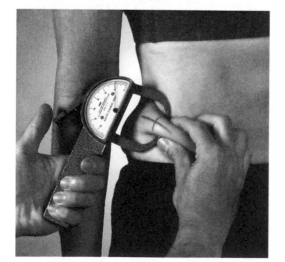

Table 6.12
Percent Body Fat Estimations for Men—Jackson and Pollock Formula

Sum of Skinfolds (mm)	Age Groups								
	Under 22	23–27	28–32	33–37	38–42	43–47	48–52	53–57	Over 57
8–10	1.3	1.8	2.3	2.9	3.4	3.9	4.5	5.0	5.5
11–13	2.2	2.8	3.3	3.9	4.4	4.9	5.5	6.0	6.5
14–16	3.2	3.8	4.3	4.8	5.4	5.9	6.4	7.0	7.5
17–19	4.2	4.7	5.3	5.8	6.3	6.9	7.4	8.0	8.5
20–22	5.1	5.7	6.2	6.8	7.3	7.9	8.4	8.9	9.5
23–25	6.1	6.6	7.2	7.7	8.3	8.8	9.4	9.9	10.5
26–28	7.0	7.6	8.1	8.7	9.2	9.8	10.3	10.9	11.4
29–31	8.0	8.5	9.1	9.6	10.2	10.7	11.3	11.8	12.4
32–34	8.9	9.4	10.0	10.5	11.1	11.6	12.2	12.8	13.3
35–37	9.8	10.4	10.9	11.5	12.0	12.6	13.1	13.7	14.3
38–40	10.7	11.3	11.8	12.4	12.9	13.5	14.1	14.6	15.2
41–43	11.6	12.2	12.7	13.3	13.8	14.4	15.0	15.5	16.1
44–46	12.5	13.1	13.6	14.2	14.7	15.3	15.9	16.4	17.0
47–49	13.4	13.9	14.5	15.1	15.6	16.2	16.8	17.3	17.9
50–52	14.3	14.8	15.4	15.9	16.5	17.1	17.6	18.2	18.8
53–55	15.1	15.7	16.2	16.8	17.4	17.9	18.5	19.1	19.7
56–58	16.0	16.5	17.1	17.7	18.2	18.8	19.4	20.0	20.5
59–61	16.9	17.4	17.9	18.5	19.1	19.7	20.2	20.8	21.4
62–64	17.6	18.2	18.8	19.4	19.9	20.5	21.1	21.7	22.2
65–67	18.5	19.0	19.6	20.2	20.8	21.3	21.9	22.5	23.1
68–70	19.3	19.9	20.4	21.0	21.6	22.2	22.7	23.3	23.9
71–73	20.1	20.7	21.2	21.8	22.4	23.0	23.6	24.1	24.7
74–76	20.9	21.5	22.0	22.6	23.2	23.8	24.4	25.0	25.5
77–79	21.7	22.2	22.8	23.4	24.0	24.6	25.2	25.8	26.3
80–82	22.4	23.0	23.6	24.2	24.8	25.4	25.9	26.5	27.1
83–85	23.2	23.8	24.4	25.0	25.5	26.1	26.7	27.3	27.9
86–88	24.0	24.5	25.1	25.7	26.3	26.9	27.5	28.1	28.7
89–91	24.7	25.3	25.9	26.5	27.1	27.6	28.2	28.8	29.4
92–94	25.4	26.0	26.6	27.2	27.8	28.4	29.0	29.6	30.2
95–97	26.1	26.7	27.3	27.9	28.5	29.1	29.7	30.3	30.9
98–100	26.9	27.4	28.0	28.6	29.2	29.8	30.4	31.0	31.6
101–103	27.5	28.1	28.7	29.3	29.9	30.5	31.1	31.7	32.3
104–106	28.2	28.8	29.4	30.0	30.6	31.2	31.8	32.4	33.0
107–109	28.9	29.5	30.1	30.7	31.3	31.9	32.5	33.1	33.7
110–112	29.6	30.2	30.8	31.4	32.0	32.6	33.2	33.8	34.4
113–115	30.2	30.8	31.4	32.0	32.6	33.2	33.8	34.5	35.1
116–118	30.9	31.5	32.1	32.7	33.3	33.9	34.5	35.1	35.7
119–121	31.5	32.1	32.7	33.3	33.9	34.5	35.1	35.7	36.4
122–124	32.1	32.7	33.3	33.9	34.5	35.1	35.8	36.4	37.0
125–127	32.7	33.3	33.9	34.5	35.1	35.8	36.4	37.0	37.6

Source: Jackson, A.S. & Pollock, M.L. (1985). *Practical Assessment of Body Composition.* Reprinted with permission of McGraw-Hill.

Table 6.13
Percent Body Fat Estimations for Women — Jackson and Pollock Formula

Sum of Skinfolds (mm)	Age Groups								
	Under 22	23–27	28–32	33–37	38–42	43–47	48–52	53–57	Over 57
23–25	9.7	9.9	10.2	10.4	10.7	10.9	11.2	11.4	11.7
26–28	11.0	11.2	11.5	11.7	12.0	12.3	12.5	12.7	13.0
29–31	12.3	12.5	12.8	13.0	13.3	13.5	13.8	14.0	14.3
32–34	13.6	13.8	14.0	14.3	14.5	14.8	15.0	15.3	15.5
35–37	14.8	15.0	15.3	15.5	15.8	16.0	16.3	16.5	16.8
38–40	16.0	16.3	16.5	16.7	17.0	17.2	17.5	17.7	18.0
41–43	17.2	17.4	17.7	17.9	18.2	18.4	18.7	18.9	19.2
44–46	18.3	18.6	18.8	19.1	19.3	19.6	19.8	20.1	20.3
47–49	19.5	19.7	20.0	20.2	20.5	20.7	21.0	21.2	21.5
50–52	20.6	20.8	21.1	21.3	21.6	21.8	22.1	22.3	22.6
53–55	21.7	21.9	22.1	22.4	22.6	22.9	23.1	23.4	23.6
56–58	22.7	23.0	23.2	23.4	23.7	23.9	24.2	24.4	24.7
59–61	23.7	24.0	24.2	24.5	24.7	25.0	25.2	25.5	25.7
62–64	24.7	25.0	25.2	25.5	25.7	26.0	26.7	26.4	26.7
65–67	25.7	25.9	26.2	26.4	26.7	26.9	27.2	27.4	27.7
68–70	26.6	26.9	27.1	27.4	27.6	27.9	28.1	28.4	28.6
71–73	27.5	27.8	28.0	28.3	28.5	28.8	29.0	29.3	29.5
74–76	28.4	28.7	28.9	29.2	29.4	29.7	29.9	30.2	30.4
77–79	29.3	29.5	29.8	30.0	30.3	30.5	30.8	31.0	31.3
80–82	30.1	30.4	30.6	30.9	31.1	31.4	31.6	31.9	32.1
83–85	30.9	31.2	31.4	31.7	31.9	32.2	32.4	32.7	32.9
86–88	31.7	32.0	32.2	32.5	32.7	32.9	33.2	33.4	33.7
89–91	32.5	32.7	33.0	33.2	33.5	33.7	33.9	34.2	34.4
92–94	33.2	33.4	33.7	33.9	34.2	34.4	34.7	34.9	35.2
95–97	33.9	34.1	34.4	34.6	34.9	35.1	35.4	35.6	35.9
98–100	34.6	34.8	35.1	35.3	35.5	35.8	36.0	36.3	36.5
101–103	35.3	35.4	35.7	35.9	36.2	36.4	36.7	36.9	37.2
104–106	35.8	36.1	36.3	36.6	36.8	37.1	37.3	37.5	37.8
107–109	36.4	36.7	36.9	37.1	37.4	37.6	37.9	38.1	38.4
110–112	37.0	37.2	37.5	37.7	38.0	38.2	38.5	38.7	38.9
113–115	37.5	37.8	38.0	38.2	38.5	38.7	39.0	39.2	39.5
116–118	38.0	38.3	38.5	38.8	39.0	39.3	39.5	39.7	40.0
119–121	38.5	38.7	39.0	39.2	39.5	39.7	40.0	40.2	40.5
122–124	39.0	39.2	39.4	39.7	39.9	40.2	40.4	40.7	40.9
125–127	39.4	39.6	39.9	40.1	40.4	40.6	40.9	41.1	41.4
128–130	39.8	40.0	40.3	40.5	40.8	41.0	41.3	41.5	41.8

Source: Jackson, A.S. & Pollock, M.L. (1985). *Practical Assessment of Body Composition*. Reprinted with permission of McGraw-Hill.

body composition. While this method of assessment has been shown to be no more accurate than skinfolds alone, it is valuable in the evaluation of girth changes that result from resistance training and provides a good check on skinfolds and other methods of assessment as body composition changes.

The two primary sources of error in measuring girth are inconsistent tape placement during repeated measures and variations in the tension placed on the tape during the measurement. You can minimize the first error by using the standardized sites described below. You can overcome the second error by using a cloth tape specifically designed for girth measurement. These tapes have a scale that standardizes the tension applied to the tape as each site is measured.

Take the measurements at these sites:

1. Chest—at the nipple line during the midpoint of a normal breath

2. Waist—at the narrowest point, below the rib cage and just above the top of the hip bones

3. Hips—with feet together, at the level of the symphysis pubis in front, at the maximal protrusion of the buttocks in the back

4. Thigh—at the crotch level and just below the fold of the buttocks

5. Calf—at the maximal circumference

6. Ankle—at the minimal circumference, usually just above the ankle bone

7. Upper arm—at the maximal circumference; arm extended, palm up

8. Wrist—at the minimal circumference; arm extended, palm up

Record the measurements for comparison each time body composition is assessed.

FLEXIBILITY TESTING AND EVALUATION

Flexibility is defined as the range of motion of a given joint. It is often associated only with muscular flexibility, the extent to which range of motion is limited by muscles and tendons surrounding the joint. But flexibility also is influenced by the amount of freedom allowed by the ligaments connecting the bones that make up a given joint. Flexibility affects both health and fitness.

Inflexibility increases risk for joint and muscle injury. Low-back inflexibility, which relates to low-back pain and injury, is a common example. For athletes to perform at optimal levels, they must be able to move through motions that are specific to their sport with ease and fluidity. Limitations to movement in sports affect both performance and musculoskeletal health.

As with strength testing, there is no single flexibility test that predicts the range of motion of other joints of the body. Each joint must be assessed individually with a specifically designed test. While it is not the purpose of this chapter to explain the assessment of multiple joints throughout the body, tests of shoulder, hip, and low-back range of motion will be highlighted.

Trunk Flexion

Trunk flexion is measured with the sit-and-reach test, which is administered with a yardstick and tape, and has well-established norms for comparison. There is a slight risk of muscle strain or pull if a forward movement is attempted that is too vigorous. Therefore, all participants should warm up with gentle stretching of the low back and hamstrings, and the test should be performed slowly and cautiously. Place the yardstick on the floor, and put a piece of tape at least 12 inches long at a right angle to the stick between the legs, with the zero mark toward the body. The client's feet should be approximately 12 inches apart and their heels aligned with the tape at the 15-inch mark on the yardstick (Figure 6.19). Have the client place one hand on top of the other, with the tips of the fingers aligned, then exhale and slowly lean forward by dropping the head toward or between the arms. The client's fingers should maintain contact with the yardstick while you keep his or her knees straight.

Flexibility Testing and Evaluation

Table 6.15
Norms for Trunk Flexibility Test (Men)

Rating	% Rating	Age (years) 18–25	26–35	36–45	46–55	56–65	66+
Excellent	100	28	28	28	26	24	24
	95	23	22	22	20	19	19
	90	22	21	21	19	17	17
Good	85	21	19	19	18	16	16
	80	20	19	19	17	15	15
	75	20	19	18	16	15	14
Above average	70	19	17	17	15	13	13
	65	18	17	17	15	13	12
	60	18	17	16	14	13	12
Average	55	17	16	15	13	11	11
	50	17	15	15	13	11	10
	45	16	15	15	12	11	10
Below average	40	15	14	13	11	9	9
	35	15	14	13	11	9	9
	30	14	13	13	10	9	8
Poor	25	13	12	11	9	8	7
	20	13	11	11	9	7	7
	15	12	11	9	8	6	6
Very poor	10	11	9	7	6	5	4
	5	9	7	5	4	3	3
	0	2	2	1	1	1	0

Source: *YMCA Fitness Testing and Assessment Manual,* Copyright 2000. Reprinted and adapted with permission of the YMCA of the USA, 101 N. Wacker Drive, Chicago, IL 60606.

The score is the farthest point reached after three trials. Scores can be compared to norms in Tables 6.15 and 6.16. The quality of the trunk flexion can be evaluated further by observing where along the spine the bend-ing is taking place while the subject is in the flexed position (Table 6.17).

Trunk Extension

The trunk-extension test evaluates the amount of backward bend (extension) available to the lumbar spine. As flexibility in the lumbar spine is lost, the risk for low-back pain and injury increases significantly. Have your client lie face down with the hands in position for a push-up (Figure 6.20). The client then pushes the upper body up while letting the lower back relax as much as possible and attempting to keep the hip bones in contact with the floor. Although this movement is commonly used as a therapeutic exercise for low-back-pain patients, it is still important to avoid injury by making sure the extension is not forced and the movement stops when the hip bones

FIGURE 6.19
Sit-and-reach flexibility test.

Table 6.16
Norms for Trunk Flexibility Test (Women)

Rating	% Rating	Age (years)					
		18–25	26–35	36–45	46–55	56–65	66+
Excellent	100	29	28	28	27	26	26
	95	24	24	23	22	21	22
	90	24	23	22	21	20	20
Good	85	22	22	21	20	19	19
	80	22	21	21	20	19	18
	75	22	21	20	19	18	18
Above average	70	21	20	19	18	17	17
	65	20	20	19	18	17	17
	60	20	20	18	17	16	17
Average	55	19	19	17	16	15	16
	50	19	19	17	16	15	15
	45	19	18	17	16	15	15
Below average	40	18	17	16	14	14	14
	35	18	17	16	14	13	13
	30	17	16	15	14	13	13
Poor	25	16	15	14	13	12	12
	20	16	15	14	12	11	11
	15	16	14	13	12	10	10
Very poor	10	14	13	12	10	9	9
	5	12	12	10	8	7	7
	0	7	5	4	3	2	1

Source: *YMCA Fitness Testing and Assessment Manual,* Copyright 2000. Reprinted and adapted with permission of the YMCA of the USA, 101 N. Wacker Drive, Chicago, IL 60606.

begin to lose contact with the floor. Note the location along the spine where the bending is taking place. Evaluate trunk extension using Table 6.18.

Hip Flexion

Hip flexion tests evaluate range of motion in the hips and hamstring tightness. Limitations to hip flexion place undue stress on the low back, increasing risk for low-back pain and injury. To assess hip flexion, have the client lie flat on his or her back. Hold the left leg down with your right hand to stabilize the pelvis, and use your left hand to passively raise the right leg to an angle of 80 to 85 degrees. Normal range of motion will allow for this amount of hip flexion (Figure 6.21). Tight hamstrings and other limitations to a normal range of motion are demonstrated when the client's leg raises to less than 80 degrees of hip flexion (Figure 6.22). All

ranges should be measured without pain in the back of the leg or bending at the knee.

To test for hip flexor length, have the client maintain a neutral spine while grasping behind the right knee and pulling

Table 6.17
Evaluation of Trunk Flexion

Flexion	Characteristics
Good	The trunk is able to move forward onto the thighs, and motion occurs at the hips and low back.
Fair	Bending forward causes some restriction in the low back so that bending occurs more in the lumbar spine.
Poor	Bending forward results in the lumbar spine remaining straight, and the bending occurs in the upper areas of the spine.

Source: Adapted from Krepton, D. & Chu, D. (1984).
Everybody's Aerobics Book. Oakland: Star Rover House.
Reprinted with permission.

**Flexibility Testing
and Evaluation**

FIGURE 6.20
Final position for trunk-extension assessment. Note where
the bending takes place.

FIGURE 6.21
Hamstrings flexibility
test: normal flexibility.

FIGURE 6.22
Hamstrings flexibility
test: tight flexibility.

the leg toward the chest. Normal length is demonstrated when the left leg stays flat to the floor (Figure 6.23). Shortened hip flexors are indicated when the left leg raises off the floor (Figure 6.24) and are often associated with low-back pain syndrome.

Shoulder Flexibility

Swimming and racquet and throwing sports all require flexibility in the shoulders for good performance and avoidance of injury. The test of shoulder flexibility measures the multirotational components of the shoulder joints. Test the left shoulder by having the client sit or stand with their right arm straight up, letting the elbow bend so the hand comes to rest, palm down, between the shoulder blades. The client should reach back with the left arm so the palm is up. Have the client attempt to touch hands (Figure 6.25). Evaluate shoulder flexibility using Table 6.19, and repeat the procedure for the opposite shoulder.

Poor shoulder flexibility also can affect a client's postural alignment. If the shoulder adductors are excessively tight, the client may assume a posture with shoulders depressed and rotated forward and the arms medially rotated, often called the "gorilla stance." To test for poor shoulder adductor flexibility, have the client lie on his or her back with knees bent, back flat, and arms overhead. Adequate flexibility is demonstrated if the arms lie flat overhead (Figure 6.26). If the arms do not lie flat (Figure 6.27), a shortness in the pectoralis major, teres major, and latissimus dorsi is indicated.

MUSCULAR STRENGTH AND ENDURANCE TESTING AND EVALUATION

Two components of muscular fitness testing are muscular strength and muscular endurance. Muscular strength is the greatest amount of force that muscles can produce in a single maximal effort. Muscular endurance refers to the muscle's ability to exert a submaximal force either repeatedly or statically over time. Adequate

muscular strength and endurance are necessary for both optimal health and athletic performance. They allow people to take part in activities of daily living without injury or undue fatigue and also enhance life at a desired level of human functioning. Strength and muscular endurance requirements for athletics vary significantly according to the requirements of each sport. Both are necessary for good performance in competitive and most recreational sports, and muscular strength training is even a subject of increased interest among distance runners.

One reason for performing fitness evaluations is to compare a client's physical ability to established standards of performance. A more useful application is to determine a client's appropriate exercise starting point

Table 6.18
Evaluation of Trunk Extension

Extension	Characteristics
Good	The hips remain in contact with the floor while the arms are fully extended.
Fair	The hips rise from the ground up to 2 inches.
Poor	The hips rise from the ground 2 inches or more.

Source: Adapted from Krepton, D. & Chu, D. (1984). *Everybody's Aerobics Book.* Oakland: Star Rover House. Reprinted with permission.

Table 6.19
Evaluation of Shoulder Flexibility

Flexibility	Characteristics
Good	The fingers can touch.
Fair	The fingertips are not touching but are less than 2 inches apart.
Poor	The fingertips are more than 2 inches apart.

Source: Adapted from Krepton, D. & Chu, D. (1984). *Everybody's Aerobics Book.* Oakland: Star Rover House. Reprinted with permission.

Muscular Strength and Endurance Testing and Evaluation

FIGURE 6.23
Test for hip flexor length: normal length.

FIGURE 6.24
Test for hip flexor length: shortened length.

FIGURE 6.25
Assessing flexibility of the left shoulder.

FIGURE 6.26
Test for shoulder flexibility: adequate flexibility.

FIGURE 6.27
Test for shoulder flexibility: muscle shortness.

and to show progressive personal improvement as a result of the training program. A basic premise of fitness assessment is to use similar exercise modes for testing and training. Although this should generally be the case, strength testing may offer occasional exceptions to the rule.

Isometric Strength Testing

Any strength test that involves movement will either underestimate or overestimate maximum force output. This is because internal muscle friction decreases effective force output during **concentric contractions,** and increases effective force output during **eccentric contractions.** To complicate matters further, faster movement speeds produce more internal muscle friction. Consequently, because **isometric** (static) strength testing entails muscle contraction without movement, it is the most accurate means for assessing actual muscle strength.

One disadvantage of isometric strength testing is that it tends to elicit a higher blood pressure response. It also requires testing at a variety of positions because effective muscle strength varies throughout the range of joint movement.

Isokinetic Strength Testing

Isokinetic strength testing measures effective muscle force output at every point in the movement range using a computer. However, for isokinetic strength comparisons to be valid, the tests must be performed with identical technique and movement speed. Even

then, the damping controls smooth out the actual force recording curves. While the data collected from isokinetic strength assessments may provide more information than isometric and isotonic testing, the necessary computer equipment is very expensive. Consequently, the accessibility of isokinetic strength evaluations may be a practical consideration.

Dynamic Strength Testing

Perhaps the most popular form of strength testing is dynamic (**isotonic**) assessments using free weights or weight-stack machines. Examples include the **one-repetition maximum (1 RM)** bench press, squat, overhead press, and dead-lift. Although these are reasonably good indicators of strength performance, it is not advisable to test beginners with maximum resistance lifts. Because most people can complete 10 repetitions with 75% of their maximum resistance, the 10-repetition-maximum (10 RM) test may be a safer means for evaluating muscle strength.

Because of momentum, isotonic strength tests must be conducted with strict form and slow movement speed. While not as comprehensive as isokinetic assessments, properly performed isotonic tests can provide valid strength comparisons at considerably less cost.

For meaningful strength assessments in men and women of different sizes, it is essential to make comparisons on a pound-for-pound basis. For this reason, it is best to use a ratio of weight lifted to body weight to accurately account for differences in body size and muscle mass.

Muscular Strength and Endurance Testing and Evaluation

Tables 6.20 through 6.23 give the one-repetition maximum ratios for men and women for one lower-body exercise, a leg press, and one upper-body exercise, the bench press. These tests were originally performed on Universal Gym® resistance-training equipment, so the data are really only valid for use on this brand of equipment. Since there are so many different brands of resistance-training equipment, one of the only options open to a personal trainer is to begin collecting data on each of your clients and determine your own percentiles based on age and gender. Undergraduate level physical education testing and evaluation texts explain how to do this basic statistical analysis (Heyward, 2002). You would need at least 30 clients of each gender to begin to have some statistical significance. As each age group reaches about 30 clients you can begin to divide the data into age ranges. You can give the results to your clients simply as per-

Table 6.20
Leg Strength (Men)

1 Repetition Maximum Leg Press
Leg Press Weight Ratio = Weight Pushed / Body Weight

				Age			
	%	<20	20–29	30–39	40–49	50–59	60+
Superior	95	2.82	2.40	2.20	2.02	1.90	1.80
Excellent	80	2.28	2.13	1.93	1.82	1.71	1.62
Good	60	2.04	1.97	1.77	1.68	1.58	1.49
Fair	40	1.90	1.83	1.65	1.57	1.46	1.38
Poor	20	1.70	1.63	1.52	1.44	1.32	1.25
Very Poor	5	1.46	1.42	1.34	1.27	1.15	1.08

Source: Adapted, with permission, from the *Physical Fitness Certification Manual*, The Cooper Institute, Dallas, Tex. (revised 2003).

Table 6.21
Leg Strength (Women)

1 Repetition Maximum Leg Press
Leg Press Weight Ratio = Weight Pushed / Body Weight

				Age			
	%	<20	20–29	30–39	40–49	50–59	60+
Superior	95	1.88	1.98	1.68	1.57	1.43	1.43
Excellent	80	1.71	1.68	1.47	1.37	1.25	1.18
Good	60	1.59	1.50	1.33	1.23	1.10	1.04
Fair	40	1.38	1.37	1.21	1.13	0.99	0.93
Poor	20	1.22	1.22	1.09	1.02	0.88	0.85
Very Poor	5	1.06	0.99	0.96	0.85	0.72	0.63

Source: Adapted, with permission, from the *Physical Fitness Certification Manual*, The Cooper Institute, Dallas, Tex. (revised 2003).

Table 6.22
Upper-body Strength (Men)

1 Repetition Maximum Bench Press
Bench Press Weight Ratio = Weight Pushed / Body Weight

				Age			
	%	<20	20–29	30–39	40–49	50–59	60+
Superior	95	1.76	1.63	1.35	1.20	1.05	0.94
Excellent	80	1.34	1.32	1.12	1.00	0.90	0.82
Good	60	1.19	1.14	0.98	0.88	0.79	0.72
Fair	40	1.06	0.99	0.88	0.80	0.71	0.66
Poor	20	0.89	0.88	0.78	0.72	0.63	0.57
Very Poor	5	0.76	0.72	0.65	0.59	0.53	0.49

Source: Adapted, with permission, from the *Physical Fitness Certification Manual*, The Cooper Institute, Dallas, Tex. (revised 2003).

Table 6.23
Upper-body Strength (Women)

1 Repetition Maximum Bench Press
Bench Press Weight Ratio = Weight Pushed / Body Weight

				Age			
	%	<20	20–29	30–39	40–49	50–59	60+
Superior	95	0.88	1.01	0.82	0.77	0.68	0.72
Excellent	80	0.77	0.80	0.70	0.62	0.55	0.54
Good	60	0.65	0.70	0.60	0.54	0.48	0.47
Fair	40	0.58	0.59	0.53	0.50	0.44	0.43
Poor	20	0.53	0.51	0.47	0.43	0.39	0.38
Very Poor	5	0.41	0.44	0.39	0.35	0.31	0.26

Source: Adapted, with permission, from the *Physical Fitness Certification Manual*, The Cooper Institute, Dallas, Tex. (revised 2003).

centiles, or you can add the descriptive "Excellent," "Good," "Fair," and "Poor" classifications. The challenge to adding the classifications is that your clients may not represent a cross-section of adults, and those in the lower categories may be unfairly labeled.

If you have access to Universal Gym® equipment you can use a 10 RM test to estimate a 1 RM weightload and determine a strength ratio using the following procedure:

1. Determine the heaviest weightload the client can perform for 10 good repetitions (10-repetition maximum weightload).

2. Convert the 10 RM weightload to a 1 RM estimation by dividing the weightload by 0.75.

3. Divide the 1 RM estimated weightload by the client's body weight to attain the strength ratio.

4. Compare the client's strength ratio to the strength fitness classifications in Tables 6.20 through 6.23.

For example, a 120-pound, 35-year-old woman who completes 10 leg presses with 120 pounds would have an estimated 1 RM of 160 pounds (120 pounds divided by 0.75). Her leg press weight ratio would be 1.33 (160 divided by 120), which places her in the "Good" category of strength fitness.

Muscular Endurance Testing

While the assessment of muscular strength can be independent of muscular endurance, the assessment of muscular endurance also measures strength to some degree. Careful consideration of client health and fitness should be made before specific muscular fitness tests are chosen. The lower-weight/high-repetition muscular endurance tests are more appropriate for less-fit clients and those with health-related exercise-strength goals, especially if they have previously been inactive. Two muscle-endurance tests that are both reliable and easy to administer are the push-up test and half sit-up test. Both measure relative muscular endurance, since their results are relative to body weight. Another

option is the bench-press test, a muscular-endurance test only. The weight used is standardized, so results do not vary as a function of body weight.

Push-up Test

The purpose of the push-up test is to evaluate muscular strength and endurance of the upper body, including the triceps, anterior deltoid, and pectoralis muscles. Men use the standard push-up position with only the hands and toes in contact with the floor (Figure 6.28a). Women use the modified push-up position (Figure 6.28b). Although the positions are different for each sex, the procedures for administering the test are similar.

Required items:

✔ Record sheet with name of the client and space for recording the number of push-ups completed

Before test day:

✔ Explain the purpose of the test to the client (to determine how many push-ups can be completed to reflect muscular strength and endurance).

✔ Review standard and bent-knee positions, making sure that the hands are shoulder-width apart.

✔ Review the test counting procedure. The push-up is complete when the chest touches the fist of a partner and returns to the start position with arms fully extended.

✔ Allow clients to practice if desired.

✔ Inform clients of proper breathing technique—to exhale with the effort (when pushing away from the floor).

Administration:

✔ Have the client assume the standard (for men) or bent-knee (for women) position while you take a position in front with your fist below the chest.*

✔ When ready, the client can begin. Count the total number of push-ups the client

* With clients with a history of shoulder problems, you may need to modify the test so that the lines formed between the elbows and shoulders do not go beyond parallel to the floor during the descent phase.

Muscular Strength and Endurance Testing and Evaluation

FIGURE 6.28
Push-up test.

a. Standard push-up position.

b. Modified bent-knee position.

Table 6.24
Push-up Norms for Men and Women by Age Groups Using Number Completed

| Age (Years) | (15–19) | | (20–29) | | (30–39) | | (40–49) | | (50–59) | | (60–69) | |
Gender	M	F	M	F	M	F	M	F	M	F	M	F
Excellent	>39	>33	>36	>30	>30	>27	>22	>24	>21	>21	>18	>17
Above average	29–38	25–32	29–35	21–29	22–29	20–26	17–21	15–23	13–20	11–20	11–17	12–16
Average	23–28	18–24	22–28	15–20	17–21	13–19	13–16	11–14	10–12	7–10	8–10	5–11
Below average	18–22	12–17	17–21	10–14	12–16	8–12	10–12	5–10	7–9	2–6	5–7	1–4
Poor	<17	<11	<16	<9	<11	<7	<9	<4	<6	<1	<4	<1

Source: *CSTF Operations Manual* (3rd ed.) Ottawa, Fitness and Amateur Sport, 1986.
The Canadian Standardized Test of Fitness was developed by, and is reproduced with the permission of, Fitness Canada, Government of Canada.

FIGURE 6.29
Half sit-up test.

a. Half sit-up test, down
   position. Head sup-
   port is optional.

b. Half sit-up test, up position.

completes before reaching the point of
exhaustion.

✔ Remind the client that rest is allowed in
the UP position only.

✔ The client's score is the total number of
push-ups performed.

You can classify your client's muscular
strength and endurance by comparing their
results to Table 6.24. For example, a 52-year-
old man who performs 18 push-ups is classified as "above average" for his age.

Half Sit-up Test

The purpose of the half sit-up test, which
was developed by the YMCA, is to evaluate
abdominal muscle strength and endurance.
Previously used sit-up tests have been unsatis-
factory because the hip flexor involvement
during sit-up motion is potentially harmful to
the low back. This is particularly true when
the feet are held motionless, since increased
stress is placed on the lumbar vertebrae. Even
though modifications to the traditional sit-up
have been instituted, including a bent-knee
position, stress to the low back is still present
during the motion. Consequently, the half sit-
up test was developed to eliminate potential
low-back problems and better assess abdominal muscle function. Additionally, the half sit-
up test remains inexpensive and easy to
administer, is valid and reliable, and affords
standards for comparing men and women of
similar ages.

The procedures for administering the half
sit-up test are as follows:

Required items:

✔ padded flooring or mat

✔ stopwatch or clock with a sweep second
hand

✔ recording sheet

✔ tape or self-adhesive Velcro

Before test day:

✔ Explain the purpose of the test to
each client (perform as many correct
crunches as possible within a one-
minute period).

✔ Review and demonstrate the half sit-up
test and allow the client to practice
if desired.

✔ Inform the client of proper
clothing requirements.

Administration:

✔ Place two strips of tape parallel to each
other and 3.5 inches (8.9 centimeters)
apart.

✔ Have the client warm-up before
taking the test.

✔ Have the client assume a supine position
with feet flat on the floor, shoulders
relaxed, and knees bent at about 90
degrees. He or she should place the
hands palms-down with fingertips touching the first strip of tape (Figure 6.29a).

✔ When ready, the client slowly curls the
upper spine until the fingertips touch
the second strip of tape (Figure 6.29b).

Table 6.25
Norms for Half Sit-up Test (Men)

Rating	% Rating	Age (years) 18–25	26–35	36–45	46–55	56–65	66+
Excellent	100	99	80	79	78	77	66
	95	83	68	65	68	63	55
	90	77	62	60	61	56	50
Good	85	72	58	57	57	53	44
	80	66	56	52	53	49	40
	75	61	53	48	52	48	38
Above average	70	57	52	45	51	46	35
	65	54	46	44	47	43	32
	60	52	44	43	44	41	31
Average	55	49	41	39	41	39	30
	50	46	38	36	39	36	27
	45	43	37	33	36	33	26
Below average	40	41	36	32	33	32	24
	35	40	34	31	32	31	23
	30	37	33	29	29	28	22
Poor	25	35	32	28	25	25	21
	20	33	30	25	24	24	19
	15	29	26	24	21	21	15
Very poor	10	27	21	21	16	20	12
	5	23	17	13	11	17	10
	0	14	7	6	6	5	5

Source: *YMCA Fitness Testing and Assessment Manual,* Copyright 2000. Reprinted and adapted with permission of the YMCA of the USA, 101 N. Wacker Drive, Chicago, IL 60606.

Table 6.26
Norms for Half Sit-up Test (Women)

Rating	% Rating	Age (years) 18–25	26–35	36–45	46–55	56–65	66+
Excellent	100	91	70	74	73	63	54
	95	76	60	60	57	55	41
	90	68	54	54	48	44	34
Good	85	64	50	48	44	42	33
	80	61	46	44	40	38	32
	75	58	44	42	37	35	31
Above average	70	57	41	38	36	32	29
	65	54	40	36	35	30	28
	60	51	37	35	33	27	26
Average	55	48	36	32	32	25	25
	50	44	34	31	31	24	22
	45	41	33	30	30	23	21
Below average	40	38	32	28	28	22	20
	35	37	30	24	27	20	18
	30	34	28	23	25	18	16
Poor	25	33	26	22	23	15	13
	20	32	24	20	21	12	11
	15	28	22	19	19	11	10
Very poor	10	25	20	16	13	8	9
	5	24	17	14	9	7	8
	0	11	7	4	2	1	0

Source: *YMCA Fitness Testing and Assessment Manual,* Copyright 2000. Reprinted and adapted with permission of the YMCA of the USA, 101 N. Wacker Drive, Chicago, IL 60606.

FIGURE 6.30
Bench press test.

a. Starting (down) position.

b. Completion of one repetition.

✔ The client then returns to the original position with the shoulders touching the mat.

✔ One half sit-up is counted each time the client's shoulders touch the mat.

✔ Count the number of repetitions completed in one minute.

Compare your client's results to Tables 6.25 and 6.26 to classify his or her abdominal muscle strength and endurance.

Bench-press Test

The bench-press test developed by the YMCA is a good method of testing the endurance and strength of the chest and shoulders. The main disadvantage of the test is that it uses a fixed weight, which places lighter clients at a disadvantage. The bench-press test should be administered as follows:

1. Use a 35-pound barbell for women or an 80-pound barbell for men. A spotter should be present during the test. If one spotter is unable to safely lift the weight, two spotters should be present.

2. Set a metronome to 60 bpm.

3. The spotter should hand the weight to the client in the down position with the elbows flexed and hands shoulder-width apart (Figure 6.30a).

4. A repetition is counted when the elbows are fully extended (Figure 6.30b). After each extension the bar should be lowered to touch the chest.

5. Up and down movements should be in time to the 60-bpm rhythm, which would be 30 lifts per minute.

6. The test is terminated when the client is unable to come to full extension or falls behind the 60-bpm rhythm.

Count the number of successful repetitions and use Tables 6.27 and 6.28 to compare the results to norms.

Follow-up

Table 6.27
Norms for Bench-press Test (Men)

Rating	% Rating	Age (years)					
		18–25	26–35	36–45	46–55	56–65	66+
Excellent	100	64	61	55	47	41	36
	95	49	48	41	33	28	22
	90	44	41	36	28	24	20
Good	85	41	37	32	25	21	16
	80	37	33	29	22	20	14
	75	34	30	26	21	17	12
Above average	70	33	29	25	20	14	10
	65	30	28	24	17	13	10
	60	29	26	22	16	12	10
Average	55	28	24	21	14	11	8
	50	26	22	20	13	10	8
	45	24	21	18	12	9	7
Below average	40	22	20	17	11	8	6
	35	21	19	16	10	6	5
	30	20	17	14	9	5	4
Poor	25	17	16	12	8	4	3
	20	16	13	10	6	3	2
	15	13	12	9	5	2	2
Very poor	10	10	9	6	2	1	1
	5	5	4	2	1	0	0
	0	0	0	0	0	0	0

Source: *YMCA Fitness Testing and Assessment Manual,* Copyright 2000. Reprinted and adapted with permission of the YMCA of the USA, 101 N. Wacker Drive, Chicago, IL 60606.

Table 6.28
Norms for Bench-press Test (Women)

Rating	% Rating	Age (years)					
		18–25	26–35	36–45	46–55	56–65	66+
Excellent	100	66	62	57	50	42	30
	95	49	46	41	33	29	22
	90	42	40	33	29	24	18
Good	85	38	34	30	24	21	16
	80	34	32	28	22	20	14
	75	30	29	26	20	17	12
Above average	70	28	28	24	18	14	10
	65	26	25	22	16	13	9
	60	25	24	21	14	12	8
Average	55	22	22	20	13	10	7
	50	21	21	17	12	9	6
	45	20	18	16	10	8	5
Below average	40	18	17	14	9	6	4
	35	17	16	13	8	5	3
	30	16	14	12	7	5	3
Poor	25	13	13	10	6	4	2
	20	12	12	8	5	3	1
	15	9	9	6	2	2	0
Very poor	10	6	6	4	1	1	0
	5	2	2	1	0	0	0
	0	0	0	0	0	0	0

Source: *YMCA Fitness Testing and Assessment Manual,* Copyright 2000. Reprinted and adapted with permission of the YMCA of the USA, 101 N. Wacker Drive, Chicago, IL 60606.

FOLLOW-UP

Consultation

When testing is completed, present the results to the client. Ideally, this consultation should take place in a private area with comfortable seating around a desk or table. The communication of test results is an art in and of itself. Try to get to know your clients so you can gauge how to effectively convey their results.

Testing

The frequency of follow-up testing will depend on the quality and quantity of exercise training and on the design of the testing and training packages offered by you or the fitness center. While many clients will begin to feel the positive effects of training in as little as one week, measurable changes will usually take about four weeks. Therefore, the first follow-up tests will usually be administered 4 to 12 weeks following the onset of training.

SUMMARY

The foundation of a well-designed fitness program is determined, in part, by the acquisition and analysis of baseline fitness information. This chapter provides you with a number of ways to test and evaluate a client's fitness level. You should assess the client's cardiorespiratory efficiency, body composition, flexibility, and muscular strength and endurance to design a quality fitness program. Most importantly, to evaluate the program's effectiveness over time, you should retest the client and measure how their results change.

Follow-up

References and Suggested Reading

REFERENCES

American College of Sports Medicine (2006). *ACSM's Guidelines for Exercise Testing and Prescription.* (7th ed.). Philadelphia: Lippincott Williams & Wilkins.

Astrand, P.O. & Rhyming, J. (1954). A nomogram for calculation of aerobic capacity (physical fitness) from pulse rate during submaximal work. *Journal of Applied Physiology,* 7, 218–221.

Golding, L.A., Meyers, C.R., & Sinning, W.E. (Eds.) (1986). *The Y's Way to Physical Fitness.* (3rd ed.). Champaign, Ill.: Human Kinetics.

Heyward, V.H. (2002). *Advanced Fitness Assessment & Exercise Prescription.* (4th ed.). Champaign, Ill.: Human Kinetics.

Jackson, A.S. & Pollock, M.L. (1985). Practical assessment of body composition. *The Physician and Sportsmedicine,* May, 76–90.

Lohman, T.G., Roche, A.F., & Martorell, R. (Eds.) (1988). *Anthropometric Standardization Reference Manual.* Champaign, Ill.: Human Kinetics.

McArdle, W.D. et al. (1972). Reliability and interrelationships between maximal oxygen intake, physical working capacity and step-test scores in college women. *Medicine and Science in Sports and Exercise,* 4, 182–186.

National Heart, Lung, and Blood Institute (1998). Clinical guidelines on the identification, evaluation, and treatment of overweight and obesity in adults: The evidence report. *Obesity Research,* 6 (Suppl. 2), 51S–209S.

Sjostrand, T. (1947). Changes in the respiratory organs of workmen at an ore melting works. *Acta Medica Scandinavia,* 128 (suppl. 196), 687–699.

Tran, Z. & Weltman, A. (1989). Generalized equation for predicting body density of women from girth measurements. *Medicine and Science in Sports and Exercise,* 21, 101–104.

Tran, Z., Weltman, A., & Seip, R. (1988). Predicting body composition of men from girth measurements. *Human Biology,* 8, 60, 167–176.

SUGGESTED READING

American College of Sports Medicine (2001). *Resource Manual for Guidelines for Exercise Testing and Prescription.* (4th ed.). Philadelphia: Lippincott Williams & Williams.

Baumgartner, T.A. & Jackson, A.S. (2000). *Measurement for Evaluation.* (6th ed.). Madison: WCB/McGraw-Hill.

Borg, G. (1998). *Borg's Perceived Exertion and Pain. Scales.* Champaign, Ill.: Human Kinetics.

Flood, D.K. (1996). *Practical Math for Health Fitness Professionals.* Champaign, Ill.: Human Kinetics.

Hassard, T.H. (1991). *Understanding Biostatistics.* St. Louis, Mo.: Mosby.

Howley, E. & Franks, D. (2007). *Health Fitness Instructor's Handbook.* (5th ed.). Philadelphia: Lea & Febiger.

MacDougall, J.D., Wenger, H.A., & Green, H.J. (Eds.) (1991). *Physiological Testing of the High-Performance Athlete.* (2nd ed.). Champaign, Ill.: Human Kinetics.

Morrow, J.R. et al. (2000). *Measurement and Evaluation in Human Performance.* (2nd ed.). Champaign, Ill.: Human Kinetics.

Nieman, D.C. (1990). *Fitness and Sports Medicine, An Introduction.* Palo Alto, Calif.: Bull Publishing.

Ross, R. M. & Jackson, A.S. (1990). *Exercise Concepts Calculations & Computer Applications.* Carmel, Ind.: Benchmark.

PART III

Principles
and Methods
of Training

Cardiorespiratory Fitness and Exercise

*Ralph La Forge, M.S., is a
physiologist and managing
director of the Duke Lipid and
Metabolic Disorder Training
Program, Duke University
Medical Center, Endocrine
Division,*

Ralph La Forge

*Durham, N.C.
He has worked
for 25 years in
clinical cardiology/endocrinology
and as an instructor of exercise
physiology at the University
of California, San Diego.
La Forge has authored more than
300 consumer and professional
publications on cardiovascular
disease management, applied
exercise science, and preventive
cardiology and is the exercise
science research editor for IDEA
Health & Fitness Source. He
has helped organize and
inaugurate cardiovascular
disease risk reduction and
preventive endocrinology
programs for more than 450
healthcare institutions and
medical groups throughout the
United States, including the
Department of Defense.*

Cardiorespiratory fitness is an essential component of physical fitness and has grown to receive equal acclaim for improving cardiovascular health in both primary and secondary prevention. For health and fitness applications, the terms cardiorespiratory fitness, cardiovascular fitness, and aerobic endurance fitness are synonymous. Cardiorespiratory fitness best describes the health and function of the heart, lungs, and circulatory system and is related to cardiorespiratory endurance, which is the ability to persist or sustain activity for prolonged periods. Cardiorespiratory fitness also describes the capacity of the lungs to exchange oxygen and carbon dioxide with the blood and the circulatory system's ability to transport blood and nutrients to metabolically active tissues for sustained periods without undue fatigue.

Benefits of

Cardiorespiratory

Fitness

BENEFITS OF CARDIORESPIRATORY FITNESS

The numerous benefits of cardiorespiratory fitness (Table 7.1) are related to a variety of adaptive physiologic responses to aerobic exercise. Physiologic responses to training—such as an increase in body-fat utilization, a decrease in **peripheral vascular resistance,** and an increase in **maximal oxygen consumption**—help decrease the risk of cardiovascular disease and diabetes by favorably modifying **risk factors** like **obesity, hypertension,** insulin resistance, and elevated **triglycerides** and **LDL cholesterol.** When such risk factors are removed from clients' health profiles, the clients can attain an acceptable level of cardiovascular health. Cardiovascular health goes beyond merely attaining aerobic fitness. It defines the status of the heart muscle, its blood vessels, and the circulatory system it serves. Acquiring and maintaining cardiorespiratory fitness is one of the primary pathways to cardiovascular health.

Likewise, aerobic endurance activities have been effective in other conditioning and clinical therapies, such as cardiac and pulmonary rehabilitation, sleep disorder treatment, diabetic treatment, prenatal/post-partum and renal dialysis conditioning, and anxiety- and depression-management programs. In clinical settings, aerobic exercise must be prescribed and managed carefully by trained exercise specialists or other qualified clinicians. Experienced and qualified personal trainers may form adjunct relationships with clinicians to effectively manage the patient. Referrals from such programs depend on your relationship and knowledge of local clinical rehabilitation programs and/or affiliated healthcare institutions.

Cardiorespiratory fitness also serves as a foundation for other fitness programs. The conditioning and health of the heart, lungs, and blood vessels are prime ingredients in the safety and performance of nearly all sports and recreational programs. Activities such as tennis, golf, skiing, dancing, skating, basketball, volleyball, boxing, and nearly all muscular strength-training programs will benefit from attaining acceptable levels of cardiorespiratory fitness. Clients with adequate cardiorespiratory fitness generally have more stamina, which translates to less fatigue and fewer risks for certain types of injuries.

Table 7.1
Reported Benefits of Cardiorespiratory Exercise Training

Health benefits

Reduction in blood pressure

Increased HDL cholesterol

Decreased total cholesterol

Decreased body fat stores

Increased aerobic work capacity

Decreased clinical symptoms of anxiety, tension, and depression

Reduction in glucose-stimulated insulin secretion

Increased heart function

Reduction in mortality in postmyocardial infarction patients

Prevention of type 2 diabetes

Adaptive physiologic responses

Increased lactate threshold

Decreased resting heart rate

Increased heart volume

Increased resting and maximum stroke volume

Increased maximum cardiac output

Increased maximum oxygen consumption

Increased capillary density and blood flow to active muscles

Increased total blood volume

Increased maximal ventilation

Increased lung diffusion capacity

Increased mobilization and utilization of fat

Reduced all-cause mortality

Decreased anxiety and depression

Decreased incidence of some cancers

Improved arterial endothelial function

Increased insulin sensitivity

Source: Modified from American College of Sports Medicine (2000). *Guidelines for Exercise Testing and Prescription* (6th ed.). Philadelphia: Lippincott Williams & Wilkins

COMPONENTS OF AN AEROBIC EXERCISE PROGRAM

It is imperative for you to understand the physiologic rationale and application of each component of the cardiorespiratory exercise program.

The essential components of the written plan are

1. Warm-up and cool-down
2. Primary cardiorespiratory activity criteria:
    a. Mode of exercise
    b. Frequency of exercise session
    c. Duration of exercise session
    d. Intensity of exercise session
3. Supportive conditioning exercise (e.g., strength and flexibility)
4. Progression plan
5. Safety and cautions

Each of these components must be discussed with the client and presented in a legible and succinct written form. Chapters 11 and 12 provide examples of formats to use in various situations.

Warm-up and Cool-down

Although most fitness professionals teach a variety of warm-up and cool-down techniques, few fully understand their physiological and psychological rationales (Table 7.2). Graduated low-level aerobic exercise is essential for maximizing safety and economy of movement during the cardiorespiratory conditioning phase of an exercise session. The warm-up should gradually increase the heart rate, blood pressure, oxygen consumption, dilation of the blood vessels, elasticity of the active muscles, and the heat produced by the active muscle groups. The warm-up should consist of two distinct components:

1. Graduated aerobic warm-up activity (e.g., walking or slow-tempo rhythmic calisthenic movements)

2. Flexibility exercise specific to the biomechanical nature of the primary conditioning activity (e.g., calf, quadriceps, and Achilles stretching prior to running or hiking).

Table 7.2
Physiological and Psychological Rationale for Warm-up and Cool-down

Warm-up

1. Permits a gradual metabolic adaptation (e.g., oxygen consumption), which enhances cardiorespiratory performance (e.g., a higher maximum cardiac output and oxygen uptake)

2. Prevents the premature onset of blood lactic acid accumulation and fatigue during higher level aerobic exercise

3. Causes a gradual increase in muscle temperature, which decreases the work of contraction and reduces the likelihood of muscle injury

4. Facilitates neural transmission for motor unit recruitment

5. Improves coronary blood flow in early stages of the conditioning exercise, lessening the potential for myocardial ischemia

6. Allows a gradual redistribution of blood flow to active muscles

7. Increases the elasticity of connective tissue and other muscle components

8. Provides a screening mechanism for potential musculoskeletal or metabolic problems that may increase at higher intensities

9. Provides a psychological warm-up to higher levels of work (i.e., increases arousal and focus on exercise)

Cool-down

1. Prevents postexercise venous blood pooling and too rapid a drop in blood pressure, thereby reducing the likelihood of postexercise lightheadedness or fainting

2. Reduces the immediate postexercise tendency for muscle spasm or cramping

3. Reduces the concentration of exercise hormones (e.g., norepinephrine) that are at relatively high levels immediately after vigorous aerobic exercise. This reduction will lower the probability of postexercise disturbances in cardiac rhythm

Source: Adapted from: McArdle, W., Katch, F., & Katch, V. (2001). *Exercise Physiology: Energy, Nutrition, and Human Performance* (5th ed.). Philadelphia: Lippincott Williams & Wilkins.

Components of an Aerobic Exercise Program

Components of an Aerobic Exercise Program

Because a warm muscle is more easily stretched than a cold muscle, the flexibility component should be preceded by five to eight minutes of low-level aerobic activity using the same muscle groups. For instance, a 10-minute walk will increase muscle temperature and circulation of the legs, thereby promoting easier and safer stretching of the same muscle groups.

Table 7.3 lists sample warm-up and cool-down activities for a variety of aerobic exercises. The intensity of the warm-up should be well below that of the primary conditioning activity. The warm-up duration depends on the level and intensity of the primary conditioning activity, as well as the fitness level of the client.

The cool-down is an integral part of the exercise program. The purpose of the cool-down is to slowly decrease the heart rate and overall metabolism, both of which have been elevated during the conditioning phase. Low-level aerobic exercise, similar to that of the conditioning exercise, is recommended (see Table 7.3). Walking, slow jogging, cycling with little or no resistance, and slow aquatic activity or swimming are good examples. Cool-down helps prevent the sudden pooling of blood in the veins and ensures adequate circulation to the skeletal muscles, heart, and brain. Cool-down may

Table 7.3
Sample Warm-up and Cool-down Activities (including Stretching Exercise)

Primary Conditioning Exercise	Warm-up/Cool-down Activity
Aerobics (group exercise)	Graduated low-level aerobic activity utilizing same muscle groups
Circuit weight training	Low-level aerobic activity (e.g., walking or cycling, and/or beginning the circuit training session with a set of relatively high-repetition, low-resistance exercises)
Hiking	Graduate from relatively flat terrain at minimal altitudes to steeper terrain and higher altitudes
Jogging and running	Walking, walk-jogging, or jogging at a slower pace
Outdoor cycling	Begin with relatively flat terrain in lower gears; gradually shift to higher gears and steeper terrain
Racquetball, handball, or squash	Walk-jog and/or graduated tempo volleying
Rope skipping	Graduated walking or walk-jogging pace and/or slow tempo rope-skipping pace
Sprinting	Jogging and graduated pace in running intervals
Stationary cycling	Start with cycling against little or no resistance at $\frac{2}{3}$ of the pedal crank rpm used in the conditioning phase
Stationary exercise devices	Begin with 50 to 60% of intended conditioning workload or speed; the duration of submaximal graduated warm-up should be proportional to the peak intensity of the conditioning work load
Stepping/standing exercise (e.g., stair climber, elliptical crosstrainer)	Low-level aerobic activity (e.g., walking or cycling and/or relatively low-tempo step exercise)
Swimming	Begin with slow crawl and gradually increase arm stroke and pace, and/or begin with short one- or two-lap slow intervals
Tennis (competitive)	Walk-jog and/or graduated tempo volleying proportional to the level of the game

aid in preventing delayed muscle stiffness and reduces any tendency toward post-exercise fainting and dizziness. For high cardiovascular risk clients, a gradual decrease in the intensity of exercise is crucial. Sudden cessation of exercise without cool-down may adversely affect cardiac function because a relatively high concentration of adrenaline remains in the blood from the conditioning exercise. Sudden exercise cessation also may adversely affect filling pressures of the heart, putting a weak heart at risk. The length of the cool-down phase is proportional to the intensity and length of the conditioning phase. A typical 30- to 40-minute conditioning phase at 70% of maximum heart rate would warrant a 5- to 10-minute cool-down. The aerobic component of the cool-down phase should be followed by several minutes of stretching those muscle groups active in the conditioning phase.

Primary Cardiorespiratory Exercise Criteria

For maximum effectiveness and safety, the cardiorespiratory exercise program must include specific instructions on the mode, frequency, duration, and intensity of exercise. Most of these criteria originate from the American College of Sports Medicine (ACSM) exercise guidelines and position statements to ensure standardization and validity in the broad field of exercise science (American College of Sports Medicine, 2000).

To avoid confusion, the exercise criteria listed in this section are those needed for measurable improvements in cardiorespiratory fitness (e.g., increase in **$\dot{V}O_2max$**). This is an important clarification because the exercise threshold criteria for health enhancement are generally lower (American College of Sports Medicine, 2000; Haskell, 1994). For instance, the minimum duration, intensity and frequency of physical activity required for health enhancement is the accumulation of 30 minutes of moderate-intensity (40–59% $\dot{V}O_2R$) activity on most days. Here, health enhancement refers to reduced risk of

degenerative disease, such as cardiovascular disease and diabetes.

Exercise Mode. Selection of the exercise mode is made on the basis of the client's **functional capacity,** interests, time availability, equipment and facilities, and personal goals. Any activity that uses large muscle groups, is rhythmical and cardiorespiratory in nature, and is maintained continuously can be used. The American College of Sports Medicine classifies **cardiorespiratory endurance** activities into three groups:

GROUP 1: Physical activities in which exercise intensity is easily maintained at a constant level, and interindividual variation in energy expenditure is relatively low. Examples are walking and cycling, especially treadmill and cycle ergometry.

GROUP 2: Physical activities in which energy expenditure is related to skill, but for a given individual can provide a constant intensity: aerobic dance, aerobic step exercise, slide exercise, swimming, skating, and cross-country skiing.

GROUP 3: Physical activities that are quite variable in both skill and intensity: soccer, basketball, and racquet sports.

Group 1 activities are recommended when precise control of the exercise intensity is necessary, as in the beginning stages of a conditioning program. These activities can be performed in a continuous or discontinuous (interval) format, depending upon the client's fitness level and personal preference, and are useful during all stages of conditioning. Group 2 activities are useful because of the enjoyment provided by group exercise and settings other than an exercise gym. Adding Group 2 exercise to a training program helps foster compliance and reduce boredom. Because of the skill and variable intensity nature of Group 3 activities, they require a base level of conditioning using Group 1 activities. Group 3 activities tend to be group- or team-sport oriented and, therefore, provide greater interest and compliance for many individuals. Group 3 activities should be cautiously

> **Components of an Aerobic Exercise Program**

considered for high-risk, deconditioned, or symptomatic individuals.

Exercise Frequency. Frequency refers to the number of exercise sessions per week included in the program. The frequency of exercise depends on the duration and intensity of the exercise session. Lower-intensity exercise performed for shorter periods can warrant more sessions per week. To improve both cardiorespiratory fitness and maintain body fat at near-optimum levels, a client should exercise at least three days per week with no more than two days between sessions. The American College of Sports Medicine recommends three to five days per week for most aerobic programs. When a client starts an aerobic exercise program, exercising every other day for at least the first eight weeks is appropriate. For those with a poor functional capacity, one to two daily sessions may be recommended. Those with an average functional capacity should exercise at least three times per week on alternate days. In general, clients who are just beginning weightbearing exercise, such as traditional aerobics, step training, and jogging, should have at least 36 to 48 hours of rest between workouts to prevent **overuse injuries** and promote adequate bone/joint stress recovery. This is especially true with those who are overweight.

Exercise Duration. Duration refers to the number of minutes of exercise during the conditioning period. The conditioning period, exclusive of the warm-up and cooldown, may vary from as little as 5 to 60 or more minutes. The duration required for cardiorespiratory benefits is dependent upon the exercise intensity. Take a given intensity of exercise, for example 75% of functional capacity, and compare it to an exercise duration of 5 minutes versus 20 minutes at this intensity. Obviously, more total energy is expended during the 20-minute exercise session.

The conditioning response to an exercise session is the result of the product of the intensity and duration of exercise (total energy expenditure). Beginners who are in the lower cardiorespiratory fitness classifications should begin with 10 to 20 minutes of aerobic conditioning. Very deconditioned individuals may be more suited for multiple sessions of short duration, such as 5 to 10 minutes. Those in the average classification should go for 15 to 45 minutes, and those in the high fitness classification can go for 30 to 60 minutes.

Intensity of Exercise. Intensity refers to the speed or exercise workload. The American College of Sports Medicine (2006) recommends an intensity range of 55/65% to 90% of **maximum heart rate,** or between 40/50% and 85% of **heart-rate reserve** or **oxygen uptake reserve ($\dot{V}O_2R$).** The $\dot{V}O_2R$ is the difference between $\dot{V}O_2max$ and resting $\dot{V}O_2$. It is important to see that the 55 to 90% of maximum heart-rate range approximates 40 to 85% of what was formerly referred to as $\dot{V}O_2max$ but now is oxygen uptake reserve ($\dot{V}O_2R$). It is important for you to understand that for any given percentage of maximum oxygen uptake, except for maximum exercise intensities, the percentage of maximum heart rate will be somewhat higher (Table 7.4).

From a physiologic point of view, this 50 to 85% of maximum oxygen uptake range is the goal for cardiorespiratory training benefits. Lower intensities, such as 50 to 60% of maximal oxygen consumption and **heart-rate maximum reserve,** are advised for beginners in the lower cardiorespiratory fitness levels. Persons with very low fitness levels, however, can benefit from training intensities as low as 40 to 50% of maximal oxygen uptake. Exercise intensities as high as 75 to 85% of maximal oxygen uptake and heart-rate reserve may be more appropriate for those who are apparently healthy and in the higher fitness classifications. Overall, the average exercise intensity for apparently healthy adults is usually between 60 and 70% of their maximum oxygen uptake.

Table 7.4 classifies and compares age-related relative exercise intensity (% of $\dot{V}O_2max$ or heart-rate max) to absolute exercise intensity (actual or estimated MET cost). This classification system is important for the personal trainer to learn because it establishes a common exercise intensity language with other trainers and healthcare professionals.

Exercise Intensity and Health-related Outcomes. Years of research on exercise and health has made it clear that such health-related outcomes as increased HDL cholesterol, decreased blood pressure, improved glucose tolerance, reduced blood clotting tendency (fibrinolysis), reduced anxiety, and decreased risk of cardiovascular disease, diabetes, and all-cause mortality can result from moderate intensities of exercise (i.e., 40 to 60% of maximum oxygen uptake). In some cases, even lower intensities are recommended (Blair et al., 1995). Employing exercise intensities as low as 30% of $\dot{V}O_2$max, the diabetes prevention program (DPP) demonstrated a 58% reduction in type 2 diabetes in glucose intolerant obese individuals (Diabetes Prevention Program Research Group, 2002). The volume of exercise attained in this three-year study was just 700–900 kcal/week.

Monitoring Exercise Intensity

Of the numerous methods for monitoring exercise intensity, five have been somewhat standardized and are recommended for the personal trainer. The method you choose will depend on your client's exercise program and level of fitness, your access to exercise test data (e.g., treadmill stress test heart rates, work loads, functional capacity), and your experience. The following are the primary methods of monitoring exercise intensity:

1. Heart Rate
   a. Percentage of maximal heart rate
   b. Percentage of heart-rate reserve
2. Rating of perceived exertion
3. The "talk test" method
4. METs

Percentage of Maximal Heart Rate. This method of monitoring intensity of exercise calculates the exercise heart rate as a percentage of maximal heart rate. Maximal heart rate can be determined by a maximal functional capacity test, using a bicycle or treadmill ergometer, or by age-predicted maximal heart-rate tables, which frequently use the 220-minus-age formula. If this method of estimating maximal heart rate is used, the following formula applies:

Training Heart Rate
= maximal measured or predicted heart rate
x 55/65% to 90%
(desired percent of maximal HR)

Table 7.4
Classification of Physical Activity Intensity

Intensity	Relative Intensity			Absolute Intensity in Healthy Adults, METs* Age			
	O_2 max§, %	Maximum Heart Rate§, %	RPE†	(20–39)	(40–64)	(65–79)	(80+)
Very light	<20	<50	<10	<2.4	<2.0	<1.6	<1.0
Light	20–39	50–63	10–11	2.4–4.7	2.0–3.9	1.6–3.1	1.1–1.9
Moderate	40–59	64–76	12–13	4.8–7.1	4.0–5.9	3.2–4.7	2.0–2.9
Hard	60–84	77–93	14–16	7.2–10.1	6.0–8.4	4.8–6.7	3.0–4.25
Very hard	≥85	≥94	17–19	≥10.2	≥8.5	≥6.8	≥4.25
Maximum	100	100	20	12.0‡	10.0‡	8.0‡	5.0‡

*Based on 8 to 12 repetitions for persons <50–60 years old and 10 to 15 repetitions for persons >50–60 years
†Borg rating of Relative Perceived Exertion (RPE), 6–20 scale.
‡Maximum values are mean values achieved during maximum exercise by healthy adults. Absolute intensity values are approximate mean values for men. Mean values for women are 1 to 2 METs lower than those for men.
Adapted from: American Heart Association's Exercise Standards for Testing and Training (2001). *Circulation,* 104, 1694.
§ACSM Guidelines

ACSM's Guidelines for Exercise Testing and Prescription, 7th ed.

Components of an Aerobic Exercise Program

For example:
A 40-year-old man for whom an intensity of 70% of maximal heart rate is desired:
220 – 40 = 180 (predicted max HR)

180 (predicted max HR)
x 0.70 (70% exercise intensity)
126 (exercise HR)

You should use caution when using age-group average maximal heart-rate tables because these tables only estimate a "rule of thumb" maximal heart rate, usually from the "220-minus-age" formula. This method has a variability of plus or minus 10 to 12 beats per minute (Durstine & Pate, 1993). In addition, women generally have a higher heart-rate response than men to the same absolute work output. Research has also demonstrated that older

individuals (older than age 65) may have significantly higher maximal heart rates than predicted by the 220-minus-age formula (Whaley et al., 1992).

It is essential for you to understand the relationship between exercise heart rate and aerobic capacity (maximal oxygen consumption). An important point is often overlooked in aerobic exercise: For nearly all levels of submaximal exercise, the percentage of heart-rate maximum does not equal the same percentage of aerobic capacity unless the heart-rate maximum reserve method **(Karvonen formula)** is used. As described in Table 7.4, for any given percentage of maximal heart rate, the corresponding percentage of maximal oxygen consumption (aerobic capacity) is 5 to 10% less.

Percentage of Heart-rate Reserve (Karvonen Formula). The heart-rate reserve method is similar to the percentage of maximal heart-rate method, except resting heart rate is factored in:

Training Heart Rate
= maximum heart rate
  – resting heart rate
  x desired intensity (40/50% to 85%)
  + resting heart rate

For example: What is the target heart rate for a 40-year-old client with a resting heart rate of 80 bpm at an intensity of 70%?
THR = (maximum HR – RHR)
      x intensity + RHR

220 – 40 = 180 (predicted maximum HR)

180 (predicted maximum HR)
– 80 (RHR)
100 (heart-rate reserve)
x 0.70 (70% intensity)
70
+ 80 (RHR)
150 (target HR at 70% of heart-rate reserve)

Note that this exercise heart rate of 150 bpm is 24 bpm higher than the straight per-

---

Maximum Heart Rate: How Useful Is The Prediction Equation?

Two methods exist for determining maximum heart rate (MHR). The most accurate way is to directly measure the MHR with an EKG monitoring device during a graded exercise test. The other way is to estimate MHR by using a simple prediction equation or formula. In 1970, the formula "220 – age" was introduced and was widely accepted by the health and fitness community. Recently, however, the validity of the formula has come under attack for several reasons. The subjects used in the study to determine the formula were not representative of the general population. In addition, even if the prediction equation did represent a reasonable average, a significant percentage of individuals will not fit the average. In fact, standard deviations of plus or minus 10 to 20 beats per minute have been observed. Consequently, basing a client's exercise intensity (i.e., training heart rate) on a potentially flawed estimation of MHR is somewhat dubious. When the training heart rate is based on an estimated MHR, it should be used in combination with the perceived exertion scale (see Table 7.5). Modify the intensity of the workout if your client reports a high level of perceived exertion, even if his or her training heart rate has not been achieved.

centage of maximum heart-rate method illustrated previously. Therefore, you must be careful when recommending exercise intensity using only the heart-rate reserve (Karvonen) method.

The physiological basis for the heart-rate reserve method is that the difference between resting and maximal heart rates for a given client represents the reserve of the heart for increasing cardiac output. Like the percentage of maximal heart-rate method, the accuracy of the Karvonen formula is somewhat compromised when the predicted maximal heart rate is estimated from tables or 220-minus-age rather than determined from an actual functional capacity test. Still, this method is one of the most popular for determining exercise heart rates.

Rating of Perceived Exertion. Exercise intensity also can be measured by assigning a numerical value (6 to 20 or 0 to 10) to subjective feelings of exercise exertion. The popular name for this method is the **ratings of perceived exertion (RPE).** Originally designed by Dr. Gunnar Borg, it is sometimes called the Borg Scale. RPE takes into account all that the exercising client is perceiving in terms of exercise fatigue, including psychological, musculoskeletal, and environmental factors. The RPE response also correlates very well with cardiorespiratory and metabolic factors such as heart rate, breathing rate, oxygen consumption, and overall fatigue. This level of perceived physical effort is assigned a rating from either of the two rating scales in Table 7.5. For instance, using the Borg Scale, an RPE of 12 to 13 corresponds to approximately 55 to 69% of maximal heart rate, or 50 to 74% of maximal oxygen consumption or heart rate reserve (see Table 7.4). An RPE of 17 would correspond to about 90% of maximal heart rate or 85% of maximal oxygen consumption or heart-rate reserve. Thus, as a rule, most clients would exercise between 12 and 16 on the Borg Scale. The Borg Scale begins at 6 because originally it was used to approximate exercise heart rate. For example, an RPE of 6 would approximate a heart

rate of 60; an RPE of 15 would approximate a heart rate of 150.

In recent years, a revised Borg Scale (see the Category Ratio Scale in Table 7.5) has made it easier to use because of its simpler 0 to 10 rating. On this revised RPE Scale, a client should exercise between an RPE of 4 (somewhat strong) and an RPE of 5 or 6 (strong) (Carlton & Rhodes, 1985). Perhaps the most appropriate use of RPE is as an adjunct to heart-rate monitoring. Ideally, the trainer or exercising client will monitor and record both intensities to ensure close observation of the cardiac and physiological exercise response.

Dishman and colleagues believe that the standard scales can be prone to error, and have been researching an alternative approach known as "preferred exertion" (Dishman, Farquhar, & Cureton, 1994). In this method, the exercisers self-select exercise intensity (e.g., power output on a stationary cycle) according to their own volition, as long as the selected intensity is within an effective exercise intensity range.

Components of an Aerobic Exercise Program

Table 7.5
Ratings of Perceived Exertion

RPE	Category Ratio Scale	
6	0	Nothing at all
7 Very, very light	0.5	Very, very weak
8	1	Very weak
9 Very light	2	Weak
10	3	Moderate
11 Fairly light	4	Somewhat strong
12	5	Strong
13 Somewhat hard	6	
14	7	Very strong
15 Hard	8	
16	9	
17 Very hard	10	Very, very strong
18	*	Maximal
19 Very, very hard		
20		

Source: Adapted, with permission, from American College of Sports Medicine (2000) *Guidelines for Exercise Testing and Prescription* (6th ed.). Philadelphia: Lippincott Williams & Wilkins

It has been suggested that complementary use of "preferred intensities" may be safer and may better promote long-term exercise adherence than a strict exercise program based on more precise physiological criteria, especially if those criteria conflict with a person's intensity preference.

The Talk-test Method. Another means of evaluating the intensity of exercise is the talk test. Like the RPE method, the talk test is subjective, but it is quite useful in determining a "comfort zone" of aerobic intensity. Clients should be able to breathe comfortably and rhythmically throughout all phases of a workout to ensure a safe and comfortable level of exercise, especially for those just beginning an exercise program. Those who progress to higher functional capacities and higher-level workouts may find this technique somewhat conservative, especially at intensities greater than 80% of functional capacity.

In summary, you can modify criteria such as the mode, frequency, duration, and intensity of exercise to suit the client's level of fitness, program goals, and schedule. As a rule, however, building a foundation of endurance at a relatively low-to-moderate intensity prior to performing higher-intensity workouts or competition is clearly justified for safety and comfort. This may mean moving the client, for the first few weeks, through gradual increases in duration, while holding intensity nearly constant until an acceptable level of endurance, such as 20 to 30 minutes, has been achieved. Within each of these criteria, you have an enormous range of choices, such as variations in modes and intensities, with which to vary the exercise stimulus and maximize the client's interest and adaptation to increasing levels of exercise.

Intensity Measured by METs. Exercise intensity can be assessed by a graded exercise test (bicycle or treadmill) (Table 7.6). Based on the time the client stays on the treadmill or bicycle ergometer, the maximal oxygen consumption (i.e., aerobic or functional capacity) can be estimated and converted to a **MET** equivalent. A MET is a multiple of resting oxygen consumption. One MET equals a person's oxygen uptake at rest, which is equal to approximately 3.5 milliliters of oxygen per kilogram of body weight per minute (3.5 mL/kg/min). The intensity of exercise may be determined as a specified percentage of the client's maximal oxygen consumption or functional capacity (e.g., 50 to 85%), and then choosing activities that are known to require energy expenditure at the desired level (Table 7.7). For example, if a client has a functional capacity of 10 METs and you recommend he or she begins at 60% of functional capacity, then 60% times 10 METs equals 6 METs beginning intensity.

Table 7.6
Training Method Selection

Cardiorespiratory Fitness Level	Aerobic Capacity (METs)	Training Method
Poor	1–3.9	Low-level (2–3 METs) aerobic interval training
Low	4–6.9	Aerobic interval training at 3–5 METs
Average	7–10.9	Aerobic interval training at 6–8 METs; continuous training at 5–8 METs
Good	11–13.9	Aerobic interval training at 9–12 METs; continuous training at 8–12 METs; aerobic composite training at 8–12 METs; moderate anaerobic interval training
High	14+	Aerobic interval training at 10–13+ METs; continuous training at 9–13+ METs; aerobic composite training at 9–13+ METs; anaerobic or Fartlek training

Table 7.7
Leisure Activities in METs: Sports, Exercise Classes, Games, Dancing

	Mean	Range		Mean	Range
Archery	3.9	3–4	Horseshoe pitching	—	2–3
Backpacking	—	5–11	Hunting (bow or gun)		
Badminton	5.8	4–9+	Small game (walking, carrying light load)	—	3–7
Basketball			Big game (dragging carcass, walking)	—	3–14
Game play	8.3	7–12+	Judo	13.5	—
Nongame play	—	3–9	Mountain climbing	—	5–10+
Billiards	2.5	—	Music playing	—	2–3
Bowling	—	2–4	Paddleball, racquetball	9	8–12
Boxing			Rope jumping	11	—
In-ring	13.3	—	60–80 skips/min	9	—
Sparring	8.3	—	120–140 skips/min	—	11–12
Canoeing, rowing, and kayaking	—	3–8	Running		
Conditioning exercise	—	3–8+	12 min per mile	8.7	—
Climbing hills	7.2	5–10+	11 min per mile	9.4	—
Cricket	5.2	4–8	10 min per mile	10.2	—
Croquet	3.5	—	9 min per mile	11.2	—
Cycling			8 min per mile	12.5	—
Pleasure or to work	—	3–8+	7 min per mile	14.1	—
10 mph	7.0	—	6 min per mile	16.3	—
Dancing (social, square, tap)	—	3–8	Sailing	—	2–5
Dancing (aerobic)	—	6–9	Scuba diving	—	5–10
Fencing	—	6–10+	Shuffleboard	—	2–3
Field Hockey	8.0	—	Skating, ice and roller	—	5–8
Fishing			Skiing, snow		
From bank	3.7	2–4	Downhill	—	5–8
Wading in stream	—	5–6	Cross-country	—	6–12+
Football (touch)	7.9	6–10	Skiing, water	—	5–7
Golf			Sledding, tobogganing	—	4–8
Power cart	—	2–3	Snowshoeing	9.9	7–14
Walking (carrying bag or pulling cart)	5.1	4–7	Squash	—	8–12+
Handball	—	8–12+	Soccer	—	5–12+
Hiking (cross-country)	—	3–7	Stair climbing	—	4–8
Horseback riding			Swimming	—	4–8+
Galloping	8.2	—	Table tennis	4.1	3–5
Trotting	6.6	—	Tennis	6.5	4–9+
Walking	2.4	—	Volleyball	—	3–6

Source: Reprinted, with permission, from American College of Sports Medicine (2006). ACSM's Guidelines for Exercise Testing and Prescription (7th ed.). Philadelphia: Lippincott Williams & Wilkins.

$$
\begin{array}{r}
10 \text{ METs (functional or aerobic capacity)} \\
\underline{\times\ 0.60 \text{ (60\% recommended exercise intensity)}} \\
6 \text{ METs (beginning exercise intensity)}
\end{array}
$$

Exercise intensity determined by METs has some disadvantages. Environmental influences such as wind, hills, heat, humidity, altitude, air pollution, and a variety of mechanical factors, such as the mechanical efficiency of a bicycle, can alter the energy cost of the activity. In addition, as the client improves cardiorespiratory endurance, higher MET levels will be required to ensure an adequate training stimulus. As a rule, training by heart rate and perceived exertion may be an easier and more accurate method for determining effective aerobic exercise.

Components of an Aerobic Exercise Program

Relative versus Absolute Intensity

Personal trainers may find it more appropriate to use a relative scale to gauge exercise intensity instead of an absolute scale. Recent research by Lee and others (2003) has demonstrated that the relative intensity of physical activity (e.g., perceived exertion) is a better predictor of health outcomes than recommending that someone exercise at an absolute intensity (e.g., a specific MET level). This research and recommendations made by the National Institutes of Health Consensus Development Panel (National Institutes of Health, 1996) and the CDC/ACSM guidelines (Pate et al., 1995) clearly de-emphasize recommending absolute exercise levels across age levels. Physical activity recommendations need to be tailored to the individual in contrast to a flat MET level for all.

Supportive Conditioning Exercise

All cardiorespiratory exercise programs must be supported by flexibility, strength, and even neuromuscular fitness exercise to enhance the efficiency of aerobic exercise (exercise economy) and minimize musculoskeletal injury. Although some of this supportive exercise, such as stretching, can be part of the warm-up and/or cool-down, it is prudent to add several separate sessions per week that improve the strength of the back, legs, and abdomen. Stretching and range-of-motion exercises are fundamental to a successful cardiorespiratory fitness program. Incorporating various neuromuscular relaxation activities into the cool-down phase of the program is appropriate for those coming from high-stress work environments who need more than just aerobic exercise. You can help your clients relax both mentally and physically by teaching them easy stretching and mental relaxation skills simultaneously. Chapters 9 and 10 describe strength and flexibility exercises in more detail.

Cardiorespiratory Fitness Goals

The goals of cardiorespiratory exercise must be clearly stated in the written exercise plan to reinforce compliance and motivation and for assessment during follow up. The client's implementation and progression plan must reflect these goals and depict means of achieving them safely and realistically. Chapter 11 contains an excellent discussion of goal formulation. The following are examples of areas that can be addressed in the formulation of cardiorespiratory exercise and activity goals:

1. Overall acquisition and maintenance of cardiorespiratory fitness (e.g., kcal/day energy expenditure, mastery of jogging, 20-pound weight loss)
2. Cardiovascular risk-factor modification
   a. Body composition
   b. Blood pressure reduction
   c. Cholesterol control
   d. Stress and anxiety reduction
3. Performance objectives
   a. Personal accomplishment (e.g., 10K run, 1-mile swim, or 6-mile hike)
   b. Increase physical stamina

Caloric Expenditure Goals

An alternative means of programming exercise is to recommend specific energy expenditure goals. Many health benefits are related to total session and weekly energy expenditure (e.g., weight loss and reduction in risk of chronic disease such as diabetes and obesity). The American College of Sports Medicine (2000) recommends 150 kcal energy expenditure in physical activity or exercise per day or 1,000 kcal per week as a *minimal* initial goal for previously sedentary individuals. Note: 1 lb of fat is equal to approximately 3,500 kcals. You must become skilled in estimating and/or calculating the energy costs of various activities. One practical method to approximate the caloric cost of exercise is to use the following equation based on the MET level of the activity:

$$\frac{(\text{METs} \times 3.5 \times \text{body weight in kg})}{200} = \text{kcal/min}$$

It is important to understand that this energy expenditure method for setting exercise goals is less precise than assigning specific target heart-rate ranges. However, it still has much utility from a health risk–reduction perspective. For a more comprehensive list of physical activities and their approximate metabolic cost, refer to *Compendium of Physical Activities: Classification of Energy Costs of Human Physical Activities* (Ainsworth et al., 2001).

Calculating Energy Expenditure. Personal trainers should be able to calculate energy expenditure for any type of cardiorespiratory assessment or activity. To calculate energy expenditure, maximal oxygen consumption (or $\dot{V}O_2$) must first be assessed. Oxygen consumption is linearly related to energy expenditure, and this provides an indirect measurement of an individual's maximal capacity to do work aerobically.

All metabolic calculations are based on direct measurements of oxygen consumption, which are typically performed in a laboratory setting where a person performs a graded maximal exercise test on a treadmill, bike, or other apparatus wearing a specialized headgear that has a non-rebreathing valve attached to it. The person mouth-breathes through the valve and the amount of oxygen and carbon dioxide is computed by a metabolic measurement cart. Maximal oxygen consumption can be calculated from the final state of exercise where the workload increases but oxygen consumption does not increase. With most standardized exercise test protocols, a person of average fitness will complete a test in approximately 10 to 15 minutes.

Since direct measurement of oxygen consumption requires specialized and expensive equipment, it is more practical to determine oxygen consumption by estimating it in a fitness setting. Numerous studies have quantified the average oxygen consumption required to maintain certain workloads on a treadmill or stationary cycle, and as a result,

equations to estimate energy expenditure have been formulated.

Since oxygen consumption is expressed in mL/kg/min, you simply need to fill in the missing values to calculate energy expenditure:

1. milliliters of oxygen ($\dot{V}O_2$ max or percentage of $\dot{V}O_2$ max)
2. weight in kilograms
3. total minutes of exercise

Conversion formulas:

Calories: 1 L of O_2 = 5 kilocalories
Power: 1 MET = 3.5 mL O_2/kg/min
Weight: 1 kg = 2.2 lbs
Volume: 1,000 mL = 1 L

Example 1
If a person weighs 175 lb, has a $\dot{V}O_2$ max of 50 mL/kg/min, and is exercising at a steady intensity of 80% of $\dot{V}O_2$ max [or heart rate reserve (HRR)] for 30 minutes, how many calories are expended during exercise?

Step 1: conversion to SI units

kg: $\dfrac{175 \text{ lb}}{2.2} = 80 \text{ kg}$

mL: 0.80 x 50 mL/kg/min x 80 kg = 3,200 mL/min

min: 30 minutes

Step 2: calculation of oxygen consumption (Note: 1 L = 1,000 mL)

$\dfrac{3,200 \text{ mL/min}}{1,000} = 3.2 \text{ L/min}$

Step 3: calculation of calories burned during the workout (Note: 1 L of O_2 = 5 kilocalories)

3.2 L/min x 5 kcal/L x 30 minutes = 480 calories

Note: the determination of energy expenditure is more accurate if the assessment used is a direct measurement, such as in a laboratory setting where a true maximal heart is obtained, and less accurate with an indirect measurement where the maximal

Components of an Aerobic Exercise Program

heart rate is estimated. Also, energy expenditure may be underestimated or overestimated if the intensity at which the person exercises varies.

Progression Plan

A written progression plan with periodic reevaluation is crucial. This plan must provide details for a graduated progression in the frequency, duration, and intensity of exercise. There must be sufficient flexibility in the rate of progression so that the plan comfortably adjusts to the client's cardiorespiratory and musculoskeletal response. The rate of progression depends upon a number of factors:

- ✔ individual level of fitness (aerobic capacity)
- ✔ age
- ✔ health status
- ✔ cardiorespiratory response to exercise
- ✔ individual preferences and goals
- ✔ social and family support
- ✔ level of exercise initiative and motivation
- ✔ access to appropriate facilities and equipment

Three stages of progression for the cardiorespiratory endurance exercise plan are identified in the American College of Sports Medicine guidelines (2000): the initial conditioning stage, the improvement conditioning stage, and the maintenance conditioning stage.

Initial Conditioning Stage. This stage usually lasts four to six weeks or longer and includes low-level aerobic activities, stretching, and light calisthenics. Exercise frequency should begin with every other day. Depending upon initial level of fitness and functional capacity, duration should start with 10 to 20 minutes and gradually increase according to the client's cardiorespiratory and musculoskeletal response. For those with low functional capacity (4 to 7 METs or less), it may be appropriate to prescribe low-level aerobic interval exercise of two to five minutes at a time. The most important thing to remember during the initial conditioning stage is

to be conservative with the exercise intensity. For example, if the individual has a 9 MET functional capacity (31.5 mL/kg/min $\dot{V}O_2$max), begin at a conservative 40 to 60% of this value, or at about 4 METs. Here, exercise heart rate should begin at approximately 40 to 60% of heart-rate reserve (Karvonen).

Improvement Conditioning Stage. This is the primary conditioning stage for most aerobic-training programs. It may last from 8 to 20 weeks, and the rate of progression in intensity is more rapid. The exercise intensity can be increased to the next highest level than that completed in the initial conditioning stage, and within the 60 to 90% of maximal heart rate (50 to 85% of $\dot{V}O_2$ max or heart-rate reserve) depending on fitness level and age. Exercise duration should be increased every two to three weeks according to the client's response and goals. It is important to periodically review progress at two- to four-week intervals during this stage, either by direct monitoring or by assessing self-report data (RPE, heart rate, symptoms, caloric expenditure).

Maintenance Stage. When clients reach their target functional capacity or primary goals, the maintenance stage begins. This stage is usually reached after the first 6 months of training, but it may be delayed as long as 12 months, depending upon goals. In any case, it is important to reassess goals at the beginning of this stage. Maintenance of a particular level of cardiorespiratory fitness can be derived from an exercise program that has similar energy requirements to that of the conditioning program. Cardiorespiratory fitness can often be maintained by regularly engaging in a variety of endurance-related sports activities that are fun and enjoyable.

Cautions

The last component of an exercise plan involves using individual information to ensure each client's exercise safety with specific precautions. List any personal or environmental information that reduces the risk of exercise injury or that may compromise exercise safety. Individualized comments such as those describing hot, humid environments or avoiding musculoskeletal symptoms specific to the client should be included. Another useful format is to list several cautions that are standard for nearly all exercise programs:

✔ Do not exercise for at least 90 minutes after a meal.

✔ Avoid continuing exercise with chest discomfort, lightheadedness, or dizziness.

✔ Reduce exercise intensity in response to very hot or humid environments or to altitudes above 5,000 feet.

✔ Avoid exercise with tenderness in a joint (for example, a knee or ankle) that tends to worsen with activity.

✔ Avoid strenuous aerobic exercise during viral infections such as the flu or upper-respiratory tract infection.

✔ If you are receiving care from a physician for a chronic medical condition (e.g., diabetes, cardiovascular disease, hypertension), you should obtain clearance from your doctor before proceeding with this exercise program.

TRAINING METHODS

Once the mode, frequency, duration, and intensity of exercise has been established, you must choose the appropriate training method. The choice provides the foundation for the exercise progression plan. Selection requires understanding the physiological response to various training methods and, preferably, personal experience with each of those methods. As with exercise intensity and progression, the training method depends on the functional fitness level and the goals of the participant. There are five major training methods (Heyward, 1984; Wells & Pate, 1988):

1. Continuous training
   a. Intermediate slow distance
   b. Long slow distance
2. Interval training
   a. Aerobic interval training
   b. Anaerobic interval training
3. Fartlek training
4. Circuit training
5. Aerobic cross training

Continuous Training

Continuous training involves conditioning-stage exercise, such as walking, jogging, cycling, swimming, and aerobic dancing. The intensity is maintained continuously between 50 and 85% of functional capacity (maximal oxygen uptake). For those with initially low functional capacities, continuous training may be initiated at 40% of functional capacity and is usually preceded by four to six weeks of interval training in the initial conditioning stage. In practice, continuous training is divided into two types:

✔ Intermediate slow distance: Generally from 20 to 60 minutes of continuous aerobic exercise—the most common type of sustained aerobic exercise for fitness improvement. Body-fat reduction, improvement in cardiorespiratory fitness, and cardiovascular risk factor management—all are responsive to this type of continuous training.

✔ Long slow distance (LSD): 60 or more minutes of continuous aerobic exercise, usually employed for athletic training in such sports as cycling and long-distance running. Cardiorespiratory and metabolic demands are great for LSD training. At least six months of successful intermediate slow distance training should precede LSD training. Increased risk of musculoskeletal injury (e.g., Achilles tendinitis) accompanies this type of prolonged aerobic training.

Interval Training

Interval training involves alternating relatively more intense bouts of cardiovascular exercise with those that are relatively less intense. Interval training has useful applications for beginning exercisers, as well as experienced,

Training Methods

conditioned clients who wish to improve aerobic power. You can use two types of interval training: aerobic and anaerobic. The following four variables should be considered when designing an aerobic or anaerobic interval training program:

- ✔ intensity of work interval (e.g., speed)
- ✔ duration of work interval (e.g., distance or time)
- ✔ duration of rest or recovery interval
- ✔ number of repetitions or repeat intervals

Aerobic Interval Training. Aerobic interval training is best suited for those beginning in the poor- or low-cardiorespiratory fitness classifications because it is less intense (Table 7.8). Generally, aerobic interval

Table 7.8
Percentile Values for Maximal Aerobic Power (mL/kg/min)

Percentile	Age				
	20–29	30–39	40–49	50–59	60+
Men					
90	51.4	50.4	48.2	45.3	42.5
80	48.2	46.8	44.1	41.0	38.1
70	46.8	44.6	41.8	38.5	35.3
60	44.2	42.4	39.9	36.7	33.6
50	42.5	41.0	38.1	35.2	31.8
40	41.0	38.9	36.7	33.8	30.2
30	39.5	37.4	35.1	32.3	28.7
20	37.1	35.4	33.0	30.2	26.5
10	34.5	32.5	30.9	28.0	23.1
Women					
90	44.2	41.0	39.5	35.2	35.2
80	41.0	38.6	36.3	32.3	31.2
70	38.1	36.7	33.8	30.9	29.4
60	36.7	34.6	32.3	29.4	27.2
50	35.2	33.8	30.9	28.2	25.8
40	33.8	32.3	29.5	26.9	24.5
30	32.3	30.5	28.3	25.5	23.8
20	30.6	28.7	26.5	24.3	22.8
10	28.4	26.5	25.1	22.3	20.8

Source: American College of Sports Medicine (2000). *ACSM's Guidelines for Exercise Testing and Prescription* (6th ed.). Philadelphia: Lippincott Williams & Wilkins. Adapted, with permission, from *The Physical Fitness Certification Manual* (revised 2003), The Cooper Institute, Dallas, Tex.

Study population for the data set was predominately white and college educated. A modified Balke treadmill test was used with V̇O₂max estimated from the last grade/speed achieved. The following may be used as descriptors for the percentile rankings: well above average (90), above average (70), average (50), below average (30), and well below average (10).

training uses exercise bouts of 2 to 15 minutes at an intensity between 60 and 80% of functional capacity (modified from Wells & Pate, 1988). Those with poor- or low-functional capacity should start with two- to three-minute exercise intervals at 60 to 70% of functional capacity. Rest intervals should take approximately the same time as a complete exercise interval. Intervals can be repeated 5 to 10 times depending on the client's response and program goals; for example, stationary bicycling for three minutes at a work load intensity of 60 to 70% of functional capacity with a two-minute "rest period" of cycling at zero resistance or load. Hypothetically, this would be repeated 5 to 10 times for a total workout of 25 to 50 minutes. Higher-intensity and longer-duration aerobic interval training (e.g., 5- to 15-minute bouts at 70 to 90% of functional capacity) should be reserved for those in higher cardiorespiratory fitness classifications seeking increased aerobic endurance and speed.

Anaerobic Interval Training. Anaerobic interval training is primarily reserved for those in the higher cardiorespiratory fitness classifications who desire to increase speed, lactate threshold, and overall aerobic power. Such training usually results in greater lactic acid concentrations in exercising muscles and is accompanied by greater muscular discomfort. Because of the relatively high metabolic and cardiorespiratory demands, beginners or those below a 10-MET aerobic capacity should refrain from anaerobic interval training. Although there are many derivations of anaerobic interval training, the training stimulus is usually between 30 seconds and four minutes at an intensity of 85% to greater than 100% of functional capacity (maximal oxygen uptake). The probability of musculoskeletal injury is greater because of high muscle contraction velocities and forces. The client, frequently an athlete, should engage in substantial low-level aerobic warm-up and stretching before vigorous activity.

Fartlek Training

Fartlek training is similar to interval training. However, the work-rest intervals are not systematically or accurately measured. Work-rest intervals and intensity are usually determined by how the participant feels. Over the years, Fartlek training has blossomed in many aerobic-training regimens, primarily to prevent boredom and to enhance aerobic endurance. One of its most useful applications is in running, where the warm up consists of running for 10 to 20 minutes, then the pace is significantly varied every 5 to 10 minutes. Like long, slow distance aerobic training, this form should be reserved for those in the average or above-average cardiorespiratory fitness levels because of the relatively high demand on the cardiorespiratory system.

Circuit Training

Circuit training takes the client through a series of exercise stations, with relatively brief rest intervals between each station. The number of stations may range from 4 to 10. Historically, circuit training was designed to enhance muscular endurance and incorporated mostly low-weight, high-repetition exercises. A circuit of 4 to 10 stations with a low-level aerobic warm-up and cool-down station (for example, the stationary bicycle) could be followed by exercise stations using either free weights and/or single-station weight machines. A good example of circuit training in a more natural environment is par course exercise, which intersperses walking or jogging with a variety of stations that feature flexibility, muscular endurance, and strength exercises.

Aerobic circuit-training programs are also popular. Between four and eight aerobic exercise stations with one to five minutes per station and a 15-second rest break between stations constitute a circuit. Stations may include stationary cycling, treadmill exercise, elliptical training, moderate stair climbing, and rowing. Depending on the number of stations, the workout provides 20 to 50 minutes of aerobic exercise. One key to success is to avoid excessive workloads at each station. Each station should be set at 50 to 70% of the client's functional capacity.

Aerobic Cross Training

Aerobic **cross training** is an individualized combination or composite of all aerobic-training methods and is characterized by a variety of intensities and modes. It is primarily for exercisers in the maintenance phase of conditioning who want variety and an intensity corresponding to how they feel during a given exercise workout. A good example is a 50-minute workout in which the client warms up by jogging 15 minutes to a nearby pool, swims for 20 minutes, and then jogs 15 minutes back home. Another example is bicycling 20 minutes to a track or running course and, after 20 minutes of running, cycling back home. Combining a group of aerobic activities into one workout at steady or various intensities is an excellent method of cross-training to fight boredom from the same daily workout mode and intensity. This method can also be applied to circuit training in a gym by combining a continuous, relatively low-level aerobic session, such as 20 minutes of stationary cycling, with 10 to 20 minutes of a variety of higher-intensity aerobic intervals on various aerobic ergometers, and concluding with a 5- to 10-minute cool-down of stationary cycling. The many obvious permutations of this method should begin and end with a continuous low-level cardiorespiratory exercise effort for effective physiological warm-up. This method instills variety and is a mini-version of a "training triathlon."

Domestic Forms of Physical Activity

Although not often thought of as a training method per se, continuous or intermittent physical movement during household chores has the capacity to generate small increases in cardiorespiratory fitness and more significant improvements in cardiovascular health. Domestic activi-

Guidelines for Cardiorespiratory Activity

ties such as yard work, cleaning, scrubbing, gardening, and repair work generate energy costs of 3 to 6 METs and are important contributors to disease prevention. While these activities do not generate the same cardiorespiratory stimulus as running or cycling, they clearly should not be viewed as insignificant contributors to weekly activity energy expenditure and cardiovascular and metabolic health.

GUIDELINES FOR CARDIORESPIRATORY ACTIVITY

The best resources for detailed aerobic activities are those that adopt sensible progression guidelines with adequate instruction for each form of exercise (e.g., American Council on Exercise, 2000; American College of Sports Medicine, 2003; Neporent & Schlosberg, 1999; Howley & Franks, 1998; Nieman, 1990). Following are guidelines for popular aerobic and sport activities.

Walking

Walking is the easiest aerobic-conditioning activity and is often preferred because of its low injury rate, relative simplicity, and adaptability to busy schedules. Although nearly anyone can incur significant health benefits from walking, several types of clients will respond particularly well to a graduated walking program:

✔ Those with low functional capacity (2 to 7 METs) who need an initial low-intensity workout

✔ Those over 60 years of age who have been sedentary and are just beginning an exercise program

✔ Those who are 20 or more pounds overweight

The energy cost of walking is relatively low compared to that of jogging because of slower speeds; however, at walking speeds of five miles per hour and faster, the oxygen and caloric cost per minute approaches that of jogging or running

(Table 7.9). There still exists an abundance of misinformation regarding the energy costs of walking versus running. Despite the long-standing claim that walking 1 mile is equivalent to running 1 mile, this is not the case, with the exception of very fast walking speeds of greater than 5 miles per hour (Howley & Franks, 1998; Howley & Glover, 1974). In general, the **net caloric cost** per mile* of walking is 50 to 60% of that for running. This is an important point if you intend to program and quantify walking mileage for weight-management purposes.

Walking is generally less intense than jogging or running, meaning that longer sessions can be maintained with less likelihood of musculoskeletal injury. When hilly terrain is gradually added to the walking program, there is greater energy expenditure. Perhaps

Table 7.9
Energy Costs of Walking (kcal/min)

Body Weight (lb)	Miles Per Hour						
	2.0	2.5	3.0	3.5	4.0	4.5	5.0
110	2.1	2.4	2.8	3.1	4.1	5.2	6.6
120	2.3	2.6	3.0	3.4	4.4	5.6	7.2
130	2.5	2.9	3.2	3.6	4.8	6.1	7.8
140	2.7	3.1	3.5	3.9	5.2	6.6	8.4
150	2.8	3.3	3.7	4.2	5.6	7.0	9.0
160	3.0	3.5	4.0	4.5	5.9	7.5	9.6
170	3.2	3.7	4.2	4.8	6.3	8.0	10.2
180	3.4	4.0	4.5	5.0	6.7	8.4	10.8
190	3.6	4.2	4.7	5.3	7.0	8.9	11.4
200	3.8	4.4	5.0	5.6	7.4	9.4	12.0
210	4.0	4.6	5.2	5.9	7.8	9.9	12.6
220	4.2	4.8	5.5	6.2	8.2	10.3	13.2

Source: Adapted, by permission, from Howley, E. & Franks, D. (2003). *Health Fitness Instructor's Handbook* (4th ed.). Champaign, Ill.: Human Kinetics.

*The net cost of exercise is the exercise energy expenditure minus resting energy expenditure. The net cost measures the energy expenditure used over that when at rest.

the safest and most effective cardiorespiratory weight-control exercise for those who are 20 to 30 pounds (9 to 13.5 kg) overweight is progressive variable-terrain walking. This walking protocol graduates from walking approximately 2 miles on flat terrain to walking up to 5 or more miles over a variety of grades, such as those found on many urban and rural park and nature trails. It is not difficult to achieve and maintain the walking intensity and duration necessary for acceptable cardiorespiratory fitness. As a general rule, achieving acceptable fitness will require at least 20 minutes (preferably 30 minutes or more) of fast-paced, flat-ground walking or slightly slower variable-terrain walking. When walking, three things are important:

1. When walking is the primary activity, footwear is important. Specialized walking or hiking shoes are available from many stores, although many walkers will prefer a good pair of running shoes.

2. Always warm up and cool down. Begin each session by walking for about five minutes and then stretch the Achilles tendons, calves, and low-back muscles. After the primary conditioning phase, cool down by walking at a slower pace and stretching the muscles that were previously stretched.

3. Give special emphasis to gradually increasing the duration—for example, from 15 to 60 minutes—over the length of the program. Progression in intensity should follow successful duration progression. Emphasize duration first, then gradually add faster-paced walking. Keep in mind that adding hilly terrain increases the intensity, so be sure that the terrain is within the client's capacity.

Adhere to guidelines for proper walking and running form when using a motor-driven treadmill. These guidelines include:

✔ Safely mounting and dismounting the treadmill
✔ Maintaining a relatively upright posture
✔ Keeping the hips tucked directly under the torso
✔ Looking straight ahead
✔ Letting the arms swing naturally

Pedometer Walking. Wearing a pedometer or step-counter to quantify walking distance as well as other domestic and recreational activities has proven to be an effective means of motivating inactive clients. Numerous health plans and health care institutions have adopted the 10,000-steps-a-day program, in part popularized by the diabetes prevention program study (Diabetes Prevention Program Research

Table 7.10
Energy Costs of Jogging and Running (kcal/min)

Body weight (lb)	Running/Jogging Speed (MPH)							
	3.0	4.0	5.0	6.0	7.0	8.0	9.0	10.0
110	4.7	5.9	7.2	8.5	9.8	11.1	12.3	13.6
120	5.1	6.4	7.9	9.3	10.6	12.1	13.4	14.8
130	5.5	7.0	8.6	10.0	11.5	13.1	14.6	16.1
140	5.9	7.5	9.2	10.8	12.4	14.1	15.7	17.3
150	6.4	8.1	9.9	11.6	13.3	15.1	16.8	18.5
160	6.8	8.6	10.5	12.4	14.2	16.1	17.9	19.8
170	7.2	9.1	11.2	13.1	15.1	17.1	19.1	21.0
180	7.6	9.7	11.8	13.9	15.9	18.1	20.2	22.2
190	8.1	10.2	12.5	14.7	16.8	19.1	21.3	23.5
200	8.5	10.8	13.2	15.4	17.7	20.1	22.4	24.7
210	8.9	11.3	13.8	16.2	18.6	21.1	23.5	25.9
220	9.3	11.8	14.5	17.0	19.5	22.2	24.7	27.2

Source: Adapted, by permission, from Howley, E. & Franks, D. (2003). *Health Fitness Instructor's Handbook* (4th ed.). Champaign, Ill.: Human Kinetics.

Group, 2002). Although there is significant inter-individual variation in the number of steps per mile, most popular step-counters record approximately 2,000 steps per mile of walking. These devices can objectively score a client's daily and weekly physical activity, which can be of great value to both the participant and personal trainer.

Jogging and Running

Jogging and running are superb cardiorespiratory-endurance activities. The essential difference between the two is that jogging is "slower running," or as some authorities define it, jogging is running slower than eight minutes per mile. For beginners, a natural sequence of progression might be:

1. Walk/jog intervals: walk 50 yards, jog 50 yards, repeat 10 to 20 times; over time, gradually increase the jogging interval to 2 or more miles

2. Jogging: gradually increase jogging distance to desired distance or energy expenditure

3. Running: as jogging endurance improves, increase stride frequency and stride length to a comfortable running style

It is not necessary to graduate to running if desired goals can be achieved by jogging. However, running is a natural progression for those who orthopedically and psychologically respond well to jogging. Table 7.10 shows the energy cost in calories per minute for jogging and running. Note that the energy cost increases proportionately with increasing speed. These proportional increases in energy cost mean that a client who runs a mile at 9 miles per hour (6.6 minutes per mile) will finish the mile twice as fast as when jogging 4.5 miles per hour (13.3 minutes per mile), but energy cost per mile is about the same. Numerous benefits can be obtained from successful jogging and running programs that are adequately balanced with appropriate muscular-strength and flexibility exercises. Some of these benefits include increased maximum oxygen uptake,

improved body composition (decrease in body-fat stores), coronary risk reduction, increased bone strength, and enhanced psychological well-being.

Four things are important when jogging or running:

1. Wear appropriate footwear. A comfortable pair of running shoes designed for distance jogging/running should have adequate sole cushion, good heel support, and sufficient sole flexibility.

2. Always accompany jogging or running exercise with appropriate flexibility exercise. Stretching the Achilles tendons, calves, hamstrings, quadriceps, feet, and low-back muscles will help improve jogging and running efficiency (see Chapter 10).

3. For beginners, jog every other day (no more than four days per week) with a day of rest between workouts to allow for adequate recovery of the weightbearing joints, ligaments, and tendons. Limit the initial duration to no more than 25 to 30 minutes per workout for the first six to eight weeks.

4. Increase jogging pace and add hills only gradually. Emphasize a gradual increase in distance at a relatively slow pace, and then slowly increase pace or speed. Aerobic interval training will facilitate a safe and gradual increase in distance.

Elliptical trainers are a relatively new form of aerobic exercise machine. With elliptical trainers, the lower-body motion is a relative combination of the cycling and stair climbing motions, except that the feet move in an elliptical (i.e., egg-shaped) pattern, as opposed to a circular movement path. Like stair climbers, elliptical motion trainers are low-impact (since the user's feet never leave the footpads) and weightbearing.

Cycling

Cycling is another excellent cardiorespiratory activity with benefits similar to jogging and running. It is a good alternative for those who do not like to jog or run or who have orthopedic limitations to weightbearing exercise. Two types are outdoor cycling and indoor stationary cycling. Both have advantages and disadvantages; however, with sufficient frequency, duration, and intensity, both can be an excellent stimulus to cardiorespiratory fitness.

Outdoor Cycling. The benefits of outdoor cycling are sunlight, fresh air, adequate cooling, and variety of terrain and scenery. And it can be a good source of inexpensive transportation. Most clients find that cycling outdoors makes it easier to prolong duration of exercise because of distances between destinations and more interesting environments. Disadvantages include inclement weather, nightfall, and some unsafe city environments. However, convenient outdoor cycling, combined with indoor stationary cycling, can be a stimulating year-round program.

Guidelines for outdoor bicycling include the following:

1. Use a bicycle with at least 10 speeds so that the cyclist can easily adapt to nearly any change in grade or wind.

2. For beginners, keep a relatively constant pedal crank speed by adjusting the gears to variable grades and headwinds. This pedal crank speed can vary depending on fitness and comfort, but will usually be between 70 and 90 rpm per leg. This will help minimize fatigue and maximize blood flow and nutrients to the legs.

3. Bicycle seat height should be high enough so that the leg that is on the downstroke is not quite completely extended when the ball of the foot is on the pedal.

4. Use toe clips, especially with significant hill climbing. Toe clips improve pedaling efficiency by delivering more muscular power to the pedal crank axis throughout the entire revolution.

5. Wear bicycling apparel. Always wear a cycling helmet. Padded shorts and gloves will increase comfort for cycling lasting longer than 45 minutes.

Indoor Stationary Cycling. The advantages of indoor stationary cycling include its convenience and relative safety. Most health clubs and fitness centers have two types of stationary cycles: those with mechanically braked flywheels and those that are electronically braked. Either type will provide a good aerobic or anaerobic workout; however, the electronically controlled cycles generally display digital workload information that may be helpful to motivate clients. On electronically controlled cycles, some beginners do not always get an adequate warm-up when selecting certain exercise programs on the display monitor. Regardless of the type of cycle, always warm up by cycling against low pedal crank resistance for at least 5 to 10 minutes. Many stationary cycles are not accurately calibrated, so there may be noticeable differences in pedal crank resistances for similarly indicated workloads between cycles.

For a thorough review of group indoor cycling refer to ACE's *Group Indoor Cycling* (Shechtman, 2000).

The following guidelines apply to stationary cycling machines:

1. Ensure proper ventilation. If necessary, a fan gives adequate cross ventilation to enable good evaporative heat loss. Cooling the body by the evaporation of sweat is necessary to prevent a rapid rise in body temperature. Unlike outdoor bicycling, indoor cycling requires adequate ventilation for prolonged exercise.

2. As in outdoor bicycling, adjust seat height for a slight bend in the knee at the downstroke position.

3. Adjust the handlebars so that the client is relaxed and leaning slightly forward.

4. Hold pedal crank speed relatively constant for beginners in the range of 70 to 90 rpm per leg.

5. Always warm up and cool down with 5 to 10 minutes of low-resistance cycling.

6. Because of the relatively intense nature of group indoor cycling, it is paramount to incorporate a more graduated warm-up and cool-down and to ensure that adequate convective cooling (i.e., cross-current ventilation) is made available.

Swimming and Vertical Water Exercise

Swimming activities are another excellent form of cardiorespiratory endurance exercise. Swimming is a good alternative for those with chronic orthopedic problems or a recent musculoskeletal injury. Relatively experienced swimmers generate a lower heart-rate response for any level of effort compared to cyclists and runners. The diminished cardiac work is due to the prone position and the effect of immersion in a relatively cool environment. This is important when determining a target heart-rate range, which may be as much as 10 beats per minute lower with lap swimming than with cycling or running. This does not mean that swimming is not a significant cardiorespiratory stimulus. However, swimming generally requires a higher level of motor skill that may take significantly longer to learn than that of cycling or running. Several factors determine swimming efficiency and early success with any swimming program, including body buoyancy, swimming skill and style, and body dimensions. Women are generally more efficient swimmers than men, partly because of greater body-fat stores and a more even distribution of body fat, which improves buoyancy. For an efficient swimmer, the energy cost of swimming 1 mile has been estimated to be more than 400 kcal. Unskilled swimmers may require twice the energy expenditure for a given velocity compared to skilled swimmers and often fatigue early.

Vertical water exercise (upright in the water) is an excellent way to develop cardiorespiratory and overall fitness without requiring swimming skills. Many clients may benefit greatly from training in the water, especially those who have problems with balance or coordination, or who need to begin exercising at a very low intensity. In addition, clients who want to achieve a relatively high-intensity workout with reduced impact can use the surrounding resistance of water as an effective exercise environment. Essentially, there are two types of vertical water exercise: shallow water exercise, which is conducted in water navel- to nipple-deep (standing position), and deep-water exercise, which is conducted in a depth where the lungs are fully submerged and the feet may be touching the bottom of the pool slightly or not at all. Flotation devices are generally used for support. Equipment that increases surface area (paddles for the feet in deep water or shoes for better traction in shallow water) may be added to progress intensity.

For a thorough review of vertical water exercise refer to ACE's *Aquatic Exercise* (Bonelli, 2001).

The following guidelines should be followed for swimming:

1. Assess swimming or aquatic exercise skill by evaluating exercise history or by observation. If skill level (i.e., stroke efficiency and style) is low, supervision and swimming lessons should precede swimming as a cardiorespiratory-conditioning exercise.

2. Keep pool temperature for lap swimming at 76 to 84°F (24 to 29°C).

3. Ideally, use a lap pool with, at the most, 80 lengths per mile to enable the swimmer to attain a reasonable stroke rhythm before turning.

4. Use interval training for the beginning swimmer. For example, swimming either the width or length of the pool one to two times may be appropriate. Each of these would constitute a set with a rest interval of walking one or two widths in waist-high water. This could be repeated 4 to 10 times, depending on skill and cardiorespiratory fitness.

5. For the beginner, include a good warm-up and cool-down exercise, such as walking the width of the pool in waist- or chest-high water for 5 to 10 minutes.

6. For those who are not comfortable in the pool and perhaps cannot swim, flotation devices can help (e.g., small life-vests, kick-boards, pull-buoys).

Rowing

Rowing machines are sometimes used in gyms and fitness centers for cardiorespiratory exercise, as well as for attaining a reasonable degree of arm, back, and thigh muscular endurance. As with any stationary aerobic exercise device, a fan should provide air circulation to facilitate sweat evaporation and prevent overheating. There are numerous manufacturers of rowing machines, some very basic and some quite sophisticated with hydraulic action of the arm movement and workload display monitors. However, most operate on the principle of coordinated effort of lower-extremity muscular work with arm rowing action. Rowing intensity (rowing motion resistance) can be varied in most machines by changing the force angle of the rowing arm of the machine, by changing the hydraulic pressure in the pressure cylinder, or via electronic programming. Intensity also can be varied by increasing the rowing rate, or number of rows per minute. Those just learning should note that several sessions are required to learn how to perform repetitive, efficient rowing motions that require synchronizing the arms, back, and legs. Several guidelines may be helpful:

1. Secure feet in the anchors on the front part of the machine.

2. Use a smooth rowing action (coordinate arm and back rowing movements with leg extensions).

3. Begin with a relatively low intensity (low resistance) with approximately 8 to 10 rows per minute for hydraulic rowers, for 5 to 10 minutes.

4. Graduate the speed to approximately 15 to 30 rows per minute and gradually increase duration to 15 to 30 minutes.

5. Gradually increase intensity according to heart rate and perceived exertion.

Stair Climbing

Stair climbing can be an effective means of attaining cardiorespiratory fitness. The client may use either a staircase or one of the electronically braked stair-climbing machines that are found in most fitness centers. The advent of computer-interactive, electrically braked stair-climbing machines brought effective and well-controlled stair climbing to the health club and fitness center. They allow for a more effective warm-up and cool-down as well as a variety of training intensities because most of these devices regulate the intensity of climbing based on step rate, depth of step, or exercise resistance. It should be noted that many people incorrectly support their weight by leaning onto guard rails, so the actual work performed is less than that indicated on the monitor. Many people find these machines challenging and fun, and they can provide an interesting addition to circuit training programs or be a primary means of attaining cardiorespiratory fitness.

Safety precaution: A fan or other means of convective cooling should always be used because of the tendency to overheat on stationary exercise machines.

Because the energy cost of actual stair climbing is largely dependent upon body weight, a large anaerobic component is possible for those who are overweight or unaccustomed to regular stair climbing. Adequate warm-up and cool-down periods must be incorporated due to the potentially large energy costs. Walking for 5 to 10 minutes on relatively flat terrain, either on a track or treadmill, usually provides adequate warm-up or cool-down. Interval-training methods are best when beginning a program with regular stairs or steps in a stadium. After warming up, repeating a sequence of walking four flights of stairs and taking a 60-second walk on flat ground 4 to 10 times is one example of an interval approach. To provide protection to your client's knee joints, instruct stair climber users to keep their knees aligned with their toes. If the knees are allowed to move far past the toes, significant stress may be placed on the anterior aspect of the knee.

Traditional Aerobics

Studies on the effects of traditional aerobics show it to be an excellent form of cardiorespiratory endurance exercise. To gain significant benefits, the client must maintain the aerobic phase for at least 20 to 30 minutes, three to four times per week. The tempo (speed or pace) should be adjusted to fit the desired intensity or heart-rate range. Like swimming, traditional aerobics requires a degree of motor skill and coordination, and may take more time to learn than walking, jogging, or cycling. For those who are significantly overweight or have a history of orthopedic injuries, this type of exercise may create undue demands on the cardiorespiratory and musculoskeletal systems.

For a thorough review of traditional aerobics refer to ACE's *Traditional Aerobics* (Bricker, 2000).

For traditional aerobics, the following guidelines apply:

1. Wear appropriate footwear that adheres to four standards: cushion, support, flexibility, and traction compatibility.

2. For beginners, recommend low-impact aerobics—a form of traditional aerobics that features one foot on the ground at all times, reducing the risk of musculoskeletal injury, and may include the use of light weights.

3. For beginners, recommend a class that will adapt appropriately to functional capacity and skill level.

4. Lower the target heart rate slightly, because traditional aerobics may elicit heart rates 10 to 15 beats per minute higher than running or cycling for the same percentage of aerobic capacity (Parker et al., 1989). This disproportionate relationship between oxygen consumption and heart rate is generally true for most aerobic-exercise routines using upper-body muscle groups.

Step Training

In the 1990s, step training gained wide popularity in fitness centers and health clubs across the United States and many parts of Asia and Europe. Available research indicates that the energy cost of step training (7 to 11 METs) is commensurate with that of traditional aerobic exercise, such as running and cycling, and is an adequate stimulus of aerobic endurance. Choices of step bench height generally range from 4 to 10 inches, with a standard stepping rate of 120 to 130 steps per minute. Advise beginners to use smaller step heights of 4 to 6 inches with a goal of 8 inches after four to eight weeks of successful training. Discourage the addition of hand-held weights for beginners and those who are coronary-prone, because of the increased blood pressure response for any given step rate and step height.

For a thorough review of step training refer to ACE's *Step Training* (Bonelli, 2000).

Tennis, Racquetball, and Handball

Tennis, racquetball, and handball are all popular sports and deserve special attention for their ability to increase cardiorespiratory fitness. Each requires various motor skills and neuromuscular coordination and the level and duration of play depend on these skills. For the beginner, racquet sports demand more from anaerobic energy systems than aerobic. However, as one becomes more skilled and efficient with movement and play, it is easier to prolong the activity and obtain more cardiorespiratory benefits. Improvements in cardiorespiratory fitness are dependent upon several factors:

✔ skill level and style of the player
✔ level of competition (intensity)
✔ total duration of each point played
✔ time interval between points and games
✔ total duration of entire exercise session

As the intensity and duration of these sports meet the criteria for cardiorespiratory endurance fitness (that is, 50 to 85% of maximal oxygen uptake for 20 to 60 minutes), they become more of a cardiorespiratory stimulus.

Racquetball and handball often are played in hot, unventilated environments, and require more attention to regular fluid intake and signs of dehydration. Generally, these racquet sports require at least average cardiorespiratory fitness and are excellent activities for developing and maintaining fitness.

Hiking and Backpacking

Hiking and backpacking activities can require high levels of cardiorespiratory endurance. Although most clients do not engage in these activities more than once a week, they are an excellent adjunct to a cardiorespiratory fitness program using fundamental aerobic activities such as jogging, cycling, or step training. The energy cost (oxygen uptake and calories expended) per minute is lower for hiking and backpacking, depending on grade, packloads, and altitude. The duration of such activity is usually prolonged (two to eight hours) and, therefore, the total energy cost is well above most routine aerobic workouts. It is important to be in at least average cardiorespiratory fitness, preferably the "above average" classification (see Table 7.8), before attempting prolonged variable-terrain hiking. One of the most important concerns with prolonged hiking is dehydration. Be sure to carry adequate water and glucose replacement on trips lasting longer than 60 minutes.

Many factors govern the cardiorespiratory and metabolic cost of hiking and backpacking. The following are among the most important:

✔ body weight of hiker
✔ duration of the hike
✔ number and size of the grades
✔ altitude at which the hike occurs
✔ speed of movement
✔ pack load
✔ air temperature

Tai Chi and Other Mind-Body Exercise Practices with an Aerobic Component

Tai chi (shorthand for tai chi chuan or t aijiquan) is just one form of the more ancient practice of qigong (Chinese health exercise). Tai chi is a "moving meditation" that has been shown to clearly increase cardiorespiratory endurance when sufficient

pace and movement sequences are learned. This aerobic benefit has been particularly demonstrated in seniors (Lan et al., 1998). Tai chi characteristically consists of more than 100 movements (Yang style). There are numerous styles of Tai chi (e.g., Chen, Yang, and Wu styles), all of which may require years of training before one becomes adequately proficient. Other mind-body exercise programs that have the capacity to increase cardiorespiratory fitness include NIA (Neuromuscular Integrative Action), Yogarobics, E-motion among others. See Appendix C for a more comprehensive discussion of mind-body fitness.

MONITORING CARDIORESPIRATORY EXERCISE

Monitoring cardiorespiratory exercise performance is necessary for assessing exercise response, regulating exercise intensity, documenting progress, and assuring safety. Essentially, three techniques are used to monitor cardiorespiratory exercise: heart rate, ratings of perceived exertion, and laboratory monitoring techniques.

Monitoring Heart Rates

As mentioned earlier, heart rate is a good guide for exercise intensity and cardiorespiratory responsiveness. The heart rate can be obtained by palpating (feeling) the pulse or by using a cardiotachometer or electrocardiogram. From a practical standpoint, palpation is the easiest method to assess heart rate. The pulse may be palpated in the neck (carotid artery), the head (temporal artery), the wrist (radial artery), or the chest (apical artery). For example, the carotid pulse may be felt by gently placing the index and middle finger over a carotid artery in the neck on either side of the larynx. It is important not to apply too much pressure, as there are carotid sensors in these arteries that are sensitive to pressure and may induce a sudden drop in heart rate. Assess the radial pulse in the wrist by placing the first two fingers (index and middle) on the underside and thumb side of the wrist. See Chapter 6 for a complete discussion of heart-rate monitoring.

Heart-rate Response to Training. There are two trends to look for when monitoring the heart-rate response to cardiorespiratory exercise training. First is the tendency of the heart rate, for any given level of exercise, to decrease with training. This tendency primarily applies to submaximal exercise, such as that between 60 and 80% of maximum functional capacity. For example, expect a decrease in heart rate for the same submaximal workload on a stationary cycle after several weeks of training. The actual decrease in exercise heart rate and the length of time required to elicit this change is variable between clients, but is primarily dependent upon age, initial level of fitness, length of the training program, and the exercise program intensity. Resting heart rate also tends to decrease with training along with the decrease in submaximal exercise heart rate. You must understand that there are other physiological reasons why resting heart rate may be low beyond that induced by endurance exercise training. A low resting pulse rate by itself is not by any means a perfect predictor of fitness.

FIGURE 7.1
Hypothetical relationship between training program duration and improvements in aerobic capacity for three cardiorespiratory fitness levels (in healthy individuals).

Required Time for Expected Increases in Aerobic Capacity

For young and middle-aged adults, the usual improvement in aerobic capacity will be 15 to 20% over 10 to 20 weeks of training (Pollock, 1973). However, aerobic capacity may increase up to 45 to 50% depending upon the following factors:

✔ initial level of fitness
✔ age
✔ frequency of training
✔ intensity of training
✔ duration of exercise and total training programs
✔ genetics (e.g., oxidative processes, muscle fiber type ratio)

Those who begin a moderately intense cardiorespiratory conditioning program with a relatively high aerobic capacity can expect little improvement in aerobic capacity compared to those with initially low capacities. Age is not a detriment to increasing aerobic capacity by itself; however, training generally shows smaller improvements in aerobic capacity because of lower exercise intensities.

Overall, you can expect greater improvements with greater intensity and/or duration of exercise up to a point. This range for aerobic improvement is reflected in the mode, frequency, duration, and intensity standards previously mentioned. For most clients, cardiorespiratory changes, including aerobic capacity, continue to take place over many months, perhaps up to 24, as depicted in Figure 7.1. This figure illustrates the relationship between initial functional capacity represented by three cardiorespiratory fitness levels and the relative difference in time required to achieve maximal or near-maximal aerobic capacity (Pollock, 1973; Saltin et al., 1977; McArdle, Katch, & Katch, 2001). This will provide you with a general estimate of expected aerobic capacity changes compared to program duration. Note that early stages of training in those with low cardiorespiratory fitness levels improve CRF relatively quickly in contrast to those who have already achieved either by training or by nature a higher aerobic capacity. Endurance performance (increasing exercise duration) may increase with little or no further increase in aerobic capacity. This is more likely to occur during the latter stages of training, such as the maintenance stage. The time required for other changes to occur, such as body-fat reduction and coronary risk modification, will vary considerably.

SPECIAL CONSIDERATIONS AND SAFETY

You are responsible for determining current health status, developing an exercise program, and following up on a variety of clients. Two areas of special importance are understanding and differentiating the various sources of cardiorespiratory exercise fatigue and maximizing exercise safety.

The ability to recognize and differentiate exercise fatigue is especially helpful when evaluating self-report progress and teaching exertion limitation and safety precautions. Chapter 1 covers the physiology of aerobic and anaerobic capacity.

This section will discuss only basic sources of endurance exercise fatigue and list their basic characteristics. These sources often overlap. For example, during longer exercise bouts, there may be heat fatigue, glycogen depletion, and lactic acid accumulation. Becoming cognizant of each source of fatigue will better enable you to understand the spectrum of exercise responses. Following are six basic sources and manifestations of fatigue observed in cardiorespiratory exercise programs:

1. Exercise fuel depletion. Liver and muscle glycogen (storage forms of carbohydrate) are at relatively low levels after 60 to 80 minutes of intense cardiorespiratory exercise, depending on the level of endurance fitness. This form of fatigue is focused in the exercising muscle groups and, if exercise continues, leads to increasing anaerobic work.

2. Large increases in lactate production and/or accumulation in working muscle is a principal cause of exercise fatigue. This usually is caused by a decreased oxygen supply and/or a substantial increase in glycolysis. This form of fatigue usually comes with overpacing at too high an intensity, usually at levels greater than 80% of maximal oxygen consumption, or as a result of inadequate warm-up. An increase in the production or accumulation of lactic acid may also occur with exercise in hot weather or exercise at relatively high altitudes (more than 5,000 feet, or 1,524 meters). This fatigue has a relatively fast onset. It is characterized by the inability to sustain a pace or intensity, shortness of breath, and transient muscular weakness.

3. Hyperthermia-dehydration. This is a gradual increase in body temperature from prolonged aerobic exercise in hot, humid conditions and/or inadequate water replenishment during prolonged exercise. Elevated body temperatures, high heart rates, inability to sustain usual aerobic exercise intensities, and mental confusion can characterize this form of exercise fatigue.

4. Musculoskeletal (orthopedic). Musculoskeletal discomfort exhibits "fatigue-like" qualities. This discomfort is often the result of overuse, with prolonged repetitive movements or unusual stress on a joint or bone from weightbearing exercise such as jogging. This form of fatigue is nearly always focused on the muscle, ligament, tendon, or joint that is stressed, and is characterized by increasing joint or muscular tenderness that tends to worsen with repeated activity.

5. General overtraining syndrome, or staleness. This syndrome refers to the final stage in a proposed continuum of increasingly severe chronic fatigue states that develop as a result of overtraining, especially high-volume endurance overtraining. Overtraining syndrome is characterized by persistent plateau or worsening in performance that is not improved by short-term rest periods or reduced training. It also is associated with disturbances in mood and sleep, loss of appetite and weight, muscle soreness, a

propensity for overuse injuries, and increased resting heart rate. Chapter 16 of this manual addresses injury prevention in much greater depth. Refer to Raglin and Moger (1999) and Raglin and Wilson (1999) for a current and detailed review of overtraining and staleness syndrome monitoring.

6. Abnormal cardiac symptoms or chest discomfort (angina). Although uncommon, this form of "fatigue" would represent a contraindication to continued exercise and justify a physician referral. This symptom usually characterizes coronary artery disease and someone who is prone to heart attack. Symptoms include chest discomfort (aching, pressure, burning, or tightness), that tends to come with physical effort and is relieved by rest. Always ensure that the client understands the seriousness of the symptoms and discontinues exercise, and require the client to report these symptoms to a physician without delay.

Maximizing Exercise Safety

You should be aware of and understand the behavioral and environmental factors that can either alter the response to exercise or predispose the client to increased risk of injury or cardiovascular complications. These factors include post-meal exercise, thermal stress, air pollutants, drugs and other substances, and the presence of unusual symptoms.

Exercise Following Meals. Vigorous aerobic exercise soon after a full meal can cause the heart to work harder, compromise oxygen and nutrient delivery to the working muscles, and cause gastric discomfort. Consequently, you should advise waiting at least 90 minutes after a full meal before beginning to engage in moderate- and higher-level aerobic exercise. The level of exercise and the amount and type of food ingested both affect the amount of time required for digestion to be completed before beginning exercise. The higher the exercise level and/or the greater the number of calories of food ingested, the longer the individual should wait between eating and exercise.

Thermal Stress. Exercise in hot, humid environments can place the client at risk for heat injury, as well as affect the usual intensity of exercise. Heat injury treatment is discussed on pages 435–436. Methods recommended by the American College of Sports Medicine (2001) can prevent thermal or heat stress.

1. Allow 10 to 14 days for acclimatization to a hot, humid environment.

2. Defer exercise if the heat index is in the "high risk" zone.

3. Avoid training during the hottest part of the day, usually between 10 A.M. and 2 P.M., during summer months.

4. Drink 17-20 ounces of fluid 2 hours before exercising, 7 to 10 ounces every 10 to 20 minutes during activity, and 16 to 24 ounces for every pound lost following exercise. Before and during exercise, replace fluid with either water or an approximately 6% glucose solution.

5. Wear loose-fitting clothing that allows for the evaporation of sweat.

6. Adjust training intensity down by monitoring heart rate.

7. Incorporate compulsory rest periods of at least 10 minutes for every 45 to 50 minutes of physical activity.

8. Closely monitor daily body weight. If losses are greater than 3% of body weight they should be replaced by drinking fluids before the next training session.

9. Give special consideration to, and use caution with, the following heat-susceptible persons: those unacclimatized to the heat, the obese, the unfit (low cardiorespiratory fitness classifications), the dehydrated, and those with a previous history of heat stroke.

Air Pollutants. The principal air pollutants that may concern those who exercise outdoors in or near big cities are ozone, carbon monoxide, and sulfur dioxide. The major factors in determining the dose are the concentration of the pollutant, the duration of the exposure, and the volume of air inhaled. Since ventilation increases with the level of exercise, the effects of the pollutant will also depend on the intensity of exercise. See the *ACSM Resource Manual for Guidelines for Exercise Testing and Prescription,* 4th edition (2001), for a more detailed description of air pollution hazards and exercise.

Perhaps the most problematic of these pollutants is ozone, or smog (not stratospheric ozone), that is formed by the reaction of a combination of ultraviolet light and emissions from internal combustion engines. The level of ozone we breathe is a function of weather patterns, traffic density, and industrial output. Ozone exposure may impair lung function during moderate aerobic exercise at concentrations as low as 0.08 parts per million, which is at or below most air quality standards.

Carbon monoxide is another common air pollutant that can substantially reduce aerobic capacity. A 10% increase in carbon monoxide in the blood results in an approximate 10% reduction in maximal oxygen consumption. Moderate submaximal exercise in healthy individuals does not appear to be significantly affected by a 10 to 15% increase in blood carbon monoxide. Cardiac and pulmonary patients are generally affected by as little as a 5% increase in this pollutant. It also is noteworthy that because of the relatively slow removal of carbon monoxide from the blood (the clearance half-time is two to four hours), exposures that occur hours before an exercise session, on crowded freeways or in smoke-filled rooms, could influence aerobic performance.

Sulfur dioxide is most frequently produced in smelters, refineries, and other stationary sources and is not a major irritant for most apparently healthy individuals. However, those persons with asthma or bronchospasm tendencies may be quite sensitive to sulfur dioxide.

Particulate matter (e.g., dust and smoke) are minute particles that are generally 3 to 10 microns in size that may arise from dust in windy conditions or smoke from burning firewood. Smaller particles of 3 to 5 microns can easily penetrate the upper respiratory

track, whereas those less than 3 microns can settle in the alveoli. Such particulate inhalation can cause bronchoconstriction (asthma symptoms) and inflammation and congestion of the lower respiratory track.

Be aware of the environmental air quality in your area. An excellent resource for local trends and standards of air quality is the county Air Quality Board or local Environmental Protection Agency. In most cities, one of these agencies or the weather bureau will periodically measure these pollutants and combine them into a Pollution Standards Index (PSI) that ranges from 0 to 500. Generally, PSI levels above 100 will affect those who are very unfit or who have cardiovascular or pulmonary disease, while levels greater than 150 will impair cardiorespiratory performance in healthy normal clients. By understanding environmental air quality standards and being knowledgeable of resources for more information, you can minimize unnecessary fatigue and respiratory distress in clients.

Drugs and Other Substances. There are a number of substances that, when combined with moderate-to-high level aerobic exercise, can increase the risk of cardiovascular complications and/or affect the response to exercise. These substances are certain prescription medications, alcohol, tobacco, strong stimulants, and over-the-counter medications. Although each is briefly discussed here, refer to a comprehensive review of drugs and substances and their effects on exercise performance in the *ACSM Resource Manual for Guidelines for Exercise Testing and Prescription,* 4th edition (2001).

Virtually all beta-blocking drugs and some of the calcium-channel blocking medications prescribed for a variety of hypertensive and cardiac disorders lower the heart-rate response to exercise (see pages 160–162). Although these medications may, in fact, increase the client's ability to perform safe exercise, it is important to understand that the heart-rate response to both submaximal

Special Considerations and Safety

and maximal exercise will be blunted. Psychological medications can have side effects that could make exercise more difficult. Some antianxiety medications, such as phenothiazines, can reduce blood pressure and cardiac output, each of which can reduce exercise capacity.

One of the most prevalent categories of drugs employed in medicine, and one that you are likely to at least occasionally observe in your clients, is antihypertensive drugs (i.e., blood pressure–lowering drugs). The major categories of antihypertensive drugs include diuretics, beta- and alpha-blockers, calcium channel blockers, and ACE inhibitors. Within limitations, all of these antihypertensive agents can make exercise safer for the patient with high blood pressure. Diuretic drugs (e.g., thiazides) can induce a relative depletion of blood volume, which can increase the vulnerability of a patient to hypotension in the postexercise period. This side effect of diuretics is of greater concern after prolonged exercise when dehydration may compound the problem.

Alcohol consumption before, during, or after exercise can impair normal exercise heat exchange during prolonged exercise in hot weather. Smoking tobacco in any form increases blood carbon monoxide levels, which will decrease the oxygen consumption of the heart and skeletal muscles. Stimulants such as nicotine, amphetamines, and especially cocaine all have the potential to induce abnormal cardiac rhythms and decrease coronary blood flow. These substances also may mask important signs of exercise fatigue that are important for the client to discern to adjust exercise intensity. Mixing these or combining any of these substances with near-maximal or maximal aerobic exercise markedly increases the risk of cardiovascular complications, even sudden cardiac death.

Over-the-counter medications such as decongestants, antihistamines, and aspirin products are not contraindications to exercise by themselves but warrant attention because of the infections or ailments for which they are taken. You should caution clients who have viral infections to abstain from prolonged and/or intense aerobic exercise because of the potential for complications and cardiac rhythm disturbances.

Unusual Symptoms. Chest discomfort, musculoskeletal pain, dizziness, lightheadedness, or malaise are indications to discontinue exercise and, in some cases, consult a physician. Exceptional chest discomfort (not necessarily chest "pain") such as aching, pressure, tightness, or burning in the chest is always an indication to consult a physician. The client should never exceed the exercise threshold necessary to cause chest discomfort.

When a client experiences overall listlessness and/or recent onset lethargy (feelings of no energy) for no apparent reason, advise the client to either abort exercise or significantly decrease exercise intensity and duration. Such vague symptoms can precede viral infections and even be an indicator of future cardiovascular complications.

Musculoskeletal pain or tenderness in a muscle or joint that tends to increase with increasing exercise intensity or duration is an indication to discontinue that particular mode and/or intensity of exercise (see Chapter 16). The beginner should be told to expect some minor muscle soreness and general postexercise fatigue. These minor symptoms usually resolve themselves in several weeks; however, those musculoskeletal symptoms that tend to reproduce themselves over the course of several weeks warrant special attention.

Exercise during viral infections, such as the flu and upper respiratory infections, may lead to complications including worsening of the infections, an increase in body temperature, and cardiac rhythm disturbances. Advise rest and the usual recuperative recommendations as long as malaise, congestion, or fever persist.

SUMMARY

Cardiorespiratory fitness, or the ability of the lungs to provide oxygen to the blood, and of the heart and circulatory system to transport blood and its nutrients to the tissues, is basic to all fitness programs. You must understand the physiology and application of each component of a cardiorespiratory exercise program: warm-up and cool-down; mode, frequency, duration, and intensity of an exercise session; importance of supporting cardiorespiratory exercise with flexibility and strength exercise; development of a written exercise progression plan that is updated on a regular basis; and information and guidance necessary to ensure each client's safety, including when to defer exercise.

You have a variety of training methods and cardiorespiratory activities with which to develop an exercise program that meets the needs of each client. You must be familiar with the application of, and the physiological response to, five basic training methods: continuous training, interval training, Fartlek training, circuit training, and aerobic composite training. You also must provide guidelines for such popular aerobic and sport activities as walking, jogging, indoor and outdoor cycling, swimming, rowing, traditional aerobics, stair-climbing, racquet sports, and hiking. These guidelines include teaching clients to monitor their exercise intensity using such self-monitoring techniques as heart rate and/or ratings of perceived exertion. Finally, you must understand the various sources of cardiorespiratory exercise fatigue, environmental considerations, and the effects of a variety of drugs and medications, and take proactive steps to maximize exercise safety for each client.

References

REFERENCES

Ainsworth, B.E. et al. (2001). Compendium of Physical Activities: Classification of Energy Costs of Human Physical Activities. In: *ACSM's Resource Manual for Guidelines for Exercise Testing and Prescription* (4th ed.). Philadelphia: Lippincott Williams & Wilkins.

American College of Sports Medicine (2003). *ACSM Fitness Book* (3rd ed.). Champaign, Ill.: Human Kinetics.

American College of Sports Medicine (2006). *ACSM's Guidelines for Exercise Testing and Prescription* (7th ed.). Philadelphia: Lippincott Williams & Wilkins.

American College of Sports Medicine (2001). *ACSM's Resource Manual for Guidelines for Exercise Testing and Prescription* (4th ed.). Philadelphia.: Lippincott Williams & Wilkins.

American Council on Exercise (2000). *Group Fitness Instructor Manual*. San Diego: American Council on Exercise.

Blair, S.N. et al. (1995). Changes in physical fitness and all-cause mortality: a prospective study of healthy and unhealthy men. *Journal of the American Medical Association*, 273, 1093–1098.

Bonelli, S. (2000). *Step Training*. San Diego: American Council on Exercise.

Bonelli, S. (2001). *Aquatic Exercise*. San Diego: American Council on Exercise.

Bricker, K. (2000). *Traditional Aerobics*. San Diego: American Council on Exercise.

Carlton, R. & Rhodes, E. (1985). A critical review of the literature on the ratings scales of perceived exertion. *Sports Medicine*, 2, 198–222.

Diabetes Prevention Program Research Group (2002). Reduction in the incidence of type 2 diabetes with lifestyle intervention or Metformin. *New England Journal of Medicine*, 346, 6, 393–403.

Dishman, R., Farquhar, R., & Cureton, K. (1994). Responses to preferred intensities of exertion in men differing in activity levels. *Medicine and Science in Sports and Exercise*, 26, 783.

Durstine, L. & Pate, R. (1993). Cardiorespiratory responses to acute exercise. *ACSM's Resource Manual for Guidelines for Exercise Testing and Prescription* (2nd ed.). Philadelphia: Lea & Febiger.

Haskell, W.L. (1994). Health consequences of physical activity: understanding and challenges regarding dose-response. *Medicine and Science in Sports and Exercise*, 26, 649–660.

Heyward, V.H. (1984). *Designs for Fitness*. Minneapolis, Minn.: Burgess Publishing.

Howley, E. & Franks, D. (2003). *Health Fitness Instructor's Handbook* (4th ed.). Champaign, Ill.: Human Kinetics.

Howley, E. & Glover, M. (1974). The caloric costs of running and walking 1 mile for men and women. *Medicine and Science in Sports and Exercise*, 6, 235–237.

Lan, C. et al. (1998). 12-month tai chi training in the elderly: its effect on health fitness. *Medicine and Science in Sports and Exercise*, 30, 345–351.

Lee, I.-M. et al. (2003). Relative intensity of physical activity and risk of coronary heart disease. *Circulation*, 107, 1110–1116.

McArdle, W., Katch, F., & Katch, V. (2001). *Exercise Physiology: Energy, Nutrition, and Human Performance* (5th ed.). Philadelphia: Lippincott Williams & Wilkins.

National Institute of Health: Consensus Development Panel on Physical Activity and Cardiovascular Health (1996). Physical activity and cardiovascular health. *Journal of the American Medical Association*, 276, 241–246.

Neporent, L. & Schlosberg, S. (1999). *Fitness for Dummies* (2nd ed.). Hoboken, N.J.: John Wiley & Sons.

Nieman, D. (1990). *Fitness and Sports Medicine: An Introduction*. Palo Alto, Calif.: Bull Publishing.

Parker, S. et al. (1989). Failure of target heart rate to accurately monitor intensity during aerobic dance. *Medicine and Science in Sports and Exercise*, 21, 230.

Pate, R.R. et al. (1995). Physical activity and public health: a recommendation from the Centers for Disease Control and American College of Sports Medicine. *Journal of the American Medical Association*, 273, 402–407.

Pollock, M. (1973). The quantification of endurance training programs. *Exercise and Sport Science Reviews*, 1, 155–188.

Raglin, J. & Moger, L. (1999). Adverse psychological consequences of physical activity: when more is too much. In: *Lifestyles Medicine*, J.M. Rippe (Ed.). Worcester, Mass.: Blackwell Scientific.

Raglin, J.S. & Wilson, G.S. (1999). Overtraining in athletes. In: *Emotion in Sports*, Y.L. Hanin (Ed.). Champaign, Ill.: Human Kinetics.

Saltin, B. et al. (1977). Fiber types and metabolic potentials of skeletal muscles in sedentary men and endurance runners. *Annals of the New York Academy of Science*, 301, 3.

Shechtman, N. (2000). *Group Indoor Cycling*. San Diego: American Council on Exercise.

Whaley, M. et al. (1992). Questioning the routine use of 220 - AGE heart rate formula. *Medicine and Science in Sports and Exercise*, 24, 1173.

Wells, C. & Pate, R. (1988). Training for performance in prolonged exercise. In: *Prolonged Exercise* (Vol.1), 357–389. D. Lamb & R. Murray (Eds.) Carmel, Ind.: Benchmark Press.

SUGGESTED READING

American Heart Association (2001). Exercise standards for testing and training. *Circulation,* 104, 1694.

Astrand, P.O. & Rodahl, K. (2003). *Textbook of Work Physiology.* (4th ed.). New York: McGraw-Hill.

Borg, G. (1982). Psychological basis of perceived exertion. *Medicine and Science in Sports and Exercise,* 14, 377–381.

Borg, G. (1998). *Borg's Perceived Exertion and Pain Scales.* Champaign, Ill.: Human Kinetics.

Franks D. & Howley, E. (1990). *Fitness Facts.* Champaign, Ill.: Human Kinetics.

Greenberg, J. & Pargman, D. (1989). *Physical Fitness: A Wellness Approach.* (2nd ed.). Englewood Cliffs, N.J.: Prentice-Hall.

Herbert, W. & Herbert, D. *The Exercise Standards and Malpractice Reporter,* 1987 to present.

Ketner, J.B. & Mekkion, M.B. (1995). The overtraining syndrome: a review of presentation, pathophysiology, and treatment. *Medicine, Exercise, Nutrition, & Health,* 4, 136–145.

Ockene, I. & Ockene, J. (1992). *Prevention of Coronary Heart Disease.* Boston: Little Brown & Company.

Pollock, M. & Wilmore, J. (2007). *Exercise in Health and Disease.* (3rd ed.). Philadelphia: WB Saunders.

Raglin, J.S. (1993). Overtraining and Staleness: Psychometric Monitoring of Endurance Athletes. In: *Handbook of Research on Sport Psychology.* R.B. Singer, M. Murphey, & L. Tennant (Eds.). New York: Macmillan.

Richie, D. (1989). Medical and legal implications of dance exercise leadership: the role of footwear. *Exercise Standards and Malpractice Reporter,* 3, 61.

Sanders, M. (Ed.) (2000). *YMCA Water Fitness for Health.* Champaign, Ill.: Human Kinetics.

Shapiro, U. & Seidman, D. (1990). Field and clinical observations of exertional heat stroke patients. *Medicine and Science in Sports and Exercise,* 22, 1.

Wilmore, J.H., Costill, D. & Kenney, W.L. (2007). *Physiology of Sport and Exercise.* (4th ed.). Champaign, Ill.: Human Kinetics.

CHAPTER 8

Muscular Strength and Endurance

Wayne L. Westcott, Ph.D., is the Fitness Research Director for the South Shore YMCA in Quincy, Mass., and the author of 15 books on strength fitness. He has served as a strength-training consultant to

Wayne L. Westcott

the YMCA of the USA, the President's Council on Physical Fitness and Sports, the American Council on Exercise, IDEA, and Prevention, Men's Health, Fitness, Club Industry, and Fitness Management magazines. Dr. Westcott has received both the Healthy American Fitness Leader Award from the President's Council and the IDEA Lifetime Achievement award for service to the fitness profession.

Every movement we make involves our muscular system. Muscles are unique in their ability to relax, contract, and produce force. In addition, this metabolically active tissue is highly responsive to training stimuli. With appropriate exercise, muscles become larger and stronger; without appropriate exercise, muscles become smaller and weaker. This chapter presents information about the benefits of sensible strength training and the recommended procedures for safe, effective, and efficient muscle development.

STRENGTH BENEFITS

Strength training is the process of exercising with progressively heavier resistance for the purpose of strengthening the musculoskeletal system. Physiologically, regular strength training results in the following positive adaptations:

✔ increased muscle fiber size
✔ increased muscle contractile strength
✔ increased tendon tensile strength
✔ increased bone strength
✔ increased ligament tensile strength

These beneficial changes within the musculoskeletal tissue have a profound influence on our physical capacity, physical appearance, metabolic function, and injury risk.

Physical Capacity

Physical capacity may be loosely defined as one's ability to perform work or exercise. Muscles utilize energy to produce movement and generate strength, functioning as the engines of our bodies. Specifically, strength training increases the size and strength of our muscle fibers, resulting in a greater physical capacity to perform work. Stronger muscles enable us to lift a heavier weight once (muscle strength) and to lift a lighter weight more than once (muscle endurance).

Research indicates that previously untrained men and women gain about 2 to 4 pounds of muscle and 40 to 60% more strength after two months of regular strength exercise. The rate of muscle gain and strength development slows down after the initial training period, but typically continues for several months.

Physical Appearance

Our skeletal muscles have a lot to do with our overall physique. Consequently, strength training can play a major role in enhancing our **body composition** and physical appearance. Consider a 114-pound woman who is 24% fat (27 pounds fat weight, 87 pounds lean weight). If she loses 4 pounds of fat and adds 4 pounds of muscle she will still weigh 114 pounds but will be only 20% fat (23 pounds fat weight, 91 pounds lean weight). Although her body weight remains the same, she has less fat and more muscle for a leaner, firmer, and fitter appearance.

Our physical appearance and capacity can be positively influenced by muscle gain or negatively influenced by muscle loss. Unfortunately, unless we perform regular strength exercise, we lose more than one-half pound of muscle every year of life after age 25. Without an appropriate training stimulus, our muscles gradually decrease in size and strength (atrophy). Strength training is essential for preventing the muscle loss that often accompanies the aging process.

Metabolic Function

Muscle is very active tissue with high energy requirements for maintenance and rebuilding processes. Even while we sleep, our skeletal muscles are responsible for more than 25% of our calorie use. An increase in muscle tissue causes a corresponding increase in our metabolic rate; likewise, a decrease in muscle tissue causes a corresponding decrease in our metabolic rate.

The gradual loss of muscle tissue in nontraining adults leads to a 5% reduction in metabolic rate every decade of life. This gradual decrease in metabolism is closely related to the gradual increase in body fat that typically accompanies the aging process. When less energy is required for daily metabolic function, calories that were previously used by muscle tissue are stored as fat. Although our metabolism eventually slows down with age, this and other degenerative processes can be markedly delayed through regular strength training.

Injury Risk

In addition to functioning as the engines of the body, our muscles also serve as shock absorbers and balancing agents. Strong muscles help dissipate the repetitive landing forces experienced in weightbearing activities such as running and aerobic dance. Balanced muscle development reduces the risk of overuse injuries that result when one muscle group is much stronger than its opposing muscle group. Jogging, for example, places more stress on the **posterior** leg muscles than the **anterior** leg muscles, creating a muscle imbalance that may cause knee injuries.

To reduce the risk of unbalanced muscle development, trainers should address opposing muscle groups such as the gastrocnemius and anterior tibialis muscles of the leg, quadriceps and hamstring muscles of the thigh, low-back and abdominal muscles of the midsection, pectoralis, latissimus dorsi and deltoid muscles of the torso, biceps and triceps muscles of the arm, and flexor and extensor muscles of the neck.

A comprehensive strength-training program that addresses all of the major muscle groups may be the most effective means of reducing the risk of injury and many degenerative diseases. Although four out of five Americans experience low-back discomfort, 80% of low-back problems are muscular in nature and appear to be preventable by strengthening the low-back muscles. Strength training also has been shown to increase bone mineral density, improve glucose metabolism, reduce gastrointestinal transit time, lower resting blood pressure, improve blood lipid levels, and ease arthritic pain.

STRENGTH PRODUCTION

When a muscle is signaled to contract, it develops tension and attempts to shorten. The resulting movement, or lack of movement, depends on the relationship between muscular forces and resistive forces.

Isometric Contraction. When the muscular force is equal to the resistive force, there is no movement. This is known as an **isometric contraction** and is most representative of one's actual strength production. For example, if Ralph can hold a maximum weight of 50 pounds at 90 degrees of elbow flexion, his effective isometric force output is 50 pounds.

Concentric Contraction. When the muscular force is greater than the resistive force, the muscle shortens, resulting in a **concentric** (positive) **contraction.** Concentric contractions are not as strong as isometric contractions because internal muscle friction decreases the effective force output by about 20%. For example, Ralph can hold a maximum weight of 50 pounds at 90 degrees of elbow flexion (isometric contraction), but he can lift a maximum weight of 40 pounds in the biceps curl exercise (concentric contraction). Ralph's actual strength production is still 50 pounds, but internal muscle friction subtracts about 20% from his effective concentric force output.

Eccentric Contraction. When the muscular force is less than the resistive force, the muscle lengthens, resulting in an **eccentric** (negative) **contraction.** Eccentric contractions are stronger than isometric contractions because internal muscle friction increases the effective force output by about 20%. For example, Ralph can hold a maximum weight of 50 pounds at 90 degrees of elbow flexion (isometric contraction), but he can lower a maximum weight of 60 pounds in the biceps curl exercise (eccentric contraction). Ralph's actual strength production is still 50 pounds, but internal muscle friction adds about 20% to his effective eccentric force output.

Prime Mover Muscles. Muscles that are principally responsible for a given joint movement are called **prime mover muscles.** For example, the biceps muscles are prime movers, contracting concentrically

Strength Production

during the lifting phase and eccentrically during the lowering phase of the biceps curl exercise.

Antagonist Muscles. Muscles that produce the opposite joint movement are referred to as antagonist muscles. For example, the triceps muscles responsible for elbow extension serve as **antagonists** to the biceps muscles. Antagonist muscles work cooperatively with prime mover muscles to produce smooth and controlled joint movements.

Stabilizer Muscles. Muscles that stabilize one joint so that the desired movement can occur at another joint are known as **stabilizer** muscles. For example, during the biceps curl exercise, the pectoralis major and latissimus dorsi muscles contract isometrically to stabilize the shoulder joint so that the desired movement can occur at the elbow joint.

Fiber Types. Muscles are composed of two primary fiber types: **slow-twitch (Type I)** and **fast-twitch (Type II).** The smaller slow-twitch fibers are better suited for aerobic energy utilization and can produce relatively low levels of force for relatively long periods of time. The larger fast-twitch fibers are suited for anaerobic energy utilization and can produce relatively high levels of force for relatively short periods of time. During a typical set of a strength exercise, both slow-twitch and fast-twitch muscle fibers actively participate in force production. The more fatigue-resistant slow-twitch fibers are recruited first. As resistive forces increase, the less fatigue-resistant fast-twitch fibers are recruited.

Motor Unit. A motor unit consists of a single motor nerve and all of the muscle fibers to which it attaches. A typical slow-twitch motor unit contains about 100 muscle fibers, and a typical fast-twitch motor unit contains about 500 muscle fibers. When activated, all of the muscle fibers in a motor unit maximally contract simultaneously. This is known as the **all-or-none principle.** Therefore, curling a 5-pound dumbbell requires only a few (slow-twitch)

motor units, but curling a 35-pound dumbbell requires many (slow-twitch and fast-twitch) motor units. Much of the performance improvement during the initial weeks of strength training is due to more efficient motor unit utilization. This is known as the **motor learning effect.**

Muscle Fatigue. The temporary muscle fatigue encountered during an exercise set is most likely due to a variety of physiological changes within the working muscle. These factors may include lactic acid accumulation, increased tissue acidity, nerve impulse interference, and chemical energy depletion. Temporary muscle fatigue and discomfort pass quickly upon cessation of the exercise.

Muscle Soreness. A more lasting form of muscle discomfort is known as **delayed onset muscle soreness (DOMS).** DOMS is usually experienced 24 to 48 hours following a demanding strength-training session. It is typically associated with eccentric muscle contractions and is most likely the result of microscopic tears in the muscle or connective tissue. DOMS indicates that a few non-training days may be required for the tissue repair and building processes that lead to stronger muscles.

STRENGTH FACTORS

We have little control over a number of factors that affect our strength performance. These include gender, age, limb length, muscle length, tendon insertion, and muscle fiber type.

Gender. Gender does not affect the quality of our muscle, but it does influence the quantity. Although male and female muscle tissue is essentially the same, men typically have more muscle than women because muscle size is positively influenced by the presence of testosterone, a male sex hormone. Because most human muscles produce approximately 1 to 2 kilograms of force per square centimeter of cross-sectional area, larger muscles are stronger muscles. However, when evaluated on a pound-for-pound basis, men and women demonstrate similar strength performance. For example, one study evaluated quadriceps strength in more than 900 men and women. The average male performed 10 strict leg extensions with 62% of his body weight, and the average female completed 10 strict leg extensions with 55% of her body weight. However, when assessed in terms of lean body weight, average strength performances for the men and women were almost identical.

Age. Recent research has revealed that men and women of all ages can increase their muscle size and muscle strength through progressive strength training. However, the rate of strength gain appears to be greater during the years of normal growth and development, generally considered to be from ages 10 to 20.

Limb Length. There are several reasons for avoiding strength comparisons with other individuals. One of these is related to limb length. Other things being equal, people with short limbs may use more exercise resistance than people with long limbs because favorable leverage factors enhance effective force output. For example, Jim and John have identical strength capacity in their biceps muscles. However, because Jim has a shorter forearm he can hold more weight at 90 degrees of elbow flexion due to his leverage advantage.

Muscle Length. Muscles are attached to bones by **connective tissue** called tendons. Relative to bone length, some people have long muscles with short tendon attachments, while others have short muscles with long tendon attachments. Other things being equal, people with relatively long muscles have a greater potential for developing size and strength than people with relatively short muscles.

Tendon Insertion. Another factor that influences effective muscle strength is the point of tendon insertion. For example, Susan and Gayle both have the same forearm length and biceps strength. However, Susan's biceps tendon attaches to her forearm a little farther from her elbow joint than Gayle's. This gives Susan a biomechanical advantage that enables her to use more resistance than Gayle in elbow flexion exercises.

Muscle Fiber Type. Most men and women have a fairly even mix of slow-twitch and fast-twitch fibers in the majority of their skeletal muscles. However, some people inherit a high percentage of slow-twitch muscle fibers, which enhances their performance potential for endurance exercise. For example, world-class distance runners are born with a preponderance of slow-twitch muscle fibers that, given appropriate training programs, enable them to be successful in their events. Other people inherit a high percentage of fast-twitch muscle fibers that enhances their performance potential for power activities. For example, world-class sprinters are born with a preponderance of fast-twitch muscle fibers that, given appropriate training programs, enable them to be successful in their events.

Although both fiber types respond positively to progressive resistance training, the fast-twitch fibers experience greater increases in size and strength (hypertrophy). Consequently, people with a preponderance of fast-twitch muscle fibers may obtain better results from their strength-training program.

STRENGTH/ENDURANCE RELATIONSHIPS

Muscle strength is defined as one's ability to perform a single repetition with maximum resistance. Muscle endurance is one's ability to perform many repetitions with a sub-maximum resistance. Muscle endurance may be evaluated at any point beyond the first repetition on the strength-endurance continuum.

Although one may train specifically for muscle strength or muscle endurance, there is an inherent relationship between these abilities. Research indicates that most

**Strength/
Endurance
Relationships**

people can perform about 10 repetitions with 75% of their maximum resistance. For example, if Kim's maximum bench press is 100 pounds, she can most likely complete 10 repetitions with 75 pounds. If she increases her maximum bench press to 120 pounds, she should be able to complete 10 repetitions with 90 pounds. In other words, Kim's 10-repetition maximum resistance changes in direct proportion to her **one-repetition maximum.**

People with a high percentage of fast-twitch (low endurance) muscle fibers typically perform fewer repetitions with 75% of their maximum resistance, whereas people with a high percentage of slow-twitch (high endurance) muscle fibers typically perform more repetitions with 75% of their maximum resistance. Because the ratio of fast-twitch to slow-twitch muscle fibers is largely unaffected by training protocol, it appears that genetics largely determines our muscle endurance with a given percentage of maximum resistance.

STRENGTH-TRAINING EQUIPMENT

There are basically four categories of strength-training equipment. These include devices that provide isometric resistance, isokinetic resistance, dynamic constant resistance, and dynamic variable resistance.

Isometric Equipment

Although **isometric (static) equipment** is frequently used for testing muscle strength, it is seldom recommended for developing muscle strength. This is because isometric muscle contractions restrict blood flow and may trigger unacceptable increases in blood pressure. Whenever possible, it is best to avoid isometric forms of strength training. However, if isometric exercises are used, encourage the client to breathe continuously during each contraction.

The advantages of isometric exercise include little equipment, low cost, space

efficiency, and time efficiency. Disadvantages include blood pressure escalation, increases in strength only at specifically exercised positions in the movement range, training monotony, and lack of performance feedback.

Isokinetic Equipment

Isokinetic equipment is characterized by a constant movement speed and a matching resistive force. That is, the amount of muscle force applied determines the amount of resistive force encountered. A greater muscle force produces a greater resistive force, and vice versa.

There are various types of isokinetic equipment, including hydraulic resistance machines and electronic resistance machines. Hydraulic machines provide resistance only during concentric muscle contractions. Some electronic machines provide resistance only during concentric muscle contractions, while others offer resistance during both the concentric and eccentric movements.

The advantages of isokinetic exercise include accommodating resistance forces, speed regulation, detailed performance feedback, and reduced muscle soreness. Disadvantages include cost of equipment, inconsistent force regulation, and lack of eccentric muscle contractions.

Dynamic Constant Resistance Equipment

Barbells are an example of **dynamic (isotonic) constant resistance equipment.** First, the amount of resistive force encountered determines the amount of muscle force applied. A greater resistive force requires a greater muscle force, and vice-versa. Second, the resistive force remains constant throughout the exercise movement. However, due to the mechanics of human movement, the effective muscle force is higher in some positions and lower in other positions. As a result, the muscle effort varies throughout the exercise movement.

The advantages of dynamic constant resistance exercise include low cost of equipment, similarity to most work and exercise activities, variety of training movements, tangible evidence of improvement, and easy accessibility. Disadvantages include the inability to train through a full range of joint motion in some exercises and inconsistent matching of resistive forces and muscular forces throughout the exercise movements.

Dynamic Variable Resistance Equipment

Dynamic (isotonic) variable resistance equipment is similar to dynamic constant resistance equipment in that the amount of resistive force encountered determines the amount of muscle force applied. It is different in that the resistive force changes throughout the exercise movement. By the use of moving levers, cams, or linkage systems, dynamic variable resistance machines provide proportionally less resistive force in weaker muscle positions and proportionally more resistive force in stronger muscle positions. Consequently, the muscle effort remains relatively constant throughout the exercise movement. Dynamic variable resistance is provided by specially designed weight stack machines and air pressure equipment.

The advantages of dynamic variable resistance exercise include the ability to train through a full range of motion on most exercises, reasonably consistent matching of resistive forces and muscular forces throughout the exercise movements and, in most cases, tangible evidence of improvement. Disadvantages include equipment expense, limited number of training movements, and lack of accessibility.

STRENGTH-TRAINING GUIDELINES

There are as many ways to develop muscle strength as there are strength trainers. In fact, almost any form of progressive resistance exercise will stimulate some degree of strength gain. Unfortunately, many strength-training programs have a high rate of injury and a low rate of muscle development.

The following exercise guidelines are essential to safe, effective, and efficient strength training. While they may not be fully representative of advanced bodybuilding or weight-lifting routines, they provide a sensible approach for achieving high levels of strength fitness.

Exercise Selection. It is important to select at least one exercise for each major muscle group to ensure comprehensive muscle development. Training only a few muscle groups leads to muscle imbalance and increases the risk of injury. The major muscle groups include the quadriceps, hamstrings, hip adductors, hip abductors, low-back, abdominals, pectoralis major, rhomboids, trapezius, latissimus dorsi, deltoids, biceps, triceps, neck flexors, and neck extensors. Other muscle groups that should be trained regularly are the gluteals, obliques, gastrocnemius, anterior tibialis, forearm flexors, and forearm extensors.

Exercise Sequence. When performing a series or circuit of strength exercises, it is advisable to proceed from the larger muscle groups of the legs to the smaller muscle groups of the torso, arms, and neck. This allows you to perform the most demanding exercises when you are the least fatigued. Another option is to group exercises into antagonistic movements or into upper-/lower-body movements. This type of exercise sequencing can provide recovery between exercises and decrease the duration of the workout.

Exercise Speed. Exercise speed plays a major role in both injury risk and strength development. Lifting at a fast pace places a high level of stress on the muscles and connective tissue at the beginning of each movement. Lifting at a slower pace requires a more even application of muscle force throughout the movement range. In addition, slow movement speeds are characterized by less momentum and less internal muscle friction. Although control is the major objective, a reasonable training recommendation is one to two seconds for

Strength-training Guidelines

each lifting movement (concentric contraction) and three to four seconds for each lowering movement (eccentric contraction).

Exercise Sets. An exercise set is usually defined as a number of successive repetitions performed without resting. The number of sets per exercise is largely a matter of personal preference. Several studies have shown similar strength gains from one, two, or three sets of exercise. Clients who prefer single-set exercise usually continue to the point of momentary muscle failure, which is referred to as high-intensity training. Those who choose multiple-set exercise typically rest one to three minutes between sets. Multiple-set training may be advisable for clients who prefer not to push themselves hard on single-set exercise routines. Regardless of the number of sets performed, each repetition should be done using proper exercise form and control.

An advantage of multiple-set strength training is the higher-calorie use for the longer exercise session. An advantage of single-set strength training is the lower time requirement for the shorter exercise session.

Exercise Resistance and Repetitions.
There is an inverse relationship between exercise resistance and exercise repetitions as you will note in Table 8.1.

Training above 85% of maximum resistance increases the injury risk and training below 65% of maximum resistance decreases the strength stimulus. Consequently, 8 to 12 repetitions with 70 to 80% of maximum resistance is a sound training recommendation for safe and productive strength development. When performed in a controlled manner, 8 to 12 repetitions with 70 to 80% of maximum resistance require about 50 to 70 seconds of high-intensity (anaerobic) muscle effort.

Exercise Range. It is important to perform each exercise through a full range of joint movement, with emphasis on the completely contracted position. Full-range exercise movements are advantageous for strengthening the prime-mover muscles and for stretching the

Table 8.1
Percent of the 1 RM and Repetitions Performed

%1 RM	Number of Repetitions Performed
100	1
95	2
93	3
90	4
87	5
85	6
83	7
80	8
77	9
75	10
70	11
67	12
65	15

Adapted, by permission, from Baechle, T.R, Earle, R.W., & Wathen, D. (2000). *Resistance training, in: Essentials of Strength Training and Conditioning* (2nd ed.). NSCA, edited by T.R. Baechle & R.W. Earle. Champaign, Ill.: Human Kinetics.

antagonist muscles, thereby enhancing both muscle strength and joint flexibility.

Exercise Progression. The key to strength development is progressive resistance. As the muscles adapt to a given exercise resistance, it must be gradually increased to stimulate further strength gains. Of course, the increase in resistance is usually accompanied by a temporary decrease in the number of repetitions performed with the heavier weightload.

A double progressive program, in which the client alternately increases repetitions and resistance, is recommended for safe and systematic muscle strengthening. The client begins with a resistance that can be performed at least eight times. When 12 repetitions can be completed, the resistance is increased by 5% or less. For example, when Mary is able to perform 12 repetitions with 50 pounds, she increases the resistance to 52.5 pounds. When she achieves 12 repetitions with 52.5 pounds, she increases the resistance to 55 pounds. Under certain circumstances it may not be practical to increase the resistance by 5% or less. Although each case must be evaluated individually, it is not advisable to increase the resistance by more than 10% between successive training sessions.

Exercise Frequency. High-intensity resistance exercise may produce tissue microtrauma that temporarily reduces strength output and causes varying degrees of muscle soreness. This is why ample rest time between successive training sessions is so important. During this recovery period, the muscles synthesize proteins and build slightly higher levels of strength. Because the muscle rebuilding process typically requires about 48 hours, strength workouts should be scheduled on an every-other day basis. Clients who prefer to train more frequently should avoid working the same muscle groups on consecutive days.

STRENGTH PROGRAM CONSIDERATIONS

These strength-training guidelines address those factors most essential for a safe and productive exercise session for presumably healthy adults. However, there are additional considerations that may affect the overall training program. For a more detailed discussion of exercise considerations when working with special populations, see *Exercise Testing and Program Design,* by Bryant, Franklin, and Conviser.

Common Training Mistakes

The most common and critical training mistakes are related to exercise technique. The tendency to use too much resistance typically results in poor form, which decreases the training stimulus and increases the injury risk. Examples of unacceptable exercise form include rebounding the bar off the chest in the bench press, bouncing at the bottom of the squat, using hip/back extension to initiate barbell curls, bending backward under barbell presses, and using momentum and fast training speeds.

Warm-up

It is always prudent to warm up prior to a strength-training workout. A few minutes of progressive warm-up exercise physiologically and psychologically prepares the body for higher levels of effort and energy utilization. Although warm-up routines may take many forms, it is advisable to include some light aerobic activity such as stationary cycling or stairclimbing. It also is important to perform stretching exercises for the major muscle groups, paying particular attention to the low-back area.

Because many clients are pressed for time, they often eliminate or abbreviate the warm-up exercises. You should encourage clients to take full advantage of a progressive warm-up to reduce their risk of injury and enhance training responsiveness.

Cool-down

Blood tends to accumulate in the lower body when a vigorous exercise session is stopped abruptly. With reduced blood return, cardiac output decreases and lightheadedness may occur. Because muscle movement helps squeeze blood back to the heart, it is important to continue lower-level physical activity after the last exercise set is completed. Easy cycling and walking are appropriate cool-down activities. A few stretching exercises are recommended at the conclusion of the cooldown. Because of possible cardiovascular complications, you must not permit clients to omit the cool-down portion of their workout. As a general guideline, the last 5 to 10 minutes of the training session should be dedicated to cool-down activity.

Circuit Training

Circuit training is a form of strength training in which the client performs a series of strength exercises with little rest between exercise stations. One popular system of circuit training involves a line of 10 to 12 exercise machines that work each major muscle group, from largest to smallest. This type of training is effective for strength development and is efficient in terms of time commitment. Generally, a 10-to-12-station strength circuit can be completed in 20 to 25 minutes. Although not the recommended means of cardiovascular conditioning, positive physiological adaptations can result from maintaining a target-zone heart rate throughout a 20- to 25-minute circuit strength-training session (e.g., 5–10% improvement in $\dot{V}O_2$ max).

Bodybuilding Routine

Some clients have the genetic potential and personal motivation to pursue competitive bodybuilding. The major objective in bodybuilding is to develop larger muscles. Bodybuilders typically perform several sets (4 to 6) of moderate repetitions (8 to 12) in each exercise, with brief rests (15 to 45 seconds) between sets. This produces blood accumulation within the muscles and is referred to as a muscle pump. Furthermore, bodybuilders generally perform three to five exercises per muscle group to maximize fiber involvement. Because bodybuilding routines are very demanding in terms of time and energy, many bodybuilders follow a six-day training schedule. For example, to provide ample rebuilding time they may train their legs, low back, and abdominals on Mondays and Thursdays, their chest, shoulders, and triceps on Tuesdays and Fridays, and their upper back, biceps, and neck on Wednesdays and Saturdays.

Weight-lifting Routine

Some clients have the genetic potential and personal motivation to pursue competitive weight lifting. The main objective in weight lifting is to develop stronger muscles, particularly those involved in the competitive lifts. Olympic lifters compete in two explosive lifts—the clean and jerk and the snatch. Power lifters compete in three slow lifts—the squat, the bench press, and the dead lift.

Because strength maximization and sport specificity require the use of relatively heavy weightloads, weight lifters usually take long rests (three to six minutes) between sets. They generally perform several sets (six to eight) of low repetitions (two to six) in the competitive lifts and a few sets of supplementary exercises. Because the training programs may be very demanding and time consuming, some weight lifters perform different exercises on different days with ample rebuilding time for individual muscle groups.

Plyometrics

Plyometrics, also known as jump training, involves stretching the muscles prior to contracting them. The Eastern Europeans first used plyometrics in the 1970s to develop greater strength and power in Olympic athletes. They based their programs on scientific evidence that stretching muscles prior to contracting them recruits the **myotatic reflex,** or stretch reflex, of a muscle to enhance the power of contraction. This prestretching of muscles occurs when jumps are performed one after the other. For example, when an individual lands from a jump, the quadriceps muscles at the front of the thighs stretch as their knees bend, and then quickly contract with the next leap. This prestretch enhances the power of the second jump.

Plyometric training has received its share of criticism due to reported cases of injury following plyometric programs of depth jumping and drop jumping, which involve jumping up to, and down from, boxes or benches that can be as high as 42 inches (106 cm). The forces sustained from these types of jumps onto hard surfaces can be as much as seven times an individual's body weight. Careful consideration of the type of jumps selected for the program, proper supervision by a competent trainer or coach, and gradual progression to more difficult exercises can make a plyometric program both safe and effective.

A safe and effective plyometric program should also stress the quality, not quantity, of jumps. Safe landing techniques, such as landing from toe to heel from a vertical jump and using the entire foot as a rocker when landing, dissipate the impact forces associated with landing over a greater surface area. When landing, individuals should avoid excessive side-to-side motion at the knee. Landing forces can be absorbed through the muscles of the lower extremity (quadriceps, hamstrings, calf muscles) more effectively when the knee bends primarily in only one plane of motion.

Spotting

In terms of performance enhancement, few things are more effective than a conscientious trainer who demands proper technique and full effort on every exercise set, and gives plenty of encouragement and just enough assistance to permit completion of a final repetition. One of your most important functions as a personal trainer is to provide protection in high-risk barbell exercises such as squats, bench presses, and incline presses. These lifts should not be performed without proper spotting, since failure to complete the final repetition could trap the client under a heavy barbell. During the squat, you should stand behind the client ready to help him or her to a standing position (arms around upper torso), if necessary. During the bench press and incline press, you should stand behind the bench ready to grasp the barbell and help lift it back to the standards when needed.

In addition to reducing the risk of injury, you can assist your clients by observing and modifying their training technique when using either free weights or machines.

Program Discontinuation

If for some reason it is necessary to discontinue strength training, one result is certain. In the absence of a strength stimulus the muscles gradually become smaller and weaker (atrophy). Although the rate of decrease may vary among individuals, strength loss occurs at about one-half the rate of strength gain. For example, during a 12-week training program Natalie gained strength at the rate of 5% per week. If Natalie discontinues her training, she will most likely lose strength at the rate of 2.5% per week until she is slightly above her pretraining level of strength. Because eating habits tend to remain rather consistent, calories that were previously utilized during strength workouts are stored as fat. Less muscle mass results in a lower metabolic rate, further reducing calorie use, and increasing fat stores. Without careful attention to diet, program discontinuation may be followed by simultaneous muscle loss and fat gain for a disappointing change in body composition, **physical capacity,** and personal appearance. Fortunately, one or two brief workouts per week are sufficient to maintain strength levels for extended periods of time. It is therefore better to schedule an abbreviated strength-training program than to discontinue strength exercise altogether.

ERGOGENIC AIDS AND SUPPLEMENTS

Protein Supplements

Muscle tissue is composed of approximately 75 to 80% water and about 20% **protein.** Protein has been emphasized as a muscle-building **nutrient,** and numerous protein supplements are available for the purpose of enhancing muscle growth. This is unfortunate for several reasons:

✔ The typical diet in modern nations provides considerably more protein than the relatively small amount required for muscle development. In fact, a 175-pound adult requires only 80 grams of protein per day (1 gram of protein for every 2.2 pounds of body-weight), which is less than 3 ounces of protein daily.

✔ Protein consumption in and of itself does not increase muscle size. After the growth years, muscles must be stimulated by progressive resistance exercise to increase their size and strength. In fact, even though

Ergogenic Aids and Supplements

American adults ingest plenty of protein, they lose more than one-half pound of muscle every year unless they perform regular strength training.

✔ Consuming too much protein can be physically harmful. Extra protein must be broken down metabolically, and the waste products must be excreted from the body, placing additional strain on the kidneys.

Vitamins and Minerals

With regard to **vitamins** and **minerals,** a balanced diet typically provides an abundance of these nutrients. Two possible exceptions are calcium and iron. However, like protein, calcium is abundant in low-fat dairy products, and iron is found in lean meats, poultry, and fish. Although a little extra protein and a daily 100% RDA vitamin/mineral pill may be advisable in some situations, a balanced daily diet is the best recommendation for meeting normal nutritional needs (see Chapter 4).

Steroids

Anabolic steroids are synthetic derivatives of the male sex hormone testosterone and are taken to increase muscle size and strength. When combined with strength exercise, anabolic steroids may enhance muscle protein synthesis and tissue-building processes. However, the physical and psychological harm that may result from anabolic steroid use far outweighs all possible benefits. The potential consequences of anabolic steroid use include increased blood pressure, decreased levels of **HDL cholesterol,** liver enzyme leakage, liver cancer, testicle **atrophy,** sterility, breast shrinkage, uterus shrinkage, and uncontrolled mood swings from depression to aggression. It is strongly recommended that anabolic steroids be avoided for medical and ethical reasons. Sensible strength training and proper nutrition are the keys to muscle development, without the risk of harmful side effects.

The following material describing three of the most popular performance-enhancing supplements—androstenedione, creatine, and DHEA—was taken, with permission, from *Exercise Testing and Program Design,* by Bryant, Franklin, and Conviser.

Androstenedione

Androstenedione is a male sex hormone produced naturally by the body, which can be converted to testosterone. It is also marketed and sold as a natural supplement under various trade names (all of which have some form of the word "andro" in their names). Androstenedione is believed to have first been used by East German sports scientists to enhance the performance capabilities of their Olympic athletes. The popularity of androstenedione skyrocketed in 1998 after it was revealed that record-setting baseball slugger Mark McGwire used the supplement.

The marketers and manufacturers of "andro" (as it is popularly called) claim that a 100-mg dose of andro can increase plasma concentrations of testosterone by a factor of four within 90 minutes. Additional claims include increases in muscle size, strength, energy, immune function, libido (sex drive), and general well-being. It has been suggested that, as with other steroids, andro improves the body's ability to rapidly recover from strenuous physical activity, allowing users to train more frequently and at higher intensities. Presumably, the result of such training would be a substantial increase in muscle size and strength.

Dr. Charles Yesalis, a leading expert on the topic of anabolic steroids, contends that andro should be placed on the list of substances covered by the Anabolic Steroid Control Act of 1990, and its use should be controlled until the long-term health effects are determined. Given its close link to testosterone, it seems logical that androstenedione has the potential to bring about the same harmful side effects associated with anabolic steroid use. Potential users should recognize that even though andro is sold legally over the counter, it has been banned by the National Collegiate Athletic Association, the International Olympic Committee, and the National Football League.

Creatine

Creatine is one of the "hottest" supplements among fitness enthusiasts. Part of the reason for its popularity is the growing evidence that suggests that taking creatine supplements may improve the ability to perform short-term, vigorous exercise.

The effect of creatine on short-term, high-intensity exercise is hardly surprising, given the relationship between creatine and skeletal muscle. All skeletal muscle tissue contains creatine, and dietary creatine is found in both meat and fish. In its phosphorylated form, creatine plays a key role in the formation of adenosine triphosphate (ATP), the body's energy source. During exercise, a portion of the muscle's creatine is depleted. Without sufficient amounts of creatine, which is manufactured in the liver and kidneys and stored in the skeletal muscles, the cycle that creates this energy is unable to produce enough ATP to meet the demand for short bursts of high-intensity exercise. Creatine supplements have been shown to increase the total creatine content (creatine and creatine phosphate) of muscle by an average of 20 to 30%.

Several studies suggest that ingestion of 20 to 25 grams of creatine monohydrate per day for five to six days improves muscular performance during activities that require short periods of high-intensity power and strength (e.g., weightlifting, sprinting). Sufficient evidence suggests that, under certain conditions, creatine supplementation can enhance performance in these activities (Williams, 1998). If individuals can train at higher intensity levels, they may be able to add strength and power at accelerated rates over time. Creatine can also lead to weight gain, but the mechanism responsible for the added weight has not

been adequately investigated. Before individuals start buying and taking creatine supplements, however, they should consider the following:

- The long-term effects of taking creatine have not been established. Most studies have examined the short-term (30 days or less) effects.
- All of the studies conducted have involved adults only. Creatine's effects on children are unknown.
- Concerns exist about possible liver and kidney damage if large quantities (>40 grams per day) of creatine are consumed.
- Stomach cramping and diarrhea have been reported as adverse side effects of creatine supplementation.
- For a 175-lb individual, approximately 20 grams per day (4 doses of 5 grams each consumed over the course of the day) should increase muscle creatine levels within 5 to 7 days.
- To encourage the storage of creatine in the muscles, 90 grams of carbohydrates should be consumed with each 5-gram dose.
- A more gradual technique would be to consume 3 grams of creatine per day for approximately one month.
- Once these levels are achieved, 2 grams of creatine supplementation per day will maintain muscle creatine levels.
- Creatine supplementation is not recommended for individuals involved in aerobic endurance activities, since accompanying increases in body mass could impair performance.
- Creatine supplementation alone, in the absence of physical training, has been shown to be ineffective.

The U.S. Food and Drug Administration (FDA) issued the following statement regarding creatine use: "Much remains unknown about whether creatine is absolutely safe for long-term use at levels currently being recommended. Both current and potential users should consult their physicians to identify any potential health problems."

Ergogenic Aids and Supplements

DHEA

Dehydroepiandrosterone (DHEA) is a substance secreted by the adrenal glands that is ultimately converted to testosterone and estrogen. As with many hormones, decreasing amounts of DHEA are produced as the body ages. DHEA production typically peaks around age 30 and steadily declines thereafter. By age 60, DHEA production is reduced to approximately 10% of what it was at age 30. Proponents of DHEA claim that it offers the following beneficial effects:

- Stops or slows the aging process.
- Stops or slows the development of Alzheimer's disease.
- Builds muscle.
- Helps individuals lose body weight and fat.
- Improves sex drive.
- May help treat cancer and AIDS.

Unfortunately, all of these claims have one thing in common: None of them have been scientifically substantiated by well-designed studies (National Institute on Aging, 1997; The Medical Letter, 1996). While a relatively large body of research on DHEA has been conducted using animals, these studies have limited value and cannot necessarily be extrapolated to human DHEA life-cycle patterns. Animals have negligible levels of endogenous DHEA. In 1996, the FDA banned the sale and distribution of DHEA for therapeutic uses until its safety and effectiveness could be reviewed. To circumvent the ban, manufacturers began marketing and selling DHEA as a nutritional supplement rather than a therapeutic drug.

The most sensible approach to take with a poorly studied supplement such as DHEA is to be extremely cautious. Because DHEA is a natural substance, the FDA has no regulatory power to control its distribution. Manufacturers are allowed to say (or not say) virtually anything they wish concerning their product. The decision to take DHEA should be based on a risk/benefit analysis. At present, few data are available to support the positive claims associated with DHEA

use. While DHEA users have reported few adverse side effects, one side effect is irreversible masculinization in women (hair loss, excessive facial hair growth, and deepening of the voice). In addition, male users of DHEA have reported irreversible gynecomastia (development of breasts in men); which may be the result of elevated estrogen levels. The long-term effects of DHEA use remain unclear. Because of its tendency to cause elevations of serum estrogen and testosterone levels, DHEA may significantly increase the risk of uterine and prostate cancer.

The potential risks associated with DHEA use appear to substantially outweigh any possible benefits. Given the lack of scientific evidence to support its performance-enhancing abilities and dismiss its potentially severe side effects, DHEA supplementation is not recommended. The National Institute on Aging (NIA) has launched an educational campaign to urge consumers to approach "anti-aging" hormone supplements with caution. Consumers can contact the NIA at 1-800-222-2225 or www.nih.gov/nia to order a free fact sheet on hormone supplements.

STRENGTH PLATEAUS

After an initial period of strength gain, most clients experience a strength plateau during which their strength level remains essentially the same. Appropriate changes in the training program usually enable the exerciser to make further progress and attain progressively higher levels of strength. The following strategies have proved useful in overcoming strength plateaus.

Training Frequency. As we become stronger, we typically perform more demanding workouts. However, more stressful training sessions may require longer recovery periods for tissue-building processes. Consequently, it is often helpful to reduce the training frequency. For example, a person who normally rests two days between training sessions may obtain better results by taking three days to recover. A person who typically trains all of the major muscle groups three days per week may make further improvement by exercising the lower-body muscles on Mondays and Thursdays, and the upper-body muscles on Tuesdays and Fridays.

Training Exercises. Because our neuromuscular system adapts to specific movement patterns, it is advisable to change the training exercises occasionally. For example, if progress comes to a halt in the bench press exercise, then the incline press, chest cross, or bar dip may serve as excellent substitutes. Although all of these exercises target the pectoralis major muscles, the movements require different muscle-fiber activation patterns that may stimulate further strength development.

Training Sets. When strength development reaches a plateau, it may be helpful to vary the number of sets performed. People who have been training with multiple sets may benefit from switching to a single-set program. Conversely, single-set trainees may benefit from a multiple-set or a pre-exhaustion protocol. Pre-exhaustion training typically involves two successive exercises for a given muscle group. For example, a set of biceps curls followed immediately by a set of chin-ups may enhance the training stimulus to the biceps muscles.

Resistance/Repetitions Relationships. The neuromuscular system adapts to specific training workloads. Occasional changes in the resistance/repetitions relationship may be beneficial. For example, if 8 repetitions with 80 pounds becomes a strength plateau, perhaps 12 repetitions with 70 pounds will produce additional strength gains. Some authorities recommend a planned program of **periodization** to enhance the strength-building stimulus (see pages 281–285). During the first month of training, for example, sets of 12 to 16 repetitions are performed. During the second month, this is reduced to sets of 8 to 12 repetitions, and during the third month, it is further reduced to sets of 4 to 8 repetitions. After a week of rest, the three-stage training program is repeated. Although some resistance/repetitions relationships appear to be more effective than others, the main objective is to avoid prolonged periods of training with the same workload.

Breakdown Training. Sometimes the training stimulus must be intensified to maximize muscle development. Breakdown training is one means of recruiting additional muscle fibers during an exercise set. For example, Claudia normally experiences momentary muscle failure after 10 leg extensions with 75 pounds. By immediately reducing the weight load to 65 pounds, Claudia can complete two or three post-fatigue repetitions. Breakdown training, although uncomfortable, enables Claudia to reach two levels of momentary muscle failure and to fatigue more muscle fibers in an extended exercise set.

Assisted Training. Assisted training is similar to breakdown training, in that the resistance is reduced in accordance with the muscle's momentary strength capacity. However, with assisted training, a partner actually helps the client perform two or three post-fatigue repetitions. For example, Susan normally encounters momentary muscle failure after 12 leg curls with 70 pounds. By receiving a little partner assistance during the lifting movement, Susan can complete a few more repetitions and fatigue additional muscle fibers. Also, by not receiving assistance during the lowering movement, Susan emphasizes the eccentric muscle contractions.

Negative Training. Because effective muscle force output is greater during eccentric contractions, negative-only training with heavier weightloads may be useful for increasing muscle strength. Lowering weights that are too heavy to lift, however, creates a higher risk of injury for the muscles and connective tissue. It is therefore recommended that negative exercises be carefully controlled and supervised by a competent personal trainer. As indicated in the previous section, assisted training is an excellent means for emphasizing eccentric muscle contractions.

Strength Plateaus

Training Motivation

Another approach to negative training is body-weight exercises such as bar dips and chin-ups. For example, Gayle steps to the top position of a bar dip (elbows extended) and slowly lowers her body to the bottom position (elbows flexed). This exercise, with careful spotting from a personal trainer, permits controlled eccentric contractions in the pectoralis major and triceps muscles.

Slow Training. Another means for making the muscles work harder is to slow the movement speed. Slower speeds reduce the role of momentum and produce greater muscle tension. A general guideline is to take 10 seconds for each lifting movement, and 4 seconds for each lowering movement. It should require only four to six slow repetitions to produce temporary muscle fatigue, and the increased muscle effort will be noticeable.

It is not advisable to perform higher-intensity training techniques during every workout. This is because higher-intensity training requires additional recovery and building time. Also, research reveals that higher-intensity strength exercise is much more productive when supervised by an attentive personal trainer.

TRAINING MOTIVATION

Though simplistic, exercise recording is an effective means for maintaining a consistent training schedule. By carefully recording each workout, you have a written progress account that provides your clients with added incentive to continue training. Record keeping is even more motivational when the workout charts are routinely reviewed and appropriate exercise modifications are implemented.

It is hard to overestimate the value of your role as a concerned and communicative personal trainer. One of the best means of motivation is performance feedback, especially when pertinent exercise information is shared in a personal and positive manner. Encouragement and posi-

tive reinforcement are highly motivational, particularly for beginners who may be unsure of themselves. To be most meaningful, reinforcing comments should contain specific information emphasizing those things that the client is doing well. Perhaps the most powerful means of motivation is the strength-fitness model. Your physical appearance, training regularity, exercise technique, and personal attitude provide an example that can significantly reduce or enhance the client's enthusiasm for strength training. See Chapter 14 for an in-depth discussion of teaching techniques for the personal trainer.

An important aspect of training motivation is maximizing the rate of improvement and minimizing the risk of injury. As a personal trainer, you should monitor each client's exercise intensity and recovery capacity to ensure optimum training results. On the one hand, clients should be encouraged to attain momentary muscle failure during each exercise set. On the other hand, clients should be discouraged from doing too much and be observed for signs of overtraining. Persistent muscle soreness, prolonged fatigue, performance inconsistency, and elevated resting heart rate are indications that the workload should be reduced or the recovery period should be increased. Also, distress symptoms that occur during a workout must be recognized and acted upon immediately. These include chest pain, blurred vision, dizziness, breathing difficulty, and nausea. See Chapter 17 for detailed information on emergency procedures.

SUMMARY

Strength training improves **functional capacity** to work and exercise, enhances physical appearance, increases metabolic rate, reduces risk of injury, decreases resting blood pressure, builds bone density, and protects against a variety of degenerative problems. To design safe and effective strength-training programs, you must understand the relationship between muscular forces and resistive forces, as well as the factors that affect strength performance. You must also be knowledgeable about the four categories of strength-training equipment: isometric, isokinetic, dynamic constant resistance, and dynamic variable resistance.

Almost any form of progressive resistance exercise will stimulate some degree of strength gain. However, many strength-training programs have a high risk of injury and a low rate of muscle development. As a personal trainer, you need to employ guidelines that ensure safe, effective, and efficient strength-training experiences for all of your clients.

Finally, you must be prepared to address the problems associated with anabolic steroids and **ergogenic aids,** implement techniques for overcoming strength plateaus, and know how to monitor and motivate clients to achieve optimal training results.

Summary

References and Suggested Reading

REFERENCES

National Institute on Aging (1997). *Pills, Patches, and Shots: Can Hormones Prevent Aging?* Bethesda, Md.: National Institutes on Aging.

The Medical Letter (1996). Dehydroepiandrosterone (DHEA). *The Medical Letter,* 38, 985, 91–92.

Williams, M.H. (1998). *The Ergogenics Edge.* Champaign, Ill.: Human Kinetics.

SUGGESTED READING

American Academy of Pediatrics (2001). Strength training by children and adolescents. *Pediatrics,* 107, 1470–1472.

American Association of Cardiovascular and Pulmonary Rehabilitation (2004). *Guidelines for Cardiac Rehabilitation Programs and Sedentary Prevention Programs.* (4th ed.). Champaign, Ill.: Human Kinetics.

American College of Obstetricians and Gynecologists (1994). *ACOG Technical Bulletin 189: Exercise during pregnancy and the postpartum period.* Washington, D.C.: American College of Obstetricians and Gynecologists.

American College of Sports Medicine (2006). *ACSM's Guidelines for Exercise Testing and Prescription* (7th ed.). Philadelphia: Lippincott Williams & Wilkins.

American Orthopaedic Society for Sports Medicine (1988). Proceedings of the conference on strength training and the prepubescent. Chicago: American Orthopaedic Society for Sports Medicine.

Baechle, T.R. & Earle, R.N. (2005). *Fitness Weight Training.* (2nd ed.). Champaign, Ill.: Human Kinetics.

Baechle, T.R. & Groves, B.R. (1998). *Weight Training: Steps to Success.* Champaign, Ill.: Human Kinetics.

Boyden, T. et al. (1993). Resistance exercise training is associated with decreases in serum low-density lipoprotein cholesterol levels in premenopausal women. *Archives of Internal Medicine,* 153, 97–100.

Bryant, C.X., Franklin, B.A., & Newton-Merrill, S. (2007). *ACE's Guide to Exercise Testing and Program Design: A Fitness Professional's Handbook.* (2nd ed.). Monterey, Calif.: Healthy Learning.

Brzycki, M. (1995). *A Practical Approach to Strength Training.* (3rd ed.). New York: McGraw-Hill.

Brzycki, M. (1995). *Youth Strength and Conditioning.* Indianapolis, Ind.: Masters Press.

Campbell, W. et al. (1994). Increased energy requirements and changes in body composition with resistance training in older adults. *American Journal of Clinical Nutrition,* 60, 167–175.

DiNubile, N.A. (1991). Strength training. *Clinics in Sports Medicine,* 10, 1, 33–61.

Durak, E., Jovanovis-Peterson, L., & Peterson, C. (1990). Randomized crossover study of effect of resistance training on glycemic control, muscular strength, and cholesterol in Type I diabetic men. *Diabetes Care,* 13, 1039–1042.

Eriksson, J. et al. (1997). Resistance training in the treatment of non-insulin dependent diabetes mellitus. *International Journal of Sports Medicine,* 18, 242–246.

Evans, W. & Rosenberg, I. (1992). *Biomarkers.* New York: Simon and Schuster.

Faigenbaum, A. (2001). Strength training and children's health. *Journal of Physical Education, Recreation and Dance,* 72, 24–30.

Faigenbaum, A. et al. (1993). The effects of a twice-a-week strength training program on children. *Pediatric Exercise Science,* 5, 339–346.

Faigenbaum, A. et al. (1996). Youth resistance training: Position statement paper and literature review. *Strength and Conditioning,* 18, 62–75.

Faigenbaum, A. et al. (1999). The effects of different resistance training protocols on muscular strength and endurance development in children. *Pediatrics,* 104, e5.

Faigenbaum, A. & Westcott, W. (2000). *Strength and Power for Young Athletes.* Champaign, Ill.: Human Kinetics.

Faigenbaum, A. & Westcott, W. (2001). *Youth Fitness.* San Diego, Calif.: American Council on Exercise.

Fiatarone, M.A., Marks, E.C., & Ryan, N.D. (1990). High-intensity strength training in nonagenarians. *Journal of the American Medical Association,* 263, 22, 3029–3034.

Fleck, S.J. & Kraemer, W.J. (2004). *Designing Resistance Training Programs.* (3rd ed.). Champaign, Ill.: Human Kinetics.

Forbes, G.B. (1976). The adult decline in lean body mass. *Human Biology,* 48, 161–173.

Frontera, W.R. et al. (1988). Strength conditioning in older men: Skeletal muscle hypertrophy and improved function. *Journal of Applied Physiology,* 64, 3, 1038–1044.

Grimby, G. et al. (1992). Training can improve muscle strength and endurance in 78 to 84 year old men. *Journal of Applied Physiology,* 73, 2517–2523.

Hagerman, F. et al. (2000). Effects of high-intensity resistance training on untrained older men. I. Strength, cardiovascular, and metabolic responses. *Journal of Gerontology. Series A, Biological Sciences and Medical Sciences,* 55, B336–346.

Harris, K. & Holly, R. (1987). Physiological response to circuit weight training in borderline hypertensive subjects. *Medicine and Science in Sports and Exercise,* 19, 246–252.

Hejna, W. et al. (1982). The prevention of sports injuries in high school students through strength training. *National Strength and Conditioning Association Journal,* 4, 28–31.

Hikida, R. et al. (2000). Effects of high-intensity resistance training on untrained older men. II. Muscle fiber characteristics and nucleo-cytoplasmic relationships. *Journal of Gerontology. Series A, Biological Sciences and Medical Sciences,* 55, B347–354.

Hurley, B. (1994). Does strength training improve health status? *Strength and Conditioning Journal, 16,* 7–13.

Kelly, G. (1997). Dynamic resistance exercise and resting blood pressure in healthy adults: A meta-analysis. *Journal of Applied Physiology, 82,* 1559–1565.

Keyes, A., Taylor, H. L., & Grande, F. (1973). Basal metabolism and age of adult man. *Metabolism, 22,* 579–587.

Koffler, K. et al. (1992). Strength training accelerates in gastrointestinal transit in middle-aged and older men. *Medicine and Science in Sports and Exercise,* 24, 415–419.

Lemmer, J. et al. (2001). Effect of strength training on resting metabolic rate and physical activity. *Medicine and Science in Sports and Exercise,* 33, 532–541.

Marino, M. & Gleim, G.W. (1984). Muscle strength and fiber type. *Clinics in Sports Medicine, 3, 1,* 85–99.

Menkes, A. et al. (1993). Strength training increases regional bone mineral density and bone remodeling in middle-aged and older men. *Journal of Applied Physiology, 74,* 2478–2484.

Messier, S.P. & Dill, M.E. (1985). Alterations in strength and maximal oxygen uptake consequent to Nautilus circuit weight training. *Research Quarterly, 56, 4,* 345–351.

Mochizuki, R.M. & Richter, K.J. (1988). Cardiomyopathy and cerebrovascular accident associated with anabolic androgenic steroid use. *The Physician and Sports Medicine, 16, 11,* 109–112.

Morganti, C.M. et al. (1995). Strength improvements with one year of progressive resistance training in older women. *Medicine and Science in Sports and Exercise, 27, 6,* 906–912.

Morris, F. et al. (1997). Prospective ten-month exercise intervention in premenarcheal girls: Positive effects on bone and lean mass. *Journal of Bone and Mineral Research, 12,* 1453–1462.

Nelson, M. et al. (1994). Effects of high-intensity strength training on multiple risk factors for osteoporotic fractures. *Journal of the American Medical Association, 272,* 1909–1914.

Outerbridge, A. & Micheli, L. (1995). Overuse injuries in the young athlete. *Clinics in Sports Medicine, 14,* 503–516.

Ozmun, J., Mikesky, A., & Surburg, P. (1991). Neuromuscular adaptations during prepubescent strength training. *Medicine and Science in Sports and Exercise, 23,* S31.

Pratley, R. et al. (1994). Strength training increases resting metabolic rate and norepinephrine levels in healthy 50 to 65 year old men. *Journal of Applied Physiology, 76,* 133–137.

Ramsay, J. et al. (1990). Strength training effects in prepubescent boys. *Medicine and Science in Sports and Exercise, 22,* 605–614.

Risch, S. et al. (1993). Lumbar strengthening in chronic low back pain patients. *Spine, 18,* 232–238.

Rowland, T. (1990). *Exercise and Children's Health.* Champaign, Ill.: Human Kinetics.

Stone, M. et al. (1982). Physiological effects of a short term resistive training program on middle-aged untrained men. *National Strength and Conditioning Association Journal, 4,* 116–120.

Taunton, J. et al. (1997). Exercise for older women: Choosing the right prescription. *British Journal of Sports Medicine, 31,* 5–10.

Trappe, S. et al. (2001). Maintenance of whole muscle strength and size following resistance training in older men. *Medicine and Science in Sports and Exercise, 33,* S147.

Tufts University (1994). Never too late to build up your muscle. *Tufts University Diet and Nutrition Letter, 12,* 6–7.

Westcott, W.L. (1991). Role model instructors. *Fitness Management, 7, 4,* 48–50.

Westcott, W.L. (1994). *Strength Fitness.* (4th ed.). New York: McGraw-Hill.

Westcott, W.L. (1995). *Strength Fitness: Physiological Principals and Training Techniques* (4th ed.). Dubuque, Iowa: Wm. C. Brown Publishers.

Westcott, W.L. (1995). High-intensity strength training. *IDEA Personal Trainer, 6,* 9.

Westcott, W.L. (1995). School-based conditioning programs for physically unfit children. *Strength and Conditioning, 17, 2,* 5–9.

Westcott, W.L. (2003). *Building Strength and Stamina.* (2nd ed.). Champaign, Ill.: Human Kinetics.

Westcott, W.L. & Baechle, T. (1999). *Strength Training for Seniors.* Champaign, Ill.: Human Kinetics.

Westcott, W.L. & Guy, J. (1996). A physical evolution: Sedentary adults see marked improvements in as little as two days a week. *IDEA Today, 14,* 58–65.

Suggested Reading

Strength Training Program Design

Douglas S. Brooks, M.S., holds a master's degree in exercise physiology and is the author of six textbooks, including Program Design For Personal Trainers *and* Effective Strength Training.

Douglas S. Brooks

Mr. Brooks frequently conducts lectures and workshops on exercise physiology, kinesiology, strength training, and personal training throughout the world and is an ACE Gold-certified Personal Trainer.

ACE would like to thank Christine "C.C." Cunningham, M.S., Ph.D. candidate, for her contributions to this chapter. Cunningham, owner of PerformENHANCE sport and adventure athlete training in Chicago, wrote the Functional Training section on pages 270–274 and the Periodization section on pages 281–283.

Resistance-training program design is crucial to a well-rounded fitness program and the overall health of your clients. The term resistance training is used to cover all types of "strength" or "weight" training. The best approach to program design is often difficult to identify because there are numerous "training systems" you can choose or create. They can be defined as any combination of sets, repetitions, and loads, and every imaginable kind of training system exists, from the light to heavy system to the bulks and super-set system. At least 27 different systems are listed by Fleck and Kraemer (1997), and this is not an exhaustive list.

Training systems can be easily understood and categorized by realizing that any system will utilize one or more of the six types of resistance training discussed in Chapters 1, 8, and 9 (Table 9.1). Furthermore, all systems fit into a specificity chart based on the number of repetitions, sets, and loads (intensity) that they use (Table 9.2). While most scientists agree on some definable parameters for effective program design, the best approach is a combination of science and art.

The defining variables in terms of results may lie in how often a person trains and how they arrange the order and number of sets, repetitions (volume), and loads (intensity), which may be the most important of these factors. Exactly how to vary the frequency, intensity, and duration within a periodization plan is the art of resistance- training program design. These factors are of little value, however, until you determine your clients' goals and understand what motivates them.

DESIGNING RESISTANCE-TRAINING PROGRAMS

The real trick in designing your clients' resistance-training programs is determining their unique needs and interests. Develop the goals of the program by first listening to what your clients think they want to accomplish, and second, acting on what you hear. Do not make the mistake of blindly adapting a program simply because it was used, for example, by a successful weight-trained athlete. There is no one optimal combination of sets and repetitions. Most systems or combinations of repetitions, sets, and loads will often produce results in spite of their design, because the body will adapt

---

Table 9.1
Six Types of Resistance Training

1. Isometric force development
2. Concentric force development
3. Eccentric force development
4. Dynamic constant external resistance*
5. Dynamic variable external resistance
6. Isokinetics

---

*Dynamic constant external resistance is often labeled as isotonic training, even though this is an imprecise term (see pages 24–25).

---

to any load to which it is not accustomed. However, results in and of themselves do not mean you have the best and safest design. Make sure the training systems you choose, or better yet develop, meet your client's needs and current situation.

Using and copying one style of training for both athletics and fitness is a common mistake when planning resistance-training programs. The needs of the general fitness enthusiast are different from those of athletes.

Training Smart: Implications for Training Your Clients

Resistance training can be
✔ planned and time efficient
✔ results-oriented
✔ functional and usable in relation to your clients' personal lifestyles
✔ directed toward health and personal wellness

The American College of Sports Medicine (ACSM) recommends resistance training at a moderate-to-high intensity that is sufficient to develop and maintain

---

Table 9.2
Training Specificity and Recovery Time

Relative Loading	Outcome	% 1 RM	Rep Range	# Of Sets	Rest Between Sets
Light	Muscular endurance	< 70	12–20	1–3	20–30 seconds
Moderate	Hypertrophy, strength	70–80	8–12	1–6	30–120 seconds
Heavy	Maximum strength/power	80–100	1–8	1–5+	2–5 minutes

Adapted, by permission, from Baechle, T. & Groves, B. (1999). *Weight Training: Steps to Success* (2nd ed.) Champaign, Ill.: Human Kinetics.

muscle mass (American College of Sports Medicine, 1990). This should be done at least two days per week for a minimum of one set of 8 to 12 repetitions that are executed to fatigue. Each session should include 8 to 10 exercises that challenge the major muscle groups.

These minimal standards influence resistance-training programming in two ways. First, they dictate the time it takes to complete a comprehensive, well-rounded program. Those that last more than 60 minutes per session are associated with high dropout rates. Second, although more frequent training and additional sets, or varied combinations of sets and repetitions, elicit greater strength gains, the difference is usually small. In fact, strength training two days per week in accordance with these guidelines produces about 80% of the strength gains seen when training three days per week. When coupled with significant results, the lower frequency may encourage adherence. Braith et al. (as reported in American College Sports Medicine, 2000) found that those who performed one set to fatigue showed a greater than 25% increase in strength. These results are favorable when compared to other, more time-intensive programs that involve more total repetitions, sets, and days of training. By training smart, you can effectively and efficiently utilize your clients' time investment to maximize their health and fitness improvements related to muscular fitness.

When designing programs for your clients, use this simple needs-analysis process. Answers to these questions will largely determine your resistance-training programming approach:

1. What are your clients' goals? Common goals include muscular hypertrophy, increasing maximal lifts, better performance in a particular sport, decreased body fat, feeling stronger, general health enhancement, personal physical independence, and increased self-esteem.

2. What are the requirements of the activities or sports your clients participate in? Based on your clients' goals, training scenarios will emerge that may require you to design programs that emphasize general health and fitness, functional strength and balance, and/or training for a competitive sport such as body building, race walking, or volleyball. Analyze activities with regard to their requirements for muscular strength and/or endurance, sport specificity with regard to requisite movement patterns, and any special training requirements such as **plyometrics.** It is necessary to weigh these considerations against the current fitness and experience base of your clients.

3. Is training dictated by the needs of the individual or the requirements of a sport? In a competitive coaching situation, athletes continue their participation based on a desire and ability to excel, often at any cost. For example, power lifting requires a full squat; the rules of the sport demand its execution regardless of the risk to the athlete. However, if your clients' needs—such as health, fitness, and well-being—are the priority, you have considerable flexibility in the approach you take to program design.

4. How much time will your clients commit? It is impossible to develop an effective resistance-training program without knowing how much available time your clients have. Part of your responsibility, based on the information that you gathered in steps one, two, and three, is to let your clients know what kind of time investment they have to make to attain their goals. For example, strength-training goals, unless connected to elite performance, can usually be accomplished as part of a workout that also includes cardiorespiratory and flexibility training components. Work to accommodate the time offered by your clients, even if it is limited, without creating unrealistic expectations. The key to success with limited client time is to help them plan independent workouts.

Designing Resistance-training Programs

**Five Program
Design Scenarios**

Overload

Muscular-strength, cardiorespiratory, and flexibility training are primary components of a balanced approach to fitness. All three require different overloads to achieve optimum results. Muscular fitness is developed by placing a demand, or overload, on the muscles in a manner to which they are not accustomed. If the overload is applied progressively and sensibly, the neuromuscular system will positively adapt to the demand.

The general guideline for change is a proper and specific overload that uses a progressive increase in resistance over time, causes the targeted muscle(s) to fatigue in about 30 to 90 seconds, and challenges all of the major movements (joint actions) to which the muscle(s) contribute.

A progressive increase in resistance provides continued improvements in muscle strength and endurance. Appropriate **intensity** (attaining momentary muscular fatigue in about 30 to 90 seconds) is necessary to optimize training results. Gradual intensity increases will reduce the likelihood of injury. All of the major movements of the body must be challenged to ensure balanced strength between all of the opposing muscle groups.

FIVE PROGRAM DESIGN SCENARIOS

The following outlines for five program design scenarios—health and fitness, functional training, bodybuilding, competitive athlete, and core training—encompass the wide range of approaches available to meet the varied and diverse needs of your clients. These approaches should not be evaluated in terms of absolute correctness, but for their appropriateness to your clients' specific training goals.

Health and Fitness Gains

Significant gains in strength and muscular endurance can be achieved with just two exercise sessions per week. For your clients, this means at least 10 exercises that target all of the major muscle groups. At least one set of 8 to 12 repetitions, completed to fatigue, should be performed to gain health benefits.

Most of your clients' health and fitness goals can be optimized by using **active recovery** between sets. For example, performing a stretching exercise or working another body part can facilitate recovery from a previous strength exercise without requiring total inactivity, and allows for more productive use of limited time.

And, because the health benefits associated with resistance training can occur at any age, it is easy to get clients, young and old, excited about resistance training (see Chapter 8).

Functional Training

Functional training involves the use of exercise specifically designed to improve a client's performance of functional activities outside of the training environment. Functional activities include movements from daily life, work, or sports, such as climbing stairs, carrying loads, or jumping. Unlike traditional strength-training exercises, which focus on the isolation of an individual muscle to maximize overload, functional strength training incorporates multiple muscles or muscle groups with an emphasis on the creation of correct movement patterns. Hence, the movements of functional training require the client to coordinate, balance, control, and time the muscle contractions in a way similar to how they might need to in a functional activity. The practice of these actions is intended to promote better neuromuscular control that will carry over to activities outside of the gym.

One of the key concepts in functional training is the **specificity of training principle,** which states that for an individual to become proficient at any given movement, that movement itself must be trained and practiced. In other words, to get better at shooting free throws or lifting a bag of groceries, you have to actually shoot free throws or lift bags of groceries. Functional strength training attempts to "cheat" the specificity principle by providing clients with the opportunity to practice parts of the functional movements or whole movements that require similar skills. This may allow clients to develop strength and movement strategies that will help them when the time comes to actually perform the goal movement.

Designing an exercise that will improve function requires you to identify the key components of a movement that can be trained in a manner the same as, or similar to, the demand of the actual movement. There are four components of resistance exercise that are key to improving functional performance: **coordination, range of motion,** type of contraction, and speed of movement (Morrissey, Harman, & Johnson, 1995; Rutherford & Jones, 1986).

Coordination

The most widely recognized component of a movement that is mimicked in functional exercises is coordination, which involves more than just the trajectory or pattern that the movement goes through. Effectively matching the coordination component requires that an exercise utilize the same muscles and contraction timing as the goal activity. In addition to similarity in the movement pattern, the exercise should require the same order of activation of both the stabilizing and motive muscle groups. **Stabilizing muscle contractions** are generally isometric contractions that act to support the trunk, limit movement in a joint, or control balance. **Motive muscle contractions** produce the actual movement at the joints and can be concentric or eccentric. Motive muscles depend heavily on the stabilizing muscles to move the body.

Core stabilization exercises challenge the abdominal and back muscles to hold the spine in the appropriate position during movement of the extremities.

Examples of core stabilization exercises include work on a stability ball, floor exercises such as the "dead bug" or "superman," and standing exercises that minimize movement in the core while moving the upper- and lower-body. Exercises that focus on movement of the core are also important components of a functional-training program because they allow the client to practice proper activation timing of those muscles during a movement. The core is involved in almost every movement made in everyday life, work, and sport. For this reason, core training, which places both stabilizing and motive demands on the abdominal and back muscles, is essential for a successful, functional strength-training program.

Challenging the balance of a client is another way to train coordination. Unstable environments such as balance boards, foam rollers, and stability balls change the order of activation of the muscles by requiring stabilizers to contract whenever needed during a movement to maintain balance. Changing the client's position or posture also affects the coordination of the movement (Wilson, Murphy, & Walshe, 1996). Being in a seated or standing position changes both the muscles that are activated as stabilizers as well as the order of activation of movers during a movement. Similarity in all aspects of coordination is an important factor that will impact the degree of performance improvement seen following participation in a functional-training program.

Range of Motion

The range of motion for a functional exercise should match the goal activity as closely as possible. In traditional training, full range of motion is emphasized. However, for functional training, exercising through a limited range is acceptable if the goal movement is also performed in a limited range. This allows the neuromuscular system to practice generating the

Five Program Design Scenarios

**Five Program
Design Scenarios**

forces necessary to start the movement from the initial position. In addition, matching the end range of motion is necessary to train the system to generate force at the appropriate joint angle to stop the movement safely and effectively. *Note: If a limited range of motion is used during functional exercises, full-range-of-motion exercises should also be included in a client's program.*

Type of Contraction

Muscle contractions can be classified as isometric, concentric, or eccentric. Research has shown that the greatest improvement in performance comes after training a muscle using the same type of contraction that the goal activity features (Morrissey, Harman, & Johnson, 1995). Concentric training has been shown to be superior to static training in producing direct changes in functional performance (Morrissey, Harman & Johnson, 1995), although the specificity principle limits the application of these findings to those functional activities that are dominated by concentric contractions. The way in which the nervous system controls an eccentric contraction is believed to be different from that of a concentric contraction (Enoka, 1997; McHugh et al., 2002). To allow for maximum practice at producing a movement, or a component of that movement, involving an eccentric contraction, an exercise should demand production of an eccentric contraction (along with the necessary coordination and range of motion). Consider similarity in contraction type when developing any functional exercise to maximize strength and performance gains.

Speed of Movement

In traditional training methods, the speed of movement is controlled to maximize the stress response of the muscle and maximize hypertrophy and strength gains while ensuring maximum safety. In accordance with the specificity principle, the speed at which the movement is trained

will determine the speed at which maximum performance gains are seen (Morrissey, Harman, & Johnson, 1995). Speed specificity is a delicate training component to address when working with most clients because of the greater potential for injury when moving at higher speeds. It is important to realize the following trade-off when designing a functional program. If speed is kept slow, then the neuromuscular system will be best suited for performing at slow speeds. Since most activities of daily life are not performed in a slow, controlled manner, it may be appropriate to train clients at speeds that match the rate at which movement is actually performed. However, faster movement speeds will increase risk of injury. To increase speed safely there are several rules that must be adhered to: (1) the load must be significantly reduced as speed is increased, (2) the client must have adequate practice at producing the movement slowly and correctly before beginning to gradually increase speed, and (3) the environment in which the movements are performed must be free from potential hazards in the event that the movement is performed incorrectly. Because spotting rapid movements, especially total-body movements, is extremely difficult, these rules must be followed carefully and diligently to minimize the risk to the client.

Adding Functional Training to a Client's Program

Due to the nature of functional strength training, it is recommended that previously untrained clients begin with a period of traditional isolated muscular training before starting functional exercises. The introductory period will allow them to become familiar with how to correctly control muscle contractions during resistance training as well as introduce them to their individual muscles and their locations. This will make it easier for the client to understand and execute instructions regarding the more complex movement patterns used in functional exercises. In addition, muscular imbalances, such as right/left or agonist/antagonist imbalances, must be eliminated before asking a client to attempt to make total-body, coordinated movements. Muscular imbalances increase the risk of injury and may be exacerbated by functional training as a client is forced to "cheat" to create movement due to weakness. Isolated muscular exercises are the best way to overcome imbalances and should be used any time an imbalance is noticed during a client's program.

Progressive overload is essential to promote increases in strength and hypertrophy. Overload can be applied during a functional exercise; however, the maximum load lifted will be limited to the ability of the smallest muscle being used during the movement. This means that many of the large muscle groups are not adequately stimulated to promote adaptations in strength and size. If this is the case, include isolated exercises in the client's program for these muscle groups if increases in strength and hypertrophy are desired.

There are several limitations to functional training to be aware of before choosing to use this type of training in place of traditional exercises. First, there is little research supporting the direct link between these types of exercises and actual improvements in function. Individual components have been studied, as mentioned above, but the exercises as a whole have not been scientifically proven to improve function. Theoretical support is available, but direct evidence has not been adequately reported. Second, due to the lack of overload that can be safely applied during a functional exercise to most of the major muscle groups, it is reasonable to question the use of functional strength training as the sole exercise mode for clients who require overload, including those at risk of **osteoporosis, sarcopenia,** or **frailty.** In these cases, traditional training may be as, if not

more, important and appropriate for the client and should be considered as the primary mode of training. Third, functional training can be more risky than traditional training because of the difficulty of spotting multi-joint movements, the use of higher speeds, and the incorporation of unstable environments to train balance and coordination. Every client should be considered an individual with regard to the risk-versus-benefit factor before including high-risk functional exercises. And lastly, the learning curve for a functional exercise is much larger than that of a traditional, isolated exercise because there are fewer restrictions to the planes of movement that the client can use. This may slow progress and create a false sense of "failure," which may increase client dropout.

Functional training has been used for years to excite, motivate, and push clients to excel and continue training. The uniqueness and "fun" factor of a correctly designed and safe functional-training program is not a benefit that should be ignored. As the drive to find ways to help clients improve their performance in everyday tasks increases, the theories and methods of functional exercise design will improve as well.

Bodybuilding

The training goal for bodybuilders centers around balanced muscular size, symmetry, and definition. Their training routines encompass a variety of exercises to promote ideal gains in size and symmetry. Generally, a moderate intensity (8 to 12 repetitions to fatigue) is used to allow for the completion of high volume, which is determined by the equation: load x repetitions x sets. A load of 8 to 12 repetitions done to fatigue seems logical as the goal of bodybuilding is not superior maximal strength. However, for maximal hypertrophy gains, research suggests training should emphasize increases in resistance as well as volume. High-intensity volume

> **Five Program Design Scenarios**

stress may be the primary stimulus to muscle hypertrophy. The order of exercises for each specific muscle group is more important than the order in which the muscle groups are exercised. Multiple or giant sets are used to accomplish volume overload. These consist of three to six sets and can go as high as 10 to 15 repetitions per exercise. Short rest periods are a distinctive feature of bodybuilding. Rests of 30 to 90 seconds seem to promote muscular definition, vascularity, and a high metabolic intensity that may help lower body fat.

Bodybuilders may work a full-body routine that targets all of the major muscle groups, or split routines, which work different body parts on alternate days. Clients should allow for two workouts per week for most muscle groups. Generally, a split routine schedule requires four to six workouts per week, and some research suggests that three full-body workouts per week may be sufficient to stimulate adaptive responses. This is important to consider since more frequent, all-out training increases the potential for overuse and poor adaptive responses to the workload.

Competitive Athlete

Are sport-specific strength-training movements (e.g., plyometrics and skill practice, which involves trying to preserve movement speed with a load) better than developing base strength traditionally and then "practicing" to see what strength carries over and is applicable to performance? While the question of specificity seems critical in designing a program for the competitive athlete, science has been unable to offer a definitive answer as to whether it is a more effective training method. You should experiment with both approaches or a combination of the two. Individual response and results will dictate the approach you follow.

Core Training

The core of the body is a major connecting link in the body's musculoskeletal chain. The trunk is the center of power for

skilled performance in both a literal and physical sense.

If you view the body as a chain, it is only as strong as its weakest link. Consider a client with very strong legs and arms, but an undeveloped lower torso or trunk. Force cannot efficiently be transferred between the upper and lower body if the midsection lacks the strength to stabilize the lower torso during movement. In other words, the body needs a strong foundation from which to direct effort so that energy that is created for movement ends up being a part of that movement, rather than wasted. Misdirected energy is not harmless; it can lead to poor performance and injury.

The midsection of the body needs to be solid and strong, and the musculature needs to be able to stabilize spinal and pelvic positioning, as well as contract dynamically. This is in contrast to a core that is deconditioned and represents something more like a blob of jelly (i.e., weak in structure), which in effect would stop the transfer of force and impede safe, efficient movement.

Adequately conditioned abdominal and back musculature represents the key "coupling" link of the body that connects movements between the upper and lower body. The strength and importance of the body's core is reflected by conditioning programs that emphasize core training as a primary objective, though not to the exclusion of other important aspects of fitness.

This power center of the body—the trunk—is the literal and physical bridge that allows for dynamic, powerful, coordinated, skillful, and integrated responses of the whole body. Core training extends well beyond vanity and into the domains of improved health and fitness and enhanced athletic performance.

For more information on training the core, refer to ACE's *Stability Ball Training* (American Council on Exercise, 2002) and Brooks' *Effective Strength Training* (2001).

PROPER INTENSITY

Results depend on proper intensity. If, in the repetition scheme suggested, you can bring the muscle to temporary fatigue (with the ability to still complete one or two repetitions with good form), exceptional results will occur. It is not absolutely necessary for you to force your clients to "true" muscle failure. Most clients will experience significant results if they are close to fatigue. The key is not how much absolute weight or resistance is used, but whether the overload is relative to the individual's current strength level and whether the muscle can fatigue within the goal repetition framework.

Intensity of effort related to strength training and best results can be demonstrated by a thorough understanding of motor units and their contribution to muscle contraction (see pages 21–22). When the nervous system commands a motor unit to contract, all the muscle fibers of this single motor unit respond together. There is no such thing as a weak or partial contraction from a motor unit—it simply fires "all-or-none." Innervation of a single motor unit does not mean stimulation of the entire muscle. If it did, you could not control movement. The way in which motor units activate fibers is crucial to skilled and/or powerful movement.

Varying the intensity of muscle contraction, or force gradation, occurs in two ways: (1) raising the number of motor units recruited for activity, or (2) increasing their frequency of discharge. By blending these two types of gradation, optimal patterns of neural discharge permit a wide variety of scaled (weak to strong) contractions (McArdle et al., 2001).

Motor units are composed of two distinct types of fibers: **fast twitch (FT)** and **slow twitch (ST)** (see page 18). During an activity involving muscular contraction, the order in which ST and FT motor units are recruited is relatively constant. It depends upon the type of activity, the force required and the position of the body. This modulatory effect is referred to as a "ramp-like recruitment effect." If a light weight is being lifted slowly, predominantly ST motor units are recruited to perform this movement. If the weight is increased or moved at a faster velocity, FT (Type IIa and IIb) motor units are recruited in addition to the continual contribution of ST units. At maximal force production, all three types of motor units will be required.

The order of recruitment holds the FT motor units, which are highly fatigable, in reserve until the ST motor units can no longer perform the particular muscular contraction. When your clients engage in high-repetition schemes, about 20 repetitions or higher, the intensity is not sufficient to significantly call the FT motor units into play. This implies that since the average participant has an equal number of FT and ST motor units, 50% of the muscle mass in the body that is especially well-suited for gains in strength and hypertrophy will not be challenged.

Motor unit recruitment order is important from a practical standpoint for several reasons (Fleck & Kraemer, 1997):

1. As previously discussed, to recruit FT fibers and achieve a training effect, the exercise must be higher in intensity.

2. The order of recruitment is fixed for a specific movement (Desmedt & Godaux, 1977, as reported in Fleck & Kraemer, 1997).

If the body position is changed, the order of recruitment can also change (Grimby & Hannerz, 1977, as reported in Fleck & Kraemer, 1997). Furthermore, the order also can change from one movement to another for multifunctional muscles. For example, motor unit recruitment order in the quadriceps is different for the performance of a seated leg extension on a machine than for a knee extension during the performance of a squat (Fleck & Kraemer, 1997). The variation in recruitment order provides some evidence to support the belief that to completely develop a particular muscle (all the motor units), it must be exercised through several different movements.

This information suggests that all training done at a slow pace, or with light force, will emphasize the use of mostly the ST fibers, inducing little training effect on the FT IIa or FT IIb fibers. Long, slow training bouts do not prepare the muscle for the demands of competition or higher forces, and do not optimize the stimulation and training effect of your clients' muscle mass.

Movement Speed

For the average client, gains in strength will be best accomplished by moving the weight slowly (about four to five seconds per repetition) through a full range of motion, and accomplishing FT recruitment by using an appropriately intense overload (Table 9.3).

Starting Resistance

A safe starting resistance for most clients is one that allows completion of at least 12 to 20 repetitions. This intensity equates to less than 70% of **one-repetition maximum (1 RM)** and is generally a safe starting inten-

---

Table 9.3
Benefits of Controlling the Speed of Movement

1. Consistent application of force
2. More total muscle tension produced
3. More total muscle force produced
4. More muscle fiber activation (both ST and FT)
5. Greater muscle power potential through high-intensity force development and, subsequently, through controlled training
6. Less tissue trauma
7. Greater momentum increases injury potential and reduces the training effect on target muscle groups

Exceptions to the above may be appropriate in sport-specific applications and when your client understands the risks.

Source: Westcott, W.L. (1991). *Strength Fitness* (3rd ed). Wm. C. Brown Publishers. Reprinted with permission.

---

sity for most people (see pages 251–252). The repetition goal range is determined by a variety of factors that include the client's current fitness level specific to resistance training, exercise history, and their stated resistance training goals (e.g., muscle endurance or muscle hypertrophy).

Initially, you may prefer not to test your clients' ability to lift their maximum weight one time (1 RM), as this places them in a high-risk, maximal performance situation for which they may not be ready. Instead, start with too little weight and gradually increase resistance when the maximum number of repetitions are performed. The focus of early workouts is not to create muscle failure, but to work on technique and allow the tissues of the body to adapt progressively to new challenges.

Recovery Between Sets

High-intensity resistance training relies primarily on the ATP-CP and lactic acid energy systems, both of which are replenished during the recovery period using the aerobic energy system. Intensity and duration of effort influences the predominance of one energy system over the other (see pages 13–14).

The complete rebuilding of the **ATP-CP energy system,** which is depleted predominantly through short bursts of maximal effort, takes about three to five minutes. That is why, for example, power and Olympic lifters take at least several minutes, usually up to five, to recover from all-out maximal lifts; the ATP-CP energy system must fully recover before these athletes can correctly and safely execute the next lift.

As maximal or strenuous efforts go beyond 10 seconds, the short-term or **lactic acid system** begins to substantially contribute to energy production in an attempt to sustain and assist in the maintenance of a high level, predominantly anaerobic effort (i.e., failure or muscle fatigue in about 30 to 90 seconds).

Half of accumulated lactic acid is metabolized within 25 minutes of recovery and almost all is metabolized within 75 minutes. It would not be practical to rest long enough between sets to completely clear lactate from the body. Fortunately, the body's musculature can sustain quality activity without a complete recovery of lactate levels. Can you imagine your clients waiting 25 minutes to an hour between sets of resistance-training exercise?

Expediting Lactic Acid Clearance

Light activity is encouraged to facilitate lactic acid removal more quickly. Rest periods that use light activity for this purpose must last at least two minutes to be effective if significant lactate has accumulated and recovery is required. The lactic acid system makes a significant energy contribution during hard workouts where sets are performed to failure in one to three minutes. Unless muscular endurance and a high tolerance to high levels of lactate is a goal, fatigue in 30 to 90 seconds is recommended. This is time efficient and will probably enhance most of your clients' health, fitness, and muscular strength and endurance goals.

Practical Implications of an Active Recovery

"Active rest" equates to accomplishing more total work in limited amounts of time. An example of active rest would be as follows: have your client perform a chest exercise, then an abdominal exercise, and then a lower-body exercise. Even though your client is continually active through all three exercises, there is sufficient recovery time for the chest musculature as the body performs the abdominal and lower-body exercises.

Adequate recovery allows your clients to prepare for and perform another quality effort or training set. Shorter recovery times do increase relative intensity. To determine whether adaptations related to shorter recovery times are relevant and useful to your clients, ask yourself:

1. Is the recovery duration appropriate for your client's program goals?
2. Is the recovery duration appropriate for your client's fitness level?
3. What is the client trying to accomplish (i.e., muscular strength, endurance, hypertrophy, and/or exercise compliance and health benefits)?

Specificity and Recovery Between Sets

Refer back to Table 9.2 and note the recommended amounts of rest between sets for light, moderate, and heavy loading by resistance. You will notice that the longest recovery period is five minutes.

Why is it not necessary to recover longer for sets of exhaustive work (i.e., 8 to 20 repetitions to fatigue in about 30 to 90 seconds) where major contributions of both the ATP-CP and lactic acid systems are prevalent? First, the question of recovery has been answered regarding the depletion of ATP-CP sources with the example of 1 RM lifts and heavy relative loading. About two to five minutes are required for complete recovery. During relatively light loading (i.e., 12 to 20 repetitions and less than 70% of 1 RM), there are not maximal contributions from either anaerobic energy system (ATP-CP and lactic acid systems). Therefore, complete exhaustion of the ATP-CP system does not occur, nor do significant accumulations of lactate via use of the lactic acid system. Short rests of 20 to 30 seconds, as recommended by the specificity chart, are usually adequate for recovery and allow for another quality set of training. Even moderate loading, which causes muscle fatigue in about 8 to 12 repetitions and 30 to 90 seconds, does not require extreme contributions from either the ATP-CP or lactic acid systems. Again, complete recovery of the anaerobic systems is not required. Rests of 30 to 120 seconds between sets is sufficient.

Always let your clients determine if more time is necessary, especially those who are looking for health returns and enjoyment from their exercise routine. In instances where they need a longer period, consider using active recovery and sequence your exercises as suggested above. Include a stretch or two after the set is completed.

In relation to program design, nothing is written in stone. It should be viewed not as an issue of right or wrong, but as a continuum of training possibilities you should operate within to maintain a scientifically valid approach. As a trainer, you have many options for maximizing your clients' training results and individual program needs.

Recovery Between Workouts

Recovery between workouts is based on the intensity of the workout and the individual recovery ability of your clients. Generally, a period of about 48 hours between intense workouts is appropriate for positive adaptations in the neuromuscular system. Adequate recovery is essential to avoid overtraining and strength plateaus, and for progressive improvements in muscular strength and endurance.

Intensity is both relative to, and dependent on, your client's current fitness level. Body-weight exercises serve as a good example. The absolute weight of a person can reflect light, heavy, or even maximal loading. For example, deconditioned clients who perform a traditional pushup may find they can only do four repetitions. This equates to a heavy 4 RM load or greater than 80% of 1 RM. These clients need a significant recovery between workouts; in this case, at least 48 hours.

More fit clients may be able to perform 50 to 100 pushups, a relatively light load representing much less than 50% of 1 RM. They probably can perform these pushup repetitions every day of the week; recovery is not required because a new workload has not been introduced. It should be noted that by performing 100 pushups, fit clients are not achieving gains in strength. If increased muscular strength is a goal,

their time could be used more effectively by progressively overloading the body's musculature in 8 to 20 repetitions.

WHEN IS THE RIGHT TIME TO CHANGE A STRENGTH PROGRAM?

When contemplating a change in a resistance-training program, it is important to consider its motivation. Is it a goal change? Is it the client? Or the trainer? A program that has plateaued in terms of results, resistance, or number of repetitions and sets may or may not be a problem. When your clients have reached their goals and are pleased with their body image and level of strength, such a program can be termed "maintenance." Maintenance is a positive state of training, wherein you keep your clients' fitness at their trained level.

Valid reasons for changing a resistance-training program include boredom, lack of motivation, lack of results, desire for change in muscle strength, hypertrophy, muscle endurance, or a change in training environment (e.g., equipment availability). Before you consider changing a program, remember that every client should have a muscle strength and endurance base. Establish this strength foundation by training your clients for at least four to six weeks.

Add Variety by Using Cross Training

If your clients are bored, disinterested, or lack motivation, cross train within the muscle strength and endurance components of fitness. This type of training is characterized by variety and the use of different exercises and equipment. Initially, try **cross training** without changing intensity. An often-overlooked variable is to change the movement pattern of an exercise, or the order of exercise, to stimulate a different pattern of motor unit recruitment (Fleck & Kraemer, 1997). This is in contrast to simply adding or subtracting the amount of resistance your clients work against.

Another first step is simply to change the sequence of exercises the clients are already doing to create variety and a new overload. It is suggested that the fatigue pattern of the involved motor units will be changed, causing your clients to adapt to the new stimulus. The next step might be to replace some or all of the exercises in the foundation routine. For each exercise, look at the joint action(s) and muscle group(s) being utilized and replace the exercise with another that targets the same group(s). For example, the bench press can be replaced by pushups, dumbbell presses, incline and decline presses, or dumbbell or elastic resistance chest flys (uses horizontal adduction only), because all of these copy elbow extension and horizontal adduction at the shoulder. Machine pullover movements can be replaced by movements that replicate shoulder extension, such as dumbbell or elastic resistance pullovers, one arm or double arm "low" rows, or straight-arm pullbacks with dumbbells or elastic resistance. These exercises help to preserve balance in the foundation routine.

Any change in movement patterns (new exercises or slight body position changes) will require a different motor unit recruitment pattern (Fleck & Kraemer, 1997). This holds true even if you are targeting the same muscle group(s) and utilizing similar joint actions. Cross training can positively affect compliance, motivation, and interest, as well as stimulate the body toward additional strength gains.

Exercise Plateau and Overtraining Challenges

Plateaus and overtraining are often the result of continuously using one training program approach. The following approaches can help minimize the possibility of either outcome. Initially, change the exercise sequence or the exercise

itself, while leaving the relative intensity the same. Next, manipulate frequency, intensity, and volume both up and down. Keep the repetitions within the 8- to 20-repetition framework if no sport-specific application is required.

Consider utilizing high-intensity training techniques (see pages 261–262). It seems that the best stimulus for increasing strength gains is to make the muscles work harder, as opposed to longer. High-intensity training may be the edge you need to move your clients who are advanced in their resistance-training gains off strength plateaus. Quality reigns over quantity.

Changing Intensity for the Well-trained Client

If your clients have been training with you two to three times per week for more than six months, performing 10 to 20 exercises per session, and are looking for additional size and/or strength gains, you should look closely at one factor: intensity.

To increase strength and/or size, intensity with an overload of resistance that keeps your clients training within anaerobic pathways must be maintained. This means that they must fatigue the musculature within a time period of about 30 to 90 seconds. In other words, the body's musculature must be presented with an intensity to which it is unaccustomed on a regular and progressive basis.

If a program remains the same (as within the maintenance phase), muscle endurance and/or the current level of strength will be maintained. This situation should not be evaluated as good or bad, but should be considered within the context of your clients' goals.

High-repetition overloads are usually not sufficient to stimulate significant strength gains (except in deconditioned clients), are rarely useful (except in sport-specific applications), and generally do not engage significant muscle mass to create a cardiorespiratory training effect. This type

When is the Right Time to Change a Strength Program?

of training also is usually ineffective in promoting any kind of health and fitness gains and, if the repetitions are redundantly high, could lead to overuse injuries, lack of results, and frustration.

For conditioned exercisers, lower the number of repetitions to 8 to 12 and/or utilize high-intensity training techniques. This intensity is safe and maximizes adaptations in the neuromuscular systems. How can you apply this information to your clients' training programs? Have your clients perform 8 to 20 repetitions to the point of temporary fatigue for each exercise set. You will have to communicate to your clients the effort and concentration that is necessary to attain this type of high-intensity training.

PRACTICAL APPLICATION THROUGH A CASE STUDY APPROACH

Do you have clients who focus on elite or advanced strength? Are you dealing with **asymptomatic** average clients or older adults? There is much confusion surrounding the number of repetitions and sets and the amount of resistance you should use with varying populations. The following case studies, one of an Olympic-style lifter and the other of an older adult (age 63), help clarify some seemingly contradictory recommendations.

Case Study 1: Olympic Lifter

Olympic lifting is a competitive sport that involves two technical and explosive lifting movements known as the "clean and jerk" and the "snatch." John is an Olympic lifter who maintains high levels of muscle strength, joint flexibility, and neuromuscular coordination. He has had years of specialized training. His goals are based on the demands of the sport: to accomplish maximal strength development and 1-repetition-maximum (1-RM) lifts. A 1-RM lift is the most amount of

weight you can lift once; a 10-RM lift is the most amount of weight you can lift 10 times with good technique. A typical protocol for Olympic lifters is as follows:

Load (resistance)	1–6 RM for max strength development
Sets	Multiple, 3–6 for each exercise
Repetitions	1–10 per set, to fatigue, for strength and power, skill development, and periodization effect
Rest/ Recovery	2–5 minutes between each set for full energy system recovery
Frequency	1–3 sessions per day, 4–6 days per week

Case Study 2: Older Adult Exerciser

Janet is 63 years old and participates in a regular walking program. She has just begun a muscular strength and endurance conditioning program. She was motivated by reports that resistance training can positively affect **osteoporosis,** increase metabolism and calorie burning, influence posture, and help maintain physical independence. Janet's program resembles the following:

Load (resistance)	12–20 RM during introduction to training; 8–12 RM after 6–8 weeks of training
Sets	1 per exercise, introduction to training; 1–2 after 4–6 weeks of training
Number of Exercises	8–10 exercises that challenge all major muscle groups
Repetitions	8–20 range per set (see Load above)

Recovery 1–2 minutes between sets, use active recovery to minimize down time

Frequency 2 times per week, for excellent gains in strength and muscular endurance

Analyzing the Case Studies

Notice that these protocols do not include how much weight either John or Janet should lift. For both clients, the load is determined by an appropriate resistance that fatigues the muscle within the stated repetition goal range. Remember, the key to strength development is high-effort anaerobic exercise. The resistance should be sufficient to fatigue the target muscle group within about 30 to 90 seconds of exercise.

Clearly, John and Janet will be training at different levels of resistance to reach muscle fatigue. But what about Joe, also age 63, who later joins Janet in the same fitness pursuit? Since their goals are similar, their exercise protocols will be the same. But this does not mean they will lift an identical amount of weight. For example, after Joe has trained for eight weeks, both he and Janet may fatigue at 10 RM. However, Janet may use a 12-pound weight for a given lift, while Joe, who has not been training as long, may use an 8-pound weight for the same exercise.

PERIODIZATION

Periodization is the systematic application of overload through the pre-planned variation of program components to optimize gains in strength while preventing overuse, staleness, **overtraining,** and plateaus. Periodization can be used to maximize the gains in muscular fitness achieved during training for any exercising client or to help athletes "peak" at the appropriate times for competitions. Research has shown periodized programs

to be superior in eliciting strength and body-mass improvements when compared to traditional methods utilizing both single- and multiple-set designs (Fleck, 1999; Kraemer et al., 2000; Marx et al., 2000; Rhea et al., 2002; Schiotz et al., 1998). In fact, periodized programs have been so successful that ACSM recommends the use of a periodized model of progression for resistance training in healthy adults (American College of Sports Medicine, 2002).

The success of periodization can be attributed to the variation in programming not commonly seen with non-periodized programs. This variation provides a constantly changing stress to the neuromuscular system, which promotes continued adaptation and prevents plateaus (Rhea et al., 2002). There are several unique characteristics of periodized programs that differentiate them from traditional training programs. They are (1) the inclusion of scheduled "rest" or periods of reduced training, (2) frequent program changes, and (3) the systematic reduction in volume when increasing intensity. There are a number of factors that can be manipulated to achieve a periodized resistance-training program. These include:

✔ Number of sets and reps
✔ Specific exercise performed
✔ Order of exercises performed
✔ Speed and type of contraction
✔ Type of resistance used
✔ Amount of rest between sets or exercises
✔ Frequency of training

To develop an effective periodized program, it is essential to understand the overall structure of such a program. Once the overall structure is clear, the process of incorporating rest, variety, and progression becomes a manageable task. The periodized structure involves a series of cycles, or periods of time, within which exercise factors are altered. Variations occur within these predetermined time frames. Three different time frames are utilized to develop a periodized strength program: **macrocycles, mesocycles,** and **microcycles.**

A macrocycle, the longest time frame, is usually designated as a period of six months to a year. Each of the other two time frames is shorter and falls within the macrocycle. The goals established for a macrocycle are long-term and generally require multiple steps to be successfully obtained. Common macrocycle goals include participating in an event (e.g., 10K running race), peaking for an athletic competition, achieving major physical transformations (e.g., significant increases in lean body mass), or establishing a long-term pattern of exercise.

Macrocylces are made up of a series of mesocycles, which are usually three to four months long. Each mesocycle has a goal to be achieved by the end of the designated time period. Common goals for a mesocycle are muscular hypertrophy, muscular power, local muscular endurance, or motor performance (developing skill). Each mesocycle goal represents a step in moving closer to achieving your macrocycle goal.

Mesocycles, in turn, are made up of a series of microcycles, which are usually one to four weeks long. The goal for a microcycle is short-term and each microcycle goal is designed to progress the client toward the successful achievement of the mesocycle's desired outcome. The goal of one microcycle may be to become proficient at new exercises, reduce a muscle imbalance, or increase the weight lifted.

As discussed, each of the three time frames have their own goals. The mesocycle and microcycle goals are carefully designed steps that move a client toward achieving the macrocycle goal. Within each of these timeframes, however, the characteristics of the periodized program are incorporated. Hence, rest, variety, and progression are programmed within each

mesocycle and microcycle, as well as across the entire macrocycle.

The simplest way to begin developing your periodized program is to determine your macrocycle time frame, then break it down into mesocycles of equal length. Finally, break each mesocycle down into microcycles of equal length. Determine your client's goals for the macrocycle and each mesocycle. Then begin specific programming at the microcycle level.

Each microcycle should incorporate a period of rest/recovery. For example, in a four-week microcycle, three weeks would involve a progressive building of exercise intensity with a reduction in volume, and the fourth week would allow for rest by reducing both intensity and volume. For a shorter microcycle (e.g., one week), the rest day could be the seventh day of the cycle. Assign volume and intensity values for each microcycle. Eventually, you will assign these values for each day.

Volume in a resistance-training program is defined as the total weight lifted in a training session.

Volume = Total Repetitions x Intensity

Intensity is determined by the amount of resistance used. You can represent resistance by the absolute weight lifted (e.g., 120 lb) or by the percent of 1 RM a resistance represents (e.g., 80%).

Intensity = Weight or %1 RM

Start each microcycle with a lower intensity and higher volume. Determine your initial intensities through strength testing for maximum or estimated maximum resistance. Choose the percent of max based on your microcycle goal. As the microcycle progresses, decrease the volume and increase the intensity until you reach the rest/recovery period. For example, start with three sets of 8 to 10 reps at 80% 1 RM, and then progress to one set of 6 to 8 reps at 85% 1 RM. The weight will increase as training progresses, but at no time should the progression be greater than 2 to 10% of 1 RM, depending on the muscle size (American College of Sports Medicine, 2002). During the rest/recovery period, both volume and intensity are reduced. Following the rest/recovery, start the next microcycle with an intensity slightly above the initial values of the preceding microcycle. This allows you to continuously move the client forward by applying overload in a comfortable stepwise fashion.

Incorporating variety into a microcycle can be achieved by manipulating any of the factors identified earlier, such as changing exercises, muscle contraction speeds or types, or exercise order. Variety within a microcycle is less important than variety between microcycles, or even better, between mesocycles. New, untrained exercisers will require less variety than trained exercisers to avoid plateaus, staleness, or overtraining. A variation on the common periodized routine, called daily undulating periodization, has been shown to be beneficial for previously trained subjects (Rhea et al., 2002). In this format, variety and volume/intensity changes are made daily instead of between microcycles.

Rest is essential for all clients, regardless of training level, to keep them motivated and free of overuse injuries. Rest should be scheduled at both the microcycle and mesocycle levels. At the mesocycle level, one cycle may have less overall volume and intensity then the preceding cycle—similar to the post-season recovery given to athletes. Including this break from the rigors of progressive overload can benefit all clients in their pursuit of long-term goals.

Periodization Model for Health and Fitness Improvement

Step 1: Set the goal(s).
- ✔ cardiorespiratory
- ✔ muscular strength and endurance
- ✔ flexibility
- ✔ other

Step 2: Determine how to achieve the goal(s).

- ✔ Assess time availability.
- ✔ Identify types (mode) of activity.
- ✔ Match training to goals.
- ✔ Choose activities that the client enjoys.

Step 3: Identify training phases.

1. *Training phases*
- ✔ Develop a yearly organizational training plan (macrocycle), or at least three to four months of mesocycles.
- ✔ Develop a three- to four-week training plan (mesocycle).
- ✔ Develop a 3- to 10-day short-term plan (microcycle).

2. *Exercise plan*
- ✔ Manipulate frequency, intensity, and duration of each activity for specific results in the body's energy/physiologic systems.
- ✔ Apply frequency, intensity, and duration to each fitness component in the general preparation phase and the goal phase.
- ✔ Control results by using proper intensity and adequate recovery.

Step 4: Plan volume and intensity.

1. *Vary volume and overload on a cyclical basis.*
- ✔ Change at least every three to four weeks, and possibly within a 3- to 10-day microcycle.
- ✔ Plan to increase or decrease volume and intensity.
- ✔ Use lower intensities and less duration during active recovery.
- ✔ Start the new mesocycle after active recovery at a slightly lower intensity than the previous cycle.

2. *Allow for the restoration/recovery process.*
- ✔ Never increase progressive overload for more than three continuous weeks.
- ✔ Follow any sustained, progressive overload of about three weeks with at least several days of active recovery activity at a lower intensity. (The effort is less

intense when compared to the last overload phase in which your clients participated.)

✔ After active recovery, start the new mesocycle at a slightly lower intensity than the previous cycle.

Step 5: Regularly evaluate the periodization planning process.

✔ Monitor results and progress.

✔ Conduct a fitness assessment (optional).

✔ Recognize goal achievement.

✔ Maintain an ongoing dialogue with your clients.

✔ Observe client compliance and enthusiasm toward the program.

Case Study: From Periodization Theory to Client Application

Jenna is a beginning exerciser whose goals are weight loss, weight management, increased strength and "muscle tone," and increased energy level. Jenna understands that a long-term plan (macrocycle) that incorporates important fitness components will help her realize her training goals.

1. Set the goals.

The first step in creating a periodized program is to assess Jenna's current fitness levels in relation to her goals of weight loss, weight management, and increased energy. Fitness testing not only accomplishes this, but also establishes a reference point for comparing fitness improvements over time and helps you evaluate the effectiveness of your program.

2. The solution: Determine how to achieve the goals.

Improvements in cardiorespiratory fitness and muscular strength and endurance will be crucial in helping Jenna attain her goals. She understands the important contribution cardiorespiratory fitness makes to calorie burning, and that if she becomes more fit, she will be able to burn more calories and fat, and develop more endurance.

Strength training will enhance Jenna's feeling of power and control. Because gains in muscle strength increase muscle endurance, she will have new energy and strength at the end of the day. Also, increases in lean muscle mass will reshape her body and increase her resting metabolic rate, which will help her lose body fat and maintain her desired weight.

3. Identify training phases.

It is usually unrealistic to plan out an entire year and expect average fitness enthusiasts to stick to this. Instead, stay focused on microcycles and mesocycles.

✔ Once the goal(s) and starting fitness level are determined, plan a menu of workouts (keeping the session length in mind) over a 3- to 10-day microcycle.

✔ Next, extend the microcycle to a planned three- to four-week mesocycle.

✔ Planning a "mini" macrocycle (long-term planning) of three to four months is the next step.

This formula will keep you ahead in the planning process and will save valuable time should events in your client's life necessitate a major change in the training program or schedule.

You now start the cycles. Since Jenna is new to fitness and her goals are set, her first 3- to 10-day microcycle will focus on a preparation phase that reflects the goals of: (1) increased overall endurance, and (2) weight management. Her program looks like this:

✔ A series of six or seven microcycles (about two months) emphasizing a basic, but progressive resistance and cardiorespiratory program. This series of microcycles is equivalent to two mesocycles.

✔ Incorporate active rest into each mesocycle by reducing the volume and intensity of one microcycle.

✔ A second mesocycle will emphasize continued, progressive increases in intensity. If Jenna is ready, exercise variety will be introduced within each fitness component.

4. Plan volume and intensity.

After the preparation phase is well established (in about eight weeks), the third mesocycle begins and progresses to the goal phase of the periodization process. This cycle will emphasize a hypertrophy phase for strength and continued challenges in duration and intensity of effort for cardiorespiratory conditioning. For example, Jenna may have progressed from a 12 to 20 repetition overload to fatigue, to an 8 to 12 repetition overload to fatigue. Progressing beyond the base of aerobic endurance built in the first two mesocycles, the third mesocycle will manipulate cardiorespiratory intensity, duration, and frequency, and utilize interval conditioning.

The goal of these specific time periods is to provide an overload that is challenging, progressive, and in sync with Jenna's new fitness gains. Microcycles and mesocycles also create goals that are reasonable, and most important, attainable in short time frames. This keeps the client motivated, compliant, and physiologically fresh.

5. Evaluate the program.

Reassessment of goals, results, client interest, and enthusiasm can never happen too often. This maintains open and fresh communication with clients, keeps you focused on their current fitness levels, and helps you anticipate your next step.

Implementing Periodized Fitness

The key to successful periodization is the ability to challenge the body with new activities and progressive overload (intensity). Three to four weeks of cycling workouts will get results. Just as the body experiences the peak benefits of one mesocycle of planned workouts and starts to adapt to it, the client moves into a whole new three- to four-week cycle that offers a completely new set of challenges.

There are several ways you can track a periodization program. One idea is to label a file folder with each mesocycle and keep each client's workout card in the file. You may have four separate file folders inside one hanging file for each client. You can do the same thing on your computer by creating a file for each mesocycle and placing the programs you create in the file.

A comprehensive, accurate planning process will draw heavily on your practical experience and knowledge of the scientific theory behind training. Periodization, planning, and program organization are not inherently complex tasks. The primary purpose of this type of training is to raise the fitness state of an individual to a higher level with a systematic approach. However, implementation does require considerable forethought and time investment. On the other hand, it is well worth it, since periodization makes both the trainer and participant accountable for results.

TRACKING GAINS WITH GOOD RECORDS

Science has not defined the "best" or "perfect" program, but variation and intensity are two of its most important factors. Make sure that you keep accurate lifting records (repetitions, sets, resistance, order of exercise, name of exercise, and periodization planning program) so that you can determine the type of program manipulation that best stimulates your clients' minds and bodies. It is likely that no two people will respond in the same manner to a given training program. Because of this phenomenon, known as individual response, your records, client feedback, strength testing if appropriate, as well as body fat and circumference measurements will help determine the program's effectiveness.

Tracking Gains with Good Records

Directing Results

DIRECTING RESULTS

Just how much control do you really have in directing results? Certain genetic factors, such as muscle fiber type, number of fibers, and neural and hormonal influences ultimately determine the outer ranges of strength and body shape. However, each person's optimal potential can best be reached by emphasizing the following:

1. Design systems with specific goals in mind.
2. Fit all systems into the specificity chart.
3. Encourage consistent, regular, and varied efforts.
4. Teach the use of proper biomechanical techniques.
5. Allow for the recovery/building process.
6. Keep accurate records.

UPPER BODY

Incline Machine Chest Press
(pectorals, anterior deltoids, triceps)

Performance recommendations

Adjust seat so hand grips are at chest level. Sit on seat with shoulders back and chest lifted. Exhale while pushing the hand grips out and up. Extend the arms until the elbows are relatively straight but not locked out. Pause and then flex the elbows, returning the weights to the starting position.

Training points to emphasize

- Keep chest lifted and maintain a neutral spine.
- Maintain alignment of the hands, wrists, and forearms.
- Lift and lower the weights in a slow, controlled fashion.

Pec Flys on Stability Ball
(pectorals, anterior deltoids)

Performance recommendations

Lie supine on the stability ball to allow free movement of the shoulders with the feet on the floor. Hold a dumbbell in each hand with the arms extended and the elbows slightly flexed. Lower the dumbbells until the elbows are at shoulder level. Pause and then raise the dumbbells back up to the starting position.

Training points to emphasize

- Lower and raise the dumbbells in arcing motion.
- Do not allow the line formed by the elbows and shoulders to go beyond the midline of the body.
- Do not let the dumbbells tilt up or down.

Standing Cable Chest Press
(pectorals, anterior deltoids, triceps)

Performance recommendations

Stand upright with a slight forward lean of the body. Maintain a neutral spine and place your feet approximately shoulder-width apart or in a staggered position. Grasp the handles so the hands are approximately shoulder-width apart and press them directly out in front of the shoulders. Pause and then return to the starting position by bringing the arms back until the line formed by the elbow and shoulder is no deeper than the midline of the body.

Training points of emphasize
- Keep the upper arms and forearms parallel to the floor.
- Keep the elbows rotated away from the body.
- Do not let the cable handles tilt up or down.

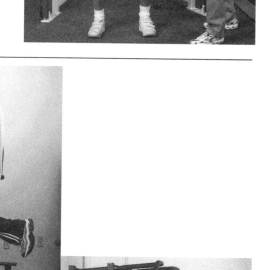

Machine-assisted Dip Movement
(pectorals, anterior deltoids, triceps)

Performance recommendations

Kneel on the machine platform with an upright posture and neutral spine. Place the hands on the support handles and slightly retract the scapula. Maintain a body position that is almost perpendicular to the floor during the descent phase. Pause and then return to the start position by flexing the shoulders and extending the elbows.

Training points to emphasize
- During the descent phase, the elbows should not flex more than 90 degrees.
- Keep the head and shoulders aligned over the hips.
- Upon returning to the straight-arm start position, depress the scapula without hyperextending the elbows.

Machine Lat Pull-down
(latissimus dorsi, biceps)

Performance recommendations

Sit facing the weight stack with knees bent under the thigh pad, feet flat on the floor, and arms extended. Grasp the bar slightly wider than shoulder-width apart with a pronated grip. Maintain a neutral spine, keep abdominals contracted, and lean back slightly so that the bar is aligned with the clavicle. Retract the scapula and pull the bar toward the chest. Pause and then return to the starting position.

Training points to emphasize

- Avoid hyperextension of the lumbar spine.
- Maintain a neutral wrist position throughout the exercise.
- Avoid performing behind-the-neck lat pull-downs, which increase the chances of injury to the shoulder joint.

Seated Cable Lat Row
(latissimus dorsi, biceps, rhomboids, posterior deltoids)

Performance recommendations

Sit facing the weight stack with knees slightly bent and feet firmly on the foot platforms. Grasp the handle with a neutral grip. Keep the chest lifted, shoulders back, and head and neck aligned with the spine. Retract the scapula and pull the handles toward the rib cage. Pause and then return to the starting position.

Training points to emphasize

- Keep chest lifted, shoulders back, and do not round the upper back when the arms extend.
- Do not initiate the pulling with the arms and shoulders—"lead with the elbows."
- Avoid hyperextension of the lumbar spine (i.e., do not arch the back).

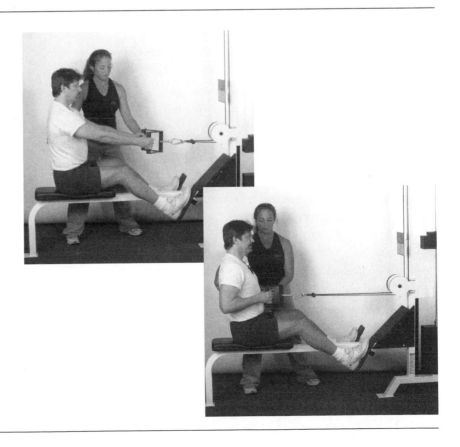

Kneeling Single-arm Dumbbell Lat Row
(latissimus dorsi, teres major, posterior deltoids, biceps)

Performance recommendations

Place one knee on the bench with the same-side hip aligned directly over it. The knee of the other leg should be at approximately the same height and slightly flexed and place the non-working hand at the front of the bench and position the upper body so that it is parallel to the floor. Slowly flex the elbow and pull the arm up until the upper arm is parallel to the floor or slightly higher and the elbow forms an approximately 90-degree angle. Pause and then slowly lower the arm back down to the starting position.

Training points to emphasize

- Keep the elbow close to the side of the body.
- Maintain neutral lumbar and cervical posture.
- Keep the chest "square" to the floor throughout the exercise movement.

Machine-assisted Pull-up
(latissimus dorsi, teres major, posterior deltoids, biceps)

Performance recommendations

Kneel on the machine platform with an upright, neutral spinal posture. Place the hands on the parallel grips overhead, with the hands directly in line with slightly flexed elbows, and using a neutral grip. Maintain a body position that is almost perpendicular to the floor. Initiate the movement by contracting the latissimus dorsi, and pull the body up until the chin is even with, or slightly above, the grips. Pause and then return to the starting position by flexing the shoulders and extending the elbows.

Training points to emphasize

- Do not allow the body to swing forward or back.
- Maintain neutral lumbar and cervical posture.
- Retract and depress the scapulae throughout the exercise movement.

Standing Cable Side Lateral Raise (medial deltoids)

Performance recommendations

Stand in a "ready" position with a neutral spinal posture. The body is upright and the hips and knees are slightly flexed. Grasp the handle with an overhand grip. With a slightly flexed elbow, raise the arm out and up until it is approximately parallel to the floor. Pause and then lower the arm back down to the starting position.

Training points to emphasize

- Keep the hand slightly in front of the shoulder with the elbow directly in line with the shoulder.
- Keep the wrist neutral with the palm oriented to the floor at the end range of motion.
- Avoid internally or externally rotating the shoulder, or supinating or pronating the elbow.
- Lower the arm back down to the starting position with control.

Dumbbell Shoulder Press (anterior deltoids, triceps, trapezius)

Performance recommendations

Sit on a bench with back erect and a dumbbell in each hand. Upper arms are shoulder height and elbows are bent to 90 degrees. Palms face forward with neutral, stable wrist position. Press the dumbbells up and toward each other overhead. Pause and then slowly return to the starting position.

Training points to emphasize

- Do not arch the back.
- Keep the shoulder blades retracted with the torso and head erect.
- Do not let the dumbbells touch at the top of the movement.
- Do not "lock out" the elbows at the top of the movement.

Prone Dumbbell Rear Pull
(posterior deltoids)

Performance recommendations

Lie prone on a bench or stability ball with the arms hanging down toward the floor. Grasp the dumbbells with the palms facing back. Keeping the elbows slightly flexed and stabilized, pull the arms up until the upper arms are parallel to the floor or slightly higher. Pause and then slowly return to the starting position.

Training points to emphasize

- Retract the shoulder blades and maintain retraction throughout the exercise movement.
- Do not let the shoulders internally or externally rotate.
- Keep the head and neck aligned with the spine.

Standing Cable Biceps Curl
(biceps)

Performance recommendations

Stand in a "ready" position with a neutral spine. The body is upright and the hips and knees are slightly flexed. Grasp the handle with an underhand grip. Bring the hands toward the shoulders and flex the elbows through their full active range of motion. Pause and then slowly lower the arms back down to the starting position.

Training points to emphasize

- Initiate the movement at the elbow (do not "swing" the handle up to lift the weight).
- Keep the wrists neutral throughout the exercise .
- Retract the shoulder blades and maintain the same shoulder position throughout the exercise.
- Do not lean forward or back during the exercise.

Seated Biceps Curl
(biceps)

Performance recommendations

Sit on a bench or stability ball with the back erect. Hold dumbbells in each hand with a neutral grip and arms extended. Bring the hands toward the shoulders and flex the elbows through their full active range of motion. Pause and then slowly lower the arms back down to the starting position.

Training points to emphasize

- Initiate the movement at the elbow (do not "swing" the dumbbells up to lift the weight).
- Keep the wrists neutral throughout the exercise.
- Retract the shoulder blades and maintain the same shoulder position throughout the exercise.
- Do not lean forward or back during the exercise.

Standing Cable Triceps Press
(triceps)

Performance recommendations

Stand in a "ready" position with feet shoulder-width apart or in a staggered stance. The body is upright and the hips and knees are slightly flexed. Grasp the handle with an overhand grip and place the elbows alongside the body. Hold the handle so that an approximately 90-degree angle is formed at the elbow. Press the handle toward the floor while simultaneously extending the elbows. Pause and then slowly return to the starting position.

Training points to emphasize

- Initiate the movement at the elbow (do not "hunch over" or pull with the shoulders).
- Keep the wrists neutral throughout the exercise.
- Retract the shoulder blades and maintain the same shoulder position throughout the exercise.
- Do not allow the elbows to flare away from the body.

Kneeling Single-arm Dumbbell Triceps Extension (triceps)

Performance recommendations

Place one knee on the bench with the same-side hip aligned directly over it. The knee of the other leg should be at approximately the same height and slightly flexed. Place the non-working hand on the front edge of the bench. Position the upper body so that it is parallel to the floor. Flex the elbow and extend the shoulder until the upper arm is parallel with the floor. Slowly extend the elbow until the forearm is parallel to the floor. Pause and then slowly lower the arm back down to the starting position.

Training points to emphasize

• Do not allow the elbow to flare away from the body.

• Keep the wrist stabilized, not allowing the top of the dumbbell to tip toward the floor.

• Retract the shoulder blades and maintain the same shoulder position throughout the exercise.

LOWER BODY

Standing Barbell Squat
(gluteals, quadriceps, hamstrings)

Performance recommendations

Use a squat rack or Smith machine. The bar should rest on the shoulder blades, off the notch of the neck. Stand with a neutral spine and feet shoulder-width apart. Slowly start the descent with hips back, keeping the weight centered over the heels or mid-foot. Lower to approximately 90 degrees of knee flexion. Pause and then slowly return to the starting position.

Training points to emphasize

- Do not allow the knees to travel past the toes during the lowering phase.
- Do not "drop" the gluteals lower than the knees.
- Avoid use of a block or board under the heels.
- Maintain a neutral spine throughout the exercise.

Seated Leg Press
(gluteals, quadriceps, hamstrings)

Performance recommendations

Sit on a leg press machine with feet hip-width apart. Hold the handles and contract the abdominals. Flex the knees to approximately 90 degrees, keeping them aligned with the ankles and keep the entire foot in contact with the foot-plate. Extend the legs until they are straight but not locked. Pause and then slowly return to the starting position.

Training points to emphasize

- Avoid hyperextension of the knee at the end of the movement.
- Push through the heels, not the toes.
- Do not allow the knees to travel past the toes during the lowering phase.

Standing Dumbbell Lunge
(quadriceps, hamstrings, gluteals)

Performance recommendations

Stand with the feet together holding a dumbbell in each hand. Take a long step forward with one foot and flex the rear knee to achieve a "fencer's" lunge position. Slowly lower the knee straight down. Push back up to the standing position in a controlled fashion.

Training points to emphasize

- Do not allow the knee of the front leg to travel forward past the toes during the descent.
- Begin with small lunges and gradually increase.
- Do not arch the back.

Modified Dead Lift
(hamstrings, gluteals)

Performance recommendations

Stand upright with the ankles, knees, and hips slightly flexed. Grasp the bar with an overhand grip, placing it at the thighs and in front of the body. Begin to lower the torso by pushing the hips back. Lower the torso until the hands are just above the knees (an approximate 30-degree hip angle). Pause and then extend the hips and slowly return to the upright starting position.

Training points to emphasize

- Make sure the spine does not flex or "round."
- Concentrate on "driving the heels into the ground" when extending the hips.
- Keep the bar close to the body and aligned with the shoulders.

Seated Leg Extension (quadriceps)

Performance recommendations

Sit on the leg extension machine with the knees at an approximately 90-degree angle. Hook the tops of the feet behind the roller pad, flex your feet, and lightly grip the handles. Extend the legs, lifting the pad upward until the knees are straight but not locked. Pause and then slowly return to the starting position.

Training points to emphasize

- Do not allow the gluteals to lift off the seat as the legs move up and down.
- Use slow, controlled movement (do not "drop or bounce" the weight stack between reps).
- Maintain alignment between the neck and spine throughout the exercise movement.

Standing Cable Hip Abduction (hip abductors)

Performance recommendations

Place an ankle strap on the outside leg and stand to the side of the cable pulley with feet shoulder-width apart and trunk stabilized. Hold on to the support bar for balance and lift the working leg out to the side. Pause and then slowly return to the starting position.

Training points to emphasize

- Do not swing the working leg to lift the weight.
- Maintain a neutral spine.
- Do not allow the hips to internally or externally rotate.

Standing Cable Hip Adduction
(hip adductors)

Performance recommendations

Place an ankle strap on the inside leg and stand to the side of the cable pulley with feet shoulder-width apart and trunk stabilized. Hold on to the support bar for balance and bring the working leg across the foot of the supporting leg. Pause and then slowly return to the starting position.

Training points to emphasize

- Do not swing the working leg to lift the weight.
- Maintain a neutral spinal posture.
- Do not allow the hips to internally or externally rotate.

Standing Dumbbell Heel Raise
(gastrocnemius, soleus)

Performance recommendations

Holding a dumbbell in each hand, stand upright with neutral spinal alignment. Slowly lift the body vertically by contracting the gastrocnemius and soleus muscles. Raise the heels up until full, active range of motion is achieved. Pause and then slowly lower the heels back down until they are almost touching the floor.

Training points to emphasize

- Keep weight on the balls of the feet.
- Keep the toes pointed straight ahead.
- To increase the exercise range of motion, stand on a block or platform and let the heels drop below the edge.

TORSO

Curl-up
(rectus abdominis)

Performance recommendations

In a supine position, place the hands or a rolled towel under the lumbar spine and flex one knee as shown. Raise the head and shoulders off the floor while maintaining a neutral spine, pause and then return to the starting position. Alternate the bent leg midway through each set of repetitions.

Training points to emphasize

- Do not flex the cervical spine by curling the neck.
- Do not elevate the head and shoulders a large distance off the floor.

Side Bridge
(quadratus lumborum, abdominal obliques)

Performance recommendations

Lie on one side as shown, bending the knees and keeping the elbow directly beneath the shoulder. To achieve this position, use the torso to lift the hips, being careful not to let the top hip rotate forward. Hold this postion for 10 to 15 seconds. Maintain a neutral neck and spine position.

Training points to emphasize

- Maintain neutral spinal alignment throughout the exercise.
- Maintain a mild contraction of the abdominal wall to help ensure spine stability.
- Extend the legs to increase the intensity of the exercise.

Birddog
(lumbar extensors—longissimus, iliocostalis, multifidi)

Performance recommendations

From an all-fours position, extend one leg and the opposite arm so that they are parallel to the floor. Hold this position for seven to eight seconds, and then repeat with the opposite arm and leg.

Training points to emphasize

- Maintain neutral spinal alignment throughout the exercise.
- Maintain a mild contraction of the abdominal wall to help ensure spine stability.
- Avoid "hiking" the hip, which twists the spine.

SUMMARY

Before you plan resistance-training programs for your clients, remember to look at their current state of psychology, personal needs, and level of fitness. When changing programs, be sure to evaluate their physiological needs and their readiness to change.

No program or exercise guideline is written in stone. Err on the side of conservatism. You must know your clients' physical limits and their perception of what is too much; intensity is relative to the individual. Do not join the ranks of trainers who create programs that are too difficult for their clients. Even if you do not injure them, you surely will defeat them. Resistance-training program design is a process that demands constant evaluation, manipulation, and change.

REFERENCES

American College of Sports Medicine (2002). Progression models in resistance training for healthy adults. *Medicine and Science in Sports and Exercise,* 34, 2, 364–380.

American College of Sports Medicine (2006). *ACSM's Guidelines for Exercise Testing and Prescription* (7th ed.). Philadelphia: Lippincott, Williams & Wilkins.

American College of Sports Medicine (1990). The recommended quantity and quality of exercise for developing and maintaining cardiorespiratory and muscular fitness in healthy adults. *Medicine and Science in Sports and Exercise,* 22, 2, 265–274.

American Council on Exercise (2002). *Stability Ball Training.* San Diego: American Council on Exercise.

Brooks, D. (2001). *Effective Strength Training.* Champaign, Ill.: Human Kinetics.

Enoka, R.M. (1997). Neural adaptations with chronic activity. *Journal of Biomechanics,* 30, 5, 447–455.

Fleck, S.J. (1999). Periodized strength training: a critical review. *Journal of Strength and Conditioning Research,* 13, 1, 82–89.

Fleck, S. & Kraemer, W. (1997). *Designing Resistance Training Programs.* (2nd ed.).Champaign, Ill.: Human Kinetics.

Kraemer, W.J. et al. (2000). Influence of resistance training volume and periodization on physiological and performance adaptations in collegiate women tennis players. *The American Journal of Sports Medicine,* 28, 5, 626–633.

Marx, J.O. et al. (2000). Low-volume circuit versus high-volume periodized resistance training in women. *Medicine and Science in Sports and Exercise,* 33, 4, 635–643.

McArdle, W. et al. (2001). *Exercise Physiology: Energy, Nutrition, and Human Performance.* (5th ed.). Philadelphia: Lippincott, Williams & Wilkins.

McHugh, M.P. et al. (2002). Differences in activation patterns between eccentric and concentric quadriceps contractions. *Journal of Sports Science,* 20, 2, 83–91.

Morrisey, M.C., Harman, E.A., & Johnson, M.J. (1995). Resistance training modes: specificity and effectiveness. *Medicine and Science in Sports and Exercise,* 27, 5, 648–660.

Rhea, M.R. et al. (2002). A comparison of linear and daily undulating periodized programs with equated volume and intensity for strength. *Journal of Strength and Conditioning Research,* 16, 2, 250–255.

Rutherford, O.M. & Jones, D.A. (1986). The role of learning and coordination in strength training. *European Journal of Applied Physiology,* 55, 100–105.

Schiotz, M.K. et al. (1998). The short-term effects of periodized and constant-intensity training on body composition, strength, and performance. *Journal of Strength and Conditioning Research,* 12, 3, 173–178.

Wilson, G.J., Murphy, A.J., & Walshe, A. (1996). The specificity of strength training: the effect of posture. *European Journal of Applied Physiology,* 73, 3, 346–352.

SUGGESTED READING

Baechle, T. & Groves, B. (1998). *Weight Training: Steps to Success.* (2nd ed.). Champaign, Ill.: Human Kinetics.

Basmajian, J. & DeLuca, C. (1985). *Muscles Alive: Their Functions Revealed By Electromyography.* (5th ed.). Baltimore, Md.: Williams and Wilkins.

Bompa, T. (1999). *Theory and Methodology of Training.* (4th ed.). Champaign, Ill.: Human Kinetics.

Brooks, D. (1999). *Your Personal Trainer.* Champaign, Ill.: Human Kinetics.

Brooks, D. & Copeland-Brooks, C. (1993). Uncovering the myths of abdominal exercise. *IDEA Today,* April, 42–49.

Brooks, D. et al. (1995). *Reebok Interval Program Manual.* Stoughton, Mass.: Reebok International, Ltd.

Brooks, D. et al. (1995). *Resist-A-Ball: Programming Guide For Fitness Professionals.* Indianapolis, Ind.: Ground Control, Inc.

Bruner, R. et al. (1992). *Soviet Training and Recovery Methods.* Pleasant Hill, Calif.: Sport Focus Publishing.

Evans, W. & Rosenberg, I. (1992). *Biomarkers.* New York: Simon & Schuster.

Hickson, R.C. et al. (1985). Reduced training intensities and loss of aerobic power, endurance and cardiac growth. *Journal of Applied Physiology,* 58, 492–499.

Kendall, F. et al. (2005). *Muscles: Testing and Function.* (5th ed.). Baltimore, Md.: Williams & Wilkins.

Komi, P.V. (Ed.) (2000). *Strength and Power in Sport.* (2nd ed.). Malden, Mass.: Blackwell Publishers.

Kraemer, W. & Fleck, S. (2005). *Strength Training For Young Athletes.* (2nd ed.). Champaign, Ill.: Human Kinetics.

McDonagh, M.J.N. & Davies, C.T.M. (1984). Adaptive response of mammalian skeletal muscle to exercise with high loads. *European Journal of Applied Physiology,* 52, 139–155.

Metveyev, L. (1982). *Fundamentals of Sports Training.* Moscow: Progress Publishers.

National Strength and Conditioning Association (2000). *Essentials of Strength Training and Conditioning.* T.R. Baechle & R.W. Earle (Eds.). Champaign, Ill.: Human Kinetics.

Ozolin, N. (1971). *The Athlete's Training System for Competition.* Moscow: Fizkultura Sport Publication.

Pate, R.R. et al. (1995). Physical activity and public health: a recommendation from the Centers for Disease Control and Prevention and the American College of Sports Medicine. *Journal of the American Medical Association,* 273, 402–407.

Siff, M. et al. (1993). *Super Training: Special Strength Training for Sporting Excellence.* South Africa: School of Mechanical Engineering, University of the Witwatersrand.

Vorobyev, A. (1978). *A Textbook on Weight Lifting.* Budapest: International Weight Lifting Federation.

Wescott, W. (1994). *Strength Fitness.* (4th ed.). Dubuque, Iowa: Wm. C. Brown Publishers.

References and Suggested Reading

References and Suggested Reading

Wilmore, J. (1991). Resistance training for health: a renewed interest. *Sports Medicine Digest,* June, 6.

Wilmore, J.H., Costill, D. & Kenney, W.L. (2007). *Physiology of Sport and Exercise.* (4th.). Champaign, Ill.: Human Kinetics.

Wilmore, J. & Costill, D. (1993). *Training for Sport and Activity: The Physiological Basis of the Conditioning Process.* (4th ed.). Boston: Allyn & Bacon.

Yessis, M. (1987). *The Secret of Soviet Sports Fitness and Training.* New York: William Morrow & Co.

Parts of this chapter are excerpted with permission from: Brooks, D. (1998). *Program Design for Personal Trainers: Bridging Theory into Application.* Champaign, Ill.: Human Kinetics and from Brooks, D. (2001). *Effective Strength Training.* Mammoth Lakes, Calif.: Moves International Fitness.

Flexibility

*Mari Cyphers, P.T., is a
physical therapist with an
extensive background in
orthopedics and sports
medicine. She is currently
a regional manager
for the Physiotherapy
Associates
clinics in the
San Francisco
Bay area and frequently
lectures for IDEA
conventions, Fitness
Associates network,
and California State
University, Hayward.*

**Mari
Cyphers**

Few would argue against the fact that flexibility is an important component of fitness and a critical factor in achieving peak physical potential. However, flexibility often is overlooked or misused. Some runners and weight lifters, for example, emphasize their cardiovascular or strength training, and pay little attention to their flexibility. Athletes and trainers who do stress flexibility often have different methods of flexibility training, and the current research does not validate or invalidate one method of stretching as being more effective than another.

While researchers have been unable to unequivocally validate the proposed benefits of flexibility training, there is evidence that indicates that flexibility training contributes to enhanced muscular relaxation, improved range

**Flexibility:
A Definition**

of motion within joints, improved muscular balance, enhanced speed of movement, reduced injury occurrence for certain activities, and improved performance of certain sport-related activities. It is important for you to include flexibility training in all your fitness programs, especially since research suggests that injuries do occur as a result of tight or stiff muscles. This chapter presents an overview of the substantial body of knowledge pertaining to flexibility training that can help your clients attain their fitness goals and decrease their risk of injury.

FLEXIBILITY: A DEFINITION

Flexibility is the range of motion within a joint along the various planes of motion. A joint itself does not move; rather, the body segments that come together within a joint move within the limitations established by the joint's properties. Within each joint and for each activity, there is an optimum **ROM** essential to peak performance that varies depending upon the activity. A number of factors can limit joint mobility: genetic inheritance; the joint structure itself; connective tissue elasticity within muscles, tendons, or skin surrounding a joint; strength of the opposing muscle group; and neuromuscular coordination. Flexibility training minimizes the factors that limit flexibility to help balance muscle groups that might be overused during physical training sessions or as a result of poor posture.

There are two basic types of flexibility: static and dynamic. **Static flexibility** can be impacted by body core temperature, body structure, muscle fiber lengths, connective tissue viscosity/elasticity, and muscle tendon attachment points. For example, a gymnast holding a split is demonstrating static flexibility. **Dynamic flexibility** involves movement through a range of motion with an emphasis on maintaining both speed and force. It is impacted by the same variables as static flexibility, but also by neuromuscular vari-

ables, balance, speed, and torque. A gymnast performing a split leap must not only possess the static flexibility of a split but also the power, coordination, and minimum tissue resistance to move to that position quickly in mid-air. Both static and dynamic flexibility are important in fitness and sports performance; therefore, it is important to become familiar with the different training methods for both static and dynamic flexibility. The benefits derived from each—full, usable, and safe ROM at various speeds of movement—include the following:

1. Increased physical efficiency and performance. A flexible joint requires less energy to move through the range of motion.

2. Decreased risk of injury. Although there is insufficient data to support this conclusion, many experts believe that increasing ROM should decrease the resistance in various tissues. Your clients, therefore, are less likely to incur injury by exceeding tissue extensibility during activity.

3. Increased blood supply and nutrients to joint structures. Flexibility training may also contribute to improved circulation and nutrient transport, allowing greater elasticity of tissues.

4. Improved nutrient exchange. Range of motion exercises may increase the quantity and decrease the viscosity, or thickness, of synovial fluid, thereby enabling better nutrient exchange. Healthy **synovial fluid** also allows greater freedom of movement and may decelerate joint degenerative processes.

5. Increased neuromuscular coordination. Studies have shown that nerve impulse velocity (the time it takes an impulse to travel to the brain and return) is enhanced with dynamic flexibility training. In attuning the central nervous system (CNS) to the physical demands placed upon it, opposing muscle groups work in a more synergistic, or coordinated, fashion.

6. Improved muscular balance and postural awareness. Flexibility helps realign soft tissue structures that may have adapted poorly

to the effects of gravity and postural habits. Realignment consequently reduces the effort it takes to achieve and maintain good posture in activities of daily living.

7. Decreased risk of low-back pain. Strong clinical evidence indicates that lumbo-pelvic flexibility, which involves the hamstrings, hip flexors, and the muscles attached to the pelvis, is critical in reducing the stress to the lumbar spine.

8. Reduced muscular tension. In general, stretching promotes muscular relaxation. A muscle in a constant state of contraction or tension may require more energy to accomplish activities.

9. Enhanced enjoyment. A physical training program must be enjoyable if a client is to stick with it. You may find that by relaxing both mind and body, flexibility training increases a client's sense of well-being and personal gratification during exercise.

Although flexibility is a valuable aspect of physical training, it is important for you to be aware of potential disadvantages associated with overtraining for excessive flexibility. How much joint flexibility is necessary varies with the activity and is highly specific to each client. Excessive flexibility often involves overstretched ligaments, referred to as ligament laxity, as well as congenital and genetic factors. With excessive flexibility, there is an increased risk of incurring injury unless the proper muscular strength and balance between muscles groups are maintained. This is sometimes seen in former gymnasts who are hyperflexible but no longer have the high levels of muscle strength to support it. Instability caused by overstretched ligaments may also lead to decreased joint-protective reflexes and neuromuscular coordination, and ultimately predispose a person to degenerative (arthritic) joint changes. For example, a severe ankle sprain overstretches the ligaments around the ankle. If the ankle is not properly rehabilitated, the overstretched ligaments can lead to additional injuries.

There may also be muscles that should not be stretched in some clients. Single-joint muscles that are placed in positions of prolonged stretch (usually due to poor postural positions) can develop a **stretch weakness** (Kendall, McCreary, & Provance, 1994). Stretch weakness may increase vulnerability to injury during even mild daily activities. These muscles need to be carefully strengthened and, if possible, allowed to return to normal resting length. These factors emphasize the need for well-balanced programs in muscular strength and flexibility to achieve greater joint stability and thus minimize the incidence of injury.

THE MECHANICS OF STRETCHING

Flexibility is enhanced by using a variety of stretching methods. It is accomplished by applying a force passively or actively to decrease tissue "stiffness" and elongate the musculotendinous unit, including lengthening of the actual muscle fiber, thereby resulting in an increased range of motion. Stretching refers to the process of elongation. It is widely accepted that the majority of resistance to stretch is not from the contractile muscle fiber itself, but rather from the connective tissue framework in and around the muscle. Therefore, understanding the mechanical properties of connective tissue under tension is essential in determining the best methods of increasing ROM and flexibility.

Connective tissue is composed of non-elastic collagen fibers and a small number of elastic fibers within a protein matrix that creates various soft tissue structures including **tendons, ligaments,** and **fascia** (Figure 10.1). Connective tissue has a very high

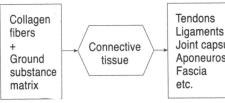

FIGURE 10.1
Organization of connective tissue structures.

The Mechanics of Stretching

tensile strength, which gives it the ability to support and protect underlying structures from injury. Organized connective tissue is **viscoelastic,** which means it has a combination of two mechanical properties related to obtaining normal flexibility: elasticity and viscosity.

An elastic stretch is an elongation of tissues that recovers when the tension is removed. It is often called temporary or recoverable elongation (deformation), and is frequently compared to a spring-like model (Figure 10.2).

A plastic stretch is an elongation in which the deformation to tissue remains even after the tension is removed. This property is termed permanent or nonrecoverable elongation and is likened to a hydraulic cylinder (Figure 10.3). If a hydraulic cylinder is pulled out, it will usually stay in the end position until another force acts upon it.

To obtain maximum results from flexibility training, you must realize that connective tissue behaves in a viscoelastic manner when stretched. That is, connec-

tive tissue exhibits both viscous (plastic) and elastic tendencies during elongation (Figure 10.4). When a soft tissue structure is stretched (in the elastic zone) and the force is removed, the tissue length recovers quickly to resting length. When a soft tissue structure is stretched in the plastic zone, a new resting length is attained, and the results are more permanent. Therefore, to produce more than temporary results, stretching techniques must be designed to increase plastic elongation (deformation).

Whether a stretch effects an elastic (temporary) or plastic (permanent) change in the tissue depends on the method and condition of the stretch. Two predominant factors in promoting permanent elongation are the force and the duration of the stretch. The degree of tissue lengthening that remains after a force is removed (plastic change) is greatest when a low-force, long-duration stretch (static) is used rather than a high-force, short-duration stretch (ballistic). It takes a minimum of 6 to 10 seconds to elicit the stretch response from the neuromuscular mechanisms.

Although different stretching methods may be appropriate in different instances, most professionals agree that a static stretch is the safest means to develop passive flexibility. The body, or in this case connective tissue, has the ability to adapt to the stresses placed upon it during physical activity by becoming stronger and better able to sustain increased and progressive levels of exercise intensity. If training conditions exceed the ability to adjust to the current levels of intensity, however, tissues will fail. According to Enoka (1994), "Whenever plastic changes are induced in a tissue, this involves a molecular reorganization and weakening of the tissue. However, this stress stimulates the tissue to adapt and the weakening is only short-term, provided training merely involves the stressing of tissue so that it adapts to a new length without any long-

FIGURE 10.2
The "spring" model, representing recoverable (elastic) deformation.

Elastic properties ⟶ Elastic stretch

Tensile force

FIGURE 10.3
The "hydraulic cylinder" model, representing permanent (plastic) deformation.

Viscous properties ⟶ Plastic stretch

Tensile force

FIGURE 10.4
Viscoelastic connective tissue has both plastic and elastic elements connected in a series.

Elastic elements   Viscous elements

Tensile force

term loss of strength." Connective tissue that is stretched too vigorously and/or for an excessive length of time can fail, leading to serious injury.

Another factor influencing connective tissue extensibility during stretching is an increase in tissue temperature. Exercise physiologists DeVries (1980) and Astrand & Rodahl (1970) concur that an elevation in core body temperature of as little as 1 to 3 degrees produces greater aerobic metabolism on a cellular level and reduced muscle fiber viscosity, increasing muscle elasticity and generally diminishing stiffness. Additional studies have shown that by raising tissue temperature, a thermal transition takes place within collagen microstructures, further augmenting viscous relaxation, and thus permitting enhanced flexibility (Sapega et al., 1981).

To summarize:

✔ A high-force, short-duration stretch performed when the tissue temperature is near or below normal will produce elastic deformation, or temporary, recoverable elongation.

✔ A low-force, long-duration stretch at slightly elevated tissue temperature will produce viscous (plastic) deformation, or permanent, nonrecoverable elongation.

THE STRETCH REFLEX

A primary component associated with the effects of stretching has a neurophysiologic basis involving reflex activity and is termed the **myotatic stretch reflex**. The sense organs or neural receptors responsible for the stretch reflex are the muscle spindles lying parallel to the muscle fiber, and the Golgi tendon organs found deep within the musculotendinous junctions. Each of these receptors is sensitive to stretch and helps protect a muscle against unnecessary injury.

In general, the muscle spindle passively mimics, or follows, the movements of its adjacent muscle fibers. That is, as the muscle fiber stretches, so does the spindle. The spindle responds to the velocity of the stretch. If the stretch is quick and extreme enough, the muscle spindle responds by sending a signal to the spinal cord, which then returns an order to create a sudden, protective muscular contraction. The spindle ceases to fire when this shortening begins, "unloading" as the muscle fiber contracts and preventing potential tissue damage (Figure 10.5a).

The reflex evoked when the patellar ligament is tapped directly below the kneecap during an examination is a classic example of the stretch reflex. By striking this ligament with a rubber mallet, the physician causes a quick stretch in the quadriceps mechanism. In turn, the muscle spindles react to this unexpected stretch by contracting the quadriceps, resulting in the knee-jerk reflex. Another example is falling

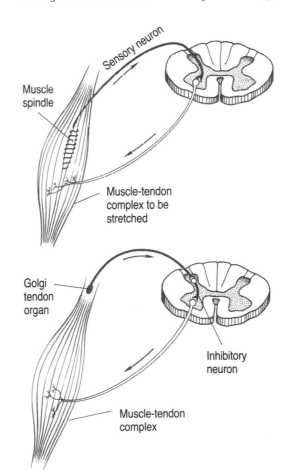

The Stretch Reflex

FIGURE 10.5
The stretch reflex and autogenic inhibition.

a. Simple muscle stretch reflex arc: The stretch of the muscle spindle causes reflex contraction.

b. Simple inverse stretch reflex arc: The stretch of Golgi tendon organ causes reflex inhibition (relaxation).

asleep in a seated position. As the head relaxes and bends forward, the muscle spindle experiences a sudden stretch, sending a message to the cervical muscle fibers, causing contraction and a sudden jerk to the upright position.

It is important to note that as the stretch reflex occurs, antagonist (opposite) muscle action is inhibited. So, when the quadriceps are stimulated with a reflex tap, the hamstrings action is automatically inhibited. This inhibitory response is called **reciprocal innervation** or **reciprocal inhibition.**

Up to a point, the harder a muscle is stretched, the stronger the reflex contraction. However, when tension becomes great enough to risk rupture, contraction abruptly stops, and the muscle relaxes. This relaxation response to extreme stretch is called **autogenic inhibition** and is chiefly dependent on the Golgi tendon organs (GTO). The GTO receptor is actually a weaker and nondominating system of muscular inhibition. Nevertheless, if all systems are overloaded as a result of excessive stretch or tension, the GTOs transmit impuls-

es to an inhibitory neuron within the spinal cord which finally overrides input from the muscle spindle, causing an immediate relaxation of the entire muscle (Figure 10.5b). A greater understanding of the stretch reflex and autogenic and reciprocal inhibition will assist you in determining the effectiveness of various types of stretching techniques used today.

In summary, three primary neural mechanisms related to the stretch reflex exist.

• *Reciprocal innervation.* When you contract a muscle, its antagonist group relaxes. This allows you to then stretch that antagonist group more efficiently when it is relaxed and its opposing muscle group is contracted.

• *Muscle spindles.* These respond to actual stretch, not speed. When a muscle fiber is overstretched, muscle spindles will fire and will cause the muscle to contract to protect itself.

• *Golgi tendon organs.* Located in the muscle tendon, Golgi tendon organs respond to tension, so that when tension is great they fire, causing the muscle to relax and reduce tension.

TYPES OF STRETCHING

There are numerous variations in flexibility exercises, but most types can be placed into two main categories: **passive stretching** and **active stretching.** During a passive stretch, the contractile components of the muscle are usually relaxed, and the portion of muscle most likely to be loaded is the connective tissue structures mentioned earlier as important in plastic elongation. The static stretch method is an excellent example of passive stretching. On the other hand, active, or dynamic, stretching has greater effects upon the elastic components: muscles, tendons, and musculotendinous junctions (Hubley-Kozey & Stanish, 1984). Because active stretching requires muscle contraction through a range of motion, it has a tendency to load, strengthen, and thus prepare these structures for the functional activities at hand.

FIGURE 10.6
Static stretching: slow, controlled elongation held for 15 to 30 seconds.

As you can see, for maximum benefits in flexibility, it is vital to include both active and passive stretching methods in your clients' training programs.

Four popular basic techniques used to increase flexibility are static stretching, ballistic stretching, proprioceptive neuromuscular facilitation (PNF) stretching, and active isolated stretching (AIS). Of these, the static stretching method is advocated by professionals as the least likely to cause injury.

Static Stretching

Static stretching involves a slow, gradual, and controlled elongation through a full range of motion. For example, a client stretching the calf (gastrocnemius) would lean (with back straight) over the forward knee until a pull is felt (without pain) in the calf and hold the position for 15 to 30 seconds (Figure 10.6). This is a low-intensity, long-duration stretch technique. Stretching in this manner physiologically suppresses the stretch reflex. As muscle spindles and the central nervous system (CNS) adapt slowly to a lengthened position, spindle discharge diminishes and muscle relaxation increases.

Ballistic Stretching

Ballistic, or dynamic, stretching employs rapid, uncontrolled bouncing or bobbing motions (Figure 10.7). This technique incorporates a high-force, short-duration stretch, stimulating muscle spindle activity and, therefore, greater reflex muscular contraction. Uncontrolled or excessive movement also can overload soft tissue structures beyond normal elastic capabilities. Consequently, many trainers, physical therapists, and physicians feel ballistic stretching is a higher risk stretching technique and should be avoided unless specifically needed to prepare for a ballistic sports activity. In this case, there may be a practical advantage to using this stretching method. **Ballistic stretching** may promote dynamic flexibility and decrease potential injury by preparing tissues for high-speed, volitional-type exercise. Since many movements in sport and exercise are ballistic in nature, a dynamic stretching technique may be appropriate when specifically training for sport competition. Technically, dynamic stretching should consist of controlled rhythmic actions meant to mimic a training activity, initially small and gradually increasing to larger ranges of motion. However, this method of stretching is not usually recommended for the general population because control may be compromised and the risk of injury increased.

Proprioceptive Neuromuscular Facilitation (PNF)

Proprioceptive neuromuscular facilitation (PNF), another common stretching procedure, was first developed by physicians and

FIGURE 10.7
Ballistic stretching: rapid bouncing or bobbing motions.

FIGURE 10.8
Proprioceptive neuro-
muscular facilitation
(PNF): contraction
followed by relaxation
and a slow, passive
stretch.

physical therapists for use in rehabilitation. PNF is a method of hastening neuromuscular responses by stimulating neural proprioceptors (Voss, Ionta, & Myers, 1985). There are many forms of PNF, each of which works with one of the three primary neural mechanisms (i.e., reciprocal innervation, muscle spindles, and Golgi tendon organs). Although PNF is extremely complicated and composed of many strategies to promote a variety of results, the aspect most commonly used in training is the contract-relax sequence of PNF. Based on the principle of reciprocal inhibition, this method requires an initial isometric contraction against maximum resistance at the end of the limb's range of motion for approximately six seconds, followed by relaxation and a slow, passive stretch at the point of limitation (Figure 10.8). This sequence is usually repeated several times, and the summation of maximum neural excitations to the muscle being stretched theoretically allows for a greater reflex inhibition and thus a greater stretch. At the end of a contract-relax stretch, it is important to slightly stimulate the antagonist (opposing muscle group) to ensure a return to neuromuscular balance. Proponents of this method claim that individuals experience

more passive mobility. However, researchers Moore and Hutton (1980) concluded that though the more complicated PNF technique was more effective than conventional stretching techniques, contract-relax was often perceived as more uncomfortable when compared to static stretching. Because PNF exercises were designed to be done with a partner, they should be performed with a knowledgeable and experienced professional.

Active Isolated Stretching

Active isolated stretching (AIS), a technique originally used with rehab surgery patients, follows a design similar to a traditional strength-training workout. Instead of holding stretches for 15 to 30 seconds at a point of resistance (i.e., mild discomfort), stretches are never held for more than two seconds. The stretch is then released, the body segment returned to the starting position, and the stretch is repeated for several repetitions with each subsequent movement exceeding the resistance point by a few degrees. Increasing the stretch a few degrees at a time allows the muscle to adjust more gradually to the stretch. The stretches are typically performed in sets of a specified number of

FIGURE 10.9
Active isolated stretching.

repetitions, with a goal of isolating an individual muscle in each set. Proponents of AIS claim that this technique targets specific muscles and prepares the body for physical activity better than static stretching can, while also protecting the joint attachments that static stretching can sometimes weaken.

To better understand AIS, consider the traditional hamstrings stretch, in which the exerciser lifts the leg onto a bench. This requires work not only from the target muscles, but also from the calf, glutes, and back muscles. This creates a passive stretch of the hamstrings, and their natural response is to contract, thereby negating the benefit of the stretch. In AIS, the quadriceps are contracted and the hamstrings are stretched in a supine position using a rope or towel as an aid (Figure 10.9). It is believed that this allows the hamstrings to relax more completely and fully benefit from the stretch. It should be noted that some experts believe that holding a stretch for only two seconds is not adequate to have an effect on the connective tissue that surrounds and runs through muscles.

FACTORS AFFECTING FLEXIBILITY

Clearly, different stretching techniques produce different results. There also are a number of additional factors specific to each client that contribute to the success or failure of a flexibility program. The factors affecting flexibility include age, gender, joint structure, muscle tendon attachments, muscle cross-sectional area, body temperature, and pregnancy.

Age and Inactivity

Several studies have indicated that there is a distinct relationship between age and degree of flexibility. Developmentally, the greatest increase in flexibility usually occurs up to and between the ages of 7 and 12. During early adolescence, flexibility tends to level off and thereafter begins to decline. After age 25, normal aging tends to accelerate, causing significant changes in connective tissue and eventually decreased extensibility. Aging increases both the diameter of collagen fibers and the number of intermolecular cross-links (Alter, 1996) (Figure 10.10). This age-related effect strengthens connective tissue bonds, further increasing the resistance to deformation. A fair amount of dehydration in and around soft tissue structures also occurs

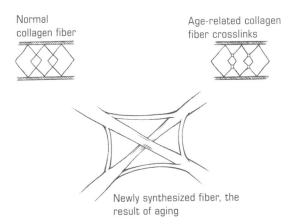

Normal collagen fiber

Age-related collagen fiber crosslinks

Newly synthesized fiber, the result of aging

FIGURE 10.10
Age-related changes in collagen fibers.

as one ages. This lack of water in soft tissue structures diminishes lubrication and the flow of nutrients to the site, ultimately creating a more fragile unit.

Generally speaking, the more active a person is throughout the aging process, the more flexible they will be. Inactivity, or hypokinesis, permits adaptive shortening within connective tissue structures. When connective tissue is not actively stretched through a full range of motion, it becomes shorter and less resilient, making it difficult to obtain the balance essential for proper alignment during activity. Regular stretching throughout one's life can enhance positive tissue adaptability and reduce natural wear and tear.

Gender

Although conclusive evidence is still lacking, there appears to be a strong gender difference related to flexibility potential. Females are generally much more flexible than males. One hypothesis for this is that, genetically, women are designed for a greater range of flexibility, especially in the pelvic region, to accommodate childbearing.

Pregnancy

Changing levels of estrogen, relaxin, and progesterone during pregnancy have various effects, including a loosening of joints, ligaments, and tendons, especially in the pelvis and lumbosacral spine. This increase in joint and connective tissue laxity may increase pregnant women's susceptibility to injury. According to Bryant, Franklin, and Conviser (2002), "The aim of flexibility programs during pregnancy should not be to improve joint range of motion, but rather to relieve muscle cramping or soreness and relax the lower-back region to alleviate the pain generated from the lordotic pressure on the spine."

Body Type and Strength Training

Many attempts have been made to relate body type and flexibility. For example, an underweight fragile body type (ecto-morph) might be thought to have greater flexibility than a heavier, overdeveloped, or massive body type (endomorph). Available research has revealed little correlation between weight and body type and the ability to achieve range of motion.

Strength training is an area where misconceptions concerning flexibility continue to exist. Many still believe that weight training causes the body to become muscle-bound and lack overall flexibility. It is true that overdeveloping muscles may encourage muscular imbalances if stretching is not incorporated into the training program, but the perception that strength training independently decreases flexibility is a myth. The 1976 U.S. Olympic weight-lifting team ranked second only to gymnasts in joint range-of-motion testing.

It is important to remember that flexibility has been consistently shown to be highly specific to the individual, to the activity, and to each joint. Since each person has different musculature, joint structure, and genetic composition, you must create programs that are individual to each of your clients. Flexibility is not necessarily an underlying characteristic of each person, but it is an essential component of physical fitness.

Warm-up

A warm-up is a slow, rhythmic exercise of larger muscle groups performed before an activity that provides the body with a period of adjustment between rest and performance of that activity. Generally, warm-up prepares the body for what is about to come. Scientists agree that by imitating an exercise activity for a period of 5 to 15 minutes before high-intensity involvement, overall performance will be heightened. This technique gradually warms tissues, increasing blood flow and nutrients to active structures. Warm-up may also fine-tune CNS receptors to improve kinesthetic awareness during activity. (That is, sensory organs within muscles, tendons, and joints facilitate our ability to know where we are in space during an activity.) This kinesthetic awareness helps prepare our bodies for activity, so that we gain a certain amount of protection and psychological readiness necessary for reducing potential injuries. Warm-up can be used to prepare soft tissue structures for the flexibility necessary for any particular activity.

PRINCIPLES OF STRETCHING

Although there is continuing controversy over which flexibility exercises are best, whether to stretch before or after exercise, or just how much to stretch, professionals currently agree on certain guidelines that should be incorporated into your clients' fitness programs. Most experts recommend stretching both before and after intense activity but each for different reasons. In preparation for activity pre-stretch is primarily active and aimed at decreasing tissue stiffness, focusing particularly on the muscles that will be used in the activity to follow. For example, a step training participant would stretch hamstrings and calves during warm-up, while a tennis player might stretch forearm and shoulder muscles as well.

With intense exercise, body temperature increases and tissues offer less resistance. Therefore, stretching for permanent elongation is emphasized later in the workout rather than at the beginning. Stretching after exercise may also enhance muscle relaxation, facilitating normal resting length, circulation to structures, and removal of unwanted waste products. Body core temperature also is found to be highest just after the aerobic or more intense portions of training programs. For these reasons, and to achieve maximum gains in range of motion, it is logical and highly recommended to include static stretching exercises at this stage.

How often one should stretch is still not fully understood. Professionals seem to agree, however, that daily stretching is best, and, at the very least, stretching should be performed before and after activity sessions. In a Swedish study, Wallin et al. (1985) found that once subjects had attained optimal flexibility, stretching just one to two times per week would maintain those ranges. However, when stretching was incorporated three to five times per week after attainment, range of motion was augmented further. Various other studies have demonstrated that increased mobility remains from only 90 minutes to 24 hours after performing stretching exercises (Alter, 1996). In other words, more frequent stretching would increase and maintain flexibility, while avoiding muscular imbalances created by daily activities or exercise.

When designing a stretching program for a client, keep the following in mind:

1. Connective tissue elongation (plastic deformation) is the primary target when stretching.

2. The two most important factors influencing stretching are intensity and duration. A low-intensity, long-duration stretch favors more lasting plastic tissue deformation. A high-intensity, short-duration stretch favors a more temporary elastic tissue deformation.

3. Elevated tissue temperature facilitates range of motion.

4. Flexibility is specific; therefore, exercises must be specific to each joint and/or muscle group.

5. Proper alignment for each stretch is critical to achieve maximum effectiveness in any one specific muscle group. By creating a good relationship between one joint and another during exercise, one biomechanically places muscles in positions to achieve maximum effectiveness in stretching, absorb shock, and decrease stress to surrounding soft tissue structures.

6. Most stretches should be held for a minimum of 15 seconds and up to 30 seconds, and repeated two to four times each.

FLEXIBILITY EXERCISES

Your clients would benefit most by regularly performing the exercises in Figures 10.11 through 10.23, which emphasize major muscle groups important in postural correction, as well as individual sports activities. If there are time constraints, your first priority should be to target a client's individual needs based on flexibility assessments (see pages 193–197). In addition, if your client has overworked a specific muscle group during exercise or daily activities, include a series of stretches addressing that area at the end of the session. Finally, it is important to include exercises addressing a client's chronically tight areas, such as hamstrings, calves, posterior neck, anterior shoulder, hip flexors, and low-back musculature.

SUMMARY

Although its role in fitness is not as well researched as other components, flexibility is an essential part of a well-balanced exercise program. To understand the effects of various stretching techniques, you need to understand the mechanics and neurophysiology of flexibility. Most professionals agree that of the major types of stretching—static, ballistic, PNF, and AIS—static stretching is overall the most beneficial and least likely to cause injury. A static stretch is a low-intensity, long-duration stretch that favors more lasting connective tissue elongation (plastic deformation). Ideally, a client should stretch daily. You also can see that your client stretches both before and after exercise sessions. Because age, gender, level, and type of activity play a role in achieving and maintaining full range of motion, it is important that you design a stretching program to meet the assessed needs of each individual client.

FIGURE 10.11
Upper trapezius stretch. Have your client apply passive pressure on the back of the head.

FIGURE 10.12
Anterior shoulder stretch (pectoralis stretch). For an effective, trainer-assisted stretch, the arm should be in a combined position of abduction, external rotation, and some hyperextension.

FIGURE 10.13
Posterior shoulder stretch. With shoulders down and relaxed, bring right arm across the chest, parallel to the floor. Place the left hand on the upper arm and apply gentle pressure toward the body. Repeat on the left side.

FIGURE 10.14
Triceps stretch. Bend the right elbow and use the left arm to bring the bent elbow up and behind the head until a stretch is felt in the back of the upper arm. Repeat on the left side.

FIGURE 10.15
Low-back stretch. On back with knees bent, gently pull both knees toward chest, lifting feet off the floor; hold and relax. This exercise may also be performed using one leg at a time.

FIGURE 10.16
Outer hip (rotator) stretch. On back, flex right knee across the body and toward the left shoulder. As a trainer, you can provide a passive over-stretch. Repeat on the left side.

FIGURE 10.17
Thoracic and lumbar spine motion exercise. On hands and knees, sag back, lifting head up. Arch back and lower head down.

FIGURE 10.18
Torso stretch. On stomach, place hands as if to do a push-up. Lift upper body, keeping hips and lower body on the floor. This stretch may also be performed while keeping the elbows on the ground. Perform this exercise in a pain-free range only.

FIGURE 10.19
Adductor stretch. The objective is to move the knees as close to the floor as possible, Clients can move the feet further from the body if needed, but should not sacrifice upper-body form and alignment.

FIGURE 10.20
Hip flexor stretch.

Begin in a forward lunge position.

Use the abdominals to tilt the pelvis posteriorly and push the hip bone of the back leg forward. To deepen the stretch, lower the knee slightly.

FIGURE 10.21

Quadriceps stretch. Using a wall or chair as support, reach back with the right hand and grasp the right foot or ankle. Be sure the hips are forward and knees are adjacent to each other. Repeat on the left side.

FIGURE 10.22

Hamstring stretch. Begin by lying on your back and looping a towel around one foot. Using the towel as a stabilizer, extend the leg by contracting the quadriceps. Repeat with the other leg.

FIGURE 10.23
Stretches for the calf.

Gastrocnemius stretch. Using a wall or chair as support, place one foot behind
the other. With front knee slightly bent, back knee straight, and heel down, lean
hips forward. Repeat on the opposite side.

Soleus stretch. Using a wall or chair as support, place one foot behind the
other. With both knees bent and heels down, lean forward from the hips.
Repeat on the opposite side.

References and Suggested Reading

REFERENCES

Alter, M. (1996). *Science of Flexibility* (2nd ed.). Champaign, Ill.: Human Kinetics.

Astrand, O. & Rodahl, K. (1986). *Textbook of Work Physiology* (3rd ed.). New York: McGraw-Hill.

Bryant, C.X., Franklin, B.A., & Conviser, J.M. (2002). *Exercise Testing and Program Design*. Monterey, Calif.: Healthy Learning.

DeVries, H. (1993). *Physiology of Exercise for Physical Education* (6th ed.). New York: McGraw-Hill Higher Education.

Enoka, R.M. (1994). *Neuromechanical Basis of Kinesiology*. Champaign, Ill.: Human Kinetics.

Hubley-Kozey, C. & Stanish, W. (1984). Can stretching prevent athletic injuries? *Journal of Musculoskeletal Medicine,* 9, 25–32.

Kendall, F., McCreary E., & Provance P. (1993). *Muscles: Testing and Function* (4th ed.). Baltimore, Md.: Lippincott Williams & Wilkins.

Moore, M. & Hutton, R. (1980). Electromyographic investigation of muscle stretching techniques. *Medicine and Science in Sports and Exercise*, 12, 322–329.

Sapega, A. et al. (1981). Biophysical factors in range-of-motion exercise. *Physician and Sportsmedicine*, 9, 57–64.

Voss, D., Ionta, M., & Myers, B. (1985). *Proprioceptive Neuromuscular Facilitation: Patterns and Techniques* (3rd ed.). Baltimore, Md.: Williams & Wilkins.

Wallin, D. et al. (1985). Improvement of muscle flexibility: A comparison between two techniques. *American Journal of Sports Medicine,* 13, 263–268.

SUGGESTED READING

Anderson, B. (2000). *Stretching* (20th Anniversary Edition). Bolinas, Calif.: Shelter Publications.

Ecstrand, J. & Gillquist, J. (1982). The frequency of muscle tightness and injuries in soccer players. *American Journal of Sports Medicine,* 10, 55–58.

Evjenth, O. & Hamberg, J. (1991). *Autostretching: The Complete Manual of Specific Stretching*. Sweden: Alfta Rehab Forlag.

Francis, P. & Francis, L. (1988). *If It Hurts, Don't Do It*. Rocklin, Calif.: Prima Publishing.

Moller, M. (1984). Athletic training and flexibility. A study on range of motion in the lower extremity. *Linkoping University Medical Dissertations*. No. 182.

Sady, S., Wortman, M., & Blanke, D. (1982). Flexibility training: ballistic, or proprioceptive neuromuscular facilitation? *Archives of Physical Medicine and Rehabilitation,* 63: 261–263.

Schultz, P. (1979). Flexibility: Day of the static stretch. *Physician and Sportsmedicine,* 7, 109–117.

Wirbed, R. (1984). *Athletic Ability and the Anatomy of Motion*. London: Wolfe Medical Publications.

PART IV

Individualized
Program Design

Programming for the Healthy Adult

*David C. Nieman, Dr. P.H.,
F.A.C.S.M., is professor
and director of the Human
Performance Laboratory
at Appalachian State
University in Boone, N.C.
He is an active researcher*

**David C.
Nieman**

*and is the
author of
several
textbooks on health and
fitness and more than 80
research articles in the areas
of sports medicine, exercise
and health, exercise
immunology, sports
nutrition, and obesity.*

As a personal trainer, you have the unique opportunity to adapt and individualize exercise workouts according to your clients' distinctive backgrounds and goals. People vary widely in their health and fitness status, motivation, goals, age, needs and desires, education, occupation, health habits, and medical background. Developing an exercise program that best meets each client's needs in a safe and effective manner requires a clear understanding of that person.

In previous chapters of this book, information is given on health screening, testing and evaluation, and training regimens for the development of cardiorespiratory and musculoskeletal fitness. In this chapter, emphasis is placed on how these components can be combined to provide comprehensive exercise programs for your clients. The intent of this chapter is to review the process whereby an individual's recommended physical activity program is designed in a systematic and personalized manner.

There are four primary steps in designing a formal, comprehensive exercise program:

1. Medical/health screening
2. Physical fitness testing
3. Selection of exercise mode
4. Design of an exercise program for total fitness

This chapter will explain the rationale for each step. You will be referred to previous chapters for specific information on conducting the various screenings and tests.

Before exploring these four steps in designing a formal exercise program, one important point needs to be addressed—the difference between exercise programs designed to develop physical fitness and those focused on health and the prevention of disease.

EXERCISE FOR PHYSICAL FITNESS vs. HEALTH AND DISEASE PREVENTION

There have always been many opinions about what is considered to be the best type of exercise. During the first half of the twentieth century, for example, muscular strength was emphasized by many fitness leaders as the primary goal of an exercise program. During the boom years of the **aerobic** movement in the 1970s and 1980s, development of cardiorespiratory fitness through high-intensity aerobic exercise was emphasized, often to the detriment of musculoskeletal fitness. The focus now is on a comprehensive approach to physical fitness in which three major components—cardiorespiratory fitness, musculoskeletal fitness, and body composition—are given balanced attention.

In 1993, the ACSM released its "exercise lite" recommendations (Table 11.1). With an emphasis on general physical

---

Table 11.1
Physical Activity and Public Health: A Recommendation from the Centers for Disease Control and Prevention and the American College of Sports Medicine: Key Statements

---

✔ The current low participation rate may be due, in part, to the misperception of many people that to reap health benefits, they must engage in vigorous, continuous exercise. Scientific evidence clearly demonstrates that regular, moderate-intensity physical activity provides substantial health benefits.

✔ Every U.S. adult should accumulate 30 minutes or more of moderate-intensity physical activity on most, preferably all, days of the week. One way to meet this standard is to walk two miles briskly.

✔ Intermittent activity also confers substantial benefits. Therefore, the recommended 30 minutes of activity can be accumulated in short bouts of activity: walking up the stairs instead of taking the elevator, walking instead of driving short distances, doing calisthenics or pedaling a stationary cycle while watching television.

✔ The health benefits gained from increased physical activity depend on the initial physical fitness level. Sedentary individuals are expected to benefit most from increasing their activity to the recommended level.

✔ Two other components of fitness—flexibility and muscular strength—should not be overlooked. Clinical experience and limited studies suggest that people who maintain or improve their strength and flexibility may be better able to perform daily activities, may be less likely to develop back pain, and may be better able to avoid disability, especially as they advance in age.

✔ If Americans who lead sedentary lives would adopt a more active lifestyle, there would be enormous benefit to the public's health and to individual well-being. An active lifestyle does not require a regimented, vigorous exercise program. Instead, small changes that increase daily physical activity will enable individuals to reduce their risk of chronic disease and may contribute to enhanced quality of life.

Source: Pate, R.R. et al. (1995). Physical activity and public health: A recommendation from the Centers for Disease Control and Prevention and the American College of Sports Medicine. *Journal of the American Medical Association,* 273, 402–407.

activity and disease prevention, these recommendations caught some people off guard. Table 11.2 provides a summary of the 2006 ACSM exercise programming guidelines for healthy adults. When the development of **cardiorespiratory endurance** is the objective, the intensity of training should range between 40/50 and 85% of $\dot{V}O_2$ **max** (or 55/65 and 90% of maximum heart rate). When improvement in health is of greater concern, the intensity can drop to 40%, and people in the general population are simply urged to "accumulate 30 minutes or more of moderate-intensity physical activity over the course of most days of the week" (United States Department of Health and Human Services, 1996).

Because these three sets of standards complement each other, you are urged to adapt these recommendations in accordance with the goals and unique characteristics of your client. ACSM released its 1993 recommendations in light of concerns that the majority of Americans had not entered the modern-day physical fitness movement because "previous public health efforts to promote physical activity have overemphasized the importance of high-intensity exercise. The current low rate of participation may be explained, in part, by the perception of many people that they must engage in vigorous, continuous exercise to reap health benefits" (American College of Sports Medicine, 1993).

For some time now, ACSM has recognized that most people prefer a less technical, more informal approach to exercise programming, and public health officials have been monitoring the response of Americans to the new guidelines. Year 2010 physical activity and fitness goals for the nation are outlined in Table 11.3. Depending on the survey, only 10 to 15% of American adults report exercising vigorously (at an intensity of at least 60% $\dot{V}O_2$ max for 20 or more minutes per session, three or more times per week), the level generally recommended for cardiovascular benefit. Approximately 25% of Americans report that they exercise moderately (at an intensity below 60% $\dot{V}O_2$ max) five or more times per week, while another 25% report living essentially **sedentary** lifestyles. The rest of Americans report exercising irregularly, which means that 35 to 40% of adults exercise fewer than three times per week, 20 minutes per session.

The biggest challenge you face as a personal trainer is motivating clients to adhere

Exercise for Physical Fitness vs. Health and Disease Prevention

Table 11.2
2006 ACSM Exercise Programming Guidelines for Healthy Adults

Component of Training Program	Frequency (sessions per week)	Intensity	Duration	Activity
Cardiorespiratory	3–5	40%/50%–85% HRR or $\dot{V}O_2$R 55%/65%–90% HRmax 12–16 RPE	20–60 minutes (or discontinuous 10-minute bouts that add up to 20–60 minutes)	Large muscle groups Dynamic activity
Resistance	2–3	Volitional fatigue (MMF) (e.g., 19–20 RPE) OR Stop 2–3 reps before volitional fatigue (e.g., 16 RPE)	One set of 3–20 reps (e.g., 3–5, 8–10, 12–15)	8–10 exercises that include all major muscle groups
Flexibility	Minimal: 2–3 Ideal: 5–7	Stretch to tightness at the end of the range of motion, but not to pain	15–30 seconds 2–4 reps per stretch	Static stretch all major muscle groups

Note: HRR = Heart-rate reserve; $\dot{V}O_2$R = Maximal oxygen uptake reserve; HRmax = Maximal heart rate; MMF = Momentary muscular fatigue; RPE = Ratings of perceived exertion

American College of Sports Medicine (2006). *ACSM's Guidelines for Exercise Testing & Prescription* (7th ed.). Philadelphia: Lippincott Williams & Wilkins.

Table 11.3
Healthy People 2010: Objectives to Increase Physical Activity in Adults

Year 2010 Goals (selected)	Best Estimate of Current Status
Increase to at least 30% the proportion of people aged 18 and older who engage regularly, preferably daily, in moderate physical activity for at least 30 minutes per day	15% (30+ minutes/5 times each wk) 31% (20 minutes/3 times each wk)
Increase to at least 30% the proportion of people aged 18 and older who engage in vigorous physical activity that promotes the development and maintenance of cardiorespiratory fitness three or more days per week for 20 or more minutes per occasion	23%
Reduce to no more than 20% the proportion of people aged 18 and older who engage in no leisure-time physical activity	40%
Increase to at least 30% the proportion of people aged 18 and older who regularly perform physical activities that enhance and maintain muscular strength and endurance	18%
Increase to at least 43% of adults aged 18 and older who perform physical activities that enhance and maintain flexibility	30%

Source: U.S. Department of Health and Human Services (2000). *Healthy People 2010* (2nd ed.). Understanding and Improving Health and Objectives for Improving Health (2 vols.) Washington, D.C.: U.S. Government Printing Office, November.

to their exercise programs. Principles of adherence and motivation are reviewed in Chapter 13. In general, to enhance long-term participation in regular physical activity, several factors should be considered, especially those that pertain to the person (gender, age, occupational status, health status, education, prior exercise experience), the exercise regimen itself (in particular, intensity and mode), and the environment (weather, community facilities, home-based programs, travel distances, time barriers, family and spousal support, employer and co-worker support, and government, economic, and public-policy support). As a personal trainer, you can do much to control these factors and reduce the barriers to long-term exercise adherence.

Design the exercise program to meet the client's needs and personal goals, whether they be health-related, fitness-related, or both. For the client who merely desires an exercise program to decrease risk of disease and feel better, a walking program with supportive calisthenics may be sufficient. For others who are seeking large increases in physical fitness for improved appearance and performance, a more formal, intensive aerobic and musculoskeletal fitness program should be designed.

Although the natural tendency of most fitness leaders is to urge clients to adopt intensive fitness programs, the ACSM's "exercise lite" recommendations will probably better meet the needs of most clients. There has been a growing shift from uniform exercise programming based on intensity, frequency, and duration to one that encourages increased levels of general energy expenditure throughout a person's day. Helping clients to increase routine or transportation-related physical activity and facilitating more convenient forms of leisure-time activity especially for those who have little interest in formal exercise programs, should now become part of your counseling skills.

As mentioned earlier in this chapter, there are four steps in establishing an exercise program for a client. These apply whether the exercise program will follow more traditional guidelines for exercise programming, or the new, more moderate "exercise lite" guidelines.

Helping Clients Manage Stress with Exercise

Stress, unfortunately, is a fact of life for most people. In general terms, stress is defined as the emotional and physical reactions individuals experience as the result of changes and demands in their lives. Some symptoms of stress, such as nervousness and irritability, are fairly obvious; other symptoms, such as neck and shoulder aches or itchy skin, are more subtle.

If a stress-induced hormonal surge occurs only occasionally, research indicates that the body is resilient enough to bounce back with few, if any, long-term negative effects. The stress response only becomes harmful when individuals are exposed to it for frequent and extended periods of time. Chronic stress, which results from repeated exposure to stress throughout the day for a period of weeks or months, appears to alter the way the body functions, primarily as the result of keeping norepinephrine and cortisol levels elevated.

Listed below are the negative effects of chronic stress on the major physiological systems of the body, as well as a basic exercise program focused on stress management.

• Musculoskeletal system: tension headache, neck and shoulder discomfort, back pain, other muscle or joint aches and pains

• Cardiovascular system: premature CAD, high blood pressure, increased platelet adhesiveness, heart attack

• Immune system: suppression of T-cell function, increased vulnerability to infections, and viral illnesses

• Central nervous system: impaired memory, neural degeneration

• Gastrointestinal system: stomach ache, nausea, constipation, diarrhea

A Basic Exercise Program for Stress Management

• Frequency of training: 3–5 days per week, preferably daily

• Intensity of training: 60–80% of maximum oxygen uptake ($\dot{V}O_2$ max), 60–80% of maximum heart-rate reserve, or 70–90% of maximum heart rate

• Duration of training: 20–60 minutes of continuous aerobic activity; limited scientific data are available regarding the effects of anaerobic-type exercise on stress

• Mode of training: Any aerobic activities that the participant finds enjoyable (e.g., walking, running, stair climbing, cycling, swimming, hiking)

STEP 1: MEDICAL/HEALTH SCREENING

As emphasized in Chapter 5, to gain a complete picture of your client's background, current medical and health status, motivation, and current goals, a comprehensive questionnaire should be completed and carefully reviewed. There are many good questionnaires available that ask about personal and family history of disease, **risk factors** and symptoms, present medications and treatment, lifestyle habits, social/demographic factors, and exercise history and attitude.

After completing the questionnaire, the client can then be classified as apparently healthy, at higher risk, or with disease. Appropriate judgments should then be made for further testing with physician supervision. According to ACSM, this "risk stratification" is important to ensure the safety of exercise testing and participation (American College of Sports Medicine, 2000). It also helps to determine the appropriate type of exercise program, identifies those in need of more extensive medical evaluation, and makes appropriate recommendations for an exercise program.

Each year, about 75,000 Americans suffer heart attacks during or after exercise. These victims tend to be individuals who are usually sedentary and at high risk for heart disease. During unaccustomed exercise, a chain of physiologic events take place in the body that lead to a heart attack. With appropriate screening and referral to medical facilities, the incidence of cardiovascular problems during exercise can be greatly reduced.

Information from the questionnaire also can be used to gain a complete background on clients so that you can better meet their needs and goals. As emphasized in the introduction to this chapter, people vary widely. The design of an exercise program for an elderly, obese female will differ greatly from one developed for a young female athlete.

STEP 2: PHYSICAL FITNESS TESTING

In Chapter 6, a complete review of physical fitness testing and evaluation is given. Before the exercise program is designed, you must know how physically fit the client is for at least four reasons:

1. To assess current fitness levels—both strengths and weaknesses
2. To identify special needs for individualized counseling
3. To evaluate progress over time
4. To motivate and educate

The testing process is invaluable and can be used to help clients learn more about themselves while establishing appropriate health and fitness goals. The very process of administering a fitness test draws attention to what is considered worthy of special attention in the lifestyle. The test results can be used to educate, motivate, and stimulate interest in exercise and other health-related topics.

Normative information on each test should be shared with every client. Research results have shown that the testing process itself often motivates people to make meaningful and lasting changes in their lifestyles.

STEP 3: SELECTION OF THE AEROBIC EXERCISE MODE

Selection of the aerobic exercise mode by the client is central to the long-term success of the exercise program. Most studies have shown that if frequency, intensity, and duration of training are similar, the cardiorespiratory training outcomes are independent of the mode of aerobic activity (American College of Sports Medicine, 2001). In other words, if different people cycle, swim, or run 5 days per week, 30 minutes per session at 70% **heart-rate reserve,** after 10 to 15 weeks, improvement in heart and lung fitness should be comparable. It should be noted, however, that some aerobic activities, like rowing and swimming, also confer considerable musculoskeletal benefits, giving more of a "total fitness" benefit when compared to running or cycling, for example. Table 11.4 summarizes the fitness benefits of selected physical activities.

Aerobic activity mode should be selected on the basis of individual interest, time and facility availability, personal goals and objectives, and fitness level. Present your client with a comprehensive list of suitable aerobic activities and discuss them thoroughly from both a practical and total fitness perspective. Next, have your client choose primary and secondary activities that they can fit into their schedule without creating undue stress and inconvenience.

"Lack of time" is the major obstacle individuals list for not continuing exercise programs, and this potential problem should be discussed from every angle to ensure long-term adherence. To improve compliance, some people like the socialization, competitiveness, and pleasure of both dual and team sports. As shown in Table 11.4, many sports can develop aerobic and musculoskeletal fitness, improving compliance for those who enjoy this type of exercise. Others enjoy various work activities such as splitting wood or shoveling dirt, feeling that while overall fitness is being improved, they also are accomplishing a worthwhile task.

National surveys show that the most popular fitness activity continues to be walking, followed by swimming, bicycle riding, and exercising with free weights. Moderate-intensity activities of longer duration are being promoted more and more by fitness leaders because these types of activities are more acceptable to the masses, increasing the likelihood of a permanent change in lifestyle. Physical activities such as brisk walking result in low rates of musculoskeletal injury and have the potential to lower blood pressure, improve the lipid profile, reduce body fat, enhance mental well-being, and reduce the risk of coronary heart disease and cancer. Walking has been found to have a higher compliance rate than other physical activities because it can easily be incorporated into a busy time schedule, does not require any special skills, equipment, or facility, is companionable, and can be undertaken by individuals of all age groups. Do not be reluctant to prescribe walking for a large proportion of your clients.

Participation in a variety of aerobic activities carries several benefits, including decreased risk of overuse injuries, reduced boredom, increased long-term compliance, and increased overall fitness. For these reasons, urge your clients to have at least one secondary activity to supplement their primary mode of exercise. Even for athletes, engaging in two or three different types of exercise modes (i.e., cross training) can help maintain fitness during the off-season, or help maintain fitness during periods of injury or when experiencing burn-out.

Step 3: Selection of the Aerobic Exercise Mode

Table 11.4
Fitness Benefits of Selected Physical Activities

Activities are rated on a 5-point scale in terms of capacity to develop aerobic fitness and muscular strength and endurance. 1=not at all; 2=somewhat or just a little; 3=moderately; 4=strongly; 5=very strongly. For muscular strength and endurance, the activity is rated high if both upper- and lower-body musculature is improved.

Physical Activity	Aerobic Fitness	Muscular Strength and Endurance
Basketball, game play	4	2
Bicycling, fast pace	5	3
Canoeing, rowing, hard pace	5	4
Circuit weight training	3	5
Golf, walking, carrying bag	3	2
Handball, game play	4	3
Lawn mowing, power push	3	3
Racquetball, squash, game play	4	3
Roller blading/skating	4	3
Rope jumping, moderate-to-hard	4	3
Running, brisk pace	5	2
Shoveling dirt, digging	4	4
Skiing, cross country	5	4
Skiing, downhill	2	3
Soccer	4	3
Splitting wood	4	4
Stair climbing	5	3
Swimming	5	4
Tennis, game play	3	3
Traditional aerobics, moderate-to-hard	4	4
Volleyball, game play	3	3
Walking, briskly	3	2
Weight training	1	5

FIGURE 11.1
A sample exercise programming form. Source: Nieman, D.C. (1996). *Fitness and Sports Medicine: A Health-Related Approach* (3rd ed.). Palo Alto: Bull Publishing. Used with permission.

The Exercise Programming Form

Stage One—Cardiorespiratory/Body Composition

1. **Warm-up**
   Purpose: To slowly elevate the pulse to an aerobic level by engaging in five minutes of slow aerobic activity.

2. **The Aerobic Session**
   Purpose: To improve the cardiorespiratory system by exercising vigorously for at least 20 to 30 minutes, three times/week, on a regular basis.

		Fitness Status		
F.I.T. Guidelines		**Low**	**Average**	**High**
F	Frequency (sessions/week)	3	3–4	≥ 5
I	Intensity (% heart rate reserve)	40–60%	60–75%	75–85%
T	Time (minutes/session)	10–20	20–30	30–60

   Mode Selection (your personal) _____

   Training HR = [(Max HR – RHR) × 0.40 to 0.85] + RHR

   _____ = [(_____ – _____) × _____] + _____

   Days of week and time of exercise sessions

   Sun _____ Mon _____ Tue _____ Wed _____ Thu _____ Fri _____ Sat _____

3. **Cool-down**
   Purpose: To slowly decrease the heart rate by engaging in slow aerobic activity for at least five minutes.

Stage Two—Musculoskeletal Fitness

1. **Flexibility Exercises** _____
   _____
   _____

   Purpose: To stretch the major muscles and joints, especially those involved in the aerobic session, using static stretching techniques.

2. **Muscular Strength and Endurance Exercises** _____
   _____

   Purpose: To build muscular endurance and strength, especially in the muscles not developed in aerobic sessions, using appropriate weight training and calisthenic exercises.

STEP 4: DESIGNING AN EXERCISE PROGRAM FOR TOTAL FITNESS

As emphasized in Chapter 6, a comprehensive exercise program addresses all components of physical fitness: cardiorespiratory endurance, muscular strength and endurance, **flexibility,** and **body composition.** Figure 11.1 is a sample exercise programming form that can be used to ensure all components are given due attention during the training session.

Notice that the exercise programming form is divided into two stages: cardiorespiratory/body composition and musculoskeletal fitness. There are many different combinations that can be used to ensure that both categories of physical fitness are developed. For example, some clients may desire a total physical fitness workout each session, while others may engage in strength training one day and aerobic training the next. Some may prefer a daily walking program supplemented with flexibility and muscular endurance calisthenics.

Once clients have selected a primary and secondary aerobic activity from Table 11.4, have them write these in the "mode selection" blank. Next, go step-by-step through each stage of the exercise programming form, explaining the basic concepts involved (see Chapters 7, 8, 9, and 10).

For the warm-up, emphasize the importance of elevating body temperature through slow aerobic activity, preferably the aerobic activity that will be utilized in the workout session. This will provide a cardiovascular and neuromuscular rehearsal for the aerobic session itself. Explain that flexibility exercises are best conducted after the aerobic session when the body is warm.

Next, circle the appropriate F.I.T. criteria based on the fitness test results. Help clients determine their personal training heart rate using the Karvonen formula, and fill in the appropriate blanks. Explain how to measure the training heart rate, and fill in the blank for the 10-second pulse count. Review the

concept of **ratings of perceived exertion** (RPE), explaining that an RPE of "somewhat hard" appears appropriate for most people. For many clients who are more concerned with health-related fitness, using just RPE is sufficient to ensure adequate exercise intensity. Explain the concept of cooling down to help the body through the transition from hard aerobic exercise to rest, especially for those who are engaging in high-intensity exercise.

Review the principles that underlie the development of joint and muscle flexibility, emphasizing the importance of stretching the muscles utilized in the aerobic session (see Chapter 10). Select at least four to six different stretching exercises and have your client complete two to three repetitions of each, sustaining the stretched position for 15 to 30 seconds.

Discuss the principles of resistance training, and develop a program based on your client's personal goals and fitness test results. Remember that a minimum weight-training program, according to the ACSM, involves at least one set of 8 to 12 repetitions of 8 to 10 different exercises conducted two days per week (American College of Sports Medicine, 2006) (see Chapter 8). There are many different weight-training regimens, and this stage of exercise programming should be highly individualized to meet your client's needs (Table 11.5). Some may prefer a calisthenic program while others may center their entire exercise program around weight training. Weight-lifting centers around five different variables (repetitions to fatigue, sets, rest between sets, order of exercises, and type of exercise), and these can be manipulated according to specific goals.

TRAITS OF A GOOD EXERCISE CONSULTANT

Establishing an exercise program for a client, and then supporting the process for the long term, is no simple task. In addition to possessing the

Traits of a Good Exercise Consultant

Table 11.5
Recommendations for Improving Muscular Strength and Endurance for the General Adult Population

	Number of Sets	Number of Reps*	Sessions Per Week	Number of Exercises	Overall Purpose
ACSM†	1	8–12	2–3	8–10	To provide basic development & maintenance of the fat-free mass
CIAR†					
Minimum	1	8–12	2	10	For strength maintenance
Recommended	2	8–12	2	10	For strength improvement
Optimal	3	8–12	2	10	For noticeable strength gains

* In all examples listed, repetitions represent maximal weight lifted to fatigue.

† ACSM = American College of Sports Medicine; CIAR = Cooper Institute for Aerobics Research

Sources: Adapted, with permission, from American College of Sports Medicine (2000). *ACSM's Guidelines for Exercise Testing and Prescription* (6th ed.). Philadelphia: Lippincott Williams & Wilkins; Cooper Institute for Aerobics Research (1990). *The Strength Connection*. Philadelphia: Lea & Febiger.

knowledge and skills of a personal trainer, it helps to adopt some of the basic traits of a good consultant.

Although no one person can fully motivate another, one can create an environment that will facilitate people to motivate themselves. Motivation comes from within and people tend to become motivated by challenge, growth, achievement, promotion, and recognition. Place emphasis on providing a proper environment for self-growth by challenging clients, giving them responsibility, encouraging them, and giving full range to individual strength. An effective personal trainer develops warm, personal relationships with each client, and regards each as worthy of genuine concern and attention.

Traits of a good personal trainer/coach include:

✔ Empathy—the ability to climb into the world of the client and communicate feelings of understanding.

✔ Respect—a deep and genuine appreciation for the worth of your clients, separate and apart from their behavior. The strength and ability of your clients to overcome and adjust are appreciated.

✔ Warmth—the communication of concern and appropriate affection.

✔ Genuineness—being freely one's self. One is sincere and not just playing a role.

✔ Concreteness—essential ideas and elements are ferreted out.

✔ Self-disclosure—revelations about self are shared at the appropriate time for the benefit of the client.

✔ Potency and self-actualization—one is dynamic, in command, conveys feelings of trust and warmth, is competent, inner-directed, creative, sensitive, nonjudgmental, productive, serene, and satisfied.

RATE OF PROGRESSION AND RETESTING

The rate of progression in an exercise-conditioning program depends on many different factors, including your client's initial fitness and health status, age, needs, motivation and personal goals, family support, and frequency and intensity of training. For example, a middle-aged, overweight, sedentary female will make greater measurable gains during the first three to six months of an exercise program than will a young, normal-weight female.

ACSM defines three progression stages (American College of Sports Medicine, 2000):

Initial conditioning stage. This stage typically lasts four to six weeks. ACSM recommends that the intensity, frequency, and duration of exercise sessions be at the lower end of the training range to help avoid muscle soreness, injury, discomfort, and discouragement. Gradual progression is urged so that clients achieve early success in coping with the change in routine and lifestyle.

Improvement conditioning stage. This stage usually lasts 8 to 20 weeks and the rate of progression is more rapid. Frequency, intensity, and duration all should be gradually increased to at least the middle of the recommended ranges, with 300 or more calories expended per exercise session. Retesting of all components of physical fitness (cardiorespiratory endurance, muscular strength and endurance, flexibility, and body composition) should take place about three months after initiating exercise, and should continue every three months thereafter to help maintain interest and motivation. After each retesting session, physical fitness objectives can be altered to allow the client to aim for a higher standard, or to maintain goals already attained.

Maintenance conditioning stage. Once the desired level of fitness is reached, the client enters the maintenance stage of the exercise program. This stage usually begins five to six months after the start of training and, hopefully, extends for a lifetime. To ensure long-term compliance, the exercise program should be enjoyable, fit into the time schedule without undue stress, meet personal needs and goals, and be adaptable to changes in weather and location.

To help maintain client interest, enthusiasm, and long-term adherence, there are many strategies you can adopt, including:

✔ encouraging group participation or exercising with a partner
✔ emphasizing variety and enjoyment in the exercise program
✔ minimizing musculoskeletal injuries with a moderate exercise intensity and rate of progression
✔ helping your client draw up reasonable goals and highlighting these in a contract to be signed by the client
✔ recruiting support from a spouse or significant other

✔ providing progress charts to document achievement of goals
✔ recognizing accomplishments through a system of rewards
✔ maximizing convenience in terms of time, travel, and disruptions in family relationships
✔ complementing fitness activities with nutrition education, stress management, and other health-promotion activities to improve the overall health of your client

Various studies support the argument that physical activity must be continued on a regular basis if benefits are to be retained (American College of Sports Medicine, 2001). Cessation of exercise training results in a rapid decrease in both aerobic and muscular power. Maintenance of physical fitness, however, is achievable even when training volume (but not intensity) is decreased by half. In other words, it appears to take more energy expenditure to increase aerobic and muscular fitness than to maintain it, as long as training intensity is sustained.

Rate of Progression and Retesting

Case History #1: A Middle-aged American Female Location: Client's Home

Data from Medical/Health Questionnaire:

Age: 45 years

Height: 64 inches (1.63 m)

Weight: 154 pounds (69.3 kg)

Desired weight: 130 pounds (58.5 kg)

Smoking status: quit five years ago

Exercise habits: sedentary both at work and during leisure for all of adult life

Family history of disease: father died of coronary heart disease at age 52

Personal history of disease: negative

Signs or symptoms suggestive of cardiopulmonary or metabolic disease: negative

Dietary habits: fruit/vegetables, two servings/day (low); cereals/grains, five servings/day (low and refined)

Personal goals: lose weight, improve appearance and muscle tone, decrease risk of heart disease

Preferred modes of aerobic exercise: brisk walking, stationary bicycling

Data from Physical Fitness Testing Session (Physician's Office and Fitness Center):
Resting heart rate: 79 bpm
Resting blood pressure: 142/93 mmHg (Stage 1 hypertension) (from two measurements on two days)
Serum cholesterol: 247 mg/dL (high risk)
HDL cholesterol: 33 mg/dL (low)
Cholesterol/HDL-cholesterol ratio: 7.5 (high risk)
Percent body fat: 35% (obese)
Estimated $\dot{V}O_2$ max: 23 mL/kg/min (low)
Sit-and-reach flexibility test: 16 inches (below average)
YMCA bench-press test: 12 (below average)

Comments

Using the medical/health questionnaire and laboratory data from recent testing, this client was classified as "at moderate risk," according to the ACSM criteria. This classification was given because she has two or more major coronary risk factors (family history, **hypertension, hypercholesterolemia,** sedentary lifestyle). Due to the number of risk factors and family history of coronary heart disease, and the client's desire to engage in moderate-to-vigorous exercise, a medical exam and diagnostic exercise test were recommended. The treadmill EKG test was negative (no evidence of ischemia or arrhythmias), and physician clearance was given for the client to begin a moderate exercise program with gradual progression. Additional physical fitness tests were conducted at a fitness center to determine body composition and musculoskeletal fitness.

Recommended Exercise Program

A home-based program using brisk walking and indoor stationary bicycling, supported with calisthenics for general muscle toning, is recommended. During the first month, have the client warm up with range-of-motion calisthenics and walking for 5 to 10 minutes, followed by 15 minutes of brisk walking and/or stationary cycling at 50 to 60% of heart-rate reserve, three days per week. After cooling down, the client should engage in static stretching activities for 5 to 10 minutes, followed by toning calisthenics for 10 to 15 minutes.

After the first month has passed, gradually increase the duration of brisk walking and/or cycling to 30 to 45 minutes per session, and the frequency to five to six days per week. The intensity of exercise can also be gradually increased to 70% of heart-rate reserve. These increases, along with careful control of dietary habits, will help ensure a steady weight loss of about 1 pound per week. Since the client has 24 pounds of body fat to lose, ideal body weight should be attained after 24 to 30 weeks of training. This degree of weight loss, combined with improvements in physical fitness, should help to bring both hypertension and hypercholesterolemia under control if improvements in dietary quality are made (i.e., less **saturated fat** and **cholesterol,** more fruits, vegetables and whole grains, less sodium and alcohol). The client has a high risk of **coronary heart disease,** and it is imperative that the risk factors be brought under control through weight loss and dietary and exercise lifestyle changes. Enlist the services of a dietitian to ensure adherence to an **anti-atherogenic diet.**

Retest every three months to help ensure motivation and attainment of goals. Long-term compliance can be enhanced by encouraging family support, goal-setting and **contracting,** establishing rewards for attainment of goals, and combating time obstacles.

Case History #2: A 30-Year-Old Male Location: Fitness Center
Data from Medical/Health Questionnaire:
Age: 30 years
Height: 70 inches (1.78 m)
Weight: 160 pounds (72.0 kg)
Desired weight: 175 pounds (78.8 kg)
Smoking status: never smoked
Exercise habits: plays golf on the weekends,

but no other formal exercise;
sedentary at work

Family history of disease: negative

Personal history of disease: negative

Signs or symptoms suggestive of cardiopulmonary or metabolic disease: negative

Dietary habits: has a healthy diet and tries to follow Food Guide Pyramid guidelines

Personal goals: increase muscle weight through weight-training program; improve aerobic fitness moderately

Preferred modes of aerobic exercise: indoor equipment, especially rowing machine and stationary bicycle

Data from Physical Fitness Testing Session (Fitness Center):

Resting heart rate: 67 bpm (average)

Resting blood pressure: 123/82 mmHg (normal) (from two measurements on two days)

Serum cholesterol: 195 mg/dL (within desirable range)

HDL cholesterol: 46 mg/dL (average)

Cholesterol/HDL-cholesterol ratio: 4.2 (average, but above optimal ratio of 3.5)

Percent body fat: 18% (average)

Estimated $\dot{V}O_2$ max: —43 mL/kg/min (average)

Sit-and-reach flexibility test: 15 inches (average)

YMCA bench-press test: 27 (average)

YMCA half sit-up test: 52 (above average)
See Tables 6.6, 6.7, 6.15, 6.16, 6.26, and 6.27 for YMCA norms.

Comments

This client has no major risk factors for disease and is, therefore, classified as "low-risk" using the ACSM guidelines. According to ACSM, a medical exam or diagnostic exercise test is not needed prior to initiating a vigorous exercise program for this type of client. Although the client has a normal body-fat percentage, his body weight is somewhat low for his height, and he desires to gain 15 pounds through a weight-training program while moderately improving aerobic fitness. He is especially interested in adding muscle bulk to improve his golf game, which is his weekend passion.

Recommended Exercise Program

The client desires an intensive weight-training program at the fitness center, three days per week, with a moderate aerobic program two days per week. Since the client has never lifted weights seriously, a gradual, progressive-resistance program should be established. During the first month, a one-set, 10-repetition-maximum (RM) program of 10 different exercises will allow the client to adapt to the weight-training program without undue fatigue and soreness (which would interfere with his weekend golf game). Over the next two to three months, gradually increase the sets to three, with the RM lowered to six to eight. On two days of the week, after 5 minutes of warm-up, the client can use the rowing machine and/or bicycle for 20 to 30 minutes at 60 to 75% of heart-rate reserve. On weight-lifting days, it is recommended that the client warm up prior to lifting for 10 minutes by rowing and/or cycling. This will allow additional aerobic training and help warm-up the muscles and joints to allow safe and effective strength training.

Establish 1 RM goal weight lifts for each of the 10 exercises, and retest every three months. Also retest aerobic fitness and body composition every three months. To facilitate a healthy gain in body weight, consult with a dietitian to provide nutrient and energy analysis of the diet every three months. The dietitian also can give recommendations to improve the energy density of the diet.

Case History #3:
An Elderly Male
Location: Client's Home

Data from Medical/Health Questionnaire

Age: 72 years

Height: 68 inches (1.73 m)

Weight: 200 pounds (90.0 kg)

Rate of Progression and Retesting

Desired weight: 175 pounds (78.8 kg)

Smoking status: quit 20 years ago

Exercise habits: walks 10 minutes after supper with wife, but no other formal exercise

Family history of disease: negative

Personal history of disease: type 2 diabetes, diagnosed one year ago

Signs or symptoms suggestive of cardiopulmonary or metabolic disease: negative, but has low energy and feels tired much of the day; feels out of breath after climbing stairs; feels weak

Dietary habits: low in fruits and vegetables (2 servings/day); low in whole grains and cereals (3 servings/day); uses whole milk and cheese; likes red meat (2 servings/day)

Personal goals: lose weight to help control diabetes; improve aerobic fitness and increase energy level; increase muscle strength moderately

Preferred modes of aerobic exercise: walking outside on good-weather days; use of a treadmill on bad-weather days

Data from Physical Fitness Testing Session (Physician's Office and Testing at Home):

Resting heart rate: 78 bpm

Resting blood pressure: 135/87 mmHg (high normal) (from two measurements on two days)

Serum cholesterol: 256 mg/dL (high risk)

HDL cholesterol: 30 mg/dL (low, high risk)

Cholesterol/HDL-cholesterol ratio: 8.5 (high risk)

Percent body fat: 36% (obese)

Estimated $\dot{V}O_2$ max: 20 mL/kg/min (low); EKG negative

Sit-and-reach flexibility test: 5 inches (poor) See Tables 6.6, 6.7, 6.15, 6.16, 6.26, and 6.27 for YMCA norms.

Comments

Using the medical/health questionnaire and laboratory data from recent testing at the doctor's office, this client was classified as an "high-risk" using ACSM criteria. This is because he was recently diagnosed with type 2 diabetes, a condition that can

often be controlled through weight loss, exercise, and improvements in the diet (especially more dietary fiber and carbohydrates). After consulting with the client's physician (who determined that the EKG results were negative), you have been given approval to put the client on a moderate-intensity exercise program. The client is considered to be at high risk for heart disease because of the presence of multiple risk factors (age, diabetes, hypercholesterolemia, obesity, sedentary lifestyle). Therefore, the physician has cautioned slow progression with retesting conducted every three months to monitor progress. Additionally, the services of a dietitian have been advised to help the client improve dietary intake.

Recommended Exercise Program

A home-based program, using walking supported with calisthenics for general muscle toning, is recommended. During the first month, have the client warm up with range-of-motion calisthenics and walking for 5 to 10 minutes, followed by 15 minutes of walking at 40 to 50% of heart-rate reserve, three days per week. After cooling down, the client should engage in static stretching activities for 5 to 10 minutes, followed by toning calisthenics for 10 to 15 minutes.

After the first month has passed, gradually increase the duration of walking to 30 minutes per session, and the frequency to five days per week. The intensity of exercise also can be gradually increased to 60% of heart-rate reserve. These increases, along with careful control of dietary habits, will help ensure a steady weight loss of about 0.5 to 1 pound per week. The client has 20 pounds of body fat to lose, which is considered critical in treating type 2 diabetes. At the same time, this degree of weight loss, combined with improvements in physical fitness, should help bring the hypercholesterolemia under control if improvements in dietary quality are made.

Individuals with diabetes tend to be at high risk for coronary heart disease, and attainment of normal serum cholesterol and HDL cholesterol is an important goal.

To ensure long-term success, seek family support for all lifestyle changes. If various goals are met during retesting sessions, organize an incentive system to improve client motivation and interest. During the entire exercise program, close communication and cooperation with the physician and dietitian is crucial.

SUMMARY

Programming for the healthy adult is one of the most important aspects of personal training. There are four basic steps in the development of a program. First, all clients must complete the medical health screening. Then, clients who qualify as apparently healthy should go through physical fitness testing that will assess their strengths and weaknesses and let you know where their training should begin. These tests will also give you a starting point to refer back to as your client progresses. The next step is to find out what exercise modes your client prefers in an effort to promote adherence. Once you have completed these three steps you are ready to design an exercise program based on the three major components of fitness—cardiovascular fitness, musculoskeletal fitness, and body composition. After you have developed and begun a training program, your client will reach three main stages of progression: the initial conditioning stage lasts 4 to 6 weeks, the improvement conditioning stage lasts 8 to 20 weeks, during which you will see the greatest amount of growth, and the maintenance and conditioning stage, which will hopefully become a part of your client's routine for the rest of his or her life. Your biggest challenge as a personal trainer is going to be motivating your clients and making sure they follow the program you design for them. One trait of a good personal trainer is the ability to create an environment that promotes growth and challenges your clients while also teaching them to motivate themselves.

References and Suggested Reading

REFERENCES

American College of Sports Medicine (2006). *ACSM's Guidelines for Exercise Testing and Prescription.* (7th ed.). Philadelphia: Lippincott Williams & Wilkins.

American College of Sports Medicine (2006). *ACSM's Resource Manual for Guidelines for Exercise Testing and Prescription.* (7th ed.). Philadelphia: Lippincott Williams & Wilkins.

United States Department of Health and Human Services (1996). *Physical Activity and Health: A Report of the Surgeon General.* Atlanta, Ga.: U.S. Department of Health and Human Services, Centers for Disease Control and Prevention, National Center for Chronic Disease Prevention and Health Promotion.

SUGGESTED READING

Baechle, T.R. (2000). *Essentials of Strength Training and Conditioning.* (2nd ed.). Champaign, Ill.: Human Kinetics.

Cooper Institute for Aerobics Research (1990). *The Strength Connection.* Philadelphia: Lea & Febiger.

Davison, R.C.R. & Grant, S. (1993). Is walking sufficient exercise for health? *Sports Medicine,* 16, 369–373.

Haskell, W.L. (1994). Health consequences of physical activity: Understanding and challenges regarding dose-response. *Medicine and Science in Sports and Exercise,* 26, 649–660.

King, A.C. (1994). Community and public health approaches to the promotion of physical activity. *Medicine and Science in Sports and Exercise,* 26, 1405–1412.

Loy, S.F., Hoffman, J.J., & Holland, G.J. (1995). Benefits and practical use of cross-training in sports. *Sports Medicine,* 19, 1–8.

Morrissey, M.C., Harman, E.A., & Johnson, M.J. (1995). Resistance training modes: Specificity and effectiveness. *Medicine and Science in Sports and Exercise,* 27, 648–660.

Nieman, D.C. (1996). *Fitness and Sports Medicine: A Health-Related Approach.* (3rd ed). Palo Alto: Bull Publishing Company.

Pate, R.R. et al. (1995). Physical activity and public health: A recommendation from the Centers for Disease Control and Prevention and the American College of Sports Medicine. *Journal of the American Medical Association,* 273, 402–407.

Robison, J.I. & Rogers, M.A. (1994). Adherence to exercise programs: Recommendations. *Sports Medicine,* 17, 39–52.

U.S. Department of Health and Human Services (2000). *Healthy People 2010.* (2nd ed.) Understanding and Improving Health and Objectives for Improving Health (2 vols.). Washington, D.C.: U.S. Government Printing Office, November.

Wilmore, J.H., Costill, D. & Kenney, W.L. (2007). *Physiology of Sport and Exercise.* (4th ed.). Champaign, Ill.: Human Kinetics.

Special Populations and Health Concerns

Scott Roberts

Scott Roberts, Ph.D., is an assistant professor in the Department of Physical Education and Exercise Science at California State University, Chico. He is the author of numerous books, including Strength and Weight Training for Young Athletes, Clinical Exercise Testing and Prescription: Theory and Application *and* Exercise Physiology: Exercise, Performance and Clinical Applications. *Dr. Roberts has also published numerous articles and book chapters on exercise, including a chapter in the* ACE Clinical Exercise Specialist Manual.

Personal trainers frequently encounter clients with special needs and health concerns. For those who work with clients of middle age or older, this will be a regular event. It is important for a personal trainer to identify health conditions that will influence exercise program development in the initial screening portion of the client-trainer interaction. As a personal trainer, you should regularly update your client screening records to identify and effectively address changes in health status as they occur.

Once you have identified that a client has a medical and/or health condition, you must obtain physician approval before proceeding with exercise program development, testing, or training. Along with physician approval, you also should request exercise guidelines and limitations from your client's physician. In many cases a physician will appoint another health professional to assist in providing exercise guidelines. This may be, for example, a nurse, physical therapist, clinical exercise physiologist, or a diabetes educator, depending on the clinical status of your client. It is important for you to obtain and follow the guidelines given and to maintain close contact with the appropriate health professional to have your questions answered and to provide status reports at predetermined intervals. An ACE-certified Personal Trainer is certified to work with clients with health challenges only after they have been cleared by their personal physician.

This chapter addresses basic guidelines for working with clients with the following health conditions and/or special needs:

Coronary artery disease
Hypertension
Stroke
Peripheral vascular disease
Diabetes
Asthma
Bronchitis
Emphysema
Cancer
Osteoporosis
Low-back pain
Arthritis
Older adults
Weight management
Children
Pregnancy

As a rule of thumb, if a client has been released to take part in independent activities of daily living (including a limited exercise program), they will probably be cleared to work with a personal trainer who can then provide guidance and motivation.

Generally speaking, clients with one or more of the above characteristics should follow a low- or non-impact, low-intensity exercise program that progresses gradually. In many cases there are specific exercises or modifications to exercises that will enhance the safety and effectiveness of the exercise program. If you train clients with special needs, it is your responsibility to enhance your knowledge and skills in this area through continuing education opportunities.

CARDIOVASCULAR DISORDERS

Cardiovascular disease is the leading cause of death in the Western world, the majority of which are attributed to coronary artery disease. **Coronary artery disease (CAD)** results from **atherosclerosis,** which is caused by a narrowing of the coronary arteries that supply the heart muscle with blood and oxygen. The narrowing may result from an initial injury to the inner lining of the arteries (due to high blood pressures, high levels of **LDL cholesterol,** elevated blood glucose, or other chemical agents, such as those from cigarettes). Once the inner lining has been damaged, the accumulation of plaque (consisting of calcified cholesterol and fat deposits) reduces the diameter of the coronary artery.

Atherosclerosis also is the underlying cause of cerebral and **peripheral vascular diseases.** Manifestations of these diseases include heart attack, **angina, stroke,** and intermittent **claudication.**

Exercise and Coronary Artery Disease

Regular physical activity reduces the risk of CAD, but how effective is exercise in treating it? In the early 1960s, physicians began experimenting with getting patients up and out of bed soon after a cardiac event, and the results were favorable. Unlike those who were advised to stay in bed, cardiac patients who stayed mobile experienced fewer clinical complications, a faster recovery, and fewer complications related to bed rest. In almost all cases, individuals recovering from a **myocardial infarction,** cardiac surgery, or other cardiac procedure, can benefit from a supervised cardiac rehabilitation program.

Exercise Guidelines for CAD

It is best if clients with a history of coronary artery disease first complete a supervised cardiac rehabilitation program before starting an exercise program with a personal trainer. Most clients who have been released to take part in activities of daily living will have been given a home exercise program and some basic activity guidelines. It is appropriate for you to inform prospective clients that cardiac rehabilitation programs are available and that they should ask their physician if participation is recommended. Exercise and activity guidelines are based on the clinical status of the client. A cardiologist or other designated health professional should provide you with an upper-limit heart rate, as well as guidelines and limitations to physical activity.

1. Low-risk cardiac clients should have stable cardiovascular and physiological responses to exercise. The term low risk is generally applied to those clients who have all of the following: (1) an uncomplicated clinical course in the hospital; (2) no evidence of resting or exercise-induced **ischemia**; (3) **functional capacity** greater than 7 **METs** three weeks following any medical event or treatment that required hospitalization, such as a heart attack, episode of angina, or open heart surgery; (4) normal ventricular function greater than 50% ejection fraction (percent of blood pumped out of the heart with each beat); and (5) no significant resting or exercise-induced **arrhythmias** (abnormal heart rhythms identified by an electrocardiogram).

2. Clients or potential clients who have two or more cardiac risk factors or a history of cardiac disease must have a physician release and referral to exercise (see Chapter 5).

3. All clients with documented coronary artery disease should have a **maximal graded exercise test** to determine their functional capacity and cardiovascular status to establish a safe exercise level.

4. Design your clients' exercise programs according to the guidelines given by their personal physicians. These guidelines will usually be based on exercise test results, medical history, clinical status, and symptoms. There are published guidelines available to assist you in working with these clients and interacting with their healthcare team (American College of Sports Medicine, 2000; American Association of Cardiovascular and Pulmonary Rehabilitation, 1999).

5. Exercise should not continue if any abnormal signs or symptoms are observed before, during, or immediately following exercise. If symptoms persist, activate the emergency medical system.

Sample Exercise Recommendation

Mode. Low-intensity endurance exercise, such as low-impact aerobics, walking, swimming, or stationary cycling, should be the primary exercise mode. Avoid **isometric** exercises because they can dramatically raise blood pressure and the work of the heart. Develop a weight-training program that features low resistance and a high number of repetitions.

Note: Any client who has had a cardiovascular event within the last month should, as appropriate, follow the exercise guidelines outlined below. If a low-risk client has been stable for at least six months, follow exercise guidelines for sedentary, healthy adults.

Intensity. **Rating of Perceived Exertion (RPE)** of 9 to 14 (6–20 scale); heart rate can be as low as 20 to 30 beats over resting heart rate and up to 40 to 75% of maximal **heart-rate reserve** (Karvonen formula).

Duration. The total duration should be gradually increased to 20 to 30 minutes of continuous or **interval training,** plus additional time for warm-up and cool-down activities.

Frequency. Three to five days per week.

HYPERTENSION

Hypertension is one of the most prevalent **chronic diseases** in the United States. According to the Centers for Disease Control and Prevention,

Hypertension

Hypertension

23% of Americans between the ages of 20 and 74 have hypertension and approximately 18,000 hypertension-related deaths occur in the U.S. each year. **Hypertension** is related to the development of CAD, increased severity of atherosclerosis, stroke, congestive heart failure, left ventricular hypertrophy, aortic aneurysms, and peripheral vascular disease.

Hypertensive individuals are at three to four times the risk of developing coronary artery disease, and up to seven times the risk of having a stroke.

Exercise and Hypertension

Exercise is now recognized as an important part of therapy for controlling hypertension. While we know that regular aerobic exercise reduces both **systolic** and **diastolic blood pressure** by an average of 10 mmHg, how it does this is not completely understood. It appears that regular physical activity reduces both cardiac output and total peripheral resistance when the body is at rest, as well as sympathetic activity.

Exercise Guidelines for Hypertension

Since many hypertensive individuals are obese and have CAD risk factors, non-drug therapy is usually the first line of treatment. This therapy will usually include weight reduction, salt restriction, and increased physical activity. Consider these factors when recommending exercise for hypertensives: (1) medical/clinical status; (2) current medications; (3) the frequency, duration, intensity, and mode of exercise the individual is currently participating in; and (4) how well the individual manages their hypertension.

1. Do not allow your hypertensive clients to hold their breath or strain during exercise **(Valsalva maneuver);** cue them to exhale on the exertion.

2. Weight training should supplement endurance training. Utilize **circuit training** rather than heavy weight lifting and keep resistance low and the repetitions high.

3. Use the RPE scale to monitor exercise intensity because medications (e.g., beta blockers) can alter the accuracy of the training heart rate during exercise.

4. Be aware of any changes in medications, which should come with written guidelines from your client's physician. Not all medication changes will require a change in an exercise program, but this should be communicated to you by your client's physician. See Appendix D for a listing of generic and brand names of common antihypertensive medications by class.

5. Exercise should not continue if any abnormal signs or symptoms are observed before, during, or immediately following exercise. If symptoms persist, activate the emergency medical system. If symptoms stop, discontinue the exercise program until your client's physician gives clearance.

6. Physicians may instruct their hypertensive patients to record their blood pressures before and after exercise.

7. Instruct your hypertensive clients to move slowly when getting up from the floor because they are more susceptible to **orthostatic hypotension** when taking antihypertensive medication.

8. Both hypertensive and hypotensive responses are possible during and after exercise for individuals with hypertension. Either of these responses should be reported, and additional exercise guidelines given as a result.

9. Carefully monitor your client's blood pressure during exercise initially, and possibly long-term. Blood pressure can be most accurately measured during lower-body aerobic activity (e.g., stationary cycling) and resistance training (e.g., leg extensions). Clients with more severe hypertension will likely be taking one or more hypertensive medications that may affect their response to exercise.

10. Individuals with hypertension may have multiple CAD risk factors, which should be considered when developing their exercise program.

Sample Exercise Recommendation

Mode. The overall exercise training recommendations for individuals with mild-to-moderate hypertension are basically the same for apparently healthy individuals. Endurance exercise such as low-impact aerobics, walking, and swimming should be the primary exercise mode. Exercises with a significant isometric component should be avoided. Weight training should feature low resistance and a high number of repetitions (initially, 12 to 20).

Intensity. The exercise intensity level should be near the lower end of the heart-rate range (40 to 65%).

Frequency. Encourage your hypertensive clients to exercise at least four times per week. Elderly clients or those with an initially low functional capacity may exercise daily for shorter duration.

Duration. Gradual warm-ups and cool-downs lasting longer than five minutes are recommended. Gradually increase total exercise duration to as much as 30 to 60 minutes per session, depending on the medical history and clinical status of the individual.

STROKE

About 600,000 Americans will have a stroke each year and 160,000 of them will die. In fact, stroke is our nation's number three killer and is a leading cause of severe, long-term disability. Every 53 seconds someone in America has a stroke. Strokes also are referred to as **cerebrovascular accidents (CVA)**. Similar to a myocardial infarction, a stroke affects the arteries of the nervous system instead of the heart. When nerve cells are deprived of oxygen because of a blockage or rupture of a blood vessel supplying blood to the brain, those cells die within minutes. The results can be devastating: speech, thought patterns and memory, behavioral patterns, and sight all may be affected and the body may become paralyzed. The risk factors for stroke include high blood pressure, heart disease, cigarette smoking, high red blood cell count, and **transient ischemic attacks (TIAs),** which are momentary reductions in oxygen delivery to the brain, possibly resulting in a sudden headache, dizziness, or a blackout.

Exercise and Stroke

There is little data on the role of exercise and stroke, as most studies have yielded mixed results. In general, because the risk factors for stroke are the same as those for CAD, exercise may lessen the risk for stroke by reducing overall CAD risk. Hypertension is a primary risk factor for strokes; therefore, exercise, because it reduces hypertension, is a primary lifestyle modification recommended for preventing strokes. Exercise also may be recommended for hypertensive individuals at risk for stroke or those recovering from a stroke. Seventy to 80% of strokes are caused by a **thrombosis,** which is the formation of a blood clot within an intact blood vessel. Exercise also may help by enhancing fibrinolytic activity, the system responsible for dissolving blood clots. For clients who are at risk for, or have experienced, a stroke, follow the same guidelines and recommendations used for coronary artery disease and hypertension.

Varied degrees of rehabilitation will follow a stroke. A minor stroke could result in very basic home guidelines given as part of the in-patient discharge instructions. Moderate and severe strokes usually require out-patient therapy. These programs are designed to assist a patient's return to an optimal level of functioning. The physical activity portion of stroke rehabilitation will usually be administered by physical, occupational, and/or recreational therapists. Ideally, your guidelines should come from this team with approval from your client's personal physician.

PERIPHERAL VASCULAR DISEASE

Peripheral vascular disease (PVD) is caused by atherosclerotic lesions in one or more peripheral arterial and/or venous blood vessels (usually in the

Peripheral Vascular Occlusive Disease

Table 12.1
Subjective Grading Scale for Peripheral Vascular Disease

Grade I — Definite discomfort or pain, but only of initial or modest levels

Grade II — Moderate discomfort or pain from which the client's attention can be diverted, by conversation, for example

Grade III — Intense pain (short of Grade IV) from which the client's attention cannot be diverted

Grade IV — Excruciating and unbearable pain

legs). Common sites for atherosclerotic lesions include the iliac, femoral, and popliteal arteries (see Figure 2.2a, page 32). Most people with PVD are older and have long-established CAD **risk factors;** it also is 20 times more common in diabetics than in non-diabetic individuals. The treatment for PVD usually involves a combination of medication (drugs to increase dilation of the arteries and veins), exercise (to improve blood flow and functional capacity), medical procedures (cleaning out the blockages), or surgery (artery bypass).

PVD is a painful and often debilitating disease, characterized by muscular pain caused by ischemia (reduced blood flow) to the working muscles. This ischemic pain is usually the result of spasms or blockages, referred to as claudication. Some people experience chronic claudication and pain even at rest. For others, activities such as walking, cycling, or stair climbing can cause painful, intermittent claudication that is usually relieved by immediate rest. Most people with PVD describe claudication as a dull, aching, cramping pain. The claudication pain scale is a subjective rating of discomfort, which can be used to regulate exercise intensity, duration, and frequency (Table 12.1).

Exercise and Peripheral Vascular Occlusive Disease

One of the primary benefits of exercise for individuals with PVD is that it helps to lower overall CAD risk (e.g., hypertension, hypercholesterolemia), as well as improve blood flow and overall cardiovascular endurance. Studies have shown that people with PVD can improve their peak work capacity with regular exercise (Regensteiner & Hiatt, 1995).

Exercise Guidelines for Peripheral Vascular Disease

Individuals with PVD should undergo a complete medical evaluation before embarking on an exercise program. Initially, focus on low-intensity, non-weightbearing activities. Because of their chronic pain, individuals with PVD often have a high anxiety level when starting out. Gradual progression can build confidence, and additional activities may be added to their program. Individuals with PVD probably do not have ambitions to run a marathon; they simply want to be able to go shopping, climb stairs, and go for a walk without a great deal of pain. In addition to exercise, other lifestyle modifications, such as diet modifications and weight management, should be encouraged in an effort to lower overall CAD risk.

1. Encourage daily exercise with frequent rest periods to allow for maximal exercise tolerance.

2. Initially, recommend low-impact, non-weightbearing activities such as swimming, rowing, and cycling. Add weightbearing activities as exercise tolerance improves.

3. Avoid exercising in cold air or water to reduce the risk of **vasoconstriction.**

4. Interval training, which may involve 5- to 10-minute exercise bouts, one to three times per day, may initially be appropriate for some PVD clients.

5. Because many PVD clients also are diabetic, they need to take excellent care of their feet to avoid blisters and other injuries that could lead to infection.

6. Ideally, individuals with PVD should be closely supervised, such as in a cardiac rehabilitation program.

7. Gradually increase the time, duration, and intensity of your PVD clients' pro-

grams. The degree of progress (absence or reduction of pain) will dictate how often and how much to increase these variables. As their functional capacity improves, increase these factors accordingly.

8. Encourage your PVD clients to walk as much and as often as they can tolerate.

Sample Exercise Recommendation

Mode. Non-impact endurance exercise, such as swimming and cycling, may allow for longer-duration and higher-intensity exercise. Recommend weightbearing activities that are shorter in duration and lower in intensity, with more frequent rest periods.

Intensity. Choose low-intensity exercises rather than high-intensity, high-impact exercises. PVD clients should exercise to the point of moderate to intense pain (Grade II to Grade III on the claudication pain scale; see Table 12.1). As functional capacity improves, gradually increase intensity.

Frequency. Daily exercise is recommended initially. As functional capacity improves, frequency can be reduced to four to six days per week.

Duration. A longer and more gradual warm-up and cool-down (longer than 10 minutes) is recommended. Gradually increase total exercise duration to 30 to 40 minutes.

DIABETES

Diabetes is characterized by reduced insulin secretion by the pancreatic beta cells and/or reduced sensitivity to insulin. **Diabetes** causes abnormalities in the metabolism of carbohydrates, protein, and fat and, if left untreated, can be deadly. This is of particular concern since the symptoms of diabetes are not always evident in the early stages.

People with diabetes are at greater risk for numerous health problems, including kidney failure, nerve disorders, eye problems, and heart disease, and are two to four times as likely to develop cardiovascular disease. Prolonged and frequent elevation of blood sugar can damage the capillaries, a condition called microangiopathy that leads to poor circulation. In addition, people with diabetes are at greater risk for permanent nerve damage.

There are two main types of diabetes. **Type 1 diabetes** is caused by the destruction of the insulin-producing beta cells in the pancreas, which leads to little or no insulin secretion. Type 1 diabetes generally occurs in childhood and regular insulin injections are required to regulate blood glucose levels.

The typical symptoms of type 1 diabetes are excessive thirst and hunger, frequent urination, weight loss, blurred vision, and recurrent infections. During periods of insulin deficiency, a higher-than-normal level of glucose remains in the blood because of reduced uptake and storage. A portion of the excess glucose is excreted in the urine, which leads to increased thirst and appetite and weight loss. Chronically elevated blood glucose levels is a condition known as **hyperglycemia.**

Type 2 diabetes is the most common form of diabetes, affecting 90% of all diabetic patients. It typically occurs in adults who are overweight and is characterized by a reduced sensitivity of insulin target cells to available insulin, called insulin resistance. Insulin resistance, a condition in which the body is unable to use its own insulin efficiently, affects approximately 60 million people in the United States, one in four of whom will develop type 2 diabetes. Unfortunately, increasing numbers of children are being diagnosed with type 2 diabetes, making the term "adult-onset diabetes" obsolete. Some people with type 2 diabetes never exhibit any of the classic symptoms of diabetes. Treatment usually includes diet modification, medication, and exercise therapy.

Type 2 diabetes also is characterized by frequent states of hyperglycemia, but without the increased catabolism of fats and protein. Because 75% of individuals with type 2

Diabetes

diabetes are obese or have a history of **obesity,** it is important to note that this condition is often reversible with permanent weight loss.

Effective Diabetes Control

Long-term regulation of blood glucose levels is necessary to effectively control diabetes. In type 1 diabetes, glucose regulation is achieved through regular glucose assessment, proper diet, exercise, and appropriate insulin medication. For type 2 diabetes, it is achieved through lifestyle changes centered around proper diet, weight management, exercise, and insulin or oral agents if needed. A combined diet and exercise regimen results in weight loss and weight control, improved circulation and cardiorespiratory fitness, a reduced need for insulin, improved self-image, and a better ability to deal with stress.

Exercise and Type 1 Diabetes

The role of exercise in controlling glucose levels has not been well demonstrated. Even so, individuals with type 1 diabetes can improve their functional capacity, reduce their risk for CAD, and improve insulin receptor sensitivity and number with a program of regular physical activity.

Exercise and Type 2 Diabetes

Exercise plays an important role in controlling type 2 diabetes, because it reduces both cholesterol levels and weight. With excessive blood glucose elevation, blood fats rise to become the primary energy source for the body. Higher-than-normal blood-fat levels put diabetics at greater risk for heart disease.

Exercise Guidelines for Diabetes

Before beginning an exercise program, clients with diabetes should speak with their physician or diabetes educator to develop a program of diet, exercise, and medication. The primary goal of exercise for type 1 diabetes is better glucose regula-

tion and reduced heart disease risk. The timing of exercise, the amount of insulin injected, and the injection site are important to consider before exercising. Exercise should be performed consistently so that a regular pattern of diet and insulin dosage can be maintained. Ideally, the diabetic client should perform a similar exercise routine every day, within one hour of consuming a meal or snack.

The primary goal of exercise for individuals with type 2 diabetes is weight loss and control, as 80% are overweight. By losing weight through diet and exercise, they may be able to reduce the amount of oral insulin medication needed. The primary objective during exercise for those with type 2 diabetes is caloric expenditure, which is best achieved by long-duration exercise. Since the duration of exercise is often high, the intensity of exercise should be kept lower.

1. Clients with diabetes should check their blood glucose levels frequently and work closely with their physicians to determine the right insulin dosage.

2. People with diabetes should always carry a rapid-acting carbohydrate (such as juice or candy) in case they develop hypoglycemia.

3. Do not inject insulin into the primary muscle groups that will be used during exercise because it will be absorbed too quickly, resulting in **hypoglycemia.**

4. Encourage your clients with diabetes to exercise at the same time each day for better control.

5. Avoid exercise during periods of peak insulin activity.

6. A carbohydrate snack should be consumed before and during prolonged exercise.

7. People with diabetes need to take very good care of their feet, which should be regularly checked for any cuts, blisters, or signs of infection. Good quality exercise shoes also are very important.

8. Physicians will usually instruct their patients to check their blood glucose level before and after exercise. Exercise should be curtailed if preexercise blood glucose is

below 100 mg/dL. With additional carbohydrate consumption, exercise may be allowed to take place. Exercise should also be curtailed if preexercise blood glucose is greater than 300 mg/dL or greater than 240 mg/dL with urinary ketone bodies. In the latter scenario, exercise would need to be postponed until the client's blood sugar is under control. Your clients with diabetes should have specific guidelines to follow in these situations. These guidelines will depend upon a client's clinical status and medical history with respect to blood glucose control.

Sample Exercise Recommendation

Mode. Endurance activities, such as walking, swimming, and cycling.

Intensity. Fifty to 60% of cardiac reserve, gradually progressing to 60 to 70%.

Frequency. Four to seven days/week. Some clients may need to start out with several shorter daily sessions.

Duration. Individuals with type 1 diabetes should gradually work up to 20 to 30 minutes per session. For individuals with type 2 diabetes, 40 to 60 minutes is recommended.

Special Precautions for Exercise and Diabetes

Individuals with type 1 diabetes face two potential problems during or following exercise: lack of insulin, which may cause a hyperglycemic effect; and rapid mobilization of insulin, which dangerously lowers blood glucose levels. Low blood glucose is referred to as hypoglycemia. One of the first rules for those with type 1 diabetes is to either reduce insulin intake or increase carbohydrate intake before exercise. If pre-exercise blood glucose is below 100 mg/dL in clients taking insulin, it is recommended they consume 20 to 30 grams of additional carbohydrate before exercise. Individuals with either type of diabetes should exercise one to two hours after a meal and before peak insulin activity. Because exercise has an insulin-like effect, insulin dosages generally should be lowered prior to exercise. Clients with diabetes should check blood glucose levels frequently when starting an exercise program and be aware of any unusual symptoms prior to, during, or after exercise.

Other potential problems associated with exercise and diabetes include autonomic neuropathy (which may blunt the HR response to exercise); peripheral neuropathy (which may cause numbness in the extremities); microvascular complication (which may cause vision or kidney problems); and peripheral vascular disease (which may cause claudication).

ASTHMA

Asthma is a reactive airway disease characterized by shortness of breath, coughing, and wheezing. It is due to (1) constriction of the smooth muscle around the airways; (2) a swelling of the mucosal cells; and/or (3) increased secretion of mucous. Asthma can be caused by an allergic reaction, exercise, infections, stress, or other environmental irritants, such as pollens, inhalants, cigarette smoke, and air pollution. Asthma is one of the most common respiratory disorders affecting both adults and children.

Approximately 80% of people with asthma experience asthma attacks during exercise (referred to as exercise-induced asthma, or EIA), which are characterized by moderate obstruction and are not life threatening. The severity of an EIA attack is related to the intensity of exercise and the ventilatory requirement of the task, as well as the environmental conditions. Inhaling cold, dry air versus warm, moist air seems to cause greater airway obstruction.

The exact cause of EIA is not well understood but is believed to be caused when the airways become dry as moisture is absorbed from the air as it passes from the nose to the lower part of the lungs. While asthma is not a contraindication to exercise, people with asthma should work with their physicians to develop appropriate exercise programs.

Exercise and Asthma

Most individuals with controlled asthma will benefit from regular exercise, which helps to reduce the ventilatory requirement for various tasks, making it easier for them to participate in normal daily activities with less shortness of breath and fewer asthma attacks. Several studies have shown that regular exercise also can reduce the number and severity of exercise-induced asthma attacks (American College of Sports Medicine, 2001).

Exercise Guidelines for Asthma

1. Before beginning an exercise program, individuals with asthma must have a medication/treatment plan to prevent EIA attacks.

2. Clients with asthma should have a bronchodilating inhaler with them at all times and be instructed to use it at the first sign of wheezing.

3. Keep the exercise intensity low initially and gradually increase it over time since exercise intensity is directly linked to the severity and frequency of EIA.

4. Reduce the intensity if asthma symptoms occur.

5. Using an inhaler several minutes before exercise may reduce the possibility of EIA attacks.

6. Use the results of pulmonary exercise testing to design an appropriate exercise program.

7. Encourage clients with asthma to drink plenty of fluids before and during exercise.

8. Individuals with asthma should extend their warm-up and cool-down periods.

9. Individuals with respiratory disorders will often experience more symptoms of respiratory distress when exercising in extreme environmental conditions (high or low temperature, high pollen count, and heavy air pollution).

10. Wearing a face mask during exercise helps keep inhaled air more warm and moist, and may minimize asthmatic responses during exercise.

11. Individuals with respiratory disorders need to be carefully followed by their physician.

12. Only people with stable asthma should exercise.

13. If an asthma attack is not relieved by medication, activate the emergency medical system.

14. Patients with asthma often respond best to exercise in mid-to-late morning.

15. Clients with asthma should avoid extremes in temperature and humidity.

Sample Exercise Recommendation

Mode. Walking, cycling, and swimming are good choices for clients with asthma. Upper-body exercises such as arm cranking, rowing, and cross-country skiing may not be appropriate because of the higher ventilation demands. Swimming may be particularly beneficial because it allows people with asthma to inhale the moist air just above the surface of the water.

Intensity. Recommend low-intensity dynamic exercise based on the client's fitness status and limitations.

Frequency. Encourage your clients with asthma to exercise at least three to four times per week. Individuals with low functional capacities or those who experience shortness of breath during prolonged exercise may benefit from intermittent exercise (two 10-minute sessions).

Duration. Encourage a longer, more gradual warm-up and cool-down (longer than 10 minutes). Gradually increase total exercise duration to 20 to 45 minutes.

BRONCHITIS AND EMPHYSEMA

Bronchitis, a form of obstructive pulmonary disease marked by inflammation of the bronchial tubes, is primarily caused by cigarette smoking, though air pollution and occupational exposure may play lesser roles. Acute bronchitis is an inflammation of the mucous membranes as well. However, an acute bout of bronchitis can develop following a cold or exposure to certain dust particles or fumes and resolve in several days or weeks. Chronic bronchitis persists for a lifetime in most cases.

Emphysema is another form of chronic pulmonary disease caused by over-inflation of the alveoli, resulting from a breakdown of the walls of the alveoli. This causes a significant decrease in respiratory function. The classic signs of emphysema are chronic breathlessness and coughing. Together, emphysema and bronchitis are referred to as **chronic obstructive pulmonary diseases,** or **COPD.**

Exercise and COPD

Individuals with COPD may or may not benefit from mild exercise training, depending on the severity of their disease. These individuals need to be carefully screened and followed by a physician. It is also important to note that many individuals who suffer from COPD also have other medical conditions, such as heart disease, which may affect exercise programming. While most people with COPD do not improve their pulmonary function, other benefits such as reduced anxiety, body weight, and stress, and an improved ability to perform daily activities can be realized through exercise. The primary goals of exercise training for individuals with COPD is to (1) increase functional capacity; (2) increase functional status; (3) decrease severity of dyspnea; and (4) improve quality of life.

Individuals with COPD who are stable and have obtained all the potential benefits from a medically supervised exercise program should benefit from participating in an exercise program that is not medically supervised. Encourage these individuals to do the best they can, because every little bit of exercise they do can result in potential health benefits.

Exercise Guidelines for COPD

1. Before starting an exercise program, individuals with COPD need to complete extensive pulmonary tests.

2. Individuals with unstable COPD should not participate in an exercise program without medical supervision.

3. Carefully choose exercise intensity and type to avoid developing shortness of breath. (For a complete review of strategies for setting exercise intensity for pulmonary patients, see *ACSM's Guidelines for Exercise Testing and Prescription*, 6th edition.)

4. Apply the exercise guidelines for those with asthma to your clients with COPD.

5. Individuals must be fully recovered from an acute bout of bronchitis before exercising.

6. Individuals with COPD should have a bronchodilating inhaler with them at all times and be instructed to use it at the first sign of wheezing.

7. Individuals with COPD should perform breathing exercises to help strengthen their respiratory muscles.

8. Initially avoid upper-body exercises such as arm cranking or rowing because of the increased strain on the pulmonary system. Upper-body resistance training may be gradually added to a comprehensive exercise program.

9. Some individuals with COPD may require supplemental oxygen during exercise as well as continuous ECG and BP monitoring.

10. Clients with COPD must not smoke.

11. Based on your clients' responses to exercise, review the type and dose of medications with their physicians.

12. If a COPD client's performance in a program lacking medical supervision worsens, encourage him or her to participate in a pulmonary rehabilitation program until signs and symptoms improve.

Sample Exercise Recommendation

Mode. Walking and stationary cycling are good choices for individuals with COPD. Upper-body exercises such as arm cranking, rowing, and cross-country skiing may not be appropriate initially because of the higher ventilation demands. Gradually add upper-body resistance exercises.

Intensity. Recommend low-intensity dynamic exercise rather than high-intensity, high-impact exercise. Adjust the intensity according to the client's breathing responses to exercise. Keep the exercise intensity below the point where any difficulty in breathing may occur.

Frequency. Encourage your clients with COPD to exercise at least four to five times per week. They may benefit from shorter, intermittent exercise sessions.

Duration. Encourage a long, gradual warm-up and cool-down (longer than 10 minutes). Gradually increase total exercise duration to 20 to 30 minutes.

CANCER

Cancer causes more than a half million deaths annually, making it the second leading cause of death in the United States. An estimated 80% of cancer cases may be prevented through appropriate lifestyle changes. For example, regular exercise, a low-fat, high-fiber diet, and not smoking all help reduce the risk of developing cancer. Dietary changes can reduce the risk of developing bowel cancer, the second most common form of cancer diagnosed, while not smoking may prevent the development of lung cancer. Thus, many types of cancers are highly preventable.

Exercise and Cancer

In general, physically inactive people are more likely to develop cancer and studies show that cancer **mortality** is higher in those who exercise the least, even after age and cigarette smoking are considered (Blair et al., 1995; Byers et al., 2002).

Exercise Guidelines for Cancer

Exercise training is generally safe and beneficial for cancer patients, as long as the patient is able and has physician approval to exercise. Regardless of the type of cancer, most studies show that cancer patients can improve their overall aerobic capacity, neuromuscular function, and quality of life as a

result of exercise. The following five questions should be asked of your client's personal physician before designing an exercise program for clients with cancer:

1. Are there any limitations in activity based on preexisting conditions or medical procedures?

2. Are there any limitations in activity as a result of nutritional and fluid deficits?

3. Are there any limitations in mobility as a result of disease or treatment?

4. Are there any limitations in oxygen delivery as a result of disease or treatment?

5. Are there any limitations based on risk for anemia, bleeding, and infections?

If individuals have any limitations based on the conditions listed above, guidelines should be given by a member of your client's healthcare team, and the exercise program should be adjusted accordingly.

OSTEOPOROSIS

Osteoporosis is a major public health threat for an estimated 44 million Americans. In the U.S. today, 10 million individuals are estimated to already have the disease and almost 34 million are at an increased risk for osteoporosis. Of the 10 million estimated to have osteoporosis, 8 million are women and 2 million are men.

After reaching its peak, bone mass declines throughout life because of an imbalance of "remodeling" of the bone. Remodeling refers to the replacement of old bone with new bone and keeps the skeletal system in peak form and helps maintain calcium **homeostasis.**

Exercise and Osteoporosis

The treatment of osteoporosis is aimed at preventing or retarding bone mineral loss. Estrogen replacement therapy is highly effective in maintaining bone mass and preventing osteoporosis in women by reducing bone reabsorption and retarding or halting **postmenopausal** bone loss. **Pre-menopausal** women should consume 1,000 to 1,500 mg of calcium per day, which appears to suppress age-related bone loss. While the role of exercise in the prevention and treatment of osteoporosis is not completely understood, it is known that physical stress determines the strength of bone. Physical inactivity is a known risk factor for osteoporosis, and exercise is recommended for its prevention and treatment because weightbearing exercise either retards the loss of, or increases, bone mass. Even individuals who have led sedentary lives can increase bone mass by becoming more active.

Exercise Guidelines for Osteoporosis

The greater the physical stress and compression on a bone, the greater the rate of bone deposition (this is why weightbearing exercise is recommended). Since most individuals who suffer from osteoporosis are elderly, refer to the exercise guidelines and recommendations for older adults that begin on page 360. Resistance training also is an important component in the prevention of osteoporosis. Additionally, individuals with osteoporosis may need to avoid:

✔ jumping, high-impact aerobics, jogging, and running

✔ spinal flexion, crunches, and rowing machines

✔ trampolines and step aerobics

✔ wood gym floors that may become slippery from sweat drops

✔ abducting or adducting the legs against resistance (particularly machines)

✔ moving the legs sideways or across the body

✔ pulling on the neck with hands behind the head

LOW-BACK PAIN

Back injuries, including sprains and strains, are the number-one disability for people under age 45. It is estimated that 80% of the population will experience an episode of low-back pain some time in their lives. Of these, 5% will go on to develop chronic low-back pain (LBP), which accounts for 10% of all chronic health conditions in the U.S., and 25% of days lost from work. LBP has been labeled the most expensive benign health condition in America.

Back injuries translate into millions of lost work days every year and cost billions for medical care, disability payments, and legal payments. Reducing back-injury rates is a top priority for all employers. In fact, the most common type of workers' compensation claim is a back strain/sprain, which accounts for up to 25% of all claims, representing annual payments of $2.5 to $7 billion, including one-half of all disability compensation payments annually.

While the cause of LBP is often elusive, four common causes have been identified: a **herniated disc** (rupture of the outer layers of fibers that surround the gelatinous portion of the disc); **spondylolisthesis** (forward sliding of the body of one vertebra on the vertebra below it); a trauma to the back (accident); and degenerative disc disease (progressive structural degeneration of the intervertebral disc). Lower-back problems are often associated with an imbalance of strength and flexibility of the lower back and abdominal muscle groups. Poor flexibility in the hamstrings and hip flexor muscles also have been linked to LBP.

Exercise and Low-back Pain

A strong correlation exists between LBP and excess body weight, smoking, and decreased physical activity. It makes sense, then, that physical fitness combined with a healthy lifestyle may help prevent LBP. In fact, many physicians feel that the major cause of chronic low-back pain is simply physical deconditioning. More specifically, low endurance in the large muscle groups, particularly the back extensors, seems to put one at a greater risk of developing LBP. Aerobic training and exercises for the low-back should be performed on a regular basis as part of the treatment and prevention of LBP.

Arthritis

Table 12.2
Exercises for the Low Back

Position	Activity
Supine with knees bent	Slowly, pull one knee to chest and hold for five seconds, then do the same with the other knee.
Supine, with knees bent and legs together	Slowly rotate knees from side to side while keeping them together.
Hands and knees	Arch your back up like a cat, hold for five seconds, and relax.
Hands and knees	Slowly sit back between your knees and then return to hands and knees.
Hands and knees	Slowly bring one knee to the chest then extend the leg straight out behind you. Repeat on the other side.
Standing against the wall; optional exercise is to place a large rubber ball behind the back	Squat down so that your lower back is pressed against the wall. Move your feet out from the wall and bend your legs to a "half-squat" and hold. Gradually straighten legs out.
Prone with legs and arms straight out	Lift one arm, hold, and relax. Alternate arms. Lift one leg, hold, and relax. Alternate legs. Lift one arm and one leg on opposite sides, hold, and relax. Alternate sides.
Supine, with knees slightly bent	Flatten your back against the floor by contracting your stomach muscles and rotating your hips backward.

Additional activities

Side stretch, abdominal curls, modified push-ups, lateral leg raises, groin stretch, hamstring stretch, calf stretch, and quadriceps stretch

Exercise Guidelines for Low-back Pain

Prevention is the key to avoiding LBP, and clients should be screened for low-back pain risk factors. If someone has experienced a recent LBP strain or injury, he or she should be cleared by a physician before starting an exercise program. In addition to aerobic and resistance training, basic core back exercises should be performed on a regular basis (Table 12.2). Clients with diagnosed low-back pain should avoid: unsupported forward flexion; twisting at the waist with turned feet, especially when carrying a load; lifting both legs simultaneously when in a prone or supine position; and rapid movements, such as twisting, forward flexion, or hyperextending.

Advise clients with low-back pain to keep in mind the following:

1. Always be aware of proper form and alignment.

2. Always maintain neutral pelvic alignment and an erect torso during any exercise movements (see pages 72–75).

3. Avoid head-forward positions in which the chin is tilted up.

4. When leaning forward, lifting or lowering an object, always bend at the knees.

5. Avoid hyperextending the spine in an unsupported position.

6. Adequately warm up and cool down before and after each workout session.

7. Most low-back pain is caused by muscle weaknesses and imbalances in the hamstrings, hip flexors, lower-back muscle groups, and abdominals. Exercise should be routinely performed to improve muscle strength and/or flexibility (see Table 12.2).

8. Advise your clients with low-back pain, or a history of chronic low-back pain, to consult with a physician and get specific recommendations for exercises.

9. If clients complain of low-back pain following exercise, have them sit or lie down in a comfortable position and apply ice to the affected area. Encourage clients to take a few days off from exercise if they experience a mild back strain.

ARTHRITIS

The most common forms of arthritis are **rheumatoid arthritis** and **osteoarthritis.** Osteoarthritis, also referred to as degenerative joint disease, is a degenerative process in which cartilage wears away, leaving

Table 12.3
American College of Rheumatology Revised Criteria for Classification of Functional Status in Rheumatoid Arthritis

Class I	Completely able to perform usual activities of daily living (self-care, vocational, and avocational)
Class II	Able to perform usual self-care and vocational activities, but limited in avocational activities
Class III	Able to perform usual self-care activities, but limited in vocational and avocational activities
Class IV	Limited in ability to perform usual self-care, vocational, and avocational activities

Note: Usual self-care activities include dressing, feeding, bathing, grooming, and toileting. Avocational activities (recreational and/or leisure) and vocational (work, school, homemaking) activities are patient-desired and age- and sex-specific.

Reprinted with permission from: Hochberg, M.C. et al. (1992). The American College of Rheumatology 1991 revised criteria for the classification of global functioning status in rheumatoid arthritis. *Arthritis and Rheumatism*, 35, 5, 498–502.

two surfaces of bone in contact with each other. Rheumatoid arthritis is caused by an inflammation of the membrane surrounding the joint, and is often associated with pain and swelling in one or more joints. More than 40 million people in the United States have some form of arthritis (one in every seven people). Osteoarthritis is a common and chronic condition affecting the joints in the elderly, aged 55 and above. Some 21 million people in the U.S. alone suffer from this degenerative joint disease. Most people over the age of 75 are affected with osteoarthritis in at least one joint, making this condition a leading cause of disability in the U.S. Rheumatoid arthritis, the most crippling form of arthritis, affects approximately 2.1 million Americans and two to three times more women than men. Further, the average onset for rheumatoid arthritis is between the ages of 20 and 45 years old.

The treatment of arthritis, which may involve medicine (corticosteroids), physical therapy, physiotherapy [transcutaneous electrical nerve stimulation (TENS) and hot packs], occupational therapy [to improve activities of daily living (ADLs)] and surgery

(joint replacement), depends on the severity and specific form of arthritis. Individuals with arthritis can be classified into four categories of functional capacity (Table 12.3).

Individuals with arthritis should not be excluded from participating in a program of regular exercise. Stronger muscles and bones, improved cardiorespiratory fitness, and improved psychosocial well-being are some of the benefits they can gain from appropriate exercise. It is contraindicated, however, during inflammatory periods because exercise can aggravate or worsen the condition.

Exercise and Arthritis

Exercise is recommended for individuals with arthritis to help preserve muscle strength and joint mobility, improve functional capabilities, relieve pain and stiffness, prevent further deformities, improve overall physical conditioning, re-establish neuromuscular coordination, and mobilize stiff or contracted joints.

Fitness programs, which should be carefully designed in conjunction with a physician or physical therapist, must be based on the functional status of the individual. For example, someone in Functional Class I should be able to perform most activities that a typical healthy person can. For those in Class II, non-weightbearing activities, such as cycling, warm water exercise, and walking, are recommended. Individuals in Class III should benefit from a cycling or warm water aquatic program. Exercise should be avoided during acute arthritic flare-ups.

Clients with arthritis may complain of fatigue and some discomfort following exercise. Exercise programs need to achieve the proper balance between rest, immobilization of affected joints, and appropriate exercise to reduce the severity of the inflammatory joint disease.

Exercise Guidelines for Arthritis

1. Encourage your clients with arthritis to participate in low-impact activities such

as stationary cycling, rowing, and water fitness classes.

2. Begin with low-intensity, frequent sessions.

3. Reduce exercise intensity and duration during periods of inflammation or pain.

4. Extend the warm-up and cool-down periods.

5. Modify the intensity and duration of exercise according to how well the client responds, any changes in medication, and the level of pain.

6. It is essential to put all joints through their full range of motion at least once a day to maintain mobility.

7. Have the individual take a day or two of rest if he or she continues to complain about pain during or following an exercise session. If a client is still experiencing exercise-associated musculoskeletal pain or discomfort more than two hours after a workout, reduce the intensity of future bouts of exercise.

8. Emphasize proper body alignment at all times. Poor posture and decreased joint mobility and strength disrupt the performance of efficient, controlled, and integrated movement. Misaligned body positions and awkward movements affect walking gait and increase fatigue. Special precautions should be taken for clients who have undergone a hip replacement (Table 12.4)

9. While pain is quite normal in people with arthritis, instruct your clients to work just up to the point of pain, but not past it. Movements that are simple for healthy people can be quite painful for individuals with arthritis.

Table 12.4
Exercise Guidelines for Individuals
with a Hip Replacement

✔ Lift knee no higher than hip level or 90° flexion

✔ Toes straight ahead, no "pigeon toes"

✔ No adduction past midline

✔ Need leg/hip abduction and lateral movements and strengthening

10. Use isometric exercises, which strengthen the joint structures and surrounding muscles while placing the least amount of stress on the joint itself.

11. If severe pain persists following exercise, clients should consult with their physician.

12. Individuals with rheumatoid arthritis should not exercise during periods of inflammation, and regular rest periods should be stressed during exercise sessions.

13. Keep in mind that clients with arthritis may be more limited by joint pain than by cardiovascular function.

Sample Exercise Recommendation

Mode. Non-weightbearing activities such as cycling, warm-water aquatic programs, and swimming are preferred because they reduce joint stress. Recommended water temperature is 83° F to 88° F (28° C to 31° C).

Intensity. Emphasize low-intensity, dynamic exercise rather than high-intensity, high-impact exercise. The exercise intensity should be based on the client's comfort level before, during, and after exercise.

Frequency. Encourage individuals with arthritis to exercise at least four to five times per week.

Duration. Encourage long, gradual warm-up and cool-down periods (longer than 10 minutes). Initial exercise sessions should last no longer than 10 to 15 minutes.

OLDER ADULT

The United States population is growing older. In fact, by the year 2030, more than 70 million Americans of our population will be over the age of 65. The most rapid population increase over the next decade will be of those over 85 years of age. This is due, in large part, to modern medicine and health-promotion activities.

But what is the quality of these extended lives? One measure of the quality of life is an individual's ability to perform activities of daily living (ADLs), such as bathing, dressing, and eating. While these tasks may become more difficult as an individual grows older, it is possible to stay healthy and lead a long, satisfying life. The things we must do to stay healthy (e.g., exercise, eat right, not smoke) become even more important as we age. Thus, while someone may be 65 years of age (chronological age), they may have a biological age of 45 based on their fitness and health status. The importance of regular exercise and health promotion cannot be emphasized enough when looking at the association of chronological versus biological age.

Physiological Challenges of Aging

Aging is a normal biological process. The signs of progressive aging are familiar to most of us and include loss of height, reduced lean body mass, gray hair, more wrinkles, changes in eyesight, and, to some extent, slightly less coordination. There are noticeable changes in the functioning of the cardiovascular, endocrine, respiratory, and musculoskeletal systems as well. To what extent these changes may be affected by exercise is not completely understood.

Heart Rate. Maximal heart rate declines with age, diminishing the accuracy of estimating training intensity based on heart rate. Other methods of monitoring exercise intensity, such as the rate of perceived exertion scale (sometimes in conjunction with heart rate), may be more effective. Even though exercise heart rate declines with age, stroke volume has been shown to increase or be maintained in healthy older subjects who exercise, thus, overcoming the effect of a lowered heart rate.

Blood Pressure. Older individuals generally display higher blood pressure readings during submaximal and maximal exercise. In addition, they may have higher myocardial oxygen consumption requirements, which can result in higher blood pressures. Endurance training can significantly reduce the mean blood pres-

sure and the systemic vascular resistance in older individuals.

Cardiac Output and Stroke Volume. **Cardiac output** (the amount of blood pumped out of the heart per minute) is typically lower in older individuals, and resting cardiac output declines 1% per year upon reaching adulthood. Resting stroke volume declines approximately 30% from the ages of 25 to 85 and, when combined with the decrease in maximal heart rate, leads to a drop in cardiac output of 30 to 60%. This effect may be countered, however, by exercise.

Maximal Oxygen Uptake. With normal aging, **maximal oxygen uptake ($\dot{V}O_2$ max)** declines approximately 8 to 10% per decade after age 30. This decline is associated with a decrease in maximal heart rate and stroke volume, and a decrease in oxygen extraction by contracting muscles. It is clear, however, that aerobic capacity can be improved at any age.

Bones. With age, bones become more fragile and porous, often debilitating fractures are common in the elderly. By the age of 90 as many as 32% of women and 17% of men will have sustained a hip fracture, and many will die of related complications. With age, the loss of calcium results in decreased bone mass, but weightbearing and resistance-training exercises are known to help maintain bone mass.

Skeletal Muscle. Muscle mass declines with age, resulting in decreased muscular strength and endurance. For each decade after the age of 25, 3 to 5% of muscle mass is lost. This is primarily attributed to changes in lifestyle and the decreased use of the neuromuscular system. Several recent studies, however, have reported significant strength gains in previously sedentary older adults following a program of regular exercise.

Body Composition. As lean body weight (muscle and bone) declines with age, body fat increases. The changes in body composition resulting from age are primarily due to a decrease in muscle mass, **basal metabolic rate,** and lack of physical activity. On average, there is a 10% reduction in basal metabolic rate between early adulthood to retirement age, and a further 10% decrease after that. Regular physical activity, which preserves lean body mass, decreases fat stores, and stimulates protein synthesis, may reverse these adverse changes in body composition that are associated with growing older.

Exercise Guidelines for Older Adults

Before starting an exercise program, older adults should first see their physician. Although the principles of exercise design are similar to those for any group, special care should be given when setting up fitness programs for older participants. A pre-exercise evaluation may need to include a complete medical history, a physical, and a treadmill test. The exercise program should combine endurance, flexibility, and balance training, as well as muscle strength and joint mobilization. For most elderly patients, low-impact exercise is advisable. Older individuals should be encouraged to become more physically active in all of their daily activities (e.g., use the stairs, walk to the store), and to bend, move, and stretch to keep joints flexible.

Sample Exercise Recommendation

Mode. Endurance exercise such as low-impact aerobics, walking, using cardiovascular equipment, and swimming should be the primary exercise mode. Recommend a program of weight training that features low resistance and high repetitions.

Intensity. Keep the exercise intensity level near the lower end of the heart-rate range (40 to 65%).

Frequency. Encourage your elderly clients to exercise at least four to five times per week. Daily exercise of shorter duration may be appropriate for certain individuals with an initial low functional capacity.

Duration. A longer and more gradual warm-up and cool-down period (greater than 5 minutes) is recommended. Gradually increase total exercise duration to 30 to 60 minutes per session, depending

on the medical history and clinical status of the individual.

Special Precautions for Older Adults

Individuals with high blood pressure, heart disease, or arthritis should take particular care when performing weight-training exercises. Incorporate an extended warm-up and cool-down period—approximately 10 to 15 minutes. You may find that your older clients have a more difficult time exercising in extreme environmental conditions, and these should be avoided. Some elderly individuals with arthritis or poor joint mobility should participate in non-weightbearing activities such as cycling, swimming, and chair and floor exercises.

WEIGHT MANAGEMENT

On any given day, at least one out of every four Americans is on a diet. Americans spend more than $30 billion annually on various weight-loss methods, most of which fail. Excess body weight is associated with numerous health-related problems including increased risk for coronary artery disease, diabetes, and **hyperlipidemia.** Unfortunately, 95% of people who lose weight are unsuccessful at keeping the weight off. In addition, an obsession with weight and weight loss can lead to practices of self-imposed starvation (anorexia nervosa), which is a serious medical problem. While maintaining a healthy body weight and eating nutritionally is important, it is not an easy task for most people.

The diagnosis and treatment of obesity can be difficult and frustrating. A detailed medical and dietary history is necessary before a physician can begin to determine the cause(s) of obesity in patients. In many cases, it is caused by complex psychosocial issues, which may require a referral to a psychologist or psychiatrist. Although caloric consumption and physical activity habits are directly related to the increased prevalence of excess weight, they are not the only causes of obesity.

Exercise and Weight Management

Exercise in combination with a sensible eating plan produces the best long-term weight-loss results. Exercise can contribute up to a 300- to 400-kcal deficit per exercise bout. With a constant food intake, an exercise program conducted three times per week (at an intensity and duration eliciting 300 to 400 kcal/session) could result in a 16-pound weight loss in one year. Exercise is important because it helps maintain **resting metabolic rate** and **fat-free mass.** Both strength training and aerobic exercise have been shown to make the greatest contribution to a weight-management program when the caloric intake does not go below 1,200 kcal per day. Regular exercise may also help control appetite and improve psychological outlook when trying to lose weight.

Sample Exercise Recommendation

Mode. Walking is a highly effective form of exercise for weight loss and control. Walking, cycling, and aerobic dance have been shown to elicit better results than swimming, although the key is to find an activity that is safe, effective, and enjoyable enough to do on a regular basis. Variety in aerobic modes has benefits in safety, effectiveness, and compliance.

Intensity. The intensity should be low initially (possibly as low as 40 to 50% of maximal heart rate). As fitness improves, increase the intensity level. The perceived exertion scale can be more useful than monitoring heart rate for determining intensity. Look for signs that a weight-management client is working at too high of an exercise intensity level: excessive sweating, higher-than-normal rate of breathing, joint pain, excessive fatigue, inability to complete an exercise session, and a flushed color.

Frequency. It is important for overweight clients to make exercise habitual; five to

six days of exercise per week is often considered the ideal. Initially, obese clients may need to start out with as few as two to three days per week.

Duration. Since most overweight clients will not be able to exercise at a high intensity level, duration is the essential exercise program variable, especially at the start of an exercise program. Generally, the longer the duration, the greater the caloric expenditure.

Resistance Training. Resistance training can help an overweight client maintain lean body mass when caloric restriction is moderate. Start beginners out with one set of 8 to 12 repetitions of 6 to 10 exercises. Some clients can progress to higher-intensity programs, while others will benefit more from a consistent and more moderate program. Regardless of intensity, variety in the exercises should be incorporated to optimize compliance and effectiveness (see Chapters 8 and 9).

Keep weight-loss goals reasonable. Significant health benefits can be realized by body-weight reductions of only 10%. According to most experts, a sensible diet-exercise approach to weight reduction tends to produce a rate of weight loss of approximately 1 to 2 pounds per week. The key to healthy weight management is consistency in both activity and healthy eating. Try not to over-focus on "weight loss"; instead, support your clients in making healthy lifestyle changes.

EXERCISE AND CHILDREN

Within the last 15 years, a great deal of research has focused on the effects of exercise in children and adolescents. It appears that children respond to exercise in much the same way as adults do. With little encouragement, most children in good health are willing to be physically active. Recent national attention on the health and fitness of American children has sparked a

---

Table 12.5
General Endurance Training Guidelines for Children

1. Although children are generally quite active, most choose to participate in activities that consist of short-burst, high-energy exercise. Encourage children to participate in sustained activities that use large muscle groups.

2. The type, intensity, and duration of exercise activities need to be based on the maturity of the child, medical status, and previous experiences with exercise.

3. Regardless of age, the exercise intensity should start out low and progress gradually.

4. Because of the difficulty in monitoring heart rates with children, the use of a perceived exertion scale is a more practical method of monitoring exercise intensity in children.

5. Children are involved in a variety of activities throughout the day. Because of this, a specific time should be dedicated to sustained aerobic activities.

6. The duration of the exercise session will vary depending on the age of the children, their previous exercise experience, and the intensity of the exercise session.

7. Because it is often quite difficult to get children to respond to sustained periods of exercise, the session periods need to be creatively designed.

---

great deal of debate over topics such as (1) how much exercise should children and adolescents be getting; (2) who is responsible for making sure children get enough exercise; and (3) what kind of exercise is important, and at what age. Many of these issues have yet to be resolved.

Millions of youth in the United States are currently at risk for developing degenerative diseases in their adult years because they are not active enough. The percentage of overweight boys and girls has more than doubled during the past two decades (National Center for Health Statistics, 2000), and of youngsters ages 5 to 15 who are overweight, 61% have one or more cardiovascular disease risk factors, and 27% have two or more (Freedman et al., 1999). Results of the 1999 California Physical Fitness Test indicate that a staggering 80%

of fifth-, seventh-, and ninth-graders tested were unable to meet minimum standards to be considered physically fit. In the United States, television viewing, "surfing" the Internet, and playing video games contribute substantially to the amount of time youth spend in sedentary pursuits. On average, young people between the ages of 2 and 18 spend an astounding four hours a day using electronic media (e.g., watching television, playing video games, or using a computer) (Kaiser Family Foundation, 1999). By high school graduation, it is likely that the average American teen will have spent more time in front of the television than in school (Strasburger, 1992).

The negative health consequences associated with childhood obesity and physical inactivity include hypertension, the development of atherosclerosis, and type 2 diabetes (formerly known as adult-onset diabetes) among children and teenagers. Furthermore, since both positive and negative behaviors established at a young age have a high probability of persisting into adulthood, it is likely that inactive kids will become inactive adults (Janz, Dawson, & Mahoney, 2000; Trudeau et al., 1999). As such, preventive health efforts that increase physical activity during childhood and adolescence will likely have favorable health benefits in later years. In the long run, health promotion strategies that ensure healthy levels of physical activity among children and teenagers could help to maintain the progress that has been made over the past few decades in reducing deaths from cardiovascular disease. The Healthy People 2010 report includes participation in physical activity as one of the nation's 10 leading health indicators (U.S. Department of Health and Human Services, 2000).

Exercise Guidelines for Children

Sufficient evidence exists that children can physiologically adapt to endurance training. However, the amount of exercise required for optimal functional capacity and health at various ages has not been precisely defined. Until more definitive evidence is available, current recommendations are that children and youth obtain 20 to 30 minutes of vigorous exercise each day (Table 12.5).

Sample Exercise Recommendation

Mode. Encourage children to participate in sustained activities that use large muscle groups (e.g., swimming, jogging, aerobic dance). Incorporate other activities, such as recreational sports and fun activities that develop other components of fitness (speed, power, flexibility, muscular endurance, agility, and coordination) into a fitness program.

Intensity. Start exercise intensity out low and progress gradually. There are currently no universal recommendations available for the use of training heart rate during exercise for children. Using the perceived exertion scale is a more practical method of monitoring exercise intensity with children.

Frequency. Two to three days of endurance training will allow adequate time to participate in other activities, and still be sufficient enough to cause a training effect.

Duration. Since children will be involved in a variety of activities during and after school, dedicate a specific amount of time to endurance training. Gradually increase endurance exercise activities to 30 to 40 minutes per session. With younger children, it will be necessary to start out with less time.

Although there are fewer resistance-training studies involving children than adults, the evidence that demonstrates increases in strength following structured resistance training in children is mounting (American College of Sports Medicine, 2001). These studies indicate strength increases in children are similar to those observed in older age groups. Furthermore, the safety and efficacy of resistance-training programs for prepubescent children has been well documented.

The risk of injuries to children participating in resistance-training programs is low. However, injuries can occur in any sport or strenuous physical activity. To minimize the risk of injury during resistance training, consider the following:

✔ Obtain medical clearance or instructions regarding physical needs.

✔ Children should be properly supervised at all times.

✔ Do not allow children to exercise unless the weight-training facility is safe for them.

✔ Never have children perform single maximal lifts, sudden explosive movements, or try to compete with other children.

✔ Teach children how to breathe properly during exercise movements.

✔ Never allow children to use any equipment that is broken or damaged, or that they do not fit on properly.

✔ Children should rest for approximately one to two minutes between each exercise, more if necessary. In addition, they should have scheduled rest days between each training day.

✔ Encourage children to drink plenty of fluids before, during, and after exercising.

✔ Tell children that they need to communicate with their coach, parent, or teacher when they feel tired, fatigued, or when they have been injured.

EXERCISE AND PREGNANCY

Numerous studies of the cardiovascular responses of pregnant women have demonstrated that women can maintain and even improve their cardiovascular, respiratory, and aerobic capacities during pregnancy (Sternfeld, 1997). Since exercise causes a redistribution of the blood flow to the working muscles, it was believed that a reduction of blood flow to the uterus might harm the fetus. However, several studies have shown that although there is a slight decrease in overall uterine blood flow during moderate exercise, blood flow to the placenta appears to be adequate.

Cardiac reserve, or the difference between resting and maximum cardiac function, is reduced in pregnant women. As pregnancy progresses, it seems the heart is less able to adapt to the increased demand, especially in the supine position, because in pregnant women the heart may already be working at a very high level due to the increased demands of pregnancy. This is why pregnant women should be discouraged from exercising at high levels or participating in activities that require sudden bursts of movement.

Many women are more flexible during pregnancy due to joint laxity. With the release of the hormone relaxin, joints become looser, increasing the risk for injury during exercise.

Pregnant exerciser must be aware of the ambient temperature prior to each workout. Exercise increases body temperature, which can be harmful to the fetus, particularly if the core body temperature exceeds 100° F (38° C). Pregnant women should be conservative when exercising in hot, humid environments since body temperature regulation is more difficult for them.

Exercise Guidelines for Pregnant Women

Most women should be able to continue exercising during their first trimester without much difficulty. While morning sickness, mild weight gain, and fatigue might sideline some, most women should be able to continue their normal exercise program. Exercise in the supine position should be performed with caution and possibly avoided after the first trimester, and some forms of exercise, such as running, may be difficult during the second and third trimesters due to increased body weight, edema, varicose veins, and increased joint mobility.

A woman should clearly understand the risks and potential benefits associated with exercising during pregnancy, and should make the decision to exercise in conjunction with her physician.

The conclusion of the American College of Obstetricians and Gynecologists (1994; 2002) that exercise during pregnancy is safe for most women is based on the recommendation that participants be carefully monitored by their physician, and that they understand and adhere to the following guidelines as appropriate:

1. Exercise goals during pregnancy should be discussed with a physician.
2. Do not begin a vigorous exercise program shortly before or during pregnancy.
3. Gradually reduce the intensity, duration, and frequency of exercise during the second and third trimesters. For example, a woman who walks or runs an average of 4 miles per day might reduce her mileage to 3 miles per day during the first trimester; to 2 miles per day during the second; and to 1 or 1.5 miles during the final trimester.
4. Avoid exercise when the temperature and/or humidity is high.
5. Try to run or walk on flat, even surfaces.
6. Wear supportive shoes while walking or running during pregnancy.
7. If running becomes uncomfortable during the second and third trimesters, try other forms of aerobic exercise, such as swimming, running in water, and bicycling.
8. Extend warm-up and cool-down periods.
9. Body temperature, which should not exceed 100° F (38° C), should be taken immediately after exercise. If body temperature exceeds 100° F (38° C), modifying intensity and duration, as well as exercising during the cooler part of the day, should help.
10. Use the rating of perceived exertion scale rather than heart rate to monitor exercise intensity. Choose an intensity that is comfortable; a pounding heart rate, breathlessness, or dizziness are indicators that intensity should be reduced.
11. Eat a small snack before exercise to help avoid hypoglycemia.
12. Drink plenty of water before, during, and after exercise.

13. Avoid overstretching or going beyond normal range of motion.

14. Any unusual physical changes, such as vaginal bleeding, severe fatigue, joint pain, or irregular heart beats, should immediately be reported to a physician.

For more detailed information regarding exercise and pregnancy, please refer to ACE's Fitness Guide, *Pre- and Post-Natal Fitness*, by Lenita Anthony.

SUMMARY

Training clients with health concerns and special needs can be very gratifying. One of the keys to success is to maintain contact with your client's physician and healthcare team. Always obtain written guidelines before proceeding with exercise training. Keep programs more conservative than you would for your clients that are without health concerns. This can be an area of tremendous professional growth for you. Investigate continuing education opportunities to maximize the safety and effectiveness of your services.

References and Suggested Reading

REFERENCES

American Association of Cardiovascular and Pulmonary Rehabilitation (1999). *Guidelines for Cardiac Rehabilitation and Secondary Prevention Programs*. (3rd ed.). Champaign, Ill.: Human Kinetics.

American College of Obstetricians and Gynecologists (1994). *ACOG Technical Bulletin #189*. Washington D.C.: American College of Obstetricians and Gynecologists.

American College of Obstetricians and Gynecologists (2002). *ACOG Committee Opinion: Exercise During Pregnancy and the Postpartum Period*. Washington, D.C.: American College of Obstetricians and Gynecologists.

American College of Sports Medicine (2006). *ACSM's Guidelines for Exercise Testing and Prescription*. (7th ed.). Philadelphia: Lippincott Williams & Wilkins.

American College of Sports Medicine (2001). *ACSM's Resource Manual for Exercise Testing and Prescription*. (4th ed.). Philadelphia: Lippincott Williams & Wilkins.

Blair, S.N. et al. (1995). Changes in physical fitness and all-cause mortality: A prospective study of healthy and unhealthy men. *Journal of the American Medical Association, 273*, 1093–1098.

Byers, T. et al. (2002). American Cancer Society guidelines on nutrition and physical activity for cancer prevention: Reducing the risk of cancer with healthy food choices and physical activity. *Cancer Journal for Clinicians, 52*, 92–119.

Freedman, D. et al. (1999). The relationship of overweight to cardiovascular risk factors among children and adolescents: The Bogalusa heart study. *Pediatrics, 103*, 1175–1182.

Janz, K., Dawson, J., & Mahoney, L. (2000). Tracking physical fitness and physical activity from childhood to adolescence: The Muscatine Study. *Medicine and Science in Sports and Exercise, 32*, 7, 1250–1257.

Kaiser Family Foundation (1999). *Kids & Media @ The New Millennium* [monograph]. Menlo Park, Calif.: Kaiser Family Foundation.

National Center for Health Statistics (2000). *Health, United States. With adolescent health chartbook*. Online at: http://www.cdc.gov.nchs/products/pubs/pudshus/tables/2000/updated/00hus69.pdf.

Regensteiner, J.G. & Hiatt, W.R. (1995). Exercise rehabilitation for patients with peripheral arterial disease. *Exercise and Sports Science Reviews, 23*, 1–24.

Stasburger, V. (1992). Children, adolescents and television. *Pediatrics Review, 13*, 144–151.

Sternfeld, B. (1997). Physical activity and pregnancy outcome: Review and recommendations. *Sports Medicine, 23*, 33–47.

Trudeau, F. et al. (1999). Daily primary school physical education: Effects on physical activity during adult life. *Medicine and Science in Sports and Exercise, 31*, 1, 111–117.

U.S. Department of Health and Human Services (2000). *Healthy People 2010: Understanding and Improving Health*. Washington, D.C.: U.S. Department of Health and Human Services, Government Printing Office.

SUGGESTED READING

American College of Sports Medicine (1993). Position stand: Physical activity, physical fitness and hypertension. *Medicine and Science in Sports and Exercise, 25*, 10, i–x.

American College of Sports Medicine (2003). *ACSM's Exercise Management for Persons with Chronic Diseases and Disabilities*. G.E. Moore & J.L Durstine (Eds.). Champaign, Ill.: Human Kinetics.

American Council on Exercise (2007). *Clinical Exercise Specialist Manual*. San Diego, Calif.: American Council on Exercise.

American Diabetes Association (1993). *Standards of Medical Care for Patients with Diabetes Mellitus. 1992–93 Clinical Practice Recommendations*. Alexandria, Va.: American Diabetes Association.

Anthony, L. (2002). *Pre- and Post-Natal Fitness*. San Diego: American Council on Exercise.

Bartram, H.P. & Wynder, E.L. (1989). Physical activity and colon cancer risk? Physiological considerations. *American Journal of Gastroenterology, 84*, 109.

Blair, S.N. et al. (1992). How much physical activity is good for health? *Annual Review of Public Health, 13*, 99.

Bonnick, S.L. (2001). *The Osteoporosis Handbook: Every Woman's Guide to Prevention and Treatment*. (3rd ed.). Dallas: Taylor Publishing Company.

Brownell, K.D. & Foreyt, J.P. (Eds.) (1986). *Handbook of Eating Disorders: Physiology, Psychology and Treatment of Obesity, Anorexia and Bulimia*. New York: Basic Books.

Campaigne, B.N. (1994). *Exercise in the Clinical Management of Diabetes*. Champaign, Ill.: Human Kinetics.

Cheung, W.Y. & Richmond, J.B. (Eds.) (1995). *Child Health, Nutrition, and Physical Activity*. Champaign, Ill.: Human Kinetics.

Christianse, C. (1993). Consensus Development Conference on Osteoporosis. *The American Journal of Medicine. 95*, 5a.

Clapp, J.F. (2002). *Exercise through Your Pregnancy*. Omaha, Nebr.: Addicus Books.

Clark, J. (1992). *Full Life Fitness: A Complete Exercise Program for Mature Adults*. Champaign, Ill.: Human Kinetics.

Danneskiold-Samsoe, B. et al. (1987).The effect of water exercise therapy given to patients with rheumatoid arthritis. *Scandinavian Journal of Rehabilitation Medicine, 19*, 31–35.

Faigenbaum, A.D. & Westcott, W.L. (2001). *Youth Fitness*. San Diego: American Council on Exercise.

Friesz, M.C. (2002). *Food, Fun 'n' Fitness: Designing Healthy Lifestyles for our Children*. Boca Raton, Fla.: Design for Healthy Lifestyles.

Frontera, W.R. et al. (1988). Strength conditioning in older men: Skeletal muscle hypertrophy and improved function. *Journal of Applied Physiology, 64*, 1038–1044.

Frymoyer, J.W. et al. (1980). Epidemiologic studies of low-back pain. *Spine, 5*, 419–423.

Gisolfi, C.V. & Lamb, D.R. (Eds.) (1989). *Perspectives in Exercise Science and Sports Medicine, Volume 2, Youth, Exercise and Sport.* Indianapolis, Ind.: Benchmark.

Gordon, N.F. (1992). *Arthritis: Your Complete Exercise Guide.* Champaign, Ill.: Human Kinetics.

Gordon, N.F. (1992). *Chronic Fatigue: Your Complete Exercise Guide.* Champaign, Ill.: Human Kinetics.

Gordon, N.F. (1992). *Diabetes: Your Complete Exercise Guide.* Champaign, Ill.: Human Kinetics.

Gordon, N.F. (1992). *Stroke: Your Complete Exercise Guide.* Champaign, Ill.: Human Kinetics.

Gordon, N.F. & Gibbons, L.W. (1990). *The Cooper Clinic Cardiac Rehabilitation Program: Featuring the Unique Heart Points Recovery System.* New York: Simon and Schuster.

Hanlon, T.W. (1995). *Fit for Two: The Official YMCA Prenatal Exercise Guide.* Champaign, Ill.: Human Kinetics.

Hiatt, W.R. et al. (1990). Benefit of exercise conditioning for patients with peripheral arterial disease. *Circulation,* 81, 602–609.

Hinson, C. (1995). *Fitness for Children.* Champaign, Ill.: Human Kinetics.

Holstein, B.B. (1988). *Shaping Up for a Healthy Pregnancy.* Champaign, Ill.: Life Enhancement Publications.

Institutes of Medicine (1995). *Weighing the Options: Criteria for Evaluating Weight Management Programs.* Washington, D.C.: National Academy Press.

Leppo, M. (1993). *Healthy from the Start: New Perspectives on Childhood Fitness.* Washington, D.C.: ERIC Clearinghouse on Teacher Education.

Miller, P.D. (Ed.) (1995). *Fitness Programming and Physical Disability.* Champaign, Ill.: Human Kinetics.

Nakamura, E., Moritani, T., & Kanetake, A. (1989). Biological age versus physical fitness age. *European Journal of Applied Physiology,* 58, 778–785.

Osness, W.H. (1990). *Functional Fitness Assessment for Adults Over 60 Years: A Field Based Assessment.* Reston, Va.: American Alliance for Health, Physical Education, Recreation, and Dance.

Paciorek, M.J. (1994). *Sports and Recreation for the Disabled.* (2nd ed.). Carmel, Ind.: Cooper Publishing Group.

Poehlman, E.T. et al. (1991). Influence of age and endurance training on metabolic rate and hormones in healthy men. *American Journal of Physiology,* 159, 66–72.

Pollock, M.L. & Schmidt, D.H. (Eds.) (1995). *Heart Disease and Rehabilitation.* Champaign, Ill.: Human Kinetics.

Pangrazi, R.P (1989). *Physical Fitness in the Elementary Schools: A Teacher's Manual* (2nd ed.). Reston: American Alliance for Health, Physical Education, Recreation and Dance.

Rickers, R. (1986). *Seniors on the Move.* Champaign, Ill.: Human Kinetics.

Rowland, T.W. (1994). *Exercise and Children's Health.* Champaign, Ill.: Human Kinetics.

Sammann, P. (1994). *YMCA Healthy Back Book.* Champaign, Ill.: Human Kinetics.

Shephard, R.J. (1990). *Fitness in Special Populations.* Champaign, Ill.: Human Kinetics.

Sinaki, M. (1989). Exercise and osteoporosis. *Archives of Physical Medicine and Rehabilitation,* 70, 3, 220–229.

Smith, E.L. (1982). Exercise for prevention of osteoporosis: A review. *The Physician and Sports Medicine,* 10, 3, 72–83.

Tipton, C.M. (1991). Exercise, training and hypertension: An update. In: *Exercise and Sport Science.* 19, 447–505. Hollozy, J.O. (Ed.) Philadelphia: Lippincott Williams & Wilkins.

Van Norman, K.A. (1995). *Exercise Programming for Older Adults.* Champaign, Ill.: Human Kinetics.

Suggested Reading

PART V

Leadership
and Implementation

Principles
of Adherence and Motivation

Abby C. King, Ph.D., is a licensed clinical psychologist, associate professor in Health Research & Policy and Medicine, and senior scientist at the Stanford Center for Research in Disease Prevention, Stanford University School of Medicine. She has written numerous articles and papers on

Abby C. King and Deborah Rohm Young

the behavioral and psychological factors influencing adherence to a variety of health regimens, is a past recipient of a National Institutes of Health research career award to study the effects of physical activity on stress-related response in older adults, and is federally funded for several research projects examining health benefits of physical activity.

Deborah Rohm Young, Ph.D., is an exercise epidemiologist and associate professor in the Department of Kinesiology at the University of Maryland. She has written articles on exercise adherence and is studying the health benefits of physical activity in community-based samples.

I n addition to providing ongoing expert advice and instruction about effective training for a client, a major part of the personal trainer's job is motivating the client to stick with a regular physical activity routine. Motivation, like other aspects of exercise, is a personal issue; what works for one client may not be successful for another. Developing strategies to keep each client interested and motivated will often be as important as designing the exercise program.

THE CHALLENGE OF MOTIVATING CLIENTS TO ADHERE TO THEIR PHYSICAL-ACTIVITY PROGRAMS

Those of us working in exercise or physical fitness find physical activity to be an integral part of our lives. Understanding what it can do for us physically and mentally, as well as the sheer enjoyment we get from working out regularly, keeps us with our exercise program regardless of inconveniences or barriers we may encounter from week to week. Indeed, many committed exercisers feel miserable if they cannot exercise; the rewards from completing an exercise session and the negative consequences of not exercising make the exercise schedule or routine a relatively simple undertaking. For such persons, regular exercise remains a high priority regardless of what life may bring.

Unfortunately, only a relatively small percentage of people in the U.S. and other Western countries share this attitude. While many acknowledge the importance of physical activity to health and well-being, a substantial proportion of the population is underactive. Current estimates suggest that approximately 30% of the American population do not engage in any leisure time activity, and only 25% are engaged in recommended levels of physical activity (Centers for Disease Control and Prevention, 2001). Citizens of other countries fare no better. The percentage of regularly active persons decreases with age as well as with educational level, and minorities are particularly likely to be inactive. Drop-out rates for those beginning an exercise program are alarming. A number of studies report drop-outs from standard exercise programs reach 50% or more by the end of the first six months (Dishman, 1991).

Why do so many people find sticking with exercise over the long haul such an arduous task? The answer is complex and multifaceted, influenced by factors associated with each client and his or her environment, the stage a person is in with respect to incorporating regular physical activity into his or her lifestyle, and characteristics of the exercise program itself.

Definition of Adherence

Adherence has been defined in a variety of ways. For the purpose of this chapter, adherence is defined as the amount of exercise performed compared with the amount of exercise recommended. Exercise refers to the specific program developed by the trainer with input from the client. Depending on the client and trainer's goals or preferences, the amount of exercise can refer to the frequency, duration (including number of repetitions), or intensity of exercise, or some combination of these three dimensions. You must consult with the client to determine adequate markers of adherence or progress toward realistic goals.

Factors Influencing Exercise Adherence

A growing body of scientific research in exercise adherence has identified a number of factors that may influence initial participation in an exercise program as well as how well someone will adhere to the program over the long term. These factors are described below.

Personal Factors. Surveys undertaken in the U.S. and elsewhere show that those most likely to begin an exercise program tend to be younger (especially when the activity is vigorous), more highly educated, white-collar workers as opposed to blue-collar, nonsmokers, whites as compared with minority groups, and not significantly overweight (Dishman, 1994). Some of these factors also are associated with how well someone may maintain an exercise program after the initial adoption period. Persons who are aware of, and believe in, the positive health benefits of exercise also are more likely to adopt a physically active lifestyle, but these factors are less influential for determining maintenance.

Smokers and overweight individuals have poorer adherence rates than their non-smoking and normal-weight counterparts. Finding ways to make the exercise program less physically demanding, such as promoting lower-intensity exercises or building frequent breaks into the exercise session, as well as using more frequent reminders concerning the physical and mental health benefits of regular exercise, may be particularly important for such clients. For smokers, pointing out how regular exercise may help counteract a number of negative symptoms and side effects associated with quitting (tension, fatigue, depressed mood, weight gain) may be especially helpful.

Other personal factors associated with exercise adherence include health status; past experiences with exercise; the actual skills (both physical and behavioral/psychological) a client has to exercise appropriately and effectively; the client's self-confidence in being able to engage in physical activity or complete an exercise program (self-efficacy); clients ratings, self-motivation, or ability to persevere without external rewards; perceptions of program convenience and enjoyability; perceptions that the activity is not overly uncomfortable or difficult; and the client's ability to resolve common barriers to exercise, such as travel, injury, illness, competing demands on time, boredom, and high-stress periods.

While some of these factors, such as smoking status or ratings of self-motivation, may be difficult to modify, others, such as self-efficacy and perceptions of enjoyability and convenience, are more amenable to change. These latter factors should be kept in mind when tackling exercise adherence issues. Assessment tools such as the exercise confidence survey may be helpful in determining early on which clients may benefit from strategies that enhance exercise confidence (Figure 13.1). McAuley et al. (1994) found that middle-aged adults who were assigned to an exercise intervention designed to increase exercise efficacy (i.e., they provided information on exercise accomplishments over time; watched videos of others with similar characteristics who were exercising and enjoying it; formed buddy groups to provide encouragement; and provided information regarding physiologic changes associated with regular exercise) had greater adherence over a five-month period compared with adults who did not receive this special training.

Program Factors. Factors related to the exercise program or regimen itself may also affect client adherence. Among such factors, convenience is particularly important to most clients in the U. S. and other Western countries. For instance, does the client have choices of time of day for training sessions and is there some flexibility in scheduling to accommodate changing circumstances? If the client is someone with a large number of time constraints, such as a middle-aged working woman who also is a wife and mother, can the personal trainer make arrangements for personal service (e.g., childcare, errand-running) to help ease competing demands? If the exercise program is held away from the client's home, is it reasonably accessible?

Other relevant program-related questions that require consideration include the following:

✔ Does the exercise mode itself require special, costly, or time-consuming preparation that could reduce participation levels?

✔ Is the exercise regimen of a sufficient intensity so that the client finds it challenging but not punishing or aversive?

✔ Does the frequency of the exercise program fit the client's expectations, lifestyle, and fitness/health goals?

✔ Is the program length acceptable to the client? In general, sessions lasting

> **The Challenge of Motivating Clients to Adhere to their Physical-activity Programs**

The Challenge of Motivating Clients to Adhere to their Physical-activity Programs

FIGURE 13.1
Instruct clients to read each of the statements and rate how confident they are of really motivating themselves to do these things consistently for at least six months. Urge them to answer every item and try to be as honest and accurate as possible in their responses.

Exercise Confidence Survey
How sure are you that you can do these things?

| **I know I can** | | **Maybe I can** | | | | | **I know I cannot** |

1. Get up early, even on weekends, to exercise.

1   2   3   4   5   6   7   8   9   10

2. Stick to your exercise program after a long, tiring day at work.

1   2   3   4   5   6   7   8   9   10

3. Exercise even though you are feeling depressed.

1   2   3   4   5   6   7   8   9   10

4. Stick to your exercise program when undergoing a stressful life change (e.g., divorce, death in the family, moving).

1   2   3   4   5   6   7   8   9   10

5. Stick to your exercise program when you have household chores to attend to.

1   2   3   4   5   6   7   8   9   10

6. Stick to your exercise program even when you have excessive demands at work.

1   2   3   4   5   6   7   8   9   10

7. Stick to your exercise program when social obligations are very time consuming.

1   2   3   4   5   6   7   8   9   10

8. Read or study less to exercise more.

1   2   3   4   5   6   7   8   9   10

To obtain your exercise self-confidence score, simply add together the eight numbers you circled above. The higher your score, the more likely it is that you may eventually discontinue a regular exercise program.

Adapted from Sallis, J. F., et al. (1988). The development of self-efficacy scales for health-related diet and exercise behaviors. *Health Education Research*, 3, 3, 283–292.

---

longer than 60 minutes are perceived as overly time consuming.

✔ Is the exercise routine varied enough to maintain interest and diminish boredom?

One of the important benefits of the one-to-one relationship between you and your client is the large amount of ongoing individualization of the exercise program that can occur. You should take advantage of every opportunity for enhancing motivation as well as shaping the actual exercise program.

Additional Factors. For many clients, environmental factors provide some powerful incentives (and disincentives) for continuing exercise. They include the general ambiance of the locale in which the exercise sessions occur and the time it takes to travel to the locale; token rewards for meeting predetermined goals; regular cues or reminders concerning the exercise training sessions, such as scheduling exercise time on the client's calendar and setting out exercise clothes the night before; weather conditions that may influence either travel to an exercise setting or willingness to exercise outside; limitation of time (either real or perceived); and the amount of support and feedback about exercise.

Ongoing support, in particular, has been found to be extremely important in promoting exercise adherence. This can come not only from you, but also from the client's spouse, family, and friends. Clients can be encouraged to talk with significant others about exercise goals and progression toward them. In addition to face-to-face contact, telephone or mail contacts, as appropriate, can remind clients about upcoming sessions and make them feel part of a larger organization. Encouragement during a time when the exercise workload is increased or when other demands are competing with exercise time can provide the client with support to carry on with the program. Lack of a group to which the client can feel they belong may be at least partially offset by using T-shirts, newsletters, or other devices to identify the client as a member of your "team."

Social support also includes finding ways to minimize negative comments from others concerning the client's attempts to exercise. For instance, negative attitudes toward a client's exercise program by their spouse, significant other, or family have a detrimental effect on attempts to stick with the program. Exploring methods to include members of the family in the exercise enterprise may be quite worthwhile. This may mean finding ways to encourage actual exercise participation on the part of the spouse or significant others, such as undertaking exercise activities at the same time as the client or simply providing that person with information about the exercise program so that they feel included. You should consider all factors when developing and carrying out exercise programming.

UNDERSTANDING MOTIVATION

Many of us have the notion that motivation is something that we are born with or that resides entirely within us. This "trait" notion of motivation suggests that whether a client succeeds in engaging regularly in an activity or not is dependent almost entirely on their personal resources, abilities, or strengths, rather than on external factors or circumstances. Faced with a nonadherent client, personal trainers subscribing to a trait notion of motivation will often place either the responsibility or the blame for nonadherence entirely on the client. By assuming that only personal factors influence adherence, they often write the individual off as lazy, incompetent, or unmotivated—in essence, engaging in what is known as "blaming the victim."

However, as noted, adherence to health regimens such as exercise is influenced by a host of environmental and situational factors in addition to personal factors. Some of these factors may be out of the client's control. Others may be factors of which the person is completely unaware. Rather than simply placing the blame for nonadherence on the client, you must view motivation as a joint responsibility shared with the client. It also is helpful to view the motivation process as something dynamic; different strategies may be needed for different clients at different stages in the program. For example, the types of strategies used to enhance adherence or attendance during the initial "critical period" of exercise (first three to six months), when many of the difficulties associated with participation typically occur, may well differ from those most useful in helping to maintain exercise over the long haul.

Because motivating the client is one of your most important and most difficult responsibilities, the ability to address the motivational needs of the client in an ongoing, effective fashion may well be the single largest measure of a trainer's success.

Leadership Qualities

Your attitudes, personality, and professional conduct are important factors in adherence and motivation. The qualities of an effective exercise leader include the following:

✔ Punctuality and dependability in scheduling sessions and communicating with the client. This includes being regularly prepared for training sessions, starting and ending sessions on time, and arranging for substitutes if you cannot attend a planned session.

✔ Professionalism in dress, behavior, and demeanor. This means treating clients with respect and letting them know (through actions as well as words) that you take the trainer-client relationship seriously. It also means respecting the client's privacy and the confidentiality of what is shared as part of the relationship.

✔ Dedication to the exercise training endeavor, demonstrated by putting continual effort into making training sessions fun, rewarding, safe, and educational. Attending workshops to keep up on the latest developments regarding exercise training, and finding out answers to questions that the client may have on exercise-related topics indicate dedication.

✔ Willingness to plan ahead for things that may interfere with a training session and preparing the client, as much as possible, for any breaks that may occur. In addition, becoming aware of upcoming events or fitness challenges, and making a plan to train for one of them may be appealing to certain clients.

✔ Sensitivity to each client's past experiences, current preferences, and current and future needs. This includes recognizing that each client is unique, customizing each exercise session to meet preferences, and working with the client to maximize each exercise session. Providing a regular means for evaluating the client's performance as well as your own and being open to suggestions and alternatives that may enhance training sessions also are important.

✔ Recognizing signs of burnout and taking steps to prevent or ameliorate it by taking time off and enlisting the aid,

advice, and support of fellow trainers. Apathy toward work and/or irritability with clients that extends beyond a few days is a sign of burnout and needs to be resolved quickly. Overuse musculoskeletal injuries also are a sign that a break is needed.

✔ Presenting oneself as a role model for exercise training and other areas of health.

✔ Taking responsibility for problems that may arise in the course of helping clients reach their exercise goals. Consider issues of motivation, the training regimen itself, and client safety and well-being. As part of this, the conscientious trainer recognizes when the client may be better served seeking assistance elsewhere, and aids the client in obtaining an appropriate referral.

✔ Forming with each client a partnership in the exercise experience, which includes having the client play an active role in developing the training program and any decisions that may be needed to pursue the exercise-training goals.

Methods for Enhancing and Maintaining Motivation to Exercise

Use the general guidelines listed on the following pages for enhancing motivation and promoting exercise adherence to develop a specific plan of action tailored to the motivational needs of each client.

1. Structure appropriate expectations at the beginning. As mentioned earlier, a client's personal beliefs about what exercise can and cannot do, as well as past exercise experiences, can influence motivation. Unrealistic expectations ("If I exercise regularly, I should be able to shed all that excess weight within a month or two," or "Exercise will completely change my life"), fueled by the media and at times a somewhat overzealous health community, currently run rampant. Such expectations,

when unfulfilled, can lead to the frustration, disappointment, or overexercise that make drop-out more likely.

You can help to structure realistic expectations by exploring what the client expects to achieve early in the program. The client should be informed about the exercise regimens you are best equipped to offer, and how the sessions will generally be structured and why. If the client currently is not a regular exerciser, starting a program at a moderate intensity level may be preferable while the client is adopting a physically active lifestyle. Explaining to the client the rationale for starting at a lower level will assist the client-trainer relationship and help to develop trust early on in the program. The use of the Borg **rating of perceived exertion (RPE)** scale can provide an excellent means for evaluating the client's perception of exercise intensity (Borg, 1970). RPE has been found to provide a useful reflection of intensity and how the client is feeling about the workout. Individuals consistently rating themselves at the upper range of the RPE, particularly early in their exercise program, may be at increased risk for nonadherence, drop out, or potential injury.

Since musculoskeletal injury is the most often cited reason for discontinuing a vigorous exercise program, starting a program slowly at a moderate intensity will allow the client's muscles, tendons, and bones to adapt to the stress of the exercise. Carroll and colleagues (1992) found that the incidence rate of injury was only 14% for adults between the ages of 60 and 79 years who engaged in a walking program, which suggests that low-impact activities may be particularly beneficial for older adults. However, most of the injuries occurred in the women, so careful monitoring of older women for proper exercise techniques, as well as adequate warm-up and cool-down periods, is warranted.

The client should be informed about the types of uncomfortable or negative

side effects that may accompany increased physical activity, such as stiffness, minor soreness or muscle pain, and some fatigue, particularly early on in the training program. These symptoms usually are transient and will dissipate over time. However, other types of symptoms, such as chest pain and undue fatigue lasting well after the exercise session, require further, and perhaps medical, attention.

2. Find out the client's preferences, needs, exercise history, and motivational readiness for exercise change. One of the advantages of being a personal trainer, as opposed to a group fitness instructor, is that usually there is time to assess your client thoroughly. Take advantage of this opportunity to find out not only what level your clients are at physically, but where they are mentally and experientially as well. This is probably best accomplished through a simple questionnaire that all clients should complete at the beginning of their program, either on their own or in an interview format. Questions of interest include the types of exercise programs clients have previously participated in (types of activities; format—with another personal trainer, in a class, or on their own; length of time of participation; reasons for drop out); reasons for seeking a personal trainer at this particular time; what expectations and goals they hope to accomplish and over what time frame; current preferences concerning specific types of exercise; past and current injuries; potential pitfalls they see ahead based on prior experiences; constraints with respect to time and other issues; and questions they would like answered concerning working with you, or concerning your particular style and strengths.

3. Work with the client to determine specific types of activities that will best fit the client's objectives, time, commitments and personal style. Based on the this information, tailor the exercise program to each client. This may mean using indoor exercises

for the client who is embarrassed to exercise in public; water exercises for clients with knee or hip problems; exercise sports for clients motivated by competitive challenges; or relaxed reading time on a reclining cycle for the stressed or exhausted executive. In addition, if a client says that in the past one of the major reasons why they stopped exercising was boredom, then building in variety within, or across, sessions, as well as varying exercise routes or locations on a regular basis, may be helpful.

Recognize that clients who are in the lower stages of motivational readiness for exercise change (i.e., those preparing to make a change) are likely to have different objectives than clients in the higher stages (i.e., current exercisers). Those in the preparation stage who are just starting to be active may have an objective to improve overall well-being that would suggest different types of activities than the regular exerciser who wishes to increase their 10K race time.

4. Set appropriate exercise goals. Once you have both determined the specific activities that will make up the client's exercise routine, the next job is to work with the client to set appropriate, realistic, and flexible goals for each portion of it. Realistic goals are important to avoid injury and maintain interest. This is particularly true in the beginning, when over-enthusiastic clients may be tempted to set goals that are unachievable given the restraints of other commitments for one's time. Short-term goals determined by the personal trainer for each exercise session, in conjunction with longer-term, monthly goals established with the client, allow for flexibility on a daily basis without jeopardizing the longer-term goals. Goals can be specific to the exercise process, such as training together a predetermined number of times combined with a certain number of individual sessions in the coming weeks, or training for a specific fitness event. Regardless of what type of goal is used, with its achievement, the next one should be discussed. Providing feedback

regarding progress toward specific goals and praising and rewarding the client when goals are reached also is a useful strategy.

Goals can be formalized in the form of a **contract** (Figure 13.2). Contracts are written agreements signed by the client and the personal trainer (and additional third parties, such as a spouse or exercise partner, if deemed appropriate) that clearly spell out the exercise goals (such as the duration, type, and/or intensity of exercise engaged in with you), preferably over a short time period (two to four weeks), and the rewards associated with achieving them. Contracts serve to increase the client's personal responsibility and commitment to the exercise program. An exercise contract should contain input from both you and the client, and the responsibilities each has in meeting its terms. The contract should specify goals that are somewhat challenging yet realistically achievable to promote success. Make certain that the client has the skills necessary to meet the terms of the contract and include precautions to ensure that they do not engage in unhealthy practices to meet contract requirements (such as exercising at a high intensity when ill). Exercise goals should be written in a manner that allows them to be objectively measured, thereby eliminating any questions regarding goal attainment. If you are responsible for delivering a contingent reward, plan ahead so it can be distributed promptly.

To summarize, a series of prudent goals should be negotiated by you and your client that focus on building the exercise habit through gradual increments rather than larger changes that, though more appealing to some clients, can lead to failure, frustration, injury, and/or dropout. During the first 6 to 12 weeks in particular, the goals may need to be focused on simply "showing up," no matter how little the client may feel like, or be able to do. Alternatively, for the zealous overachieving client, goals can aid efforts to diminish overexertion and injury. The important

My Responsibilities:

1. To attend all of my scheduled exercise sessions (three times per week) over the next four weeks.

2. For any sessions that I have to miss due to illness or other unavoidable reasons, I will:

   a. Call my trainer to let them know the reason(s) why I had to miss (Trainer's telephone number = _____).

   b. Plan to make up the missed session by (specify): _____.

3. To reward myself at the end of each week that I attend all of my scheduled sessions by engaging in thirty or more minutes of reading for my own enjoyment.

My Helper's Responsibilities:

My designated helper is: _____ . They have agreed:

   a. To prompt me during work to attend my exercise sessions.

   b. In return, I will prompt them concerning a behavior of their choice, as desired.

This contract will be evaluated on _____ .
                                        (date)
Signed:

_____   _____
(participant)   (date)

_____   _____
(helper)   (date)

_____   _____
(trainer)   (date)

FIGURE 13.2
Sample four-week contract.

thing is to match the goals to the needs and preferences of each individual.

5. Whenever possible, offer choices. While some structure is typically welcomed by clients attempting to adopt or maintain a behavior such as exercise, many will benefit from being offered some choice of alternatives within the general structure of the program. Doing so helps to stave off boredom that often creeps into an exercise program. Choices may be made available with respect to the exercise regimen itself (types of activity engaged in, frequency, intensity, and/or duration factors), or the types of goals, **feedback,** and/or incentives used to enhance adherence. An increasingly flexible view is being taken by national organizations regarding types of physical activity and the frequency, intensity, and duration suitable for obtaining reasonable health benefits.

Over the last decade, researchers have reevaluated the scientific evidence linking physical inactivity with a variety of chronic diseases. These analyses suggest that the intensity or dosage of exercise needed to achieve health-related benefits is probably less than that required to improve fitness (Pate et al., 1995; United States Department of Health and Human Services, 1996). Accordingly, frequent bouts of moderate-intensity activity (e.g., brisk walking, household chores, gardening, recreational sports) can be as effective as vigorous exercise, provided that the daily energy expenditure is comparable (Gordon et al., 1993). In other words, the desk-bound executive who regularly jogs may not be any better off than the person who does periodic moderate-intensity activity throughout the day.

Research studies have confirmed that a lifestyle approach to physical activity can be as effective as a traditional exercise program (Pate et al., 1995; United States Department of Health and Human

Services, 1996; Pollock, Gaesser, & Butcher, 1998). These findings are encouraging in that they support a wide range of choices for physical activity. Specific suggestions may include taking several flights of stairs instead of the elevator and walking to the store instead of driving.

To assist your clients in tracking their daily activities, you might recommend that they consider buying a pedometer. These are easy to use and can be worn on the belt, at the midline of the thigh. The base models just count steps, whereas the newer electronic versions (which range from about $25 to $35) convert steps to miles and calories burned and include a built-in stopwatch. The conversion: 2,000 steps is roughly 1 mile or 100 Calories.

How much exercise is enough? Inactive people take 2,000 to 4,000 steps per day, moderately active people take 5,000 to 7,000 steps per day, and active people take at least 10,000 steps per day. And, glancing down at the pedometer and checking progress can provide the client with the motivation to go for an extra walk when they are short of their daily goal.

Although lifestyle exercise is not being suggested to replace more traditional workouts, it's a wonderful complement to any health and fitness program. Exercise professionals should consider broadening their clients' recommendations from the traditional frequency, intensity, duration, and mode of training that are associated with structured exercise programs to promoting increased activity in daily living.

6. Remember that exercise, like other behaviors, is strongly influenced by its immediate consequences. Often the immediate feelings and consequences surrounding actions, rather than more abstract or long-term beliefs or views, have the most powerful effect on daily activities. Despite the best of intentions, if the immediate or short-term benefits of exercise do not outweigh the time and effort required, it is likely that a relapse to being sedentary

will result. You must work with the client to identify short-term benefits (feelings of accomplishment, stress reduction, better sleep), rather than focusing only on long-term outcomes (better health, reduction in cardiovascular risk, weight loss). While weight control is certainly an important by-product of regular aerobic exercise, for many clients weight loss through increased exercise alone is a slow process. In addition, in at least some individuals, the loss in fat weight is often compensated for by an increase in lean weight (muscle) resulting in no change on the scale. Periodic measurements of parts of the body might, for some clients, be a better gauge of progress. For those clients who are regular exercisers, you can reinforce how the workout meets goals or assists in achieving long- or short-term goals.

7. Increase the immediately rewarding aspects of the behavior and decrease the negative or punishing aspects. Analyze both the positive and negative aspects of the exercise session itself to increase enjoyability and decrease discomfort and boredom. For some, providing a means of distraction from the chore of exercise through social interaction, music, or an interesting exercise routine is important. Modify the regimen by regularly monitoring how clients are enjoying the session (using a simple six-point rating scale, with one equaling "extremely unenjoyable," and six equaling "extremely enjoyable"). For instance, if a client dislikes a particular portion of the exercise routine you can substitute a different exercise to achieve the same results. Because what is rewarding or punishing about an exercise program differs from person to person, it is important to individualize strategies for enhancing enjoyment.

For some clients, modifying the exercise session to increase enjoyment will not be enough, especially for those just beginning an exercise program. For them, the uncomfortable aspects of increased exertion (sweating, increased heart rate, sore muscles) may outweigh any positive outcomes. Such clients may need external incentives, such as earning points toward a desirable reward once the goal has been reached. For some clients, an external incentive system can be set up in the form of an achievement club, or related activities, with formal recognition in the form of pins, T-shirts, certificates, or other rewards for achieving training goals.

Teaching clients how to successfully monitor their own intensity levels can help them maintain an enjoyable workout. Beginning exercisers should be encouraged to exercise at an intensity that allows them to talk comfortably without undue sweating. Knowing how to accurately monitor their heart rates, through regular pulse taking or the use of a portable heart monitor, is another method of monitoring intensity. The RPE scale previously described also provides information regarding the client's perceived intensity of a workout and can be used to gauge how a client is responding to a new routine.

8. Provide feedback whenever possible. Regular feedback that is specific and relevant to the client can be an extremely powerful reinforcer or incentive, particularly early in the exercise program when more intrinsic benefits from exercising, such as an increase in muscle tone or reduction in tension, may not yet be present. Feedback can take many forms. Physiologically based feedback may include changes in resting or exertional heart rate or RPE. Use of a standardized submaximal exercise test, such as the step-test or 12-minute distance test (Cooper, 1968), administered at the beginning of the exercise program and at regular intervals, can provide useful information to both you and the client. The objective of this test is to jog/run the greatest distance in the allotted time period. Testing clients every three months or so should provide them with enough feedback to reinforce current activities and motivate future adherence. However, if the client has had to lay off

training, it is preferable to allow them to build back up to a reasonable intensity before initiating further testing. Testing during a plateau or down period in the client's training program can lead to discouragement and frustration, which in turn can result in either dropping out or overtraining. It also is important to determine if testing is preferable to an individual client; some may be opposed to regular testing or find the procedures or results to be unmotivating.

Behaviorally based feedback can include regular recordings of the amount of activity (frequency, duration, number of repetitions, distance covered), as well as periodic completion of an exercise balance sheet in which the client lists both the positive and negative aspects of regular exercise. Through completing such a sheet, clients are often reminded of the reasons they decided to exercise in the first place. For those clients who are amenable to it, regular logging of exercise behavior serves as an immediate, visual record of their session-by-session accomplishments. If the exercise activity is walking, running, or hiking, pedometers can be worn to log the distance traveled. Logging of exercise behavior helps to bridge the gap between the exercise sessions and more distant rewards of changes in **body composition,** endurance, or strength, and earning something tangible such as a T-shirt. Having clients maintain their own records also helps to drive home the point that they share responsibility with you.

9. Teach the client how to use **prompts** and reminders to set the stage. Exercise can be one of a long list of activities vying for one's time and attention. To keep exercise prominently placed in the client's list of priorities, set up a system of prompts or reminders, about the exercise sessions. This may involve writing the sessions into a daily schedule book or providing the client with a calendar to be prominently displayed on the refrigerator or other

suitable place in the home or at work. Encouraging the client to ready their exercise apparel the evening before a scheduled exercise session, and to display it in a prominent place, may help get them to a class or group.

10. Model the appropriate behaviors for the client. Appropriate and consistent **modeling** of exercise-related behaviors can provide motivation in the early as well as later stages of participation. When modeling the actual exercise routines or activities, perform them slowly, both as a demonstration as well as along with clients during their execution of the activity. Breaking complicated routines into easily learned segments will help the client increase his or her self-confidence in performing the routine. Remember that, as a health professional, you are in an excellent position to serve as a role model for other important health behaviors by not smoking or abusing alcohol and by maintaining healthy dietary patterns and prudent weight-control activities.

11. Foster self-management of the exercise regimen. To help clients establish exercise as a lifelong habit, foster a sense of personal responsibility and commitment to exercise. It is critical to realize that we must take charge of our exercise as a lifelong goal, rather than as a time-limited commitment that ends when certain goals have been reached or temporary setbacks occur. To do this, train clients in the use of self-management strategies that will help them keep the exercise habit going when circumstances interfere with their usual routine. This may mean equipping clients with strategies to keep them exercising during those periods, such as business travel, vacations, or changes in work hours, when they are unable to make normally scheduled exercise sessions. For a client who will be traveling, this may include packing appropriate exercise attire, being aware of exercises that can be undertaken in a hotel room, and/or making

arrangements to stay in a hotel that has in-house exercise facilities. Because anticipated breaks from an exercise schedule can lead to drop out, planning for them ahead of time can increase the probability of subsequent resumption of the exercise program.

When unplanned breaks in the exercise regimen occur, it is important to first let clients know that you care, and then encourage them to get back into the regimen as soon as possible. Expect that many clients will feel at least some level of guilt (that they have let you, as well as themselves, down), in addition to frustration and discouragement. Such feelings breed drop out. Research shows that even a brief supportive, nonjudgmental telephone call during such a period can help clients maintain their exercise programs (Buckworth & Dishman, 2002).

12. Prepare the client for inevitable **lapses.** Clients should be fully informed about the pitfalls that are often encountered when people attempt to exercise regularly. These may include unplanned breaks in the exercise regimen due to illness, work schedule, unplanned travel, holidays, and the like, or failure to observe further gains following a period of significant progress. Preparing clients ahead of time for particularly high-risk situations, when breaks in the exercise regimen are likely, may help prevent the full-blown drop out often seen following such unplanned breaks. By encouraging the client to also exercise on his or her own, you will provide the confidence needed to exercise without supervision when a scheduled class must be missed. An additional strategy is to promote an abbreviated workout during busy times.

13. Help clients identify barriers to behavior change, including time constraints (real or perceived) and negative moods or thoughts. Help them see the critical relationship between saying, "I just don't feel like exercising today; I'll do it

tomorrow," and ultimately giving up their behavior-change goals altogether.

Teach and refine problem-solving skills to help clients effectively anticipate and negotiate these barriers. By defining the problem, generating potential solutions, and evaluating the effectiveness of each solution during your time together, you can model the usefulness of this approach. Demonstrate your belief in the process by spending a reasonable percentage of time in each session systematically working through problems. Problem solving also effectively reduces the emotional shame clients experience when they fail to follow through with set goals.

14. Create a hierarchy of experiences to enhance your client's sense of self-efficacy—an individual's belief or expectation that they are able to behave in a certain manner in a specific situation. Self-efficacy has been observed to be a consistent predictor of exercise behavior and can be modified to alter activity levels in the short term. Sense of self-efficacy is thought to influence both one's choice of activities and selection of environments. For example, most persons avoid activities and situations they believe exceed their coping capabilities, but readily engage in activities and environments that they believe they are capable of handling. Thus, to bolster their confidence, help a client identify activities he or she has previously enjoyed or are likely to master in the beginning (e.g., a walking program). The overall approach is to first help clients feel competent as an exerciser, and then assist him or her in expanding the choice of activities.

The best way to enhance self-efficacy is through mastery experiences. Short-term success enhances a person's belief in his or her ability to handle situations. Thus, early in your work together, ensure the goals you have developed with your client maximize the likelihood for short-term success. Structure experiences each week that build upon previous gains to further bolster confidence.

Self-efficacy also is enhanced when an individual experiences a setback, then recovers. Recovery from a setback provides evidence that the person has the skills needed to cope, further reinforcing self-efficacy.

15. Prepare the client for changes in trainers. Perhaps the most disruptive event for many clients is the loss of the regular trainer, even for a brief period. Unfortunately, little, if anything, is typically done to prepare clients for this often unsettling circumstance. Planned transition periods (pregnancy leave, travel, permanent relocation) can be smoothed immensely by preparing clients well ahead of time and, if possible, introducing the trainer who will be stepping in well before the regular trainer takes leave. Having the regular and new trainers team-teach several of the exercise sessions can go a long way to allay fears and prevent clients from dropping out. Even the most healthy trainers will have days when they are unable to work, so all trainers should plan for substitutes and, if possible, introduce them to clients ahead of time. If a substitute is not available, following up with clients by telephone may help to keep them from feeling abandoned, betrayed, or discouraged.

16. Utilize as many types of social support as possible. Ongoing social support, in all of its many forms, is invaluable both in the early and more advanced stages of an exercise program. While the face-to-face support provided during the session itself can be invaluable for many clients, do not overlook other potentially important avenues that can complement your personal instruction. These include telephone contacts following missed sessions; regular newsletters or other mailed items that can both educate and motivate continued participation; and the encouragement of support on the part of family members or co-workers through mailed newsletters or other informational pieces.

17. Look for opportunities to promote an overall healthy lifestyle. Exercise does not occur in a vacuum, but rather is only

Summary

one of a number of activities clients engage in throughout the week. Because for many of us our exercise program has a major impact on the rest of our lives, we often assume that those who exercise regularly will automatically change other health behaviors, such as smoking and dietary practices. Unfortunately, very little scientific evidence supports this widely held belief. Many people who exercise maintain a regular smoking habit or eat a diet high in saturated fats and sugar. Indeed, some maintain the inaccurate belief that regular exercise will protect them against the other negative health habits. We must help clients recognize that exercise alone is not a panacea for health, but, rather, only one of a number of behaviors that comprise a healthy lifestyle.

As a trained health professional, you are in an excellent position to provide basic, accurate information and encouragement for the development of a healthy lifestyle beyond exercise. Most trainers are deluged with questions on diet, weight control, and other health regimens by those concerned about their health and confused by the mixed messages currently being promulgated by the media and by special-interest groups. Regular contact with clients interested in improving their health provides an invaluable opportunity for educating them in a manner not available to many other types of health professionals. The trainer who stays abreast of current scientific information and developments in health promotion can help ensure that health information is responsibly disseminated. Refer to Chapters 4 and 12 for useful information about nutrition and weight control, and consider becoming an ACE-certified Lifestyle & Weight Management Consultant.

A healthy lifestyle also involves participating in physical activities beyond the scheduled training session. Encourage clients to look for opportunities to be more active as a way of life (by walking instead of driving, or by using stairs instead of elevators or escalators). Increasing lifestyle-type activities such as these is being promoted as a way to accumulate 30 minutes per day of moderate-intensity activity and provide health benefits (American College of Sports Medicine, 2006). Including these types of activities in one's regular routine may also help clients maintain a high energy level when more vigorous activities are not possible. Such activities are particularly important for the older client, as well as other subgroups, such as those who are overweight or those who have been unable to give up the smoking habit. By encouraging physical activity in all of its forms, you can serve as an important teacher and role model for achieving a healthy lifestyle.

SUMMARY

Drop-out rates for those beginning an exercise program can reach 50% or more after only six months. Instead of blaming the client, you must view motivation as a shared responsibility. By analyzing each client's preferences, habits, and circumstances to anticipate blocks to success, you can design a specific approach to motivate each client to achieve mutually determined goals.

Factors affecting adherence to a health regimen can be complex and interrelated. Motivation is a dynamic process and requires the use of a variety of techniques that will help a client achieve and maintain a healthy lifestyle. These techniques range from structuring appropriate expectations and goals, identifying short-term benefits, and providing specific feedback, to serving as a positive role model and training clients in self-management strategies. Understanding and applying the principles of adherence and motivation will make you a more effective teacher and health professional.

REFERENCES

American College of Sports Medicine (2006). *ACSM's Guidelines for Exercise Testing and Prescription* (7th ed.). Philadelphia: Lippincott Williams & Wilkins.

Borg, G. V. (1970). Perceived exertion as an indicator of somatic stress. *Scandinavian Journal of Rehabilitation Medicine,* 2, 92–98.

Buckworth, J. & Dishman, R.K. (2002). *Exercise Psychology.* Champaign, Ill.: Human Kinetics.

Centers for Disease Control and Prevention (2001). Physical activity trends—United States, 1990–1998. *Morbidity and Mortality Weekly Report,* 50, 166–169.

Carroll, J. F. et al. (1992). Incidence of injury during moderate- and high-intensity walking training in the elderly. *Journal of Gerontology: Medical Sciences,* 47, M61–M66.

Cooper, K.H. (1968). A means of assessing maximal oxygen uptake. *Journal of the American Medical Association,* 203, 3, 135–138.

Dishman, R.K. (1991). Increasing and maintaining exercise and physical activity. *Behavior Therapy,* 22, 345-378.

Dishman, R.K. (Ed.) (1994). *Advances in Exercise Adherence.* Champaign, Ill.: Human Kinetics.

Gordon, N.F. et al. (1993). Life style exercise: A new strategy to promote physical activity for adults. *Journal of Cardiopulmonary Rehabilitation,* 13, 3, 161–163.

McAuley, E. et al. (1994). Enhancing exercise adherence in middle-aged males and females. *Preventive Medicine,* 23, 498–506.

Pate, R.R. et al. (1995). Physical activity and public health: A recommendation from the Centers for Disease Control and Prevention and the American College of Sports Medicine. *Journal of the American Medical Association,* 273, 402–407.

Pollock, M.L., Gaesser, G.A., & Butcher, J.D. (1998). The recommended quantity and quality of exercise for developing and maintaining cardiorespiratory and muscular fitness, and flexibility in healthy adults. *Medicine and Science in Sports and Exercise,* 30, 975–991.

United States Department of Health and Human Services (1996). *Physical Activity and Health: A Report of the Surgeon General.* Atlanta, Ga.: US Department of Health and Human Services, Centers for Disease Control and Prevention, National Center for Chronic Disease Prevention and Health Promotion.

SUGGESTED READING

American College of Sports Medicine (2006). *Resource Manual for Guidelines for Exercise Testing and Prescription.* (5th ed.). Philadelphia: Lippincott Williams & Wilkins.

Annesi, J.J. (1996). *Enhancing Exercise Motivation.* Los Angeles: Fitness Management.

King, A.C. et al. (1992). Determinants of physical activity and interventions in adults. *Medicine and Science in Sports and Exercise,* 24, S221–S226.

Sallis, J.F. & Owen, N. (1998) *Physical Activity and Behavorial Medicine.* Thousand Oaks, Calif.,: Sage Publications.

References and Suggested Reading

CHAPTER 14

Communication and Teaching Techniques

Amy P. Jones, M.Ed., L.P.C., is a licensed psychotherapist and leads the organizational capability practice for The Feld Group, a firm specializing in Information Technology

Amy P. Jones

transformation in Fortune 500 companies. In addition to working with executive teams in leading organization change and transformation efforts, much of her time is spent coaching and training executives in interpersonal communication, leadership development, and organizational effectiveness. She was formerly the director of programs for the Cooper Fitness Center in Dallas, Texas, for 12 years, served on the American Council on Exercise Board of Directors, and was a technical advisor to the National Aerobic Championship.

A personal trainer's relationship to a client is clearly the helping relationship of educator to student. Helping relationships differ from most other kinds of relationships encountered in daily routines. Most ordinary experiences are dialogues in which both individuals seek personal enhancement or the mutual exchange of ideas or information. In the helping relationship, one person temporarily sets aside personal needs to help another person. The focus of the relationship is on the client's needs and on goals that will lead to new behavior. Simply put, helping is enabling another person to change. Instead of encouraging dependence, the purpose of helping is to enable the client to take more control and become self-sufficient. Helping is an active process of advising, informing, correcting, and directing.

There are many kinds of helping relationships. Because there is usually a fee for service in personal training, you can be classified as a structured, professional helper, like social workers, teachers, school counselors, and legal advisors. In contrast to this professional level are unstructured levels of helping such as friendships and family relationships.

Your role is complex, as you will function as a teacher, coach, advisor, supporter, counselor, and negotiator.

Teacher: Explaining to clients what they need to know and must do (e.g., outlining and explaining an aerobic exercise program).

Coach: Training clients in desired skills (e.g., coaching during a free-weight workout).

Advisor: Telling clients the wisest course of action (e.g., warning about potential dangers associated with nutritional supplements containing ephedra).

Supporter: Encouraging clients as they work on specific lifestyle changes (e.g., providing emotional support for a client who has stopped smoking).

Counselor: Helping clients sort through personal problems (e.g., listening to a client's frustrations regarding problems at work).

Negotiator: Bargaining with clients to reach an acceptable agreement (e.g., negotiating an exercise contract with a client for a period of travel).

These roles are described only in a general sense. You should be acutely aware of your limitations and must not exceed the professional parameters of offering advice or counseling about personal problems. You can obviously listen and offer support, but you should know when to refer clients to other qualified professionals.

STAGES OF THE PERSONAL TRAINER/CLIENT RELATIONSHIP

There will be distinct stages in your relationships with clients and they form a general model or frame-

work for the divisions and related skills of the helping relationship (Figure 14.1). They may not always occur in this exact sequence, nor are all stages always present. Their length also may vary from client to client. Generally, the initial contact between the personal trainer and client is made in the **rapport** stage. The process of gathering information after the relationship has begun forms the investigation stage. This gives way to the planning stage in which the client's goals and steps toward them are mapped out. Finally, the action stage begins when the actual training process starts.

Each stage requires specific skills and techniques. In the beginning, for example, attentive listening skills can build the working relationship; the following stages require more decision-making and behavioral-change skills. Developing these skills can increase your effectiveness as a personal trainer. Because the personal trainer/ client relationship is dynamic and ever-changing, these stages and skills overlap and may not occur in the exact order given. The specific stages and required skills are outlined as follows:

Stage 1: Rapport—interpersonal communication skills

Stage 2: Investigation—information-gathering skills

Stage 3: Planning—problem-solving or decision-making skills

Stage 4: Action—behavioral change skills (e.g., feedback, contracting, modeling)

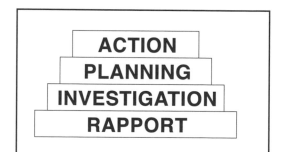

FIGURE 14.1
Stages of the personal trainer/client relationship.

RAPPORT STAGE

The **rapport** stage is the foundation for the entire relationship between you and your client. Rapport means a relationship of mutual trust, harmony, or emotional affinity. Establishing it entails building a certain level of comfort or shared understanding into a relationship. The rapport stage begins at first contact. Whether in person or on the telephone, the client is "checking out" the personal trainer and answering the question, "Can this person help me?" Confidence or trust in your skills must be established early because only then will the client be willing to receive guidance.

According to Rogers et al. (1967), people in the helping profession need to communicate three basic attributes or qualities for the helping relationship to be successful. These three primary qualities are (1) **empathy,** (2) warmth, and (3) genuineness. The importance of these qualities has been demonstrated repeatedly in research by Truax and Carkuff (1967) and others. They are the foundation for a successful helping relationship and are key factors during the rapport stage.

Empathy is the ability to experience another person's world as if it were one's own. It is understanding the client's point of view or where the client is "coming from." The empathetic personal trainer will be able to respond appropriately to the client's covert feelings and verbal messages by communicating perceptions to the client. The absence of empathy may lead the client to think the trainer does not understand what they are experiencing and, therefore, will block the entire helping process.

Warmth is an unconditional positive regard or respect for another person regardless of their individuality and uniqueness. It bridges professional distance through friendliness and consideration regardless of a "liking" for another person.

Warmth is about caring and understanding rather than judging and impersonalizing. This quality will convey a climate that communicates safety and acceptance to a client, even when they are making mistakes.

Genuineness can be defined as authenticity or being honest and open without putting up a front. It is a state in which the helper's words and actions are congruent. For example, when you greet a client with "I'm glad to see you're here today," your body language must be consistent with the words of welcome. Genuineness is the ability to relate to people without hiding behind a clipboard or white coat. It is not necessarily being fully self-revealing, but rather being committed to a responsible honesty with others.

Empathy, warmth, and genuineness are paramount in establishing trust in a working relationship. At first glance, they may seem simplistic because they are the outgrowth of ordinary effective human qualities. However, relevant research and cumulative experience points out the necessity for continuous monitoring of the timing and amount of conditions that facilitate the development of these qualities.

Interpersonal communication skills are the primary skills needed to establish rapport and thereby build a relationship. They are not only important during the rapport stage, but are necessary throughout the relationship. Interpersonal communication skills can be broadly categorized as nonverbal and verbal. The nonverbal category includes such behaviors as attending and perceiving nonverbal and verbal messages. The verbal category includes paraphrasing, reflecting, and clarifying. Many of these skills are natural for anyone genuinely involved in helping another person, but specific communication skills can be learned, practiced, and continuously mastered.

Nonverbal Behaviors

Listening is the primary nonverbal

communication skill. It is a complex concept and is not the same as hearing, which is the perception of sound through the ear. Listening obviously involves the physiology of hearing, but also is a more complex psychological procedure of involvement with the other person that includes skills in attending, perceiving verbal and nonverbal messages, and even verbal responding. All of these skills overlap and are difficult to treat separately.

Attending. **Attending** behaviors are exhibited by the listener to put the speaker at ease and entail being attentive or giving physical attention to them. Instead of interrupting, the listener gives nonverbal acknowledgments during the conversation through posture, eye contact, and gestures. Verbal responses also are a form of attending. The listener may say, "Yes, I see," to encourage the speaker to continue.

Effective attending can build trust and can work wonders in human relationships. Conversely, nonattentive behavior can be

FIGURE 14.2
Trainer working in a client's intimate space.

devastating. For example, when you are speaking to someone who appears bored and whose eyes are continually distracted to other things, you may feel ignored and not encouraged to continue the conversation. The trainer interested in developing good attending behaviors or skills needs to be aware of the following:

1. Posture: When you and your client are seated, specific postures can communicate your interest. To show involvement, face the client squarely at eye level and lean toward them in a relaxed manner. Avoid expressing defensiveness by maintaining an open position with arms and legs uncrossed. This posture says, "I am interested in you and am ready to listen." Research has shown that these postural behaviors demonstrate to the client the traits of empathy, warmth, and genuineness.

2. Positioning: Position yourself at an appropriate distance from the client to demonstrate a respect for his or her personal space. Hall (1966) describes an 18-inch (46 cm) or less distance between two people as "intimate space," an 18-inch to 4-foot (46 cm to 1.2 m) distance as "personal space," a 4-foot to 12-foot (1.2 to 3.7 m) distance as "social distance," and beyond 12 feet (3.7 m) as "public distance." Most normal conversation will occur in the personal space. However, the very nature of your working relationship demands at times that you enter the client's intimate space (Figure 14.2). Because of this intimate positioning, be sensitive to the client, particularly when hands-on work is being done. Early in the relationship you may want to ask permission to touch the client and should take care that the client does not misconstrue your touching or presence in his or her personal space.

3. Mirroring: Another technique you can use to establish rapport is mimicking or **mirroring.** Mirroring may be either conscious or unconscious, but its purpose is to establish rapport with another person. The technique of mirroring involves sensitively matching the posture and gestures of the

other person, and may include matching voice tone and tempo and breathing patterns. These techniques often occur naturally as people interact.

4. Eye Contact: Eye contact is a key vehicle for indicating interest in a person. Good eye contact is not a fixed stare but rather a relaxed focus on the client's eyes, face, and body gestures. It enables the client to feel safe and comfortable and conveys your interest at the same time.

5. Gestures: Appropriate body movement is essential in attending. Try to use relaxed motions instead of appearing rigid and unmoving. Nervous mannerisms such as playing with objects, jingling pocket change, waving to others, and drumming fingers should be avoided.

6. Environment: Since much of the personal training process takes place in a gym that is usually full of talking people, blaring music, and clanging weights, a quiet place is preferable for effective communication. Pleasant surroundings facilitate conversation, so initial sessions should be conducted in a nondistracting environment. To give someone your undivided attention when distractions are present is difficult. Distractions may consist of a blaring TV or radio, a ringing telephone, people stopping by to talk, uncomfortable room temperature, and inappropriate lighting. Another type of distraction is seating arrangement. Sitting behind a desk not only puts up a physical barrier, but can be an interpersonal barrier as well. Attempts should be made to limit environmental distractions so that the client's thoughts are not interrupted and effective communication can take place.

Perceiving Nonverbal Messages. The saying "actions speak louder than words" is especially true in communications. Mehrabian (1972) determined that 93% of communication is nonverbal, leaving only 7% for actual content of spoken words. A person's expressions, gestures, posture, and other actions provide a constant source of information.

Therefore, improving your interpretation of body language is a valuable communication skill. Nonverbal messages are usually a means of expressing emotions. We search someone's face to determine feelings of anger, sadness, or disgust. Nonverbal messages tend to be more reliable than verbal messages and are essential to understanding many of the most important things others are trying to communicate to us (Table 14.1).

Table 14.1
Examples of Nonverbal Cues

Feature	Nonverbal Cues
Head	Nodding, cocked to side, thrown back, motioning a direction
Facial expression	Frowning, grimacing, animated, distracted
Eyes	Squinting, wide open, closed, winking, blinking, rolling, teary
Mouth	Smiling, pursed lips, lip licking, lip biting, open, closed
Skin	Blushing, paleness, perspiration, rashes
Body posture	Relaxed, rigid, stooped shoulders, leaning forward, leaning backward, chest extended out
Hands/arms	Fidgeting, tapping, laced fingers, fisted, pointing, touching, crossed arms
Feet/legs	Foot tapping, legs crossed, legs open, knee knocking

Although voice intonation is verbal and explained in more detail later, it is appropriate to mention it as a nonverbal behavior. The sound of the voice communicates beyond the specific words. The words spoken may be fast, slow, high-pitched, loud, or whispered. The voice tells much about the mood of the speaker. For example, some people may speak very rapidly or at a high pitch when they are nervous or fearful.

General appearance also is a nonverbal cue. The way in which a person grooms and dresses is a statement to others.

One aspect of interpreting body language is noting discrepancies between verbal and nonverbal messages. It is easy to note incongruence in a person who says he is not angry while slamming his fist on the table. When you note a difference between words and nonverbal behavior, it may be helpful to search for the meaning of both. Body language can have multitudes of meanings and should be interpreted in context. A single gesture does not stand alone, but should be seen in relationship to other body movements and related to a person's words.

Misunderstandings often occur when listening only to words or observing only body language. Clarify the accuracy of your interpretation with the client.

Perceiving Verbal Messages. To understand verbal messages, you must be able to recognize both the apparent and the underlying content. The apparent or cognitive content is composed of the actual words and facts of the message. Cognitive messages are more easily recognized because they are stated and usually involve talking about things, people, or events and may include one or more themes or topics. The underlying or affective content is composed of emotions, attitudes, and behaviors. Affective messages are communicated both verbally and nonverbally and are more difficult to perceive and interpret. The client may not even be aware of their own feelings and might be surprised when you reveal your perceptions of what they are saying. Generally, emotions can be grouped into four major categories—sadness, anger, fear, and happiness—and a feeling from one category may often cover up a feeling from another.

Discriminating between cognitive and affective messages will allow you to respond appropriately to the client. Many cognitive themes may be communicated at once, but hearing the emotional message will help you to establish priorities for cognitive topics. It seems listeners will often respond to the most recent verbal theme instead of the most important one.

To illustrate, a client says to a personal trainer in their first meeting, "There is so much going on right now. I have gained 25 pounds since starting school. I'm about to flunk chemistry and if I do, my dad said he would take me out of school. I can't concentrate and I'm not sleeping at night. It seems I just keep gaining weight." In this situation, it is necessary for the personal trainer to listen to the whole message and prioritize the cognitive themes. It may be helpful for this client to learn some stress-reduction techniques from a qualified professional even before being put on a weight-control and exercise program.

Verbal Behaviors

Verbal responses are a form of listening and they demonstrate to the client an understanding of what he or she is saying and feeling. Appropriate responses will encourage the client to continue talking and will allow for more exploration. The following are commonly used verbal responses:

✔ Minimal encouragers—brief words or phrases that allow the client to continue speaking. These verbal prods let him or her know that you are following what is being said. Examples of minimal encouragers are "Mmm-hmmm," "I see," "Yes," and "Go on."

✔ Paraphrasing—a response that concisely restates the essence of the speaker's content. For example:
Client: I didn't sleep well and don't feel like working out.
Personal Trainer: You're tired today.

✔ Probing—an attempt to gain more information. Statements such as, "I'm wondering about ..." and "Let's talk about that" will help reveal more information.

✔ Reflecting—restating feelings and/or content in a way that demonstrates understanding. You can reflect stated or implied feelings, nonverbal observation, specific content, and even what has been omitted. Examples of reflecting are: "You're feeling uncomfortable about starting an exercise program," and "Sounds like you are angry at your husband for insisting that you come today."

✔ Clarifying—an attempt to understand what the client is saying. "I'm confused about ..." and "Could you please explain that again?" are examples of clarifying statements.

✔ Informing—sharing factual information, as when you explain the pros and cons of a particular piece of exercise equipment.

✔ Confronting—providing the client with mild or strong feedback about what is really going on. Confrontations are more easily heard when communicated with "I" messages such as "I feel you really don't want to be here today." Another example of confronting is "It seems to me you say ... and yet you do ... "

✔ Questioning—asking for a response. Questions may be closed or open. Closed questions direct the client to give a short response such as "yes" or "no." Open questions provide space for them to explore their own thoughts without being hemmed in. "What's on your mind today?" is an example of an open question.

✔ Summarizing—recapping what has been communicated and highlighting major themes. Effective summarizing can tie loose strands of a conversation together at its conclusion. A summary might begin with "Let's recap what we've discussed so far."

As mentioned earlier, the way in which we speak is often more important than

what we actually say. An effective communicator is aware of the quality of delivery of the message. The elements of voice in delivery are intensity, pitch, and pace. The intensity, or force, is an important factor in delivery. Some personal trainers speak so softly that they cannot be heard, while others speak with such volume that they become annoying. Delivery should be loud enough to be heard, while reserving a range to emphasize important points. When working in the weight room, you may find an unusual amount of interference from others talking, background music, and weights clanging. This situation provides you with a challenge to determine an effective intensity for your voice. Decreasing voice volume in a noisy situation can actually increase the attentiveness of the other person. For example, instead of shouting to a client in a noisy gym, you can experiment with lowering your voice volume to encourage him or her to listen more intently. This technique also will reduce vocal stress.

Pitch is the general level of the voice on the musical scale. Everyone has a characteristic pitch. Some speak in a singsong fashion while others speak in a monotone. Some people may end their sentences with an upward inflection while others end with a downward inflection. A noticeable rise in pitch level may decrease effective delivery because it usually denotes incompleteness of thought or indecisiveness. Experienced personal trainers cultivate a wide range of pitch, which they use effectively during delivery.

Rate means the speed of the utterance, or the number of words spoken per minute. Most people speak at the rate of 115 to 150 words per minute. Variations in rate depend upon such factors as the importance of the material, the desire for emphasis, and the mood of the content. Speaking too quickly reduces clarity and can be confusing for those listening. Even though speaking at a slower rate allows others time to absorb what is being said, speaking too slowly may bore the listener. Pausing gives people time to think about what is being said and can accentuate important information.

The rapport stage, which begins at first contact, is critical to establishing a good working relationship between the personal trainer and client. Sometimes a level of comfort may be quickly established, while at other times more time and energy may have to be expended to win a client's trust. Interpersonal communication skills can be learned and mastered. Merely reading about these skills does not necessarily improve application to everyday situations; they must be continuously practiced. Even though the rapport stage is presented as the first stage, there is really no end to it. The primary qualities (empathy, warmth, and genuineness) and the interpersonal communication skills are important and valuable throughout the entire personal trainer/client relationship.

INVESTIGATION STAGE

The goal of the investigation stage is to gather information about your client's present fitness level, personal goals, and physical and psychological limitations. This may begin in the initial interview, when the client is encouraged to talk about desires and expectations for training. The health history and lifestyle questionnaires discussed in Chapter 5 will yield a wealth of information. Additional data can be gathered from fitness assessments (Chapter 6). Historically, health history and lifestyle questionnaire forms are filled out by the individual client. However, you are encouraged to ask these questions orally. This method requires more time, but it can be valuable in establishing rapport. In addition, clients will probably reveal more about themselves when they observe your interest. At a minimum, you and your client should discuss his or her

written responses to the questionnaire. During the discussion you can probe, question, and clarify to gain more information. After all the information is gathered, you and your client can begin planning by setting goals and making decisions about how to achieve them.

PLANNING STAGE

Up to this point, most of your time with your client has been spent building rapport and gathering appropriate information regarding lifestyle behaviors and current fitness level. In the planning stage, the personal trainer and client begin setting goals according to the client's needs and desires. Because there are usually several ways to reach any goal, you must make use of decision-making skills to determine the best course of action. The outcome will be more effective if the process is done together than if you dictate to the client what to do each step of the way.

Decision-making occurs frequently as we go about our daily activities; we must constantly decide how we will spend our time, money, and energy during any given day. Many of these decisions are second nature for us, so we do not consider the process we go through in determining what is best in a particular situation. Even though there are many decision-making models, the basic process for the personal trainer/client relationship consists of the following steps:

1. Setting goals
2. Generating alternatives
3. Exploring the alternatives
4. Making the decision
5. Formulating a plan
6. Evaluating the implementation

Setting Goals. Clients will seldom approach you with neatly stated goals. They are usually expressed in vague statements, such as, "I want to be in better shape," or "I want to lose some weight." It is your responsibility to translate these general aims into precise goals.

Effective goals must be SMART, which means they are

Specific—The goals must specifically tell what is to be accomplished. They must be easily understood and unambiguous.

Measurable—The goals must be measurable so there is no question of attainment. Examples of measurement would be percent body fat, number of pounds, or a specific fun run.

Attainable—The goals must be attainable, not too difficult or too easy. Easy goals do not motivate and overly difficult ones may frustrate.

Relevant—The goals must be relevant or pertinent to the particular interest, needs, and abilities of your client.

Time-bound—The goals must be time-bound with specific deadlines for completion.

It is difficult to know when a client has obtained a goal that is expressed in terms such as "I want to get in better shape." However, both parties would know when the goal is attained if it is stated as, "I want to be able to walk three miles in 45 minutes by March 31st," or "I'd like to drop 20 pounds by the end of the year." According to Dick, Carey, and Carey (2000), one method of clarifying a broad goal is to follow these steps:

1. Write the goal down.

2. Write down things the client can do to demonstrate they have achieved the goal (e.g., lose 20 pounds, drop to 12% body fat, fit into a size 10 dress they have not worn in three years).

3. Sort through the statements and pick out the ones that best represent the original goal.

4. Rewrite the original goal to include your new statements or make smaller goals.

Express the goals in terms of client actions rather than personal trainer actions. A goal stated as, "the trainer will get me in shape," does not give the client ownership of or responsibility for the goal.

The goals must also be attainable. It would not be attainable for a nonrunner client to say, "I want to run a 10K next week." Attainable goals will help ensure the client's success. Finally, setting both short- and long-range goals will be helpful. For example, a female client who is 30% body fat may have a long-range goal of reaching 20% body fat in six months. The short-range goal might be to reach 27% in the next six weeks. Setting a time line, or date of completion, often creates a sense of urgency for both the client and the personal trainer and can be effective in overcoming client procrastination. You also can help the beginner client create behavioral goals that will remove intimidating evaluation procedures like body-fat tests, tape measures, and weight scales. For example, a behavioral goal can be stated as, "I want to exercise three times per week, for 30 minutes of aerobic training, 20 minutes of strength training, and 10 minutes of stretching, for 12 consecutive weeks starting January 1st." In this example, the personal trainer and client are establishing positive lifestyle changes rather than strictly emphasizing physiological changes.

Generating Alternatives. This step in the decision-making process involves proposing all possible alternatives for reaching the goal. This brainstorming process gives the client more choices. For example, a client might define his or her goal as, "I want to get my thighs stronger for the upcoming ski season." In exploring alternatives to reach this goal, you and your client might generate the following:

a. I could increase my thigh strength by riding the stationary cycle.

b. I could increase my thigh strength by performing squats with free weights.

c. I could increase my thigh strength by climbing stairs.

d. I could increase my thigh strength by stepping up and down on a bench.

Planning Stage

The client now has several viable options for obtaining their goal.

Exploring Alternatives. After brainstorming the list of options, the next step is to weigh or rank them. Evaluate the alternatives for implementation realities and hypothesized consequences. Some options may immediately be thrown out because they are impractical, making it easier for the client to prioritize the remaining alternatives. From the previous example, a client may discard option b because of its relative inconvenience. With your help, he or she may then rank the rest of the alternatives according to interest, availability, and time.

Making the Decision. You and the client now decide on one or more of the alternatives. Choose the most effective strategy or a combination of the options for this person at this time. For example, our skier may choose to train for skiing by doing squats with free-weights at the gym at least two days a week. In addition, he or she can climb stairs at home when there is no time to get to the gym.

Formulating a Plan. At this point you and the client determine a specific sequence of action that likely will result in the accomplishment of the goals. Formulating an action plan includes determining who needs to do what, when, where, what materials are required, and so forth. This step is further developed as exercise programming, which is covered in Chapters 11 and 12.

Evaluating the Implementation. This step measures accomplishment in relation to the predetermined goals and may occur in a formal setting where the client's fitness level is reassessed. The appropriate fitness assessments are described in Chapter 6. The evaluation process may also occur informally during the training sessions as both client and trainer report progress. Either way, together you determine the accomplishment and, if necessary, a new set of action steps.

ACTION STAGE

Once rapport has been established, information has been gathered, and goals have been set, the action stage, or actual training, begins. You coach the client toward his or her goals. As a teacher or tutor, you may use many methods of education. In a broad sense, personal training is similar to an individual approach to direct instruction, which is essentially active learning. It consists of the personal trainer explaining a new concept or skill to the client. Afterward, the client demonstrates understanding by practicing under the personal trainer's direction, while the trainer encourages him or her to continue to practice until the skills become natural. The climate of direct instruction is task-oriented and is high in expectations. The client will be more motivated to learn in areas they find interesting and may actively resist learning in areas they do not. You can increase motivation by teaching information that meets the needs and desires of the client. Once an area of interest is discovered, you can use a variety of teaching techniques to help the client feel successful with learning. According to Wlodkowski (1998), an initial small success can lead to greater confidence in the learning process, improved self-esteem, and increased motivation to learn new things. Your selection of techniques will depend upon your style and that of the client. What works well for one client may not work for another. Having a variety of teaching techniques is essential to the success of the trainer/client relationship.

Multisensory Input

Clients gather information through their senses (visual, auditory, kinesthetic, smell, taste) and this creates a pathway for information to be received and processed. Pathways often overlap with clients showing a "preference" for gathering information in one pathway over others. Approximately 60% of the population prefers a primary visual pathway, while 20% accesses information auditorily and another 20% prefers to kinesthetically receive data. Even though a client may enjoy charts and pictures because he or she prefers to gather information visually, the client is still able to gather information verbally, although it is not their dominant pathway.

You can identify which pathway the client prefers by observing actions during learning situations and by listening for clues in language (Table 14.2). For example, a personal trainer is discussing basic anatomy with a client using an anatomy chart on the wall. The visual learner may focus directly on the chart and may walk right up to it while the trainer is talking. The auditory learner may ignore the chart and focus directly on the trainer's words. The kinesthetic learner may touch the chart or touch and move the corresponding muscles as the trainer describes them.

If you can identify the learning pathway that the client prefers, you can match your words and behaviors to that preference (see Table 14.2). This not only enhances learning, but it also allows you to maintain rapport with your client.

"Tell, Show, Do"

> *I hear and I forget*
> *I see and I remember*
> *I do and I understand*
> —Confucius

This proverb is at the heart of day-to-day personal training. As early as the 1930s, John Dewey advocated "learning by doing." Probably the most effective systematic method of teaching a skill is by explanation, demonstration, and execution, also known as "tell, show, do." It involves observing how something is done correctly and then performing it under the supervision of an instructor (Figure 14.3). The instructor provides an auditory, visual, and kinesthetic learning experience, thus stimulating all learning pathways.

Explanation. The explanation should be a concise verbal description of the skill that gives a clear understanding of what is to be accomplished. A simple skill may only require one sentence while a more complex skill may require more detail. During this time, the client should be told what to watch for during the demonstration. For example, the trainer might say, "I'm now going to show you how to perform a biceps curl. Watch how I control the movement and do not use momentum to help lift the weight."

Demonstration. The demonstration is the visual presentation of the skill. It is critical that it be an accurate representation of the desired action. Therefore, you must be keenly aware kinesthetically so that proper form is communicated to the client. If you have just explained that there should be no use of momentum or swinging during the biceps curl, then you must perform the curl with complete control without using momentum for the lift.

Table 14.2
Learning Pathways

	Visual	Auditory	Kinesthetic
Client actions	Watches intently Prefers reading	Listens carefully Prefers hearing	Touches or holds Prefers to be spotted
Client statement	"Oh, I see" "Let me see that again"	"Yeah, I hear you" "Say that one more time"	"I feel that" "This does not feel right"
Strategy	Demonstrations	Question and answer	Hands-on supervision

FIGURE 14.3
"Tell, Show, Do."

Trainer explaining hamstring stretch.

Trainer demonstrating hamstring stretch.

Trainer watching client perform hamstring stretch.

Demonstrating the movement slowly will help the client see what is happening. Repeating the demonstration at normal speed while reiterating the main points also will aid learning. The explanation and demonstration steps can be effectively combined to save time.

Performance. The performance is the client's opportunity to practice the skill. Carefully monitor and supervise the client's performance to correct errors and encourage proper form. Constructive feedback and more practice time complete the learning loop. The problem in many teaching programs is that all the above steps are not followed. Often the explanation or "tell" step is not followed by the "show" and "do" steps. Telling a person exactly how to perform a skill does not ensure that he or she will be able to do it correctly. Simply telling a client to "stretch the hamstrings after you jog" does not ensure that he or she will perform the stretch effectively. To complete the process, the client should be shown how to perform a hamstring stretch properly, and then given an opportunity to practice it while you coach proper form and execution.

You must decide if a skill should be taught as a whole or if it should be broken into parts. These methods of teaching are often referred to as the whole approach and the parts approach, respectively. Less complex skills are usually taught as a whole to establish a general idea and feel for the movement. Practicing the biceps curl from start to finish is an appropriate application of the whole approach. More complex exercises that require much attention may be demonstrated by you as a whole movement and then broken down into lower-torso and upper-torso movements so that the client may master each part of the skill. Breaking down race walking into individual parts makes it easier to perform the activity in its entirety.

Association. You can also help the client learn by creating links or bridges between old and new information. By discovering what the client already knows, beginning in the rapport stage, you can build on pre-existing knowledge. Each client will have unique personal experiences to draw from. For example, when working with a client who skis, you can redirect the feet during a standing calf stretch by cueing to "point both skis downhill." By using an association, you allow clients to place meaning to the instruction, and, ultimately, they learn more deeply and are more likely to make a lasting improvement on performance.

Modeling

Humans want to identify with other humans. We look at others and imitate traits we would like to have. The concept of emulating another's behavior or attitudes is called modeling and the individual demonstrating the behavior is known as the model. We see many examples of modeling in our daily lives. Children adopt parent's language patterns and nonverbal cues and they can learn aggressive behavior from watching television. Celebrity models have a profound impact on clothing and dress, hair styles, music, and food. According to Bandura (1977), modeling is probably the most efficient and effective form of learning a new behavior. This places both enormous opportunity and responsibility on the personal trainer.

Two forms of modeling are identified by Good and Brophy (1999). The first is simply imitation, or "monkey see, monkey do." The observer adopts the behavior of the model. The second is more complex because the observer must infer attitudes, values, beliefs, or personality characteristics as a result of watching the model. The observer draws his or her own conclusions and, over time, may change a behavior. This is a common occurrence in the personal trainer/client relationship. As a result of observing your dedication to a healthy and fit lifestyle, the client may choose a healthier alternative to the regular Friday afternoon happy hour. In this form of modeling, people often communicate atti-

tudes unconsciously and are unaware of the effects. Students constantly observe a teacher's approach to a subject, studying the teacher's attitudes and beliefs. They watch the way the teacher interacts with other students and colleagues and the student may then make inferences regarding the learning process. The way in which a teacher responds to a student's question can affect the learning climate. The response, "I don't know ... let's find out," models enthusiasm for learning and makes not knowing the answer acceptable. This form of modeling is both subtle and powerful.

There are several factors that influence modeling. The first is the state of the learner. The more uncertain a learner is, the more significant the effects of the model will be. Therefore, a client is more susceptible to the effects of your modeling at the beginning of the relationship. A second factor that influences modeling is the status of the model in the eyes of the learner. Students are more likely to adopt the behaviors of a teacher they like and respect than of one they do not.

You cannot escape being a model. However, you can decide what kind of model you will be. Who a personal trainer is and what he or she does sends loud and clear messages to the client about what is important and how the program is really supposed to work. In other words, the way you behave is just as important as what you say. The personal trainer who advocates doing what he or she is unwilling to do will more than likely be unconvincing. For example, it is fruitless for a personal trainer to tell clients that steroids are bad for their health when it is known that the trainer uses steroids. "Do as I say, not as I do" has no place in the personal trainer/client relationship. The client views you as an expert and will generally believe everything that you say and do with regard to fitness. Therefore, it is critical that you be aware of your influence. Be competent and wise in fitness matters and obtain at least a level of fitness that corresponds to

Action Stage

Action Stage

the level of teaching. Going beyond mere competence is even more desirable.

Contracting

Contracting finds its roots in the behavioral theory of reinforcement that says rewarded behavior tends to be repeated. Contracting systematically arranges the rewards so that the probability of the desired response is increased. Most behavioral **contracts** are verbal or written agreements between two or more people and consist of two primary parts (Figure 14.4). The first part is specifying the behavior to be achieved. The second part is stating specific reinforcements that will reward the desired behavior. It may take the form of, "If you will do _____ , I will do _____ ." A contract does not necessarily require involving other people. It is possible to make an agreement with oneself by preparing a self-contract (Figure 14.5).

All helping relationships have implied contracts or understandings that both people will have responsibilities to carry out. Verbal or informal contracts are used when there is little chance of a misunderstanding of the conditions. The written contract is used to prevent those misunderstandings and to add impact by having the client sign to indicate a commitment.

Several features are necessary for an effective contract. The terms should be explicitly stated so that the expectations are clearly understood by all parties. An example of an unclear contract statement is, "I agree to lose some weight so I may do something I enjoy." A more clearly stated contract term might be, "I will lose 5 pounds and then I'll be permitted to buy that new dress." Many contracts fail because of impossible terms, so they should be feasible and reasonable. "I will lose 50 pounds this month so I can buy that new dress," is an unreasonable goal. "I will lose 1 to 2 pounds a week for the next two months," is a more reasonable goal. Composing the contract in positive rather than negative terms will encourage a more

favorable attitude toward the contract. "If you do not quit smoking, I will not work with you," is a negative approach. A more positive approach would be to determine a reward given upon smoking cessation.

To ensure satisfactory results, contracts need to be evaluated frequently and perhaps renegotiated. This renegotiation can occur any time or during the formal evaluation process. What appeared to be fair and reasonable initially may not be so later. If a client discovers he or she cannot meet a specified commitment, you should discuss the difficulty and a new contract can be negotiated, drafted, and signed. This evaluation process will help ensure that the contract remains effective.

The following questions will help you trouble-shoot while writing contracts:

1. Are the terms of the contract clear?
2. Is the contract fair?
3. Is the contract positive?
4. Is the target behavior clearly specified?
5. Does the contract provide for immediate reinforcement?
6. Is the reinforcement frequent and in small amounts?
7. Does the client understand the contract?
8. Is there a time specified for evaluation?

Feedback

Feedback is a powerful contributor to effective learning and client performance. It is any information about current or past behavior that can be used to improve performance and can be given verbally or nonverbally. It usually occurs after a client has asked a question or done something related to the exercise session. Feedback informs the client of the correctness of performance and recognizes effort. You will naturally respond and react to clients' behaviors, and they are greatly influenced by the way you behave toward them. They monitor their personal trainers' reactions and adjust their performance in accordance with what they interpret.

I, the undersigned, agree to the following conditions, which I will follow to the best of my ability.

From _____ to _____, for a period of one week, I will choose to eat at meal time only.

From _____ to _____, for a period of one week, I will eat foods recommended by the American Heart Association and the American Dietetic Association.

At the end of the week, as a reward for fulfilling the above conditions, I will attend a movie or other social function with my husband.

Date _____

Signature of wife _____

I, the undersigned, agree to take my wife to a movie when the above conditions are met.

Date _____

Signature of husband _____

FIGURE 14.4
Example of an exercise contract between two people.

I will walk in my target zone a minimum of _____ minutes _____ times per week.
I will record my progress in my personal log.
The following people will help me reach my goal:

_____

Person	Method
1. _____	1. _____
2. _____	2. _____
3. _____	3. _____
4. _____	4. _____

I will reward myself for adhering to the above for _____ weeks with the following:

_____
_____
_____

I will begin the program __(date)__ and will reevaluate it on __(date)__ .

FIGURE 14.5
Example of a personal exercise contract.

For feedback to be effective, a clearly defined standard of performance must be given. For example, a personal trainer defines the standard of performance for proper placement and movement of the arms in race walking during their explanation and demonstration of the skill. The client's performance is then measured and corrected according to the demonstrated criteria. The performance standard may need to be set at frequent intervals during instruction by continuing to explain and demonstrate. For the feedback to be effective and learning to occur, there must be a practice session that gives the client an opportunity to correct performance and reach the preset standard.

Research indicates that effective feedback has three characteristics: (1) it is specific; (2) it is contingent on performance; and (3) it provides corrective information for the learner. Specific feedback is clear about what was right and/or wrong. You may watch a client incorrectly perform a lat pulldown on the weight equipment and then exclaim, "That's not right, Susie!" Your response does not aid Susie's understanding of the performance, it only lets her know that it was wrong. By contrast, you might respond, "Not quite Susie. Let's reverse the position of your hands." Corrective feedback helps the client know what was wrong with the performance and what to do to get back on track. The number of different cues is infinite, and striving for unique ones will require your creativity and committed practice.

Feedback should not be given for every single move because too much of a good thing can have a negative effect; people tend to disregard excessive compliments. The feedback should match the achievement and specifically relate the response to the performance. For example, a personal trainer observing a client performing a biceps curl might respond with, "That's good," which is only a statement of general praise. However, an even more

effective response would be, "That's it John, you're really isolating the biceps muscle now." This response gives the client specific information as to why the performance is correct. To maximize the effect, cues can be personalized by using a client's name, for instance, "That's the right idea, Jennie." Typical verbal cues are

Good	Excellent
Right	Correct
All right	OK
Very good	Fine

These words are less effective because they have been overused. Examples of other, more effective cues that you might use are

That's an effective thought.
You've got it.
You're on the money.
You are really with it today.
I'd give that move a 10.

Nonverbal feedback is far more effective than verbal feedback. Clients tune into facial expressions and gestures. When used properly, nonverbal cues are the epitome of personalization. How else can a "thumbs up" signal and a generous smile be interpreted? Nonverbal positive feedback interactions include

Smiling	Making an "Okay" sign
Nodding	Patting on the back
Shaking hands	Touching
Clapping	Winking
Thumbs up	Applauding

Nonverbal negative feedback interactions include

Frowning	Thumbs down
Shaking head	Drumming fingers
Looking away	Rolling eyes
Grimacing	

A final and important point needs to be made regarding verbal and nonverbal feedback. As in all interpersonal communication, when both verbal and nonverbal cues are given, they must be congruent. For example, if you frown while telling a client that they are doing a great job, the two behaviors are incongruent and the conflicting messages are confusing. The client will receive a mixed message and will probably believe the frown rather than the words. On the other hand, when verbal and nonverbal cuing are congruently combined, you can have a powerful influence on the client.

STAGES OF LEARNING

Understanding the various stages of learning will help you teach more effectively. One of the most commonly cited learning models was developed by Fitts and Posner (1967), who theorized that there are three stages of learning for a motor skill: cognitive, associative, and autonomous. Within the **cognitive stage of learning,** learners make many errors and have highly variable performances. They know they are doing something wrong, but they do not know how to improve their performance. At this stage, participants seem terribly uncoordinated and consistently perform exercises incorrectly. Those in the **associative stage of learning** have learned the basic fundamentals or mechanics of the skill. Their errors tend to be less gross in nature and they can now concentrate on refining their skills. During this stage, exercise participants are able to detect some errors and the instructor needs to make only occasional corrections. During the **autonomous stage of learning** the skill becomes automatic or habitual. Learners can now perform without thinking and can detect their own errors. Driving a car, for example, is a very complex motor skill that over time is performed in the autonomous stage. The driver often is concentrating elsewhere and

is able to recognize when mistakes are made. The type and amount of information that exercise participants can understand depends on their current stage within the learning process. An awareness of your client's stage of learning will enable you to employ the appropriate teaching strategy for each individual.

SUMMARY

Your relationships with clients are helping relationships throughout the stages of establishing and building rapport with them, gathering vital information, developing fitness goals, and implementing a plan to accomplish them. As a helper, you create conditions and use techniques that will help bring about the desired outcomes for the client. Merely possessing a fit body, technical skills, and a wide-based knowledge of health and fitness does not ensure your success. Probably the most crucial factor for determining a positive climate for the working relationship is the trainer's repertoire of communication skills. These skills include both verbal and nonverbal behaviors, such as attending, perceiving nonverbal messages, perceiving verbal messages, and verbal responding. These interpersonal communication skills can be learned, practiced, and mastered, and are important not only in the first stage of establishing rapport, but throughout the entire process.

Personal training is about behavioral change, which is the true measure of a successful trainer/client relationship. Every personal trainer is unique and brings into the relationship his or her own personal experience and opinions about what brings about lifestyle changes in people. Each client also is uniquely different. Therefore, you must be flexible in matching teaching techniques and changing strategies to meet the goals, needs, and personality of the client. A technique that is successful for one client does not ensure the same achievement or

Summary

change for another. A skilled personal trainer will get to know the client and apply various techniques with wisdom, while another may resist to the point of discontinuing the relationship.

The flexibility required to do your job sometimes demands that you be deeply personal and at other times remain an objective observer. Being able to move freely along the full range of interpersonal skills and teaching techniques will permit you to respond appropriately at various stages of the relationship. On one hand, the process of sizing up and assisting a client toward a healthy lifestyle is naturally intuitive, but, on the other hand, it needs to be a deliberate, rational process.

REFERENCES

Bandura, A. (1977). *Social Learning Theory.* Englewood Cliffs, N.J.: Prentice Hall.

Dick, W., Carey, L., & Carey, J.O. (2000). *The Systematic Design of Instruction* (5th ed.). New York: Addison-Wesley Publishing.

Fitts, P.M. & Posner, M.I. (1967). *Human Performance.* Belmont, Calif.: Brooks/Cole.

Good, F. & Brophy, J. (1999). *Looking in Classrooms* (8th ed.). Needham Heights, Mass.: Allyn & Bacon.

Hall, E.T. (1966). *The Hidden Dimension.* Garden City, Calif.: Doubleday.

Mehrabian, A. (1972). *Nonverbal Communication.* New York: Walter de Gruyter.

Rogers, C.R. et al. (1967). *The Therapeutic Relationship and Its Impact.* Madison: University of Wisconsin Press.

Truax, C.B. & Carkuff, R.F. (1967). *Toward Effective Counseling and Psychotherapy.* New York: Walter de Gruyter.

Wlodkowski, R. (1998). *Enhancing Adult Motivation to Learn.* San Francisco: Jossey-Bass.

SUGGESTED READING

Bolton, R. (1986). *People Skills.* Carmichael, Calif.: Touchstone Books.

Boothman, N. (2000). *How to Make People Like You in 90 Seconds or Less.* New York: Workman Publishing.

Carkhuff, R.R. & Anthony, W.A. (1999). *The Skills of Helping.* Amherst: Human Resource Development Press.

Covey, S.R. (2004). *The Seven Habits of Highly Effective People: Powerful Lessons in Personal Change.* New York: Simon & Schuster.

Covey, S.R. & Merrill, A.R., & Merrill, R.R. (1996). *First Things First.* New York: Simon & Schuster

Csikszentmihalyi, M. (1991). *Flow: The Psychology of Optimal Experience.* New York: HarperCollins.

Goleman, D. (2006). *Emotional Intelligence: When It Can Matter More Than Your I.Q.* New York: Bantam Books.

Jacobson, D., Kauchak, D., & Eggen, P.D. (1992). *Methods for Teaching: A Skills Approach.* (4th ed.). New York: Macmillan College Division.

Kauchak, D.P. & Eggen, P.E. (2002). *Learning and Teaching: Research-based Methods.* (4th ed.). Needham Heights, Mass.: Allyn & Bacon.

Krumboltz, J. (1966). *Stating the Goals of Counseling* (Monograph No. 1). Fullerton: California Personnel and Guidance Association.

Malouf, D. (1999). *Power Up Your People Skills: Communication in the New Millennium.* Australia. Australian Print Group.

Martens, R. (2004). *Successful Coaching.* (3rd ed.). Champaign, Ill.: Human Kinetics.

Mosston, M. (1966). *Teaching Physical Education: From Command to Discovery.* Columbus: Merrill.

O'Connor, J. & McDermott, I. (2001). *Way of NLP.* London. Thorsons Publishing.

Okun, B.F. (2001). *Effective Helping: Interviewing and Counseling Techniques.* Belmont, Calif.: Wadsworth Publishing Company.

Rogers, C. (1995). *On Becoming a Person.* New York: Houghton Mifflin.

Vernacchia, R. et al. (1996). *Coaching Mental Excellence.* Portola Valley, Calif.: Warde Publishers.

CHAPTER 15

Basics of Behavior Change and Health Psychology

Glen D. Morgan, Ph.D., completed his doctorate in clinical psychology from Washington University in St. Louis. He was full-time faculty at the Wyoming Valley Family Practice Residency, with an appointment in the Department of Family & Community Medicine, Pennsylvania State University College of Medicine, for 14 years. He joined the National Cancer Institute of the National Institutes of Health in 1998. He oversees tobacco use treatment research and the Transdisciplinary Tobacco Use Research Centers.

Glen D. Morgan

Health psychology is concerned with psychology's contribution to the promotion and maintenance of health, the prevention and treatment of illness, as well as the identification and evaluation of the factors that optimize health. It developed as a result of a growing body of research that pointed to the interdependency of psychological and behavioral processes and health. This chapter will identify and address specific behaviors related to physical activity and health.

Disclaimer: This chapter was written in a personal capacity and does not represent the opinions of the NIH, DHHS, or the Federal Government.

The last 20 years have witnessed a dramatic evolution in the conceptualization of disease, health, and behavior. Advances in public health and pharmacology have largely eliminated or controlled diseases that were the leading causes of death through the early part of the twentieth century. Behavioral factors, particularly tobacco use, diet and activity patterns, alcohol consumption, sexual behavior, and avoidable injuries are among the most prominent contributors to mortality (McGinnis & Foege, 1993). Lifestyle factors, in fact, significantly contribute to more than half of the annual deaths in the United States (Goldstein et al., 1990). There has been a dramatic increase in the understanding of the importance of exercise and physical activity for preventing disease and maintaining health. According to the *Surgeon General's Report on Physical Activity and Health,* regular physical activity that is performed on five or more days of the week reduces the risk of developing some of the leading causes of illness and death in the United States (U.S. Department of Health and Human Services, 1996). Despite common knowledge that exercise has health benefits, more than 60% of American adults are not regularly active and 25% are sedentary (Jones et al., 1998). Nearly half of American youth are not vigorously active on a regular basis (U.S. Department of Health and Human Services, 1996). The modification of all of the above-mentioned behavioral risk factors may prevent or reduce the symptoms of many diseases.

Scientists are not the only ones to recognize the link between health and behavior. The public's interest in, and demand for, information on health, wellness, risk factors, and disease prevention has skyrocketed over during the last two decades. Not only are health articles regularly featured in daily newspapers and popular magazines, books on health and health behaviors often top the best-seller lists.

The evolving landscape of healthcare is also changing how people look at health and lifestyle. Healthcare reform not only involves medical care but is also an economic, political, and social phenomenon. The prevailing motivating factor in the development of health maintenance organizations (HMOs) is cost control. Managed-care systems project that keeping enrollees healthy will reduce medical visits, hospital admissions, and medication use. Consequently, many programs provide incentives both to practitioners (to encourage risk-factor reduction) and to enrollees (to stay healthy by adopting healthier lifestyles).

These converging factors—healthcare reform, growing public awareness of health issues, their desire to maintain health, and the economics of healthcare—have provided new opportunities in two related areas: exercise and weight management. An irony of HMOs is that primary care health practitioners are expected to see more patients in less time, while concurrently providing the additional services of preventive care. Consequently, patient education and lifestyle change counseling is becoming increasingly difficult during medical visits. Fitness professionals have a unique opportunity in this growing marketplace to play an important role in helping clients achieve their exercise and fitness goals.

DETERMINANTS OF BEHAVIOR

Most behaviors have multiple intertwined determinants. Cigarette smoking is an example of the interaction of psychological, social, economic, and biological factors. Most individuals begin smoking at the urging of a close friend; nicotine is not only highly addictive, but is also known to have psychoactive effects; the billions spent yearly on marketing cigarettes induce teens to initiate smoking and influence established smokers to switch brands; finally, research shows genetic predisposition to nicotine dependence (Fisher et al., 1990). Exercise and physical activity are no less complex. An individual's behavioral patterns are usually the result of several variables: learned behavior, moods, habits, social models, and environmental triggers. Furthermore, these factors can influence each other. Being out of shape may contribute to a poor self-image that, in turn, leads to negative predictions of one's ability to establish a regular fitness program.

Health Belief Model

The **Health Belief Model** provides an explanation of health-related behaviors (Glanz, Rimer, & Lewis, 2002). This model suggests that individuals adopt (or do not adopt) healthy behaviors based largely upon their appraisal of their susceptibility to an illness combined with their perception of the probable severity of the consequences of having the illness. A second part of this model is the person's view of the benefits of the behavior change as contrasted with the difficulty of changing. The final section of the model refers to internal, environmental, and social cues to action. For example, a client is unlikely to try losing weight or begin exercising if they do not feel prone to disease (susceptibility), perceive it as minor (severity), or see behavioral change as too difficult (costs).

Social Factors

Social factors play a significant role in the acquisition, maintenance, and cessation of behaviors. Family members and friends can be sources of assistance and support, as well as stress or sabotage. For example, sedentary individuals whose social network is composed of others who are inactive may feel less social pressure to exercise. They are also less likely to observe modeling of healthier exercise patterns. Conversely, if one's social network is made up of friends and family who enjoy an active lifestyle, there will be more

social influences to modify exercise patterns. Encouragement (not nagging) and reinforcement from friends, family, and co-workers can be powerful incentives for initiating and maintaining behavior change (Morgan, 1996).

Stages of Change

Obviously, an individual's motivation or readiness for change is an important factor in determining whether efforts at change will occur. Change does not occur as a discrete event; rather, it is a process that develops over time. The **stages-of-change model** is useful for understanding lifestyle modification (Prochaska & Goldstein, 1991). According to this model, people go through distinct, predictable stages when making lifestyle changes. These stages are precontemplation, contemplation, preparation, action, and maintenance. The process is not linear; individuals may move back and forth between stages (Prochaska, DiClemente, & Norcross, 1992).

During precontemplation the individual is not intending to change soon (i.e., within six months). Clients in the precontemplation stage may be unaware of, or denying the need for, lifestyle change. They might be pessimistic about either their abilities to change or about the effectiveness of change methods. In this stage, they are likely to selectively filter information that justifies their decision to maintain their unhealthy lifestyle. Smokers who deny the health risks and refuse to consider stopping are obvious precontemplaters.

During contemplation the client weighs the costs (effort, treatment effectiveness, finances, time) and benefits of lifestyle modification. They may, for example, be considering starting a fitness program in the near future. This stage is often characterized by ambivalence about changing. Individuals can remain in this stage for months or years, vacillating between approaching readiness to make an effort at change and distancing themselves from it.

Individuals who have decided to initiate an effort to change within a month's time are in the preparation stage. This is marked by observable efforts on their part to begin the change process. Clients in this stage may have set up an appointment with a fitness professional, or have begun walking or jogging.

Individuals in the action stage are in the process of changing their behavior; they are walking regularly for exercise, going to the gym, and/or reducing caloric consumption. During this stage, individuals are at greatest risk for relapse.

Maintenance is the stage of successful, sustained lifestyle modification. Though individuals in this stage may not be active in changing their behavior, they continue to actively utilize methods to monitor and control their behavior. The person who has been exercising regularly for a year illustrates this stage. Additionally, people in the maintenance stage might modify or engineer their environments to reduce the probability of relapse to old habits. You can play a vital role here by working with clients to help keep their routine fresh, interesting, and challenging.

PRINCIPLES OF BEHAVIOR CHANGE

Habits are stable behaviors formed by constant repetition of the same pattern over time, to the point where they are automatic and may even be unconscious. Horace Mann, a well-known educator, once said: "Habit is a cable. We weave a thread of it each day, and at last we cannot break it." Though most behaviorists would disagree with Mann (habits can be broken), there would be no argument of the strength of habits and the difficulty of changing them. Habits can be so ingrained in daily life that they become automatic. Just as habits are formed by learning process, changing them requires learning as well. Though "breaking" is a common term regarding changing habits, the process may be more akin to "unweaving."

Behavioral scientists view behavior as following certain orderly or lawful relationships between it and the environment. There are several basic principles of behavioral psychology that are important to understand to effectively help others change their health habits.

Antecedents

Behaviors have **antecedents** (stimuli that precede the behavior) and **consequences** (stimuli that follow the behavior). Antecedents are sometimes referred to as cues or triggers and can be events, situations, thoughts, or feelings. A ringing phone, anxiety, or finishing a meal are all examples of potential antecedents for smoking a cigarette. Initially these cues are neutral; they elicit no behaviors when encountered. The desire to smoke or eat, or another behavioral response, comes only after repeatedly pairing the specific behavior and the environmental stimulus over time. If people habitually eat popcorn at movies, for example, they will want popcorn even if they have just finished a substantial meal.

Consequences

Consequences may be either positive or negative. Positive consequences tend to increase the probability of the behavior recurring in a similar situation in the future, while negative consequences have the opposite effect. Examples of positive consequences are praise, money, affection, dessert, or gifts. Negative consequences might be rejection, guilt, punishment, or a hangover.

Antecedents and consequences become tied to the behavior with each successive repetition (Taylor, Ureda, & Denham, 1982). For the out-of-shape client, working out intensely from the outset can lead to extreme muscle pain. This unpleasant experience can lead to negative associations with exercise. In contrast, having a vigorous workout that is stimulating and fun can be extremely rewarding. This is, then, a positive reinforcer and strengthens the chances of continuing exercise. Habits become stronger with each repetition of the antecedent-behavior-consequence cycle.

Behavioral Chains

It is not unusual for behaviors to be preceded by a series of other behaviors, each one in some way connected to its predecessor. Skipping a workout and eating fast food, for example, may be followed by feelings of guilt or self-reproach. Subsequent irritability may lead to an argument with a significant other and then to eating two bowls of ice cream (another misstep for the person seeking to increase fitness). This series of connections is often referred to as a **behavioral chain** and highlights the complexity of most behaviors. Along with explaining the behavior, it provides useful information concerning changing it. The terminal behavior will not occur if any links in the chain are broken. It is usually easier to alter behavior earlier rather than later in the chain. Buying cheesecake at a bakery on Tuesday may be an initial link in a chain that ends with bingeing on four pieces of it on Thursday. Intermediate links might include a trying day at work, fatigue, and frustration. Not buying cheesecake in the first place would be an easier link to break than battling an urge to binge when feeling frustrated and tired.

Shaping

Shaping is the reinforcement of successive approximations until a desired goal is reached. This principle is used daily by teachers. When children learn to print their name, they are first taught to hold a pencil, then to form the outline of the first letter, and then practice. Each behavioral repetition brings them closer to their final goal. This principle has applications for setting objectives in a step-wise fashion leading up to the final goal. With clients who have never exercised, for example, the trainer might be careful to begin with a very easy (and short) exercise regimen, and then slowly progress as the client's health and technique improve.

Observational Learning

The social environment provides models for behavior. In other words, individuals are influenced by how friends, family, and co-workers behave. Seeing others exercise can serve as both an example and a prompt to change behavior. The influence of a positive model for health increases when the model shares similarities with the client. Encourage clients to seek out friends or family members who model the goal behavior to support them in their efforts.

Cognitions and Behavior

The above examples illustrate how behavior may also be influenced by current thoughts (**cognitions**) or feelings. Cognitions can function either as antecedents or consequences for overt behaviors, influencing the person's actions in a manner similar to environmental events. Missing a workout or two may be accompanied by the thought, "I should never miss a workout—I blew it." This might be followed by guilt, which may make it even harder to make it to the next workout.

BEHAVIORAL CHANGE STRATEGIES

Several principles of behavioral change are prominent in exercise and physical activity interventions. Some strategies (e.g., self-monitoring) have dual functions as both an assessment tool and a behavior change vehicle. Decisions regarding appropriate strategies should be based on behavioral change objectives as well as client variables (Table 15.1).

Table 15.1
Behavioral Change Strategies

Stimulus control methods
Behavioral contracts
Rewards
Cognitive methods
Self-monitoring

Stimulus Control Methods

Stimulus control methods, sometimes called "cue extinction," are a means to break the connection between events or other stimuli and behavior. For the overeater, this might involve limiting the locations in the house or times when eating takes place. Over time, the triggers lose their power and the target behavior "extinguishes." These same methods, though, can be utilized to establish and strengthen new behaviors. For exercising, it is best to establish a routine in which one exercises on specific days, at the same time, in the same place. The more one practices this routine, the more these cues will become associated with exercise. An associated feature, of course, is that this behavior pattern becomes integrated into one's daily routine.

Contracts

Many clients respond well to written agreements specifying the target behavior, the frequency, and the timeline. These can be very useful for the fitness professional and their clients. They can specify frequency and duration of training, and the time when the plan will be reassessed and modified. It is helpful to establish that the objectives and plan are consistent with the client's ability level, time availability, and level of motivation. It is better to start slowly—and then build.

Rewards

Rewards from a significant other can be powerful reinforcers in a client's efforts at behavioral change. Rewards are positive consequences, such as those mentioned earlier: praise, money, affection, dessert, or gifts. It is also reasonable for clients to plan their own self-rewards to coincide with reaching objectives in the program. Not only can rewards have extrinsic value, they are symbolic of making progress. Often, the acknowledgment from others in the form of a reward is more influential than the reward itself. Rewards can be for staying on track for a specific number of weeks and reaching a fitness goal (e.g., being able to jog a mile).

Cognitive Methods

Cognitive behavior therapy proposes that emotional reactions are not direct responses to environmental events but are mediated by thoughts (cognitions). That is, instead of an event leading directly to an emotion, an event leads to a thought, which, in turn, leads to an emotion. Seeing a dog may produce fear in people who say to themselves, "Dogs are dangerous." Seeing the same animal may produce no fear in a dog owner, who might think, "That dog looks just like mine." Different individuals may have disparate cognitions associated with the same event. For example, upon running a mile and feeling winded, one person might think, "That's great—I have never done that before," and feel wonderful; another might think, "I should not be breathing this hard," and feel discouraged. These two different thoughts, of course, lead to two entirely different emotional consequences/reactions.

"Cognitive quicksand" is irrational or overly negative thinking that causes emotional distress. Cognitions concerning events play a large role in determining reactions to those events (past, present, or future). These are the "shoulds," the "musts," and the "have tos." They can lead to guilt, anxiety, and worry. A specific example of such negative cognitions is **dichotomous** or **"light-switch" thinking.** This is when one looks at events as being all positive or all negative—there is no neutral ground. When clients view events in this manner (they are either fit or fat, smart or stupid, successful or a failure), they may be perfectionistic, high-strung, miserable to others, and riding an emotional roller coaster. A key seems to be whether people exclusively link their self-worth to their achievements.

You can assist clients in identifying and altering maladaptive, unrealistic, or extreme thinking patterns. For the exceedingly self-critical client, it helps to ask them if they would be as judgmental of their best friend if he or she behaved similarly. While in reality missing a workout may be only a minor diversion, a perfectionist client may see it as representative of no motivation, predictive of continued failure, and as leading to further failure. Perfectionism manifests itself in exercise patterns, such as overly extreme exercise routines, inflexible schedules, rigid nutritional regimens, and obsessive attention to outcomes such as percentage of body fat.

IMPLEMENTING BEHAVIORAL CHANGE

Health psychologists and clinical psychologists have predominantly used health behavior psychology techniques. The last 15 years, though, have witnessed a broadening of the applications of scientific findings in health psychology. Physicians, nurses, and other health providers are using health psychology techniques and scientific findings in patient education and in primary and secondary interventions. Interventions, across disciplines, may be directed to an individual, a group, or an entire community (e.g., through a televised health awareness and screening program).

BASIC TEACHING METHOD

The basic teaching method was developed to be straightforward and useful across a range of lifestyle health behaviors, and applicable in both clinical and nonclinical settings. There are three fundamental steps: assessment, teaching, and evaluation (A.T.E.). It is grounded in the principle that a major determinant of health lifestyles is learned behavior and that the principle method in fostering behavioral change is teaching. The term "teaching" is preferable to intervention, which generally occurs in healthcare settings.

Assessment

Assessment of client characteristics is essential to developing appropriate, effective exercise programs. A general rule of thumb is that more useful and valid information can be acquired when a greater variety of assessment methods are employed. Comprehensive assessment includes a review of demographic (e.g., age, number of children in the home), health (e.g., presence of medical problems, tobacco use), and behavioral variables (Table 15.2).

Initial assessments usually begin with an interview. It is also efficient to first gather information using questionnaires, and then clarify and focus upon specific points during the interview. Review the following variables with each client: type and extent of historical and current physical activity and the types of activities they like and dislike. Exercise history is useful to ascertain what worked well (as well as what did not) in the past. It is often helpful to build on past successes.

A basic behavioral assessment tool is self-monitoring (e.g., using a chart or exercise record), in which clients record the type of exercise, resistance/duration, reps, etc. Determination of clients' readiness to change is also essential. Precontemplators will not be amenable to developing a behavioral change plan. If they do, it is unlikely to be successful. Generally, people

Basic Teaching Method

Table 15.2
Behavioral Variables Used for Assessment

Stage of change
Expectations
Health beliefs
Previous behavior change attempts
Exercise history
Family history
Mood

Basic Teaching Method

in this stage of change will not even make it to an assessment session. They often attend only at the urging of their doctor or spouse. This is an opportunity for you to explain the health risks of sedentary behavior and briefly describe physical activity and exercise options. Instruct the client to wait until he or she is ready to change before returning. Beginning an exercise program with an insufficiently motivated client increases the probability of poor outcome and the client scapegoating you or the program. Determining the clients' health beliefs (belief in disease susceptibility) may provide another view of variables affecting motivation.

Finally, it is important to assess client expectations for the program (expectations for change). Are their predictions or hopes for outcome reasonable? Do they anticipate an amount of effort and time for change that is consistent with the program requirements? Unrealistic expectations will either lead to self-attribution of failure or seeing the program as being ineffective. It is time well spent to clarify client expectations and compare them to a realistic outcome for the program.

Careful, comprehensive assessment is the cornerstone of fitness programming. It is critical for developing strategies that are tailored to the client's specific background, needs, and psychosocial features. When carefully done, it will guide you to optimal programming and favorable outcomes.

Teaching

Teaching and learning are dynamic, interdependent processes. During this interaction, the client is constantly integrating information and beginning behavioral change. Continually modify your instruction based on observation and verbal feedback from the client. This process works in a cyclical manner (from assessment to teaching to evaluation and back to teaching).

The first step in the teaching process is setting goals. It is important to have realistic, attainable expectations for short-, moderate-, and long-term goals. It is common for clients to wish to achieve more in less time with less effort than is feasible. You might consider cutting the client's goals by half or a third to ensure success. It is important to separate the ideal from the real. It helps to explain that, since most behaviors are learned over time, it takes time to change them. Ideally, goals should include behavioral, psychological, physical, and physiological measures. It is typical for progress to occur in different spheres at different times. Having more than one focus may keep your clients from becoming discouraged about their rate of progress in one area.

Development of the behavioral plan should be a collaborative effort by you and your client. The plan must require enough effort to cause behavioral change but not so much as to discourage your client. For example, a program that requires several hours a day will be difficult to maintain in both the short and long terms. Negotiation may be necessary to come to a mutually agreed upon plan and set of goals, which will more likely lead to satisfying outcomes.

Previous assessment will reveal a variety of potential behaviors that should be addressed during programming. The initial step in program development is to identify those goals and objectives that will be addressed. The plan should be systematic, progressive (step by step), concrete, and cohesive. Pre-exercise program assessment may reveal opportunities to integrate exercise into activities of daily living or into a busy lifestyle. For example, exercise could replace sedentary activities like watching television or browsing the Internet. Initially, it may be useful to focus on very brief, frequent exercise sessions that are more easily integrated into the client's schedule. As this happens, new variations can be introduced.

In the 1980s, behavioral management research for health risk factor modification focused upon developing more powerful programs that would increase outcome rates. Most sought to achieve this by combining strategies that had been successful when used alone. A review of these studies suggests that these multicomponent programs often did not have substantially better results than simpler approaches. Clients might reach a saturation point regarding the number of strategies they can effectively employ. A parallel interpretation is that adherence decreases with increasing program demands. Thus, this research raised the point that focused, rather than broad, programming might yield better outcomes. Consequently, you must be attuned to your client's saturation point and remember that adding program requirements may backfire. This, of course, may vary over the course of treatment, based on normal expected fluctuations, environmental stressors, or time constraints. It is better to keep program demands flexible and in tune with your client's time and energy constraints, rather than rigidly conform to objectives or challenge the client's motivation. It is critical to involve the client as an equal participant in program adjustments.

It is useful, however, to employ a variety of methods to prevent boredom. New strategies can be introduced as "experiments" for the client to "try out" to see if they are effective for them. Since the strategies are meant to change behavior, they interrupt the client's daily patterns and will be moderately difficult at first.

Behavior change is difficult, requiring substantial effort. People would not seek out help if they had been successful on their own. You play the role of educator, guide, and coach, but never drill sergeant. Reassurance about your clients' progress and praise for their efforts are powerful positive reinforcers. When a strategy or objective appears out of reach for a client,

remember the principle of shaping, which works best when the final objective can be reduced to component parts that the client can address one step at a time. The metaphor of walking to the top of a stairway is a useful way to explain this process. Often, clients feel they must simply change all at once. They may see their failure to change seen as reflective of poor motivation or insufficient ability. This is akin to leaping to the top of the stairs in a single bound. Poorly conditioned clients, as an illustration, should not begin running a mile or two daily. Instead, they should begin their exercise program by walking 10 to 15 minutes, gradually increasing their pace and distance. This, then, is congruent with taking the stairs step by step. While the final objective is the same, the means to reach the objective differs.

Social Support. During behavioral change efforts, encourage your clients to ask significant others for help. Clients will exercise more regularly when they have a buddy to accompany them. Self-help and support groups have played a prominent role in many health-related and lifestyle-management programs. Being part of a group with a common goal can combat isolation, increase optimism about personal change, and enhance motivation. This is part of the appeal of group fitness classes for many people. Not only is there a schedule to adhere to, the clients may feel that their exercise companions expect them to attend. They are more likely, then, to show up even when they may be feeling tired or rushed. Friends, family members, and co-workers can encourage clients to stay on track, compliment them on their efforts, and remark on their success.

Cognitive Strategies. It is not unusual to observe clients engaging in light-switch thinking when they are setting objectives or are frustrated with their progress. You might ask them to identify those components of

Basic Teaching Method

the program they have successfully completed. This keeps them from viewing several bad days, or a difficult time with one task, as indicative of their entire effort. This process helps develop a more realistic appraisal of behavioral changes and the progress that has been made. This, combined with your periodic reviews, usually is sufficient to reassure the client.

Try to be objective and accurate or the client might view you as patronizing. Also, your client may be addressing real problems that might require refinement of the lifestyle management plan. Sometimes, clients are putting in less effort than they are capable of. Recognition of this on their part is essential to getting back on track. It is up to both you and your client to jointly review progress and agree upon a plan or resolution.

Independent Practice. Individuals must practice a behavior to change a behavior. Often, people wait for inspiration or motivation before trying a new behavior. Simply meeting with a personal trainer and thinking about changing is not sufficient to alter behavioral patterns. Breaking old habits while establishing new ones requires both planning and repetitive practice. Communicate this concept with the following statement: "It is easier to act yourself into a new way of feeling rather than feel yourself into a new way of acting" (Morgan, 1996). The misconception that behavior change is accomplished only through talking can be addressed by assigning homework tasks at each session. This also clarifies that behavior change is ultimately the responsibility of the client, not the personal trainer.

Independent practice can take many different forms, from generating objectives to keeping a log of efforts. Self-monitoring is an effective, standard assignment because it provides continuous feedback and the opportunity for self-correction. Other assignments to consider are experimenting with new strategies, writing down

objectives for specific behaviors, clarifying expectations, finding sources of social support, brainstorming alternative behaviors for particularly difficult situations, generating a plan for how the standard plan could be altered for special occasions, or making a list of personal rewards for reaching short-term goals.

Evaluation

Evaluation is a continuous process. Throughout the program, you should determine the effectiveness of the strategies, your client's level of effort, compliance with behavioral tasks, and degree of satisfaction. Educators refer to this ongoing tracking of progress as **formative evaluation.**

Multiple objectives, using multiple assessment methods, provide advantages over single-method assessment. There is greater accuracy when behavioral, psychological, physical, and physiological measures are utilized. For developing tailored exercise programs, these might include client satisfaction, feedback from significant others, weight change, change in clothing size or measurements, subjective reports of "feeling better," fitness measures, blood pressure changes, or changes in medication needs.

Self-monitoring, in addition to being an excellent initial assessment method, is a useful formative evaluation tool. It provides you with feedback regarding your clients' adherence to the treatment plan and enhances their awareness of their behavior by providing immediate feedback. As such, it often provokes behavior change. Furthermore, it is a useful tool when modifying the exercise program.

Follow-up. Follow-up is useful for several different reasons. First, you may learn how well your client has been able to maintain his or her behavior change. It also gives you the opportunity to make simple suggestions to the client regarding staying on track, as well as provide you with outcome data for the effectiveness of the program.

Finally, follow-up communicates to your client that you are committed to helping them. Follow-up often serves as a prompt for the client to recommit himself or herself to the behavior change effort and may result in several booster sessions. Though face-to-face meetings are most useful, contact by e-mail, phone, or mail can also be valuable. Frequency of follow-up is best individualized to the needs of the client. Most clinical research programs evaluate outcome in 6- and 12-month periods. Earlier follow-ups, though, might help to catch clients before they begin to slip.

Relapse Prevention. Relapse is the opposite of maintenance and generally refers to baseline behavior. It is not unusual for clients to drift off track a bit. This is sometimes referred to as a slip or a lapse. During behavioral change efforts, fluctuations are normal and should be expected. Your role is to encourage and redirect the client. Relapses should be viewed as opportunities for fine-tuning. Clients may experience some frustration or disappointment that they are not doing better. They may perceive themselves as failing and be ready to give up. This is an opportunity to explain that learning is a process that does not usually occur at a constant rate and direction. Slips are normal, not reflections of failing, and should be viewed as learning opportunities. There are two metaphors that might prove useful when discussing the challenges of behavior change. One is of a baby learning to walk. They need a lot of help, and they fall a lot. Their efforts, though, are consistently reinforced. No one would think of telling the child, "Forget it—you will never walk." Another metaphor that nicely illustrates the process of behavioral change is that of a football game. All football teams experience gains and losses in yardage during a game. The short-term goal may be to get a first down; the moderate—to score; the long term—to win the game. Giving up after a few slips in a behavioral change effort would be like a football team leaving the

field in the first quarter after losing yardage. Slips are occasions for you to address some of the cognitive quicksand issues that inevitably arise during lifestyle modification efforts utilizing the cognitive approaches outlined earlier in this chapter.

Compliance Difficulties. It is common in medical practices for patients to take medicines inappropriately or inadequately follow their physician's advice. Estimates of noncompliance range from 4 to 92%, and average from 30 to 35% for medical therapies. A difficulty with the term "noncompliance" is that it suggests that all of the fault lies with the patient and that it is reflective of poor motivation or laziness. Failure to follow a physician's advice (even this phrase blames the patient) is, as this chapter has illustrated, the result of an equation of intertwined determinants. Your task is to evaluate adherence issues utilizing multiple assessment techniques and address the following questions:

✔ Are there specific situations or times when behavior occurs or does not occur?
✔ Can antecedents and consequences be identified?
✔ What are the barriers to change?
✔ Is the client overloaded?
✔ Does he or she feel there is not enough time?
✔ Does he or she perceive themselves as failing and that it is their own fault?
✔ Has he or she lost confidence in their ability to change?
✔ Is he or she frustrated?

There are two important guidelines when addressing adherence issues. First, always attend to those things the client is doing well (not just the problem areas). Second, be sure that both you and your client have realistic expectations. Less than optimal adherence is an opportunity to further refine and tailor the treatment program to fit the client. Your primary objective is to optimize your client's chance for a successful experience.

> **Basic Teaching Method**

WHEN TO ASK FOR HELP

Probably one of the most disconcerting circumstances for anyone to be in is the sudden recognition of "being in over your head." Everyone has limitations to their abilities, no matter the endeavor. Awareness of personal limitations and the development of a protocol for consultation or referral are essential to conducting a quality, safe exercise program.

It is often prudent and sometimes essential to either consult or correspond with your client's family physician when initiating an exercise program. In addition to securing medical clearance, communication with physicians can provide a valuable perspective on the client's motivation, readiness, and previous attempts at lifestyle change. Collaborative efforts with health professionals enhance the opportunity to design optimal programming for each client.

Clients should always consult with their physician or other health professional if their health status changes. In the case of significant or sudden changes, suspend the exercise program until medical clearance is obtained.

Psychological disorders or conditions may prevent your client from participating successfully in an exercise program. If psychological problems are suspected, it is important to consider consulting a psychologist, psychiatrist, or family physician. There are several problem areas that you may encounter. Eating disorders **(anorexia nervosa** and **bulimia nervosa)** affect between 1 and 4% of young women, and they are marked by the following features:

 ✔ Body-image disorder (they see themselves as much fatter than others do)
 ✔ Marked (overly rapid or severe) weight loss
 ✔ Excessive concern with weight and appearance
 ✔ Extreme fear of gaining weight
 ✔ Compulsive exercising

 ✔ Purging (vomiting, or laxative or diuretic use to control weight)

Low self-esteem is common in people with eating disorders and can be a barrier to behavioral change. Here, clients may exhibit persistent dissatisfaction about their efforts and progress, be excessively self-critical, and be very resistant to your suggestions of alternative interpretation. Similarly, distorted or unrealistic thinking that endures and interferes with adherence to the program is reason for referral.

Distorted thinking, especially self-criticism, helplessness, and hopelessness, are common in depression. Other features of depression include loss of interest in people or activities, fatigue, energy loss, insomnia, sadness, guilt, and irritability. Anxiety is also common in today's society. Symptoms of anxiety disorders include irritability, fears, panic attacks (palpitations, dizziness, fear of dying or going crazy, trembling, chest pain, and shortness of breath), muscle tension, restlessness, apprehensiveness, concentration difficulties, and difficulty falling asleep. The clinical features, prevalence, and diagnostic criteria for the above disorders are thoroughly described in the Diagnostic and Statistical Manual of Mental Disorders-IV (American Psychiatric Association, 1994).

A negative change in your client's adherence or satisfaction with the program may be indicative of psychological distress. Gently inquire about concerns, thoughts, and feelings. If you suspect the possibility of psychological difficulty, express your concern and ask the client if he or she would consider talking to a physician or psychologist. This sensitive and personal area is best dealt with in a direct and compassionate manner.

Your feelings are often an effective tool in working with clients. If you feel uneasy or think that the client's needs might exceed your expertise, this is reason enough to evaluate your concern further. In short, if you feel you are in over your head, you probably are. Carefully attend to the impression that you are exerting greater effort than the client. This is often a reflection of poor motivation, or perhaps your client has reverted to a stage of contemplation rather than action. In this case, the rule could be: "If you are working harder than the client, you are probably working too hard" (Morgan, 1996). It is also an opportunity to review your client's plan and evaluate if there is an opportunity to improve its tailoring, or fit, to the client.

When there are concerns about a client's progress or suspicions of significant problems, begin by carefully reviewing the assessment data. This may yield directions for modification. It is then useful to discuss the circumstances with a colleague, who may suggest different approaches or reinforce a decision for consultation or referral with a health professional.

SUMMARY

Health psychology provides guiding principles and scientific support for exercise program development. Exercise programs must be grounded in the science of health psychology and utilize a variety of strategies tailored to each client's individual needs. Health behaviors are complex and have multiple determinants. This chapter presented a three-step protocol for behavioral management/lifestyle management consulting: assessment, teaching, and evaluation. Assessment is essential for thorough understanding and guidance in planning programs. Teaching encompasses objective and goal development, identification of behavioral strategies, and management plan implementation. Evaluation is an ongoing process throughout the program that allows revision and refinement, as well as periodic follow-up after program termination. Finally, evaluation yields data regarding program effectiveness and provides directions for program improvement.

Summary

References and Suggested Reading

REFERENCES

American Psychiatric Association (1994). *Diagnostic and Statistical Manual of Mental Disorders.* (4th ed.). Washington, D.C.: American Psychiatric Association.

Fisher, E.B. et al. (1990). State of the art: Smoking and smoking cessation. *American Review of Respiratory Diseases,* 142, 702–720.

Glanz, K., Rimer, B.K., & Lewis, F.M. (2002). *Health Behavior and Health Education: Theory, Research and Practice.* San Francisco: Jossey-Bass.

Goldstein, M.G. et al. (1990). Behavioral Medicine for Medical Patients. In: Stroudmire, A. *Clinical Psychiatry for Medical Students*, Philadelphia: Lippincott.

Jones, D.A. et al. (1998). Moderate leisure-time physical activity: Who is meeting the public health recommendations? A national cross-sectional study. *Archives of Family Medicine,* 7, 285–289.

McGinnis, J.M & Foege, W.H. (1993). Actual causes of death in the United States. *Journal of the American Medical Association,* 270, 18, 2207–2212.

Morgan, G.D. (1996). Health Behavior Psychology. In: Cotton, R. (Ed.) *Lifestyle and Weight Management Consultant Manual,* San Diego: American Council on Exercise.

Prochaska, J.O., DiClemente, C.C., & Norcross, J.C. (1992). In search of how people change: Applications to addictive behaviors. *American Psychologist,* 47, 1102–1114.

Prochaska, J.O. & Goldstein, M.G. (1991). Process of smoking cessation. *Clinics in Chest Medicine,* 12, 727–735.

Taylor, R.B., Ureda, J.R., & Denham, J.W. (1982). *Health Promotion: Principles and Clinical Applications.* Norwalk, Conn.: Prentice-Hall.

U.S. Department of Health and Human Services (1996). *Physical Activity and Health: A Report of the Surgeon General.* Atlanta, Georgia: U.S. Department of Health and Human Services, Public Health Service, CDC, National Center for Chronic Disease Prevention and Health Promotion.

SUGGESTED READING

Bolton, R. (1986). *People Skills.* Carmichael, Calif.: Touchstone Books.

Boothman, N. (2000). *How to Make People Like You in 90 Seconds or Less.* New York: Workman Publishing.

Carkhuff, R.R. & Anthony, W.A. (1999). *The Skills of Helping.* Amherst: Human Resource Development Press.

Covey, S.R. (2004). *The Seven Habits of Highly Effective People: Powerful Lessons in Personal Change.* New York: Simon & Schuster.

Covey, S.R., Merrill, A.R., & Merrill, R.R. (1996). *First Things First.* New York: Simon & Schuster

Csikszentmihalyi, M. (1991). *Flow: The Psychology of Optimal Experience.* New York: HarperCollins.

Goleman, D. (2006). *Emotional Intelligence: When It Can Matter More Than Your I.Q.* New York: Bantam Books.

Jacobson, D., Kauchak, D., & Eggen, P.D. (1992). *Methods for Teaching: A Skills Approach* (4th ed.). New York: Macmillan College Division.

Kauchak, D.P. & Eggen, P.E. (2002). *Learning and Teaching: Research-based Methods* (4th ed.). Needham Heights, Mass.: Allyn & Bacon.

Krumboltz, J. (1966). *Stating the Goals of Counseling* (Monograph No. 1). Fullerton: California Personnel and Guidance Association.

Malouf, D. (1999). *Power Up Your People Skills: Communication in the New Millennium.* Australia. Australian Print Group.

Martens, R. (2004). *Successful Coaching.* (3rd ed.). Champaign, Ill.: Human Kinetics.

Mosston, M. (1966). *Teaching Physical Education: From Command to Discovery.* Columbus: Merrill.

O'Connor, J. & McDermott, I. (2001). *Way of NLP.* London. Thorsons Publishing.

Okun, B.F. (2001). *Effective Helping: Interviewing and Counseling Techniques.* Belmont, Calif.: Wadsworth Publishing Company.

Rogers, C. (1995). *On Becoming a Person.* New York: Houghton Mifflin.

Vernacchia, R. et al. (1996). *Coaching Mental Excellence.* Portola Valley, Calif.: Warde Publishers.

Injury
Prevention
and First Aid

Musculoskeletal Injuries

Denise Fandel is the executive director of the National Athletic Trainers' Association Board of Certification (NATABOC). Ms. Fandel

Denise M. Fandel

served for 15 years at the University of Nebraska at Omaha, where she managed the athletic training service and education programs. She is also a contributing author to numerous textbooks on athletic training, sports medicine, and athletic injuries.

Musculoskeletal injuries are probably the most common injuries that occur in active individuals. They also are one of the most common reasons people stop being active. To help prevent musculoskeletal injuries, you must focus on the following areas when developing a total fitness program for your clients: strength, flexibility, muscular endurance, and balance. Even when programs are designed properly, injuries can happen. However, a properly conditioned client can rehabilitate an injured area quickly and more completely.

TYPES OF TISSUE

Four tissues of the body are of concern when discussing musculoskeletal injuries: muscle, **tendon, ligament,** and bone. Each has individual characteristics that, when understood, can help you prevent musculoskeletal injuries.

Muscle Tissue

Muscle tissue is elastic and able to withstand an enormous amount of stress. Muscle tissues act as springs for the body by absorbing a tremendous amount of shock. They also facilitate movement. Preventing injuries to the muscles and the joints is dependent upon a muscle being strong and flexible. Flexibility in any exercise program is important for preventing injuries.

An injury to muscle tissue is called a **strain.** Strains are classified as mild, moderate, or severe. A severe strain may be called a rupture or complete tear. These injuries heal with scar tissue, known as **collagen** tissue, that is not elastic. The collagen tissue goes to the injury site and is laid down in an unorganized pattern. If left in this unorganized state, the tissue will be very weak. Therefore, it is important that some stretching be initiated to help the collagen tissue organize. Stretching and the gradual addition of strengthening exercises will cause the tissue to "line up" in the direction of the surrounding muscle fibers. This organization increases the strength of the collagen tissue. However, even in an organized state, this tissue will not be as strong or flexible as the surrounding uninjured tissue.

Tendon Tissue

Another part of a muscle group that can be injured is the tendon, which connects muscle to bone. The tendon area of muscle is supplied with less blood than is the belly of the muscle. Because of this anatomical difference, injuries to tendons heal more slowly.

Ligament Tissue

Ligaments are made up of nonelastic tissue designed to connect bone to bone. They are found around joints, and when injured, they do not contract as muscle tissues do to protect the area. Once stretched, the ligaments allow for unwanted motion at the joint, thereby necessitating increased strengthening of surrounding muscle tissues.

Joint capsules, larger versions of ligaments that surround joints, provide stability. They may be injured in more severe **sprains** and can result in serious dislocations and **subluxations.**

Bone Tissue

Bone is the only tissue in the body that, when injured, repairs itself with exactly the same type of tissue. Bone can develop cracks from abnormal types and amounts of stress, resulting in stress fractures. Complete breaks in the bone also are called fractures. They result from excessive stresses and usually involve a large amount of trauma. When a client complains of pinpoint pain over a bone, or of hearing or feeling a "snap," you should consider the possibility of a fracture and refer him or her to a physician. It is not true that "if you can move it, it isn't broken."

TISSUE REACTION TO INJURY—INFLAMMATION AND THE HEALING PROCESS

When tissue is injured or damaged, the body immediately begins the repair process, beginning with inflammation, which acts as a protective, as well as a healing, mechanism. Some relate the process to an army fixing a weak spot in a line that has been penetrated by the enemy. The body's main transportation system is the circulatory system. It transports the foot soldiers, the white blood cells, to the area of injury. Here, the white blood cells encircle the injury containing it and thereby preventing damage to other tissues.

Injuries can often be recognized by the swelling, black and blue color (ecchymosis), pain, and decreased range of motion that accompanies them. These are just a few of the signals that the body is defending itself from the injury and is repairing the damage. You must recognize these signs and symptoms and provide proper referral to a medical professional. In addition, if appropriate, you must provide the proper instruction for participation in exercise that will not make the injury worse.

Signs and Symptoms of Inflammation

The body is a predictable machine when handling injuries. Tissue that is injured relies on the inflammatory reaction for its early defense and to begin the healing process. It is important for you to be able to recognize the following signs and symptoms of inflammation:

Increased temperature is the result of an increase in blood flow to the injured area due to damaged blood vessels and the need to supply the area with increased numbers of white blood cells. Much as the body develops a generalized fever when ill, an injury to a soft tissue of the body causes a "local fever." This is why heat, hot packs, or hot soaks, are not used on a new injury. Why turn up the heat under a boiling kettle?

Redness is due to the increase in blood flow to the area.

Swelling also is due to the increase in blood flow to the area. Additionally, damage to the cells, small capillaries, and lymphatic vessels in the area may allow the leaking of some fluid.

Pain is often due to pressure on nerve endings from increased swelling.

Loss of function is caused by swelling in the area and "guarding" of the muscles surrounding the injury. This also produces an increase in pain.

ACUTE TREATMENT OF MUSCULOSKELETAL INJURIES

Acute Treatment of Musculoskeletal Injuries

The acronym RICE is the most common method of describing the **acute** treatment for musculoskeletal injuries. This acronym stands for Rest, Ice, Compression, and Elevation, the four steps of the accepted first aid standard for the treatment of these types of injuries.

Though swelling is a key protective mechanism and a part of the healing process, it is still important to reduce swelling. Little can be done to stop initial swelling, but the RICE principle can be applied to reduce secondary swelling, which occurs when injuries are not properly treated. Secondary swelling slows the healing process and decreases one's ability to safely participate in activity.

Remember that it may not always be prudent to actually apply treatment to an injury. Check with local governing associations for the most current standards for providing emergency treatment. Of course, the more education you have in first aid and injury management, the more comfortable you will feel if an injury situation develops. Therefore, the guidelines for RICE are included below:

Rest	Avoid continuing the activity that has caused injury or will make the injury worse.
Ice	Ice should be applied for 20 to 30 minutes. There should be some sort of insulating layer between the skin and the ice to prevent frostbite. Never apply ice to an already numb area.
Compression	Elastic bandages can help prevent or reduce excessive swelling. The elastic bandage should always reach from the largest muscle area below the injury to the largest muscle group above the injury.

Elevation

The force of gravity can reduce swelling. After applying the first three steps, raise the injured area as high as possible while still being comfortable. The injured areas should be raised at least level with, or slightly above, the heart.

Flexibility and Musculoskeletal Injuries

Flexibility is described by some as the key to longevity. A flexible muscle is better able to absorb shock and periodic overstretching than an inflexible muscle. Unfortunately, some believe that if a little **flexibility** is good then more must be better. When it comes to injury prevention, however, this is not always the case.

A client's flexibility should be compared to that of the average population. If their measurements fall below what is considered normal for flexibility (hypoflexible), they should be instructed in a solid, well-designed flexibility program. These clients are more prone to muscle injuries, strains, and ruptures. Conversely, if their measurements are above normal (hyperflexible), their program should place more emphasis on strength development (Anderson, Hall, & Martin, 2000; Pfeiffer & Mangus, 1998). These clients are at increased risk of joint dislocations and **subluxations**. Guidelines for the development of the flexibility program are discussed in Chapter 10.

EXERCISE TECHNIQUE AND PRE-EXISTING JOINT INJURIES

Working with clients who have pre-existing joint injuries is often a challenge. Postural conditions such as "knock-knee" and "sway back" often make certain activities difficult. Clients who are loose-jointed or have joint injuries may not be able to perform all exercises using traditional methods and body positions. It is critical that you strictly reinforce the importance of proper technique for these clients. Correct exercise technique is essential to a safe, effective, and enjoyable exercise experience.

PRE-EXISTING CONDITIONS AND EXERCISE SELECTION

You may have a client who has had previous injuries, which makes it a bit more difficult to design safe and effective personalized programs. The medical history form each client completes should list any previous injuries, surgeries, or conditions that have made exercise difficult in the past. The medical staff working with the client will dictate when it is safe to begin exercising again.

FIGURE 16.1

Impingement of bursa and supraspinatus under the coracoacromial arch with abduction movement.

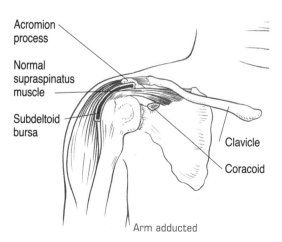

Acromion process

Normal supraspinatus muscle

Subdeltoid bursa

Clavicle

Coracoid

Arm adducted

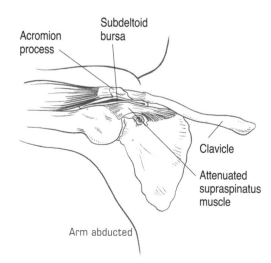

Acromion process

Subdeltoid bursa

Clavicle

Attenuated supraspinatus muscle

Arm abducted

They may provide additional information or suggestions for the exercise program. With this information and guidance, you can design a safe, effective, and personalized program for your clients.

Upper-extremity Conditions

Impingement syndrome makes it difficult to perform exercises that require the arms to be above the head for extended periods of time (Figure 16.1). Exercises such as overhead presses, military presses, lat pulldowns, and incline presses may aggravate this condition (Anderson, Hall, & Martin, 2000; Starkey & Ryan, 2001; Pfeiffer & Mangus, 1998). It is up to you to substitute nonaggravating exercises.

Individuals with dislocating shoulders are usually more susceptible to injury when the shoulders are in an abducted and externally rotated position, such as the starting position of a lat pulldown or behind-the-neck overhead press. Most commonly, the front, or anterior, ligaments of the shoulder have been stretched. When the client places their shoulder in this position, the shoulder is more likely to "slip" forward and recreate the dislocation.

Avoiding these positions is critical. You may want to "block" the full range of motion for these individuals. For example, a client can perform the bench press on a machine where the trainer can place a pin in the weight stack after the handle has been lifted up to a safe position. A second pin can then be used to set the desired weight. This will protect the shoulder from excessive abduction and external rotation.

Lateral epicondylitis and medial epicondylitis are similar conditions (Figure 16.2). They most commonly result from a lack of flexibility and overuse of the flexor and extensor groups of the forearm, especially when beginning a new exercise. "Tennis elbow" is a common name for lateral epicondylitis. The pain is located at the elbow on the radial, or thumb, side. "Little League elbow" is the common name for

Inflamed extensor tendon

Lateral epicondyle of humerus

Extensor muscles of forearm

FIGURE 16.2
Lateral epicondylitis, or "tennis elbow."

medial epicondylitis and describes the inflammation on the opposite side of the elbow. Both conditions respond well to conservative treatment by medical professionals. You should understand these conditions and implement appropriate flexibility exercises for these muscle groups. In addition, refrain from any activities that may aggravate the condition.

Carpal tunnel syndrome (CTS), a peripheral neuropathy caused by entrapment of the median nerve, is most commonly seen as an occupational illness (Figure 16.3). It is usually seen in persons who do repetitive, fine-motor tasks, such as

Musculocutaneous nerve

Radial nerve

Ulnar nerve

Median nerve

FIGURE 16.3
The nerves of the wrist, highlighting the median nerve. (Source: *Human Anatomy*, 3rd ed., by Martini, F.H., Timmons, M.J., & McKinley, M.P. Copyright 2000. Reprinted by permission of Pearson Education.)

typing or working on a cash register. It also can result from resistance training and other athletic activities (Anderson, Hall, & Martin, 2000; Starkey & Ryan, 2001; Pfeiffer & Mangus, 1998). Individuals with CTS may complain of numbness in the middle fingers of their hands, usually after doing some kind of repetitive work using the wrist and finger flexor muscles. Clients with CTS should avoid resistance training during periods of acute flare-up. They should also avoid wrist flexion, forearm supination, and pressure to the base of the palm such as when leaning on the handle bars of a piece of aerobic exercise equipment. Once again, flexibility plays a key role in preventing and treating the symptoms of carpal tunnel. The flexor group should receive extra flexibility attention to prevent this injury. Physician referral may be necessary if symptoms persist.

Lower-extremity Conditions

Ankle sprains, one of the most common athletic-related injuries, may be prevented through the proper use of proprioceptive training, proper footwear, and ankle bracing.

The most common ankle injury is a sprain of the ligaments on the **lateral** side, or outside, of the ankle (Figure 16.4). Sprains to the **medial** side, or inside, of the ankle are relatively rare. Because the lateral aspect of the ankle is more frequently injured, you should focus on strengthening the peroneal muscles to prevent, or reduce the severity of, an injury.

Proprioceptive training can be as simple as rope skipping. Many footwork drills also can increase ankle **proprioception.** If an ankle has been recently sprained, basic proprioceptive training may be as simple as having the client stand on the injured ankle and try to maintain balance.

Research has confirmed that the use of ankle braces may decrease the incidence of ankle sprains without sacrificing speed or agility (Bot & van Mechelen, 1999). However, convincing clients of this may prove difficult if they have had a negative experience or have no experience with bracing.

Knee ligament injuries are often the most feared among active individuals. The knee is an inherently unstable joint and depends heavily on muscular strength for its dynamic support. Muscle strength should be balanced so the hamstrings have 60 to 70% of the strength of the quadriceps.

The medial collateral ligament (MCL) is located on the inside, or medial aspect, of the knee (Figure 16.5). The medial side is the major weightbearing side of the knee. A sprain of the MCL can lead to varying degrees of disability, so you must take care not to stress it when performing activities such as squats, multidirectional lunges, slide board, and lower-extremity flexibility exercis-

FIGURE 16.4
Lateral ankle sprain.

Shin bone (tibia)
Fibula
Anterior talofibular ligament
Ankle bone (talus)
Calcancofibular ligament
Heel bone (calcaneus)

Femur
Anterior cruciate ligament
Lateral meniscus
Splint bone (fibula)
Posterior cruciate ligament
Medial collateral ligament
Medial meniscus
Shin bone (tibia)

FIGURE 16.5
Knee joint anatomy depicting the anterior cruciate ligament (ACL), the medial collateral ligament (MCL), and the medial and lateral menisci.

es (Anderson, Hall, & Martin, 2000; Starkey & Ryan, 2001; Pfeiffer & Mangus, 1998).

Anterior cruciate ligament (ACL) injuries are the most dreaded of the knee injuries (see Figure 16.5). The importance of a healthy ACL in an active individual has been demonstrated by the large number of athletes who have been able to rehabilitate an injury to it completely and return to pre-injury form. You must have solid communication with the client's orthopedic surgeon and certified athletic trainer or physical therapist to determine the limitations of activity for the client. No two surgeries are exactly alike. Also, no two surgeons or therapists will use the same rehabilitation protocol. You will most likely be supervising upper-body strengthening and cardiovascular training early in the rehabilitation process, and lower-extremity and functional activities as the process moves into the later months (Anderson, Hall, & Martin, 2000; Pfeiffer & Mangus, 1998).

The knee cap joint, also called the patellofemoral joint, is a common site of pain (Figure 16.6), which has been referred to by different terms, such as runner's knee and jumper's knee. It is generally caused by two things: decreased hamstring and calf flexibility, or improper tracking of the patella (kneecap) in the femoral groove. You can work with the client on hamstring and calf flexibility exercises to reduce the stress on the quadriceps. If there is a tracking problem, this will be diagnosed by a medical professional. Physical therapists or certified athletic trainers will work with the client on the specifics of this problem. Generally, there will be a substitution for knee extension exercises.

Eccentric strength training should be stressed for clients who seem predisposed to injuries in this area. The patellofemoral joint is under constant eccentric stress during **ballistic** activities such as running and jumping. This stress is similar to that placed on a car's brakes. The quadriceps muscles are constantly absorbing shock and decelerating the leg. If the muscles are not trained eccentrically, they will fatigue earlier. This fatigue can lead to changes in the client's movements and sometimes a substitution of other muscles to absorb the shock to the lower extremity. Unfortunately, it is not a common practice in most conditioning programs to do

Pre-existing Conditions and Exercise Selection

FIGURE 16.6
Injuries of the patella. The roughened area on the undersurface marks the region of chondromalacia and patellofemoral pain syndrome. The frayed area is the region of patellar tendinitis.

Kneecap (patella)

Patellar tendon

FIGURE 16.7
Shin splints. The darkened area marks the most common region of pain.

Tibialis anterior

eccentric training of the quadriceps group. A complete conditioning program should emphasize some of this type of training.

Shin splint syndrome is a term often used to describe any pain in the lower leg (Figure 16.7). Shin splint syndrome may be the result of decreased flexibility of the Achilles tendon and posterior muscles of the calf, decreased strength of the anterior muscles of the lower leg, fallen arches, or flat feet. Once again, the lower leg is the initial shock absorber during activities. If the shock-absorbing system begins to fail, the client may begin to experience pain. Shin splint syndrome pain will decrease when the aggravating activity is stopped (Anderson, Hall, & Martin, 2000; Starkey & Ryan, 2001; Pfeiffer & Mangus, 1998). It is important that the client be referred to a medical professional to rule out the possibility of a stress fracture. The medical professional will often prescribe flexibility and strengthening exercises for the lower leg and/or shoe orthotics for corrective support.

Stress fractures are commonly seen in the lower extremities (Figure 16.8). The most common sites are the lower one-third of the medial tibia and the third, fourth, and fifth metatarsals of the foot.

Stress fractures are the result of excessive stress on the bone that causes the outer lining of the bone, the periosteum, to crack. The periosteum is one of the most sensitive structures in the body, and cracking is the initial cause of pain. Small cracks will initially produce pain only with activity, but as the stress fracture progresses, the pain will occur outside the activity.

Some biomechanical and postural considerations can contribute to the healing of stress fractures. Clients with "knock-knee" or flat feet have decreased shock absorption ability. These conditions must be evaluated by a medical professional.

The spine is another common site of injury. The lower back is often injured due

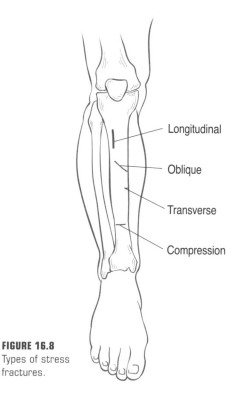

FIGURE 16.8
Types of stress fractures.

Longitudinal

Oblique

Transverse

Compression

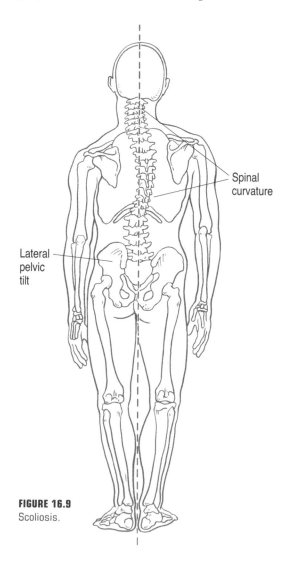

Spinal curvature

Lateral pelvic tilt

FIGURE 16.9
Scoliosis.

to excessive stress, such as using improper techniques when lifting objects. Poor posture also can contribute to low-back pain.

You may have a client who has a predisposing condition such as **scoliosis** (Figure 16.9). This is an abnormal lateral curvature of the thoracic spine that places abnormal stress on the muscles of the upper back. The muscles on the side away from the curvature are stretched while the muscles on the opposite side are pinched. You may have to work with the client to balance strength and flexibility. If the client has problems with the upper spine, he or she should be evaluated by a medical professional before significantly modifying the strength program.

Another spine condition that you may see, especially in older clients, is **kyphosis** (see pages 74–76). This is sometimes called a "hunchback" or a dowager's hump. It is an excessive posterior curvature of the upper thoracic spine. This condition places increased stress on the upper trapezius, cervical spine, and rhomboids. You should work in close communication with the client's physicians to determine the best exercises for the condition.

The final, and probably most common, spinal condition is excessive **lordosis.** This is an abnormal or excessive curvature of the lower back, sometimes called "swayback." Weak abdominal muscles and poor posture contribute to pain in this area, so emphasizing abdominal strengthening and hamstring flexibility is important.

If a client complains of low-back pain, encourage him or her to be evaluated by a physician. A condition that can mimic some of the common muscular pain patterns of the lower back is **spondylolysis.** This is a stress fracture of the vertebrae of the spine. Those who do heavy lifting as a part of their jobs and athletes and active people who perform squats or Olympic-style lifts can develop spondylolysis. Strengthening for these clients may demand a creative approach to protect the lower back during exercise.

ENVIRONMENTAL IMPACT ON INJURIES

One of the caveats of human physiology is that the body is constantly in search of balance or **homeostasis.** Environmental conditions can wreak havoc on the body (Anderson, Hall, & Martin, 2000; Starkey & Ryan, 2001; Pfeiffer & Mangus, 1998). Encourage clients to maintain a proper hydration level to prevent adverse reactions to the environment.

To ensure that there is an adequate amount of water in the body, an active individual should consume a minimum of 8 to 10 8-ounce glasses of water each day. If this is done, the color of the urine in an active person who is not taking any supplements will be clear. Supplements and some medicines will make the urine appear a dark yellow to orange, no matter how much water is consumed.

When an active individual loses too much water, one of three conditions related to heat illness, or **hyperthermia,** are likely to occur: heat cramps, heat exhaustion, or heat stroke. Heat stroke is the most serious of the three and is considered a true medical emergency.

Recognizing the signs and symptoms of heat illness is important. **Heat cramps** are usually seen in the dominant, active muscles such as the gastrocnemius and abdominals. A person who is suffering from **heat exhaustion** may look pale, and have cool, clammy skin and a rapid, weak pulse. They may sweat profusely, yet exhibit a normal body temperature for an active individual. The person suffering from **heat stroke** will most likely have hot, red, and dry skin. Their core body temperature will be elevated, sometimes as high as 105° F (40.6° C). They are usually not sweating because the body is trying to conserve body fluids.

Immediate care for the victim of a heat-related condition is simple. Stop the exercise session, remove the client from the hot environmental conditions, activate

Environmental Impact on Injuries

EMS, and, if conscious, give fluids until proper medical assistance arrives. For the client with heat cramps, stretching can be helpful.

If a client is exercising in a cold environment, be mindful of the possibility of **hypothermia** (low core body temperature) and/or frostbite. Attention to proper clothing can prevent many cold-related injuries. Layering clothes and using hats, mittens, ear protection, and nose covering will prevent the majority of injuries related to cold.

A person who is the victim of hypothermia will initially display signs or symptoms of the physiologic response to decreasing body core temperature (i.e., shivering and cold extremities caused by the shunting of blood to the body core to conserve heat). As the core temperature continues to fall, all bodily functions are progressively depressed (e.g., heart rate and respiratory rate decrease, reflexes become slower, speech becomes slurred). First aid for those suffering from mild hypothermia is to remove them from the cold environment, warm them as quickly and gently as possible, and, if conscious, give warm fluids. Frostbite occurs as a consequence of the body's attempts to prevent heat loss. Vasoconstriction in the skin causes reduced blood flow, so the skin rapidly cools. This reduced blood flow, combined with the lack of oxygen and nutrients, causes the skin tissue to die. Moderate to severe cases of hypothermia require treatment under the direction of a physician and should be handled as an urgent medical emergency. Those with frostbite should not rub or massage the frozen tissue. This will only cause more significant tissue damage.

RECORD KEEPING FOR THE PERSONAL TRAINER

Prevention of injuries comes from expecting the unexpected. If you have some knowledge of the medical history of a client, you will be, at the minimum, more prepared. The use of medical history forms and emergency in-

formation forms is essential in case of an emergency or injury. For any conditions noted on the medical history form, ask the client for additional information. When possible, note any musculoskeletal injuries and ask for information from the client's medical professionals.

These documents are, of course, confidential and should be kept in a secure location and never released without the permission of the client.

It also is pertinent that you keep detailed records of your conversations with, and observations of, those clients who have known injuries or illness while under your supervision. These notes should be completed daily and include the client's level of activity and progress toward recovery. Keep these records in a secure location.

SUMMARY

You will most likely deal with clients who have sustained, or will sustain, musculoskeletal injuries in the course of their activities, supervised or unsupervised.

Avoid exercises that aggravate pre-existing conditions. An understanding of how the body reacts to injury and the resulting repair will help you plan an appropriate program. Recognizing the signs and symptoms of inflammation and knowing the proper steps in acute injury care can help the injured client recover more quickly.

It also is important for you to know the common injuries associated with activity. The ability to design a program for a client that will avoid injury is critical to the success of the program.

Receive as much training as is available in first aid and injury recognition. This will increase your confidence in dealing with your clients in these types of situations.

REFERENCES

Anderson, M.K, Hall, S.J., & Martin, M. (2000). *Sports Injury Management.* (2nd ed.). Philadelphia: Lippincott Williams & Wilkins.

Bot, S.D. & van Mechelen, W. (1999). The effect of ankle bracing on athletic performance. *Sports Medicine,* 27, 3, 171–178.

Pfeiffer, R.P. & Mangus, B.C. (1998). *Concepts of Athletic Training.* (2nd ed.). New York: Jones & Bartlett.

Starkey, C. & Ryan, J. (2001). *Evaluation of Orthopedic Athletic Injury.* Philadelphia: F. A. Davis.

SUGGESTED READING

Arnheim, D. & Prentice, W. (2005). *Principles of Athletic Training.* (12th ed.). St. Louis: Mosby.

Booher, J. & Thibodeau, G. (1999). *Athletic Injury Assessment.* (4th ed.). St. Louis: Mosby.

Galaspy, J. & May, J. (2001). *Signs and Symptoms of Athletic Injuries.* New York: McGraw-Hill.

McComas, A.J. (2005). *Skeletal Muscle: Form and Function.* (2nd ed.). Champaign, Ill.: Human Kinetics.

Street, S.A. & Runkle, D. (2000). Athletic Protective Equipment. New York: McGraw-Hill.

Taber's Cyclopedic Medical Dictionary. (2001). (19th ed.). Philadelphia: F. A. Davis.

Watkins, J. (1999). *Structure and Function of the Musculoskeletal System.* Champaign, Ill.: Human Kinetics.

Whiting, W.C. & Zernicke, R.F. (1998). *Biomechanics of Musculoskeletal Injury.* Champaign, Ill.: Human Kinetics.

References and Suggested Reading

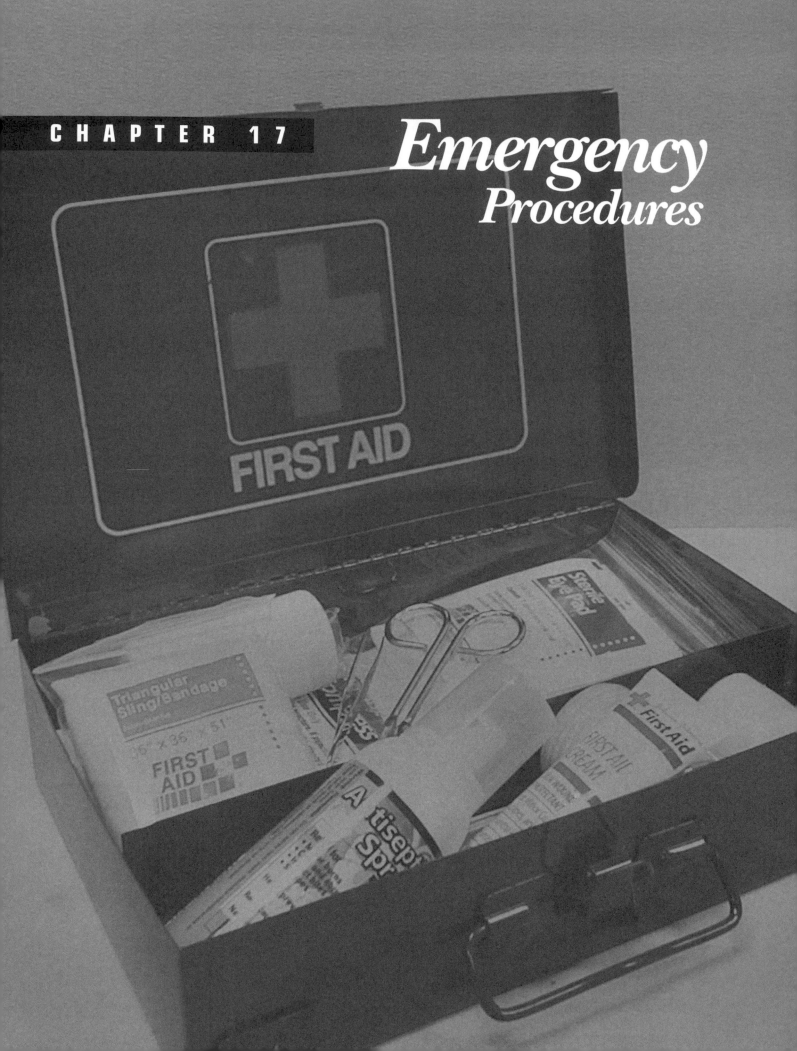

Emergency
Procedures

FIRST AID

Kathleen M. Hargarten

Kathleen M. Hargarten, M.D., F.A.C.E.P., is an assistant professor at the Medical College of Wisconsin, is the medical director of the Watertown Memorial Hospital in Wisconsin, and has served as medical director for paramedic and emergency medical technicians in Southeast Wisconsin. She is board certified in emergency medicine and is a fellow of the American College of Emergency Physicians. She is a past member of the American Council on Exercise's group fitness instructor and personal trainer examination committees.

As a personal trainer, you encourage your clients to realize a healthier lifestyle through exercise and improved nutrition, minimizing the risk of injury. However, no matter how knowledgeable you are or how well-designed your program, a medical crisis or acute injury may occur. Although most people who actively engage in regular physical activity are healthy adults with no serious medical problems, some may have an underlying disease that has not yet manifested itself. Appropriate health screening and fitness testing before an exercise program begins will help identify these persons. You can then simply refer them to their physicians for medical clearance, thereby forestalling emergency conditions. But what if the unforeseen happens? Knowing what to do during those first critical moments, or how to access the emergency medical system, can make the difference between life and death, between temporary and permanent disability, between rapid recovery and a long hospital stay.

This chapter will familiarize you with several procedures for preventing and coping with emergencies. Although the following information is a good overview of first-aid procedures, it is not comprehensive nor is it a substitute for formal training in first aid. As a personal trainer, you should take a first aid and basic injury prevention and treatment course (www.acefitness.org/calendar/aha_events.aspx). You also are required to take a course and become certified in airway management and cardiopulmonary resuscitation (CPR). Should injury or medical conditions arise, refer clients to their physicians for diagnosis and medical advice.

EMERGENCY EQUIPMENT AND EMERGENCY MEDICAL SERVICES

Whether you work in a health club, out of a home, or in clients' homes, you need a telephone and first-aid kit nearby. Rapid access to a telephone is vital for contact with emergency medical personnel if they are needed. The first-aid kit should be sys-

tematically maintained and stocked with the following supplies:

For airway management:
✔ CPR microshield or pocket mask with one-way valve for protected mouth-to-mouth ventilations (Figure 17.1)

For assessing circulation:
✔ sphygmomanometer (blood pressure cuff)
✔ stethoscope
✔ penlight or flashlight

For general wound management:
✔ personal protective equipment, including latex gloves, mask, and eye protection
✔ sterile gauze dressings (medium and larger sizes)
✔ adhesive tape (1- and 2-inch sizes)
✔ bandage scissors
✔ liquid soap (if soap is unavailable in the workplace)

For suspected sprains or fractures:
✔ splinting material (see Fractures, page 455)
✔ chemical cold pack, or ice and plastic bag
✔ compression wrap

You should check the first-aid kit at least every three months to replace outdated items and become familiar with the contents. Any items used from the kit should be immediately replaced. Tape a list of contents to the inside cover so that nothing will be inadvertently omitted during restocking.

Automated External Defibrillators

Automated External Defibrillators (AEDs), portable electronic devices used to restore normal heart rhythms in victims of sudden cardiac arrest, have become increasingly common in health clubs and fitness centers. When used correctly, AEDs can be key to survival. Survival rates as high as 90% have been

FIGURE 17.1
Mouth-to-mask ventilations: A mask with a one-way valve prevents contact with a victim's face during mouth-to-mouth resuscitation. Small pocket masks (below) are effective, inexpensive, and convenient.

reported if defibrillation is achieved within the first minute of a sudden cardiac arrest, with time being of the utmost importance. For every minute that passes without defibrillation, the victim's chance of survival drops by 7 to 10%. After 12 minutes, the survival rate can be as low as 5% (American College of Sports Medicine & American Heart Association, 2002).

You should seek training and certification in the proper use of AEDs to increase the overall safety of your clients and of your workout environment (please check www.acefitness.org/calendar/aha_events.aspx for more information regarding AED training in your area). See page 473 for information on the legal issues surrounding the use of AEDs.

Accessing the Emergency Medical Services System

Every personal trainer needs a well-thought-out plan of action, for any emergency, that takes into account services available in the community. When an emergency occurs, you must know how to activate the **emergency medical services (EMS) system** and who to call for immediate stabilization of a person in critical condition. Most cities have a 911 telephone number that will automatically set the EMS system in motion. Note: If possible, it is better to call 911 from a land line rather than a cell phone. From a land line, the operator is able to access the address, phone number and the person's name to whom the phone is billed. When someone dials 911, a dispatcher trained in recognizing emergencies will answer the telephone and ask questions that help determine which medical unit is needed. You must be prepared to provide the name, address, and telephone number of your location. The dispatcher will ask questions about the sex and approximate age of the victim, the nature of the illness or injury (for example, level of consciousness, respiratory difficulty, location of pain, presence of trauma or bleeding), and past medical history that may affect the victim's condition.

This information becomes important for the dispatcher so that the appropriate emergency medical unit can be sent. There are several types of pre-hospital personnel that may respond to the emergency at hand. Emergency medical technicians (EMTs) are trained to recognize the nature and seriousness of a patient's illness or injury and to provide basic care to sustain life and prevent further injury. This basic care includes splinting fractures, handling simple wounds, controlling bleeding, maintaining open airways, and administering CPR. Some EMTs also are trained in **defibrillation,** which involves delivering an electric shock to a victim in cardiac arrest in an attempt to restart the heartbeat. Some may be trained in inserting an advanced airway, administering epinephrine (EpiPen) for serious allergic reactions and glucagon shots for insulin reaction. Paramedics, on the other hand, are specially trained to administer advanced care and work under direct physician supervision, usually by radio. With approximately 1,000 hours of training, they are qualified to perform many lifesaving procedures, such as interpreting heart rhythm, managing advanced airways, starting intravenous fluids for shock, administering multiple medications, and performing simple lifesaving surgical procedures. Clearly, any victim of a potentially life-threatening emergency needs a paramedic's services immediately. When in doubt about which help is needed, contact the EMS to be safe.

EMERGENCY ASSESSMENT

Most injuries or illnesses allow enough time for you to obtain a history, perform a brief examination, obtain assistance from emergency systems, and provide reassurance to the victim. Unfortunately, a few situations require prompt action to save a life. Any condition that prevents the victim from breathing adequately or getting enough oxygen could cause death. A few basic principles will help you to identify these situations and act appropriately.

Oxygen, the basic fuel for sustaining life, is required by the cells of all the body's organs to carry out their functions. The three vital organs that must function to sustain life are the heart, lungs, and brain. The heart is a muscle that acts as a pump, supplying oxygen-rich blood to the cells through the arteries, and then returns oxygen-depleted blood back to the lungs through the veins. The brain coordinates most of our functions, including movement, sensation, emotion, speech, wakefulness, sleep, and thought. The lower brain level coordinates body functioning, as well as life-support systems, such as respiration and arterial blood pressure. Important for sustaining life, these brain cells are so sensitive to oxygen depletion that they will die within minutes after circulation to the brain stops.

Although many types of injuries and medical emergencies may occur, anything affecting your client's airway (A), breathing (B), or circulation (C) must be promptly acted on. The most obvious example is a person who suffers a cardiac arrest. An asthma attack, airway obstruction, injury to the trachea, heart attack, or heavy hemorrhage from a wound has the potential to be just as serious a threat to life. When assessing an injury or illness, ask the ABC questions:

A. Does this person have a compromised **A**irway?
B. Is this person **B**reathing adequately?
C. Is **C**irculation preventing blood and oxygen from getting to their heart, lungs, or brain?

Once you have identified a true emergency, you must respond rapidly and appropriately.

You need two skills to determine the nature of an emergency: (1) the ability to extract key information from the victim and other people around; and (2) the ability to assess the condition of the victim. If

the victim is awake and responding, you may ask what problems he or she is experiencing and whether these problems have occurred before. Usually, the victim can talk about what is wrong: "My asthma is acting up again," "I'm having chest pain that feels the same as my last heart attack," "I think I broke my ankle," or "I'm having an insulin reaction." The victim may even give information about the help needed: "My inhaler is in the locker room," "If you could get my nitroglycerine pills from my purse, I think I'll be fine," or "I need some sugar to reverse my insulin reaction."

Unfortunately, it is not always this easy. If the victim is unconscious, cannot breathe easily, or has never experienced these symptoms before, you must rely on physical assessment of the victim for answers. The **primary assessment** includes rapid examination to identify life-threatening or disabling circumstances. When help is on the way and the victim is out of immediate danger—breathing without assistance, bleeding controlled, pulses present—you can proceed to a more complete **secondary assessment.**

Primary Assessment

The purpose of the primary assessment, which may take only one or two minutes, is to identify any threats to life or limb that need immediate attention. This examination provides not only enough information to start first aid, but also valuable information for the EMS dispatcher, the paramedics, or a physician.

The first moments after an emergency occurs can be so frightening that logic and experience are insufficient; to be able to respond appropriately and rapidly enough, you need to follow a systematic approach to assessing the victim. You may recruit other people on the scene to summon the EMS once an emergency has been identified, freeing yourself to continue assessment and apply first aid.

Begin with the ABCs of basic life support. Although the canned question from the Basic Life Support (BLS) course, "Are you OK?" may seem trite, asking the victim a simple question can give an assessment of the ABCs in less than five seconds. If the victim can answer, the airway is open, breathing is sufficient to sustain life for the moment, and circulation is adequate to supply the brain with oxygen. If the victim is unable to answer a simple question, you must individually assess airway, breathing, and circulation by physical examination.

1. Assess the airway. If the victim is not breathing or is making "snoring" respirations, the airway may be obstructed. You should establish an open airway by using the head tilt–chin lift (Figure 17.2). With anyone who has sustained an injury above the clavicle (collar bone), you should suspect cervical spine injury and avoid extension of the neck. Excessive movement of the neck could convert a cervical spine fracture without neurological damage into a fracture dislocation with paralysis.

2. Look to see whether the victim's chest rises and falls. If the chest does not move, and if exhaled air cannot be felt coming from the mouth or nose, begin mouth-to-mouth or mouth-to-mask ventilations at 10 to 12 breaths per minute (see Figure 17.1).

3. Initially, give two slow breaths using a pocket mask. Allow for exhalation between breaths.

4. Look quickly for signs of bleeding, and control hemorrhage with direct pressure over the wound. Victims who are bleeding profusely will not get enough oxygen-rich blood to vital organs. Even when they are alert at first, they will go into shock and quickly lose consciousness if appropriate measures are not taken.

Secondary Assessment

Once the life-threatening needs of the victim have been addressed (airway, breathing, and circulation) and help is on the way, you can conduct a more thorough evaluation. Again, a systematic approach will prevent you from missing a subtle but

Emergency Assessment

FIGURE 17.2
The chin-lift maneuver: Tilt the head back and lift the chin to move the tongue away from the back of the throat. Check for breathing by looking at the chest and listening and feeling for breath.

important injury. The simplest method is to survey the victim from head to toe.

1. Look at the victim's general appearance. Does he or she look sick or seriously injured? Is he or she having obvious respiratory difficulty?

2. Look at the skin. Skin color and condition can give clues about amount of pain, amount of bleeding, and underlying injuries. A victim who is sweating excessively may be in severe pain. Pale, cool, clammy skin may indicate significant blood loss. Any break in the skin (lacerations, bruises, swelling, or deformity) may reveal an underlying injury.

3. Check the head and face. Look for lacerations (cuts), hematomas (bumps), or bruises, and then ask whether the victim is having pain in the neck. If any evidence of head or neck injury appears, you should immediately immobilize the victim's neck to prevent spinal-cord damage and permanent disability.

4. Observe the chest for injury. The chest should rise and fall evenly with each respiration, and the chest should be symmetrical. Look for lacerations or bruising.

5. Ask whether the victim has abdominal pain. Look for signs of obvious trauma such as bleeding or breaks in the skin.

6. Protect the spine if a fall has occurred. You can assess spinal injury by simply asking if the victim is in pain. If the person cannot answer or is unconscious, you must assume a spinal injury until proven otherwise. The victim should not be turned over

for examination but should be kept on his or her back and prevented from moving until a physician can perform an examination and order X-rays. Do not move a victim who falls in a side-lying position and is having back pain. Wait for help to arrive so the victim can be properly positioned on a backboard to immobilize the spine. Your actions may prevent permanent paralysis.

7. Check for injury to arms and legs. If swelling, discoloration, or deformity are present, prevent the victim from moving until help arrives. If the victim must be moved because of a long delay in getting help or a dangerous situation, immobilize the limb with a simple splint.

8. Perform a more thorough neurological examination. Now that the more urgent problems have been addressed, you can take a moment to ask whether the victim is noticing any weakness, numbness, or "pins-and-needles" feeling in their extremities. If the victim complains of these symptoms, you should prevent unnecessary movement and then report the symptoms to the emergency medical personnel so that they can take precautions against spinal injury. You may also reevaluate the victim's level of consciousness by repeating the same simple question asked during the primary assessment: "Are you OK?"

9. Check the respiratory rate. This vital sign provides valuable information about the severity of respiratory problems.

COMMON MEDICAL EMERGENCIES AND INJURIES

Y ou may encounter a variety of injuries and medical emergencies over the course of your career as a personal trainer. Here are some of the most common, along with guidelines for treatment.

Dyspnea (Difficult Breathing)

Labored breathing that persists after an exercise session may have several causes. The sudden feeling of **dyspnea** may result from

emotional excitement, airway obstruction, emphysema, **asthma** attack, or acute metabolic abnormalities. Victims may feel they cannot get enough air (air hunger) and may display an anxious expression. Their breathing may be audibly labored and their nostrils flared, or their neck and chest muscles may retract with each breath, indicating their distress. **Cyanosis,** a bluish discoloration, may appear around the lips and fingertips. Breathing may be rapid and shallow. If left untreated, the condition may progress to respiratory arrest. Following are basic first-aid procedures you should use with someone who is having respiratory difficulty:

1. Stop all activity immediately. Have the victim sit down in a comfortable position. Never urge a victim to lie down if they are resisting; the supine position may make the symptoms worse.

2. Question the victim about any history of medical problems. However, a victim in severe respiratory distress needs energy for the work of breathing and may not be able to respond to extended questioning.

3. If properly trained to do so, administer oxygen if it is available. Allow the victim to take inhaled medication.

4. Administer mouth-to-mouth or mouth-to-mask ventilations if the victim is unconscious and has no spontaneous respirations.

Asthma. Many asthmatics are active people who do not need to restrict their activities, but some may need occasional modifications to their exercise schedule. During an asthma attack, the smooth muscles surrounding the airway go into spasm. Mucous plugs or excessive secretions in the airway also contribute to respiratory difficulties. Most attacks result from allergic reactions to things in the environment, such as mold, pollen, dust, trees, grass, animals, and certain foods. Some people suffer asthma attacks that are influenced by the type, intensity, and duration of exercise. Some also suffer asthma attacks or more intense symptoms if they inhale cold air. During a typical asthma attack, the victim wheezes, breathing with a musical or "whistling" quality. Severe breathing difficulties will produce retracted neck and chest muscles, flared nostrils, cyanosis, and the inability to speak. A victim who cannot speak in complete sentences because of the struggle to breathe needs immediate treatment and rapid transport by paramedics. A breathing treatment via an albuterol nebulizer or advanced airway maneuvers may be necessary and delay could mean the difference between life and death.

The asthmatic client can easily manage mild symptoms by decreasing the intensity of the workout. Other asthmatics may need to use their inhalers to reverse the symptoms quickly. If the symptoms resolve, the client can continue exercising as before. Here are some steps to prevent an asthma attack:

1. Use a prolonged warm-up to prevent or reduce the symptoms of **exercise-induced asthma.**

2. Decrease the intensity and increase the duration of the aerobic phase to avoid asthma symptoms while maintaining the cardiovascular benefits of the exercise.

3. Using a medicated asthma inhaler such as albuterol before beginning exercise may prevent an asthma attack. The client should consult with a physician before using this strategy.

4. Urge clients to comply with prescribed medication and follow up with a physician to maintain an active lifestyle while controlling asthma symptoms.

Chest Pain

Chest pain can originate from any structure in or near the chest, such as the esophagus, aorta or other large blood vessels, muscles, cartilage, lungs, or heart. The most common cause of chest pain is **coronary artery disease,** which is still the number-one killer of adults in the United States. Each year, approximately 2 million people in the U.S. will be diagnosed with symptoms of coronary artery disease and 1.5 million will actually have a heart attack, of

which 500,000 will die. Half of these deaths will occur suddenly, within the first hour of the onset of symptoms. With the population of physically active older adults growing, more personal trainers may find themselves providing first aid to clients complaining of chest pain or other signs and symptoms of a heart attack.

Coronary Artery Disease. The coronary arteries supply blood rich in oxygen to the myocardium (heart muscle). When plaque build-up or a spasm of the artery wall impedes blood from flowing through the arteries, the victim will feel chest pain. This pain originating from the heart is called **angina.** Someone who has coronary artery disease may experience angina during or immediately following physical exertion. The pain generally goes away when the victim dissolves a nitroglycerine pill under the tongue. However, if the myocardium continues without enough oxygen for a prolonged period, or if complete blockage of the artery stops flow to the heart, the muscle will die. This permanent damage to the myocardium is called a heart attack, or **myocardial infarction.**

Victims of a myocardial infarction will complain of pain in the middle or on the left side of their chests. Frequently, they describe this pain as a pressure sensation over the anterior chest. Others have described this pain as "vise-like," "heavy," or "squeezing." The pain may radiate to the shoulders and arms, up the neck, or around the back. In addition, victims commonly have shortness of breath, nausea and vomiting, palpitations (heart pounding), and lightheadedness. You may observe excessive sweating, difficult breathing, and an anxious expression in the victim.

About half of all cardiac deaths occur within one hour after the onset of symptoms, often before the victim reaches the hospital. Immediate recognition of symptoms and effective treatment within the first few moments are crucial to the victim's survival. Upon observing cardiac symptoms, you should immediately activate the EMS system or recruit a bystander to assist with this task. Paramedics are needed because they are trained in advanced life-support and can begin treatment immediately. If the victim has a cardiac arrest, paramedics or EMTs trained in defibrillation (EMT-Ds) can use electric stimulation to convert an erratic heartbeat into a functional rhythm. Paramedics also have been trained to perform advanced airway procedures and administer intravenous medications to resuscitate the victim. Before paramedics arrive, these first- aid measures should be followed:

1. Have the victim stop all activity immediately.

2. Place the victim in a comfortable position. Victims frequently ask to sit up, especially if dyspnea (breathing difficulty) accompanies the chest pain.

3. Allow the victim to take prescribed medication (nitroglycerine) if they request it.

4. If properly trained to do so, administer oxygen if available. The myocardium is not getting enough oxygen for the demands made on it.

5. Keep the victim still until help arrives, thereby avoiding excessive exertion and increased demands on the heart. Reassurance that help is on the way will reduce stress and anxiety.

6. If the victim is unconscious, check their airway, breathing, and circulation. Begin CPR as needed.

Syncope (Fainting)

Fainting, or **syncope,** is a transient state of unconsciousness during which the person collapses from lack of oxygen to the brain. Some common causes of syncope include rapid or irregular heartbeat, vasovagal reaction, heat illness, and insulin reaction (hypoglycemia). Anything that causes a relative decrease in blood volume, such as excessive blood loss or severe dehydration from vomiting or diarrhea, also can cause fainting.

Angina or a heart attack may disrupt the normal electrical activity coordinating the heartbeat. The resulting rapid or erratic heart rhythm can cause the victim to collapse. If the heart loses its ability to pump, quivering instead, the brain may incur irreversible damage within four minutes, and death may occur.

The most common and least serious form of fainting results from an increase in vagal nerve tone combined with dilation of the arteries, a vasovagal reaction. Such an attack typically occurs with the victim in a standing position, and follows an unpleasant or anxiety-provoking event, such as pain, fright, or the sight of blood. The victim typically experiences profuse sweating, loss of skin color, nausea, and restlessness. Heart rate and blood pressure drop dramatically, decreasing flow to the brain so that the victim loses consciousness. These symptoms resolve rapidly when the victim lies down.

Insulin Reaction
(Insulin-induced Hypoglycemia)

Hypoglycemia occurs when there is a deficiency of sugar in the blood. The most common cause of hypoglycemia is an insulin reaction in a person with **diabetes.** Insulin, the antidiabetic hormone secreted by the pancreas, is necessary for the utilization of glucose (blood sugar) by the cells and for maintenance of proper blood-sugar levels. Inadequate production or utilization of insulin leads to improper metabolism of glucose and fats for energy production and brings on diabetes. Diabetes, a chronic disease resulting from poor insulin production or utilization, is characterized by high blood sugars and excretion of glucose in the urine. A person with diabetes can control the symptoms and prolong life by using insulin injections and by closely monitoring blood sugars.

A hypoglycemic episode may be the result of too much insulin, too much exercise, or insufficient food. The episode produces fatigue, excessive sweating, headache, trembling, slurred speech, and poor coordination.

The victim may feel faint, lose consciousness, or have a seizure. Other physical symptoms, such as pale moist skin, full rapid pulse, tremors, and elevated blood pressure, may also appear. Many people with diabetes are aware of early symptoms and can quickly reverse the process by simply consuming candy, fruit juice, or some other food rich in simple sugars. Other people may have no warning and go into insulin shock suddenly. Your prompt response may prevent hospitalization or serious complications. Basic first aid for someone experiencing a hypoglycemic reaction includes the following steps:

1. If the victim is conscious, prevent injury by having them lie down or sit while someone gets help.

2. Give the victim sugar in the form of fruit juice or soft drinks sweetened with sugar.

3. Prevent the victim from resuming activity after the insulin reaction.

4. Encourage the victim to eat a meal and consult a physician to prevent further reactions.

If the victim loses consciousness, first-aid treatment changes. Following is a list of procedures in order of priority:

1. If the victim is unconscious, check the airway, breathing, and circulation. Artificial ventilations may be started as needed. Protect the victim's cervical spine if a fall has occurred.

2. Protect the victim and prevent injury if they have a seizure. During a seizure, avoid restraining the victim. Place a soft object (towel, jacket, blanket) under the head to keep it from banging on the floor during violent muscular contractions.

3. Activate the EMS system. Paramedics or EMTs certified to start IVs can administer intravenous glucose that will quickly reverse a potentially life-threatening insulin reaction.

4. Do not give anything by mouth. An attempt to give sugar by mouth to an unconscious person could cause aspiration of the substance and airway or respiratory compromise. If the victim vomits, turn the victim onto his or her side to prevent aspiration (Figure 17.3).

Adapting a Training Regimen for Clients with Diabetes. Most physicians today encourage their patients with diabetes to exercise because of the many physical and psychological benefits. In consultation with their physicians, experienced and knowledgeable individuals can safely embark on a training program, maintain good diabetic control, and avoid hypoglycemic reactions. The following methods will help athletes with diabetes:

✔ Athletes on insulin may need to reduce their doses by 20 to 40% when beginning an exercise program. People with diabetes need to work closely with their physicians during this process to ensure the appropriate dosage of insulin.

✔ Individuals with diabetes respond best to exercises that have a predictable duration, intensity, and frequency. Some examples of exercise that allow consistent and predictable energy expenditure include aerobic activities such as walking, running, cycling, traditional aerobics, step training, and cross-country skiing.

✔ People with diabetes should avoid injecting insulin into exercised extremities. The increased circulation in the exercised limb may cause the insulin to be absorbed too rapidly, causing hypoglycemia. Abdominal sites may be safer for insulin administration.

✔ During sustained exercise, a quick source of energy containing 10 grams of **carbohydrates** should be taken every 15 to 20 minutes. This could include ½ cup of a soft drink with sugar, or ¼ cup of gelatin dessert.

✔ Several hours before competing in an athletic event, people with diabetes

FIGURE 17.3
Side position for unconscious victim: Placing the victim on his or her side prevents airway blockage in case vomiting occurs. This position allows fluids to drain from the nose and mouth.

should eat a meal high in carbohydrates and relatively low in **fats** and **protein.** Within one hour before prolonged strenuous exercise, a mixed snack containing 15 to 20 grams of carbohydrates should be consumed. This could consist of ½ cup of milk and two or three crackers.

✔ Individuals with diabetes must take responsibility for their own care by closely monitoring blood sugars, taking insulin as recommended, eating properly, exercising regularly, and keeping all medical appointments.

Heat Illnesses

Hot climates present serious health hazards to athletes. Runners, especially enthusiastic novices, are particularly vulnerable to heat illness. Runners may attempt to finish a race by exceeding their training levels or running too fast for their level of fitness. The normal metabolic processes of the body continuously produce heat that is dissipated to a cooler air temperature.

Normal body temperature is about 98.6° F (37° C). When the body gains excess heat—from increased metabolism during exercise, a hot environment, impaired dissipation of heat to the environment, or a combination of these—the brain's temperature regulatory center, the hypothalamus, activates several cooling mechanisms. Sweating, the most important method the body has to release excess heat during exercise, produces heat loss through evaporation. Also, the superficial veins in the

skin dilate, losing heat through convection (transfer of heat to air currents), and radiation. The amount of evaporation and heat loss depends on the air temperature, humidity, and wind speed. When humidity is high and the air is still, evaporation will diminish or cease completely. Convection of heat will cease when the air temperature approaches 100° F (38° C).

Anyone who exercises in a hot, humid environment, indoors or outdoors, runs a risk for heat illness. Injuries from heat occur in three forms: **heat cramps, heat exhaustion,** and **heat stroke.** Although the following descriptions separate them, they overlap a great deal. A person with heat illness may display a combination of these symptoms.

Heat Cramps. The mildest heat illness, heat cramps typically occur during or after strenuous physical activity. This disorder is characterized by painful muscle spasms affecting those muscles worked the hardest. For example, runners most often feel heat cramps in their calf muscles, while racquetball players are more likely to have them in their arms. It is not clear what causes heat cramps, although they appear to be related to profuse sweating accompanied by loss of body salt (sodium). Hyperventilation and accumulation of lactic acid in the muscles also may contribute to the condition. The heat-cramp victim exhibits painful muscle cramps, sweating, and a normal body temperature. Treatment consists of drinking a commercially available electrolyte solution and massaging the affected muscle. If the cramps do not respond to these simple measures, the victim should be transported to a hospital for intravenous fluids and, possibly, muscle-relaxing medication.

Heat Exhaustion. The most common heat illness that occurs in athletes, heat exhaustion typically follows intense exercise in a hot, humid environment. Profuse sweating with resultant fluid and electrolyte loss and inadequate fluid replacement may produce a dramatic drop in blood pressure. The victim's temperature may be normal or slightly elevated, and they will be sweating profusely. Other signs and symptoms may include early fatigue, lightheadedness, nausea, vomiting, severe headache, decreased coordination and staggering, hypotension (blood pressure lower than 90 mmHg systolic), tachycardia (heart rate higher than 100 beats per minute), and syncope (fainting).

A victim of heat exhaustion needs rest and fluid replacement. Follow these simple first-aid measures:

1. Move the victim to a cool place to reduce further sweating and fluid loss.

2. Immediately apply cold compresses to areas of increased blood flow—the groin, underarms, and neck.

3. Apply cool water to the skin surface and then fan the victim by hand or machine to increase evaporation.

4. If the victim begins shivering, remove the cold compresses and use only cool sponging. Intense shivering increases metabolism and promotes heat production. Note: If victim becomes unresponsive initiate CPR.

5. If the victim is profoundly hypotensive (blood pressure lower than 90 systolic), call paramedics to transport the victim to the hospital.

6. If the victim is alert and mildly hypotensive (blood pressure 90 to 100 systolic), offer the victim an oral electrolyte solution until help arrives. The victim can be more effectively rehydrated in the hospital with intravenous saline.

7. Victims of heat exhaustion should avoid activity for at least 24 hours following

the condition and be sure to drink adequate amounts of fluids during that time. Furthermore, they should refrain from exercising in the heat for at least one week because they are especially susceptible to repeat episodes within that period.

Heat Stroke. The least common but most serious heat illness, heat stroke results from heat overload and impairment of the body's ability to dissipate heat. A true medical emergency, it may result in significant complications or death. The three classic symptoms of heat stroke are high body temperature [106° F (41° C) or higher], altered consciousness, and dry skin because of a lack of sweating. However, in heat stroke induced by exertion, dry skin is not a reliable sign because the victim may be sweating from exercise. People affected by heat strokes have commonly been exercising in hot, humid weather. The conditions that predispose someone to heat stroke include:

✔ old age
✔ exercise and exertion
✔ hot, humid weather
✔ dehydration
✔ obesity
✔ heavy clothing
✔ infection and fever
✔ certain drugs: alcohol, amphetamines, diuretics, beta blockers, and anticholinergics
✔ cardiovascular disease
✔ poor acclimatization
✔ hyperthyroidism

Older people and those who have been using drugs (including alcohol) may not be able to protect themselves from a high environmental temperature, leaving them susceptible to heat stroke. Alcohol dilates the blood vessels, making it easy for the body's temperature to increase if the air temperature is higher than the body's. Any condition that increases metabolism can increase heat production and susceptibility to heat stroke. This includes any exercise

Common Medical
Emergencies
and Injuries

or exertion, infections, and stimulants such as amphetamines, and the excess thyroid production seen in people with hyperthyroidism.

Acclimatization refers to the body's ability to adapt to heat stress over time, resulting in an increased capacity to work in hot, humid conditions. On the first day of rigorous exercise in a hot environment a person may experience severe fatigue, elevated body temperature, and a heart rate near maximum. Over the next four to eight days of similar exposure, the body will compensate by improving blood distribution and increasing blood volume, sweating at a lower temperature to improve heat loss, reducing urination to preserve body fluids, and reducing salt concentration in the sweat glands. People with inadequate acclimatization tolerate heat poorly and are more susceptible to heat stroke.

Anyone who is dehydrated, has cardiovascular disease, or takes diuretics or beta blockers may have reduced skin circulation. Adequate skin circulation is needed to dissipate heat. Anticholinergic drugs, such as certain medications prescribed for depression, can impair the body's ability to sweat and thus impair cooling from evaporation. Many other drugs that affect mood and thinking can also impair the brain's temperature-regulatory center.

Once heat stroke is suspected, the victim needs rapid treatment aimed at lowering the body temperature by whatever means are available. For immediate first aid you should:

1. Activate the EMS system. At the same time, move the victim to a cool area and remove excess clothing to expose the skin to air.

2. Immediately apply cold compresses to areas of increased blood flow—the groin, underarms, and neck.

3. Apply cool water to the skin surface and then fan the victim by hand or machine to increase evaporation.

4. If the victim begins shivering, remove the cold compresses and use only cool sponging. Intense shivering increases metabolism and promotes heat production. Note: If victim becomes unresponsive initiate CPR.

After transportation to an emergency room, the victim will receive care to minimize the damage from prolonged and intense heat to various organ systems.

Prevention of Heat Illness. All heat illnesses may be prevented with proper planning and common sense. To minimize risk of problems with heat, you should:

✔ Avoid training clients in extreme heat and humidity.

✔ Urge clients to wear sensible, porous, light-colored, loose-fitting clothing while exercising in the heat.

✔ Train clients for competition in heat by acclimating them slowly, increasing the intensity and duration of exercise over eight days.

✔ Help your client avoid **dehydration** by urging them to drink adequate amounts of water before, during, and for 24 hours after vigorous exercise. Commercially prepared **electrolyte** and glucose solutions are unnecessary except for long periods of exertion in the heat, as in running a marathon. In fact, excessive salt intake can cause stomach cramps, weakness, and high blood pressure. Use of solutions containing too much glucose can retard absorption from the gastrointestinal tract by keeping the solution in the stomach longer.

✔ Encourage clients to use table salt more liberally the day before prolonged exercise (eight hours or more) in heat. Plenty of fluids should be consumed before the event (8 ounces,

20 to 30 minutes ahead), in anticipation of fluid loss through sweating and breathing. A **hypotonic** electrolyte solution containing less than 0.9% concentration of sodium chloride (salt) should be consumed every 10 to 15 minutes during a long event. A commercially made or homemade solution consisting of ¼ teaspoon of salt dissolved in a quart of water, can be used. Salt tablets should be avoided.

✔ Recognize the early symptoms of heat stress: dizziness, cramps, clammy skin, and extreme weakness.

✔ Have your client take more frequent rest periods and find a cool, shaded area for these breaks.

✔ Encourage clients to avoid drugs (including alcohol) that may predispose them to heat injury.

Seizures

A **seizure,** or convulsion, originates from the brain and causes disturbances in movement, behavior, sensation, or consciousness. Symptomatic of another condition, a seizure can result from an irritation in the brain from trauma, infection, blood clot, or hemorrhage. Other causes include decreased blood supply to the brain from cardiac or respiratory disturbance; metabolic abnormalities in sodium, calcium, magnesium, or glucose (hypoglycemia); poisons; alcohol withdrawal; high fever (especially in children); and complicated pregnancy. Epilepsy is a seizure disorder without an underlying cause. Epileptic seizures usually appear during childhood and recur spontaneously throughout life. With the use of an anticonvulsant medication, epileptics can lead normal lives and control their symptoms.

A major motor seizure, called a **grand mal seizure,** causes violent and uncontrollable muscular contractions. It can be frightening to see for the first time. It has four phases:

✔ The aura, when an unusual sensation of smell, taste, or sound warns a person that a seizure is imminent.

✔ The tonic phase, in which the victim loses consciousness, becomes rigid with all extremities extended, and holds their breath. As a result of not breathing, they appear cyanotic.

✔ The clonic phase, in which the muscles alternate between contraction and relaxation, making the victim appear to jerk.

✔ The postictal phase, in which the victim is comatose and their muscles become flaccid (limp). Consciousness returns slowly, with some initial confusion, headache, and extreme fatigue.

First Aid For Seizures. Your first task is to protect the victim from injury that might result from the flailing head and extremities. The simplest method is to put something soft under the victim's head and move all objects out of the way. Never attempt to hold the victim's arms or legs down, because this restraint may inadvertently cause a fracture or dislocation. Facial muscle spasms may cause the victim to bite his or her tongue. You should avoid placing fingers or any object into the victim's mouth for fear of damage. The jaw muscles are creating an enormous force that has the potential for serious injury.

It is important not to panic or attempt to force open the jaw during the tonic phase, when the victim may stop breathing and look cyanotic. This phase will pass and the clonic phase will bring renewed breathing and improved skin color.

During the postictal phase, the victim's muscles will become flaccid. A snoring sound during respiration usually indicates an airway obstruction. If the victim has fallen to the floor and has noisy respirations, you can make a big difference by protect-

Common Medical Emergencies and Injuries

ing the neck from further movement and controlling the airway with the jaw-thrust maneuver (see Figure 17.2). Call an ambulance to immediately transport the victim to a hospital emergency department.

Soft-tissue Injuries

Tissues, such as skin, muscles, and nerves, are composed of groups of cells that act together for a specific function. Bone, the hardest connective tissue in the body, is discussed later in this chapter. This section will present identification and first aid for common wounds, sprains, and acute strains.

Wounds. A break in continuity of the soft tissue, a wound can be open or closed. An open wound is manifested by broken skin, while a closed wound involves injury to underlying tissues without a break in the skin. Types of open wounds are:

- ✔ **Abrasion**—a scraping away of the skin or mucous membrane. Bleeding from an abrasion may be minimal, perhaps just a little oozing. However, abrasions still have potential for contamination and infection.
- ✔ **Incision**—a cut in the skin, typically from contact with a sharp object. The amount of bleeding depends on the size, depth, and location of the incision.
- ✔ **Laceration**—a jagged, irregular cut or tear in the soft tissues, usually caused by a blow. Bleeding may be brisk in a laceration and tissue destruction is greater than with an incision. A laceration has great potential for contamination and resulting infection.
- ✔ **Puncture**—a piercing wound from a sharp object, such as a nail, pin, or wood splinter, that makes a small hole in the skin. If external bleeding is minimal, the risk of infection is high. Bleeding flushes the area and assists in removing dirt and bacteria. A puncture wound over the trunk (chest, back, abdomen) can damage the

underlying organs, causing internal bleeding.

- ✔ **Avulsion**—a forcible tearing away of tissue from the body. Damage may be small, as when a minor accident tears away a little skin, or extensive, as when a crushing injury tears a limb from the body. In more serious avulsion injuries, significant bleeding may occur and infection may develop if precautions are not taken.

Hemorrhage Control. Wounds usually result from external physical forces, such as falls or mishandling of equipment. First aid for open wounds emphasizes controlling bleeding and reducing the risk of infection. If an open wound is bleeding profusely, bleeding control takes precedence over infection control. Once the dressing has been applied and the bleeding is under control, the dressing should not be removed until the victim reaches the hospital. You should attend to the most life-threatening condition first. Following are some simple techniques you can take to control bleeding.

1. Apply direct pressure over the bleeding point, using a gloved hand over a gauze dressing (Figure 17.4). If bleeding is brisk and gauze dressings are not readily available, firm pressure with a small towel over the wound may be used.

2. Place a victim who has lost a significant amount of blood, looks pale and sweaty, and has a weak pulse in the shock position (i.e., elevating the legs above the level of the heart). This position assists venous return of blood to the heart.

Direct pressure and the measures discussed above will control nearly all bleeding wounds. A tourniquet shuts off the down-stream blood supply to the extremity. All viable tissue will die. Medical personnel may consider using a tourniquet *only* under life-threatening conditions, bearing in mind that its use means saving a life at the cost of losing a limb.

Caution: A tourniquet can be dangerous and should only be used by medical personnel.

Preventing Infection. Contamination of a wound leads to infection, and open wounds are vulnerable to contamination from several sources, including the object that inflicted the injury, air-borne bacteria and particles, and normal skin bacteria. To minimize the risk of infection, you may take several measures:

1. Remove all debris, such as wood splinters, pieces of glass, clothing particles, or dirt by gently flushing the wound with warm water. For a superficial wound, you may remove embedded particles by gently brushing them off with a cotton swab or pulling them out with tweezers. Particles embedded deep in a wound should be left for a physician to remove, because pulling them out could disrupt an artery or sever a tendon or nerve.

2. Encourage the victim to wash a superficial wound with mild soap and warm water, rinsing thoroughly with warm, running tap water. The wound may be blotted gently with a clean towel or sterile piece of gauze and covered with a dry sterile bandage. If signs of infection develop—redness, warmth, swelling, tenderness—the victim should seek medical attention.

3. Obtain immediate medical attention for any wound that may need stitches. Delay in closure of the wound increases infection risk.

4. Place a dressing over any open wound to protect it from additional contamination. The dressing may be secured with tape or a gauze strip.

First Aid for Closed Wounds. Closed wounds typically result from external forces, such as a fall or a blow from a blunt object (a racquetball hitting the body or a free-weight falling onto it, for example). Even when the skin has no visible break, injury may still occur to underlying skin and other organs, muscles, tendons, ligaments, and bones. Internal bleeding may produce a contusion (bruise), hematoma (collection of blood),

FIGURE 17.4
Direct pressure for hemorrhage control.

or bleeding within the body cavity. Closed wounds are much less susceptible to infection than open wounds because the skin keeps out environmental bacteria. Although most closed wounds heal by themselves, some may involve deep structures with significant internal bleeding. Here are some tips for managing a closed wound:

1. If the wound is minor, apply ice to the area to reduce swelling and slow bleeding within the tissues.

2. If the victim has no outward signs of injury but complains of pain and tenderness, suspect an internal injury. **Call paramedics immediately if any of the following signs and symptoms appear:**

✔ Pale, cool, and clammy skin; rapid and weak pulse; complaints of lightheadedness. These may be signs of shock from internal bleeding.

✔ Extreme pain and tenderness over the injured area.

✔ Vomiting or coughing up blood, or blood in the urine or feces. These may be signs of significant injury to the chest or gastrointestinal tract.

✔ Rapid, painful, or difficult breathing (dyspnea). Breathing difficulty may result from injury to the chest wall (ribs, cartilage, muscles) or to the respiratory system.

3. Examine the victim's extremities for swelling, discoloration, or deformity that might indicate a fracture or dislocation. If these indications are present, avoid moving that body part. Keep the victim quiet and wait for help to arrive. The limb may be immobilized using simple splinting techniques if the victim must be moved before EMTs or paramedics arrive (see Fractures, page 455).

Sprains. When the ligaments that normally stabilize a joint tear, the resulting **sprain** can range from a simple twist that causes minimal symptoms to a complete tearing of the ligaments that produces an unstable joint, severe pain, and swelling. The ankle is the most commonly sprained joint, typically from an inversion injury (turning in of the foot) caused by landing off balance or exercising on an irregular floor surface. When a joint is sprained, the victim may hear a popping sound if a significant tear has occurred. Pain, swelling, discoloration, or the inability to bear weight also may be present. It is often difficult to distinguish between a sprain and a fracture without X-rays. Treatment of a sprain consists of RICE (rest, ice, compression, elevation). If a sprain is suspected, you should:

1. Stop all activity immediately and have the victim rest the injured extremity.

2. Apply an elastic bandage and ice to the injury. Elevate it to minimize swelling.

3. If pain or swelling is severe, do not allow the victim to walk. Immobilize the extremity with simple splinting maneuvers, and arrange for transportation to a hospital where the limb can be examined for fracture or other disabling injury.

Muscle Strains. A tear in a muscle or its tendon, a muscle strain is often called a "pulled muscle." This injury can be minor, involving less than 5% of the muscle fibers, or it can be severe, with complete disruption of the muscle or its tendon. There are several causes. The muscle may have been warmed up insufficiently before vigorous use, or it may have been overtrained and fatigued. It also could have been weakened by a previous injury. A tense muscle or tendon may be injured in movements that demand flexibility. And muscles exposed to cold weather have less capability of contracting than normal. The following are symptoms of a muscle strain:

✔ At the moment of injury, a sharp pain is felt; contracting the injured muscle reproduces this pain.

✔ Localized tenderness and swelling may occur over the damaged muscle or tendon.

✔ Pain may inhibit the muscle from contracting if it is partially torn; the muscle will not be able to contract at all if completely torn.

✔ Bruising and discoloration may appear 12 to 24 hours after the injury.

Treatment of minor muscle strain consists of RICE. If the injury affects the leg and walking causes discomfort, the victim should use crutches until a medical evaluation can be obtained.

Fractures

A fracture, or break in a bone, may be closed or open. A closed (simple) fracture has no opening from outside the skin to the broken bone. An open (compound) fracture, which is more serious, results when the broken ends of the bone pierce the skin, or when a sharp object penetrates the skin and fractures the underlying bone. In either case, the opening between the skin and the injured bone brings a high risk of infection. A fracture is a serious injury not only because the bone is broken, but because of the potential injury in the surrounding soft tissue. Tendons, ligaments, muscles, nerves, and blood vessels may be damaged, with a threat of permanent disability. Fractures may result from a direct blow or a more indirect cause, such as a fall. Following are signs of possible bone fracture:

✔ audible snap at the time of injury
✔ abnormal motion or position of the injured limb
✔ inability to bear weight on the limb (stand or walk)
✔ swelling
✔ deformity
✔ discoloration
✔ pain or tenderness to the touch

First Aid for Suspected Fracture. Immediate care for a victim with a suspected fracture involves controlling hemorrhage, preventing further injury to the bone and soft tissue, and providing first aid for shock, if necessary. If you suspect a fracture, take the following steps:

1. Keep the victim quiet; do not allow them to move the injured part or attempt to put weight on it.

2. Remove or cut away clothing that covers the injury. This step allows more thorough assessment and prevents contamination of an open fracture.

3. Cover an open fracture with a sterile gauze dressing or clean cloth to prevent further contamination. Activate the EMS system immediately and keep the victim lying down if there is significant bleeding to improve circulation to the heart and brain until help arrives. Apply gentle pressure to slow or stop the bleeding, using care not to disturb the fractured site.

4. Leave the protruding ends of bone where they are. Attempting to push them back in place will increase risk of infection and further injury to soft tissues.

5. If the victim must be transported, splint the limb to immobilize it. However, if the extremity is grossly deformed and splinting may be difficult, merely prevent the injured limb from moving until medical help arrives. An untrained person's attempts to move a fractured limb can convert a closed fracture into an open one, or cause nerve and vascular injury in an uncomplicated fracture.

Splinting Techniques. Splinting or immobilizing a fractured limb protects it against further injury during transportation, reduces pain, and prevents bone fragments from injuring arteries or other tissues. Many household objects or pieces of equipment in a health club may be converted to emergency splints—any object that provides support and prevents movement. Some examples include heavy cardboard, newspapers, rolled blankets or towels, exercise mats, and straight sticks. The splint should simply be long enough to extend past the joints above and below the suspected fracture and should be padded to prevent pressure injuries from hard surfaces or sharp edges. A first-aid course will teach you the how to splint an extremity.

Figures 17.5 and 17.6 illustrate properly applied splints of the forearm and ankle, using materials commonly found in the home or health club.

Head Injuries

Typically the result of a blow or fall, head injuries are less common than extremity injuries, but their complications can produce long-term disability. Thus, it is important for you to be able to identify a potential head injury and take appropriate precautions. When the skull accelerates or decelerates suddenly, the brain can move within the skull, and its impact on the skull may injure the brain. Bleeding may occur within the brain tissue, as in cerebral contusions (bruising of the brain) and hematomas (collection of blood). Bleeding also may occur from vessels between the membranes covering the brain. Because the skull is a rigid bony structure filled with brain tissue, it contains little room for expansion. Any bleeding or tissue swelling exerts compression force against the brain cells, and can result in serious neurological damage.

Symptoms of head injury may be fairly minor, such as headache, dizziness, nau-sea, and vomiting. They may be severe, including speech disturbance, partial or complete paralysis, seizures, and coma. A force strong enough to cause a temporary loss of consciousness is strong enough to cause serious complications or death. **Any victim of head injury who loses consciousness, however briefly, needs immediate transportation to a hospital emergency department for neurological evaluation.**

Visible signs of trauma to the head or face are further clues that hidden injury to the brain may have occurred. A laceration or large hematoma of the scalp (collection of blood under the scalp that feels like a large bump) needs a physician's attention. Signs of a possible skull fracture include discoloration and swelling around the eyes (raccoon sign), visible blood in the ear canals, and clear fluid draining from the nose or ears. This seepage may be cere-brospinal fluid, the fluid that surrounds the brain and spinal cord. A fractured skull needs further evaluation that may include a radiological scan or observation in the hospital. The excessive force re-quired to fracture the skull may also have produced injury to the underlying brain.

Head injuries seldom occur in isolation. Damage to the cervical spine (neck) ac-companies 15 to 20% of head injuries, so it should always be considered when caring for the victim, especially someone with altered mental status, unconsciousness, or any of the visible signs listed previously. You must take precautions to immobilize the neck, thereby preventing disabling injury. When in doubt, always protect the cervical spine until the victim is thorough-ly examined by a physician and X-rays are taken. Paramedics are needed immediately to open the airway and transport the vic-tim to the hospital.

Neck and Back Injuries

Airway Compromise. Blunt force against the front of the neck, the face, or the jaw can produce airway compromise. For exam-

FIGURE 17.5
Splinting the forearm: The bone has been immobilized by news-paper that has been rolled up, padded with a towel, and tied with strips of material to hold the splint in place. Using a sling in combi-nation with the splint will immobilize the joints below the frac-ture (wrist) and above the fracture (elbow). The sling also elevates the hand slightly above the elbow to minimize swelling.

FIGURE 17.6
Splinting the ankle: Check circulation and sensation. Splint the ankle using a rolled blanket (or exercise mat), applying it around the ankle and sole of the foot and tying it into place with cloth strips.

ple, a client may bench press too much weight, become fatigued, and drop the barbell on the front of their neck. Extensive swelling may occur around the trachea, or the larynx may fracture, either of which may result in airway obstruction. Time is critical and paramedics should be summoned immediately for rapid transport to a hospital, where a surgically made airway (tracheotomy) may be necessary. If the victim sustains a respiratory arrest, you should begin mouth-to-mouth or mouth-to-mask ventilation while waiting for help to arrive.

Spinal Cord Injury. Injuries to the vertebral column occur most frequently when excessive force is applied from the top or bottom, as in a fall or a dive into a shallow pool. The resulting fractures or dislocation of the vertebrae disrupt the ligaments that hold the bones in place. The spinal cord, normally protected within the vertebral canal, may be injured, the blood supply to the cord interrupted, and neurological dysfunction with paralysis may result.

It is extremely important to keep in mind the possibility of vertebral injury for any victim of head trauma, or for someone with several areas of trauma. It is easy to overlook the neck during the initial assessment when, for example, a large laceration or bone deformity may distract one's attention. However, many victims of multiple trauma also have spinal cord injuries. For the purpose of first aid, anyone with one or more of the following signs should be considered to have an injured spinal cord:

✔ altered level of consciousness
✔ obvious numbness, tingling, weakness, or paralysis
✔ a fall or injury that might have injured the spinal cord
✔ head or facial injury
✔ pain or tenderness over the spine
✔ swelling or deformity over the spine

Emergency Response to Neck and Back Injury. Initial management of a neck or back injury is extremely important to the long-term outcome. Improper management may turn a simple bone injury into permanent neurological disability and paralysis. Following are techniques you can use to protect the spinal cord while help is on the way:

1. Handle the victim carefully, avoiding movement of the head and neck or bending of the neck. Simply hold the head and neck stationary to prevent the victim from moving until help arrives (Figure 17.7).

2. Do not attempt to reposition or move the victim until an ambulance arrives with trained EMTs equipped with spinal immobilization devices.

3. If the victim's airway is compromised, or they require artificial respirations, you may need to roll the victim onto his or her back, keeping the entire spine straight as a board to protect the neck and back ("log roll"). The victim will then be in a position conducive to establishing an airway.

PROTECTION AGAINST BLOODBORNE PATHOGENS

There are many bloodborne diseases that you could be exposed to while caring for an injured client. These include non-A hepatitis, non-B hepatitis, hepatitis B, and delta hepatitis. Other diseases transmitted through blood include

FIGURE 17.7
Immobilization of the head and neck: Kneel at the victim's head, place your hands on either side of the head and neck, and hold them firmly in place. Keep the victim quiet and prevent movement of the head. Do not try to reposition the victim.

syphilis, malaria, and human immunodeficiency virus (HIV). Of these, the most common and serious diseases are hepatitis B and HIV.

Hepatitis B

Hepatitis B virus (HBV) is one of the most common bloodborne hazards you may face on the job. Hepatitis is defined as an inflammation of the liver ("hepatic" = liver, "itis" = inflammation). Among healthcare workers alone (e.g., nurses, doctors, laboratory technicians) more than 8,000 persons become infected with hepatitis annually, resulting in approximately 200 deaths.

Some of the signs and symptoms of HBV are similar to the flu, and may include abdominal pain and vomiting severe enough to necessitate hospitalization. Some persons have no symptoms at all, but their blood, saliva, and other body fluids may be infected.

Acquired Immunodeficiency Syndrome (AIDS)

The first reported case of AIDS in the United States occurred in 1981. Initially, it was considered a "gay" disease because most individuals who contracted AIDS were homosexual. As more cases were discovered in the population at large, it became clear that AIDS did not discriminate against certain populations. AIDS has now gained recognition as being an epidemic due to the alarming number of new cases discovered each year.

HIV attacks the body's immune system causing the AIDS disease. This weakens the body's ability to fight off infections from bacteria, viruses, and parasites. The HIV may remain inactive for years in some individuals, and the person infected may be completely asymptomatic.

When the virus becomes active, the person infected may begin to experience headaches, fatigue, swollen lymph glands, night sweats and fever, nausea, diarrhea,

loss of appetite, skin rashes, and sores in the mouth, nose, or anus. AIDS is the last stage of HIV infection and causes such diseases as pneumonia, infections of the brain, Kaposi's sarcoma (a rare skin cancer), severe weight loss, and eventual death.

Universal Precautions

An individual may be infected with HIV or HBV and not show visible signs or symptoms. Some clients may be carriers without knowing it and a careful history or examination may not pick up those who are infected. You cannot afford to risk exposing yourself to these communicable diseases. All human blood and certain body fluids should be handled utilizing universal precautions. It is possible to reduce your risks from bloodborne pathogens by understanding the facts and taking the following precautions:

✔ Contaminated razors, broken glass, or other sharp objects should be carefully placed in a disposal container that is puncture-resistant and leak-proof.

✔ If infected material gets on your hands, wash them immediately with soap and running water.

✔ Personal protective equipment such as gloves, masks, gowns, faceshields, protective eyewear, and CPR protective mouthpieces should be used when appropriate. The type of protective equipment you use will depend on the type of exposure that is anticipated when assisting a client or responding to an emergency.

✔ If personal protective equipment or street clothes become contaminated, remove them as soon as possible and place them in the designated area for disposal or washing.

✔ If you are at risk of exposure to HBV on the job, your employer will make the hepatitis B vaccination available to you at no cost. Currently, there is no vaccine to prevent AIDS.

SUMMARY

A s a personal trainer, you may work closely with clients of various ages and fitness levels. This requires you to have (1) a basic knowledge of common injuries and medical emergencies, and (2) a well thought-out plan of action for all emergencies. This chapter is not comprehensive, but it has presented most of the common medical emergencies you might encounter and first-aid procedures for responding to them. You should be competent in CPR and take additional training in first aid. A well-stocked and systematically maintained first-aid kit should always be near at hand, whether you work in a health club or in a client's home. Your ability to recognize a true emergency, as well as your ability to respond correctly, can play a critical role in the ultimate outcome of an illness or injury. Immediate treatment for such common injuries as sprains and strains can reduce pain and swelling and shorten a client's recovery time. By familiarizing yourself with the signs of a heart attack, insulin shock, or seizure, you may be able to save a life. Finally, it is important to remember that you should never attempt to provide medical advice. Instead, your responsibility is to provide immediate first aid, refer injured clients to their physicians and, when necessary, call for emergency assistance.

Summary

References and Suggested Reading

REFERENCE

American College of Sports Medicine & American Heart Association (2002). Joint position statement: Automated external defibrillators in health/fitness facilities. *Medicine & Science in Sports & Exercise,* 34, 3, 561–564.

SUGGESTED READING

American Diabetic Association (1998). *Medical Management of Type 1 Diabetes.* (3rd ed.). Alexandria, Va.: American Diabetes Association.

American Heart Association (2005). *Heartsaver First Aid with CPR and AED.* Dallas, Tex.: American Heart Association.

American Heart Association (2005). *Heartsaver AED for the Lay Rescuer and First Responder.* Dallas, Tex.: American Heart Association.

American Red Cross (2006). *Community First Aid and Safety.* Washington, D.C.: American Red Cross.

Perrin, D.H. (1998). *The Injured Athlete.* Philadelphia: Lippincott, Williams & Wilkins.

Peterson, L. (2001). *Sports Injuries: Their Prevention and Treatment.* (3rd ed.). Champaign, Ill.: Human Kinetics.

PART VII

Chapter 18 Legal Guidelines and

Professional Responsibilities

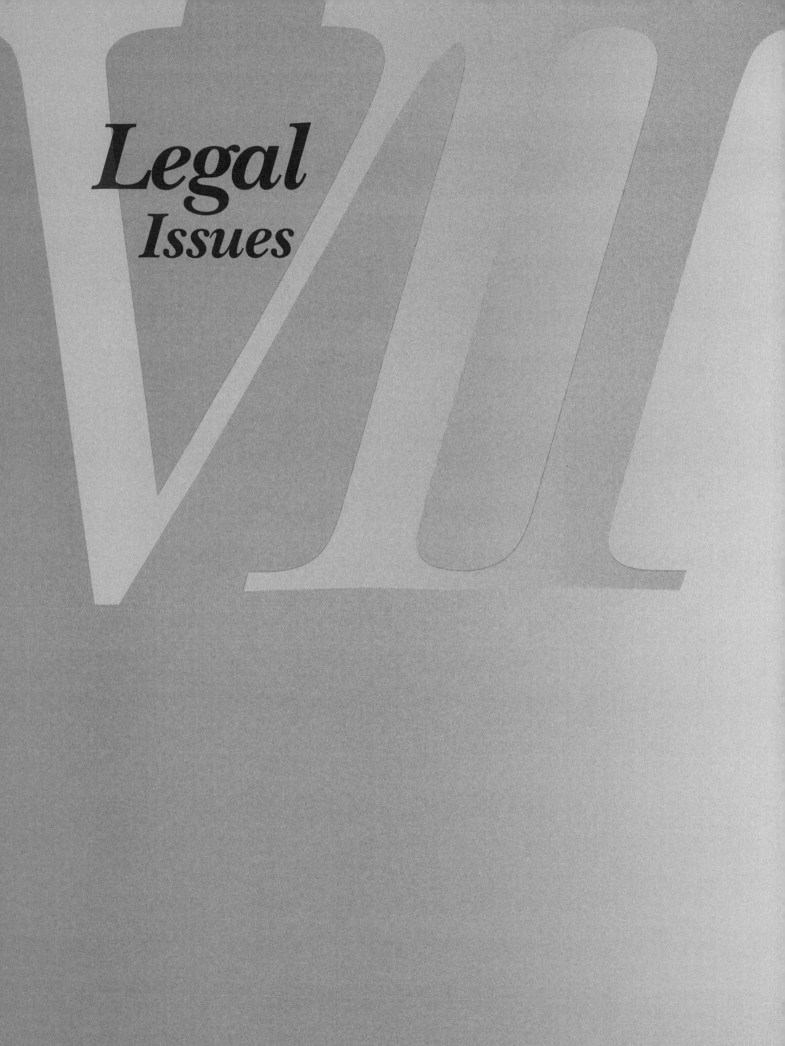

Legal
Issues

VII

CHAPTER 18

Legal Guidelines
and Professional Responsibilities

David K. Stotlar, Ed.D., teaches sport management and sport law and is a professor of sport management in the School of Exercise and Sports Studies at the University of Northern Colorado.

David K. Stotlar

He is a consultant, author, and lecturer, has contributed to numerous publications, and conducts management seminars throughout the world.

Although the majority of personal trainers may be well trained and comfortable with their responsibilities for designing exercise programs and working with clients, they may be far less comfortable with legal concepts important to running a fitness business. This chapter is intended to increase your comfort level and to address some of the legal and business concerns you may have as a personal trainer. It also will describe the scope of practice in personal training and summarize your legal responsibility as a personal trainer. The guidelines offered here, while based on sport law and the experience of fitness professionals, are not intended as legal advice, but rather as guidance. You should always consult lawyers in your own state for specific legal questions and problems.

INDEPENDENT CONTRACTORS vs. EMPLOYEES

Personal trainers who work in clubs are either **independent contractors** or **employees,** while self-employed personal trainers are usually independent contractors. This term evolved from the concept of a leased employee. For example, a homeowner might hire a bulldozer and an operator to move some dirt in their backyard. The bulldozer operator would not legally be considered the homeowner's employee, but rather an employee of the bulldozer company. The driver merely came along with the equipment, making the bulldozer company responsible for any **negligent** actions of the driver. Similarly, clients who hire personal trainers do not usually intend to hire them as employees, but prefer to lease their services for a brief period of time.

Some owners of fitness clubs use independent contractors, thereby avoiding the expense of training, medical benefits, social security withholding, worker's compensation, or unemployment coverage for these workers. However, most clubs still require independent contractors to follow club rules. Clubs also may prefer to deal with independent contractors because it is legally more difficult to fire an employee than it is to simply not renew a contract.

As a personal trainer with independent contractor status, you would enjoy the following benefits:
- ✔ Choosing when and where to work
- ✔ Charging variable fees for different situations
- ✔ Having professional freedom in conducting work

These freedoms must be weighed against the disadvantages of not having training, benefits, or equipment provided for you.

Legal Tests

Both independent contractors and club employees must be certain that all details of their agreements are clear from the beginning of their professional relationship with a club or fitness center. Often the legal nature of the relationship is ambiguous, and people have filed lawsuits attempting to collect worker's compensation or unemployment insurance from clubs that consider them independent contractors. Personal trainers, whether as employees or as independent contractors, are often left without health benefits or insurance coverage. In addition, trainers quickly discover the penalties of neglecting payments to tax and social security accounts if they assume that the clubs they worked for were paying into the accounts for them. Clubs only do this for people they consider employees, not for independent contractors.

Court cases have established 10 legal tests for determining whether someone is an employee or an independent contractor.

1. How much control can the employer exercise over the details of the work? The right to control indicates an employer-employee relationship.

2. Are people paid by the hour or by the job? People paid regularly by the hour or by the week are generally considered employees. On the other hand, people who receive a single payment for services rendered more easily qualify as independent contractors.

3. How long has the person been working in this establishment? People hired for short periods (a few days or weeks) are more easily defined as independent contractors than people employed over several months or years.

4. How much training does the person require? If the worker brings specialized or technical skills to the employer, the worker typically may be considered an independent contractor. On the other hand, if the employer provides training to a recently hired person, the court usually considers

that person an employee.

5. Does the person provide service to more than one client or business? If so, this person may be seen more easily as an independent contractor. If the person provides services for only one business or client, he or she would probably be considered an employee.

6. Who provides the equipment? In general, independent contractors provide their own equipment. However, using the club's or client's equipment, in itself, would not disqualify a trainer from independent contractor status.

7. Is the work integral to the business? If so, the worker will more likely be considered an employee. Supplemental services are more likely to support the status of independent contractorship.

8. In other clubs, is the work traditionally performed by an independent contractor or an employee? Current practices in the field may help determine if a trainer is an employee or an independent contractor.

9. What did the club and the trainer intend when they made their agreement? If the trainer believed they were hired as an independent contractor, as did the club, the court would attempt to enforce their original intent.

10. Is the employer engaged in business? If a client hires a trainer to perform personal training, the court will probably consider the trainer an independent contractor. The intent is to protect clients from being misconstrued as employers.

All of these questions have arisen in court cases over employment status, each with varying degrees of authority. Both you as a personal trainer and the clubs you work with must understand these issues when you initiate an agreement.

CONTRACTS

To perform your work, get paid for it, and avoid costly legal battles with clients and employers, you need to understand legal **contracts.** Whether you work as an independent contractor or as an employee of a club or fitness center, you must be aware of basic contract law. The following elements are necessary for a binding contract:

✔ An offer and acceptance with a mutual agreement on terms
✔ Consideration—an exchange of valuable items, such as money, for services
✔ Legality—acceptable form under the law
✔ Ability of the parties to enter into a contract with respect to legal age and mental capacity

For example, you may talk to a prospective client and mention the services you can provide, such as designing individualized exercise sessions to meet their goals. You and your client also may agree on dates and times for exercise sessions. This negotiation constitutes an offer and an acceptance. Stating a fee of $50 per hour for services sets up an exchange of consideration (i.e., training services for money). Once these negotiations are settled, you should prepare a written contract by filling out a basic contract form or by having one specifically written for each agreement. In either case, you should consult legal counsel to ensure that the written form is valid under contract law. This document becomes a valid contract when signed by both you and the client, if both of you are of legal age to enter into contracts.

Some personal trainers beginning in business may feel that written contracts are unnecessary, that a brief chat and a handshake are enough. However, in case of a misunderstanding or injury, legal complications can arise from such a simple oral contract, which can be enforceable under law. Business matters are less likely to lead to problems when the parties put the contract in writing, spelling out details to avoid potentially expensive misunderstandings. It is useful to pay for the services of a

Contracts

lawyer to develop the basic agreement. You can then personalize this agreement for each client and avoid additional legal fees. Whether the contract is to be used with clients or with a fitness club, you and your attorney should address the following considerations in developing it:

✔ Identification of the parties to the contract, such as you and the client or club
✔ Description of services (fitness training and consultation)
✔ Specification of compensation, payment method, or rate of compensation per hour, day, or month
✔ Confidential relationship—an agreement by each party not to divulge personal or business information acquired through the relationship
✔ Business or employment status
✔ Term and termination—defining the length of the contract and the conditions under which termination will be allowed by either party

BUSINESS STRUCTURE

Early in your professional life, you must decide whether you are acting as an individual, as a corporation, or as an employee of fitness centers. If you conduct business independently from a fitness center or club, you have three types of business structures available: **sole proprietorship, partnership,** and **corporation.**

Sole Proprietorship

As the name implies, a sole proprietorship is a business owned and operated by one person. This person owns all assets and is responsible for all income, losses, and liabilities. Forming a sole proprietorship establishes a legal right to conduct a business and gives the owner legal title to it. The owner—the personal trainer, in most cases—has sole control over decisions and profits. This business structure

offers the advantages of ease and low cost when the business is started. Furthermore, profits are taxed at the owner's individual rate, which is typically lower than a corporation rate. The owner reports income and taxes on a schedule that is attached to the personal income tax form instead of a separate business tax return. Government regulation is minimal compared to other business structures.

The risk of **liability,** however, is a drawback that often convinces people to choose other business structures. In sole proprietorships, the owner is completely responsible for all liabilities, court awards, or damages incurred by the business. An injured person who sues the owner and wins a sizable judgment can be awarded, if necessary, the proceeds from seizure of the owner's personal savings and property, such as house and auto. If the owner's business liabilities exceed their personal assets, the owner could be paying for today's problems years into the future.

Another disadvantage of sole proprietorships is the difficulty of getting away for vacations, illness, or emergencies. It may be impossible to find someone to watch the shop with the same care and interest as the owner. Often, the owner does not recognize these pressures in the early days of establishing the business, but later, the stress and pressure of successful operation may suggest a break from daily routine.

Partnership

Two or more people who agree to operate a business and share profits and losses may form a partnership. Two personal trainers, for example, could form a company, or a trainer could become part owner of a club. Although partnerships may be loosely created without legal documents, serious business relationships benefit from a partnership agreement that establishes rules of operation. This agreement should lay out the structure for authority, the partners' rights, expected performance and contributions from each partner, buy-out clauses, income distribution, and responsibility for debts. The agreement also should stipulate whether the business is a general or limited partnership.

General Partnership. In a general partnership, all partners are fully liable for the actions of the business. For example, suppose you and a friend go into business together. You will be the personal trainer and your friend will run the office as well as do the marketing and promotion. Because the business was your idea, you will put up $50,000 to get started; your friend agrees to work at minimum wage until things get rolling. Early on, a video company approaches your friend to produce and sell videotapes to your clients as part of the fitness package. Your friend agrees to a deal for $25,000, payable in 90 days. Shortly thereafter, your friend suffers a breakdown, gets a divorce, squanders all personal assets, and stops managing the business. After 90 days, the video company can legally collect from you all the money owed. It makes no difference that you owned only 50% of the business, or that you had an agreement that each partner would be responsible for only 50% of all debts. You also are liable for all debts if a court judgment is entered against your partner for activities of the business. You could sue your partner to try to recover your losses, but you might never benefit from your suit.

Limited Partnership. To avoid such devastating personal liability, limited partnerships allow certain partners, usually those who have invested in the business, to limit their liability to the amount of money they have contributed. The law usually prevents limited partners from taking an active role in managing the business. Although it might seem intriguing to limit financial liability by organizing a business with only limited partners, the law also requires that at least one person be designated as a general partner. The general partner may be anyone in the business, typically the person who runs the day-to-day operations. General partners are personally liable, while limited partners risk only their original investment.

All partnerships have the same tax advantage as sole proprietorships: profits are taxed at personal rates. This advantage makes partnerships attractive to investors because the partnership passes on to them the tax losses, credits, and deductions, while providing the limited partners with many of the legal protections they would only find in corporate structures.

Corporations

Regulated by state laws, corporations exist as legal entities and are independent of their owners. They are taxed separately from their owners, and corporate assets may be easily sold or transferred. In most cases, any number of people may own the corporation through shares issued by the business. Typically, the shareholders elect a board of directors to represent their interests. If you intend to form a corporation, you must first choose a company name that has not been previously registered. Then you should file a notice of incorporation with your state, paying the appropriate fees and designating a registered agent as a contact for the state. You may want to retain an attorney to guide you through this process, or simply call your secretary of state directly. Often a friendly and knowledgeable state clerk can talk applicants through the incorporation procedures, saving them hundreds of dollars in legal fees.

Many businesses form corporations to limit the financial liability of their shareholders. Creditors can attach the assets of a corporation if it owes money or has a judgment against it, but the personal assets of the corporate officers, board, and shareholders are typically not at risk for liabilities of the corporation. Taxes, however, can be more burdensome in a corporate structure. As an independent legal entity, a corporation must pay taxes, usually at a rate higher than for individuals. In addition, all corporate profits after taxes are paid as dividends to the shareholders, who in turn must declare them as income and pay taxes on them. This double taxation may be avoided if shareholders play an active part in the corporation management and draw salaries as managers. These salaries may offset the corporate profits, eliminating a tax on corporate earnings. The Internal Revenue Service requires that the salaries be reasonable for the work performed. The salaries, of course, are subject to individual tax as earned income.

A second method of avoiding double taxation, known as the S corporation, may be a better choice for personal trainers just starting out. This structure passes its profits through to shareholders, where the income is taxed at the individual rate. S corporations have certain restrictions, such as limiting the number of shareholders to 35.

Table 18.1 offers a brief summary of the advantages and disadvantages of each of the business structures just discussed. Few personal trainers will choose to take on the complicated tax structure, government regulations, and legal procedures necessary to begin and maintain a corporation. Most will simply register at their county courthouses as sole proprietors. In most cases, it is helpful to consult a lawyer when making this choice.

SCOPE OF PRACTICE

Whether you work as an employee in a fitness club or as an independent business person, you will find that clients ask for your advice on a variety of problems. Not only is it important for you to be well-educated and familiar with your own discipline, but it also is important for you to understand the limitations of your practice. Personal trainers are not usually licensed or qualified physicians, physical therapists, dietitians, marriage counselors, or social workers. You should avoid practicing these disciplines without appropriate training (Table 18.2).

Personal trainers should note, however, that many of these allied health professionals can provide meaningful information and services to their clients. Establishing a network of counselors, dietitians, physicians, and physical therapists can be valuable. Clients who need the specialized services of these healthcare professionals should be referred for treatment and counseling. In turn, your network of professionals may refer clients to you who need or desire personal training.

Health Assessment

According to fitness law experts Herbert and Herbert (2002), wellness-assessment documents should be utilized for the determination of an individual's level of

---

Table 18.1
Advantages and Disadvantages of Sole Proprietorships, Partnerships, and Corporations

Sole Proprietorships and Partnerships
- **Advantages**
  - ✔ Easily formed under the law
  - ✔ Low costs of formation
  - ✔ Typically can operate in different states
  - ✔ Owners pay taxes, but business does not
  - ✔ Minimal government regulation
- **Disadvantages**
  - ✔ Unlimited liability (except limited partners)

Corporations
- **Advantages**
  - ✔ Limited liability for corporate acts
- **Disadvantages**
  - ✔ Complicated legal requirements
  - ✔ High costs of formation
  - ✔ Must be registered in each state where business is conducted
  - ✔ Both corporation and owners are taxed, except for S corporation
  - ✔ Extensive government regulation

Table 18.2
IDEA Personal Fitness Trainers' Scope of Practice

Fitness Professionals DO NOT:	Fitness Professionals DO:
diagnose	• receive exercise, health, or nutrition guidelines from a physician, physical therapist, registered dietitian, etc. • follow national consensus guidelines for exercise programming for medical disorders • screen for exercise limitations • identify potential risk factors through screening • refer clients to an appropriate allied health professional or medical practitioner
prescribe	• design exercise programs • refer clients to an appropriate allied health professional or medical practitioner for an exercise prescription
prescribe diets or recommend specific supplements	• provide general information on healthy eating, according to the USDA Food Guide Pyramid • refer clients to a dietitian or nutritionist for a specific diet plan
treat injury or disease	• refer clients to an appropriate allied health professional or medical practitioner for treatment • use exercise to help improve overall health • help clients follow physician or therapist advice
monitor progress for medically referred clients	• document progress • report progress to an appropriate allied health professional or medical practitioner • follow physician, therapist, or dietitian recommendations
rehabilitate	• design an exercise program once a client has been released from rehabilitation
counsel	• coach • provide general information • refer clients to a qualified counselor or therapist
work with patients	• work with clients

Source: IDEA Health & Fitness Association's Opinion Statement: Benefits of a Working Relationship Between Medical and Allied Health Practitioners and Personal Fitness Trainers, *IDEA Health and Fitness Source*, September 2001. Reprinted with permission.

fitness, never for the purpose of providing or recommending treatment.

As a personal trainer, you should use the health history form to screen the client for appropriate placement in a fitness program. In cases where any significant risk factors are indicated, you should refer the client to a physician for clearance before the program begins. If you were to use this form to recommend treatment, you could be accused of practicing medicine without a license. It is far better to have a physician sign the form, indicating the types of training suitable for this client, or clear the client for exercise by writing a letter on their letterhead. Some trainers prefer a physician's letter to avoid the possibility of

a client forging the doctor's signature on a fitness form. However, if a client fakes a physician's signature to obtain acceptance to a fitness program, the trainer probably would not be held liable.

You must understand how to use the information collected on the health history form, asking only those questions you know how to interpret and apply. If you request information about the types of medications your client is taking, you may be held responsible for knowing the biochemical and physical reactions to these drugs. You must read and fully understand the answers to other questions as well. One sports administrator required all participants to complete health and physical appraisal forms, and then filed them without reading them. When a participant who had noted his heart defect on his form died, the sports administrator had little legal defense in the ensuing lawsuit.

Nutritional Counseling

According to the American Dietetic Association, more than 40 of the 50 states regulate or license dietitians or nutritionists. In one case in Ohio, a personal trainer was prohibited from providing nutritional counseling without a license. The plaintiff centered his case around the titles he was using: nutritionist or registered nutritionist. The court determined that, regardless of his title, he was not a registered dietitian (RD) and was in violation of Ohio law by practicing dietetics without a license. This included advising his client to use nutritional supplements. Several professional associations have also cautioned practitioners when recommending nutritional supplements. If you are not a registered dietitian or healthcare professional, you should avoid making specific recommendations and refer your client to a registered dietician or physician. (See Appendix E for ACE's position statement on nutritional supplements.) In one situation, charges were filed against a personal trainer who recommended that his client take over-the-counter supplements that contained ephedrine. According to the materials filed in the case, the personal trainer had been informed that the client was taking medicine for her hypertension, yet he still prescribed the nutritional supplements. Unfortunately, the client died of a massive cerebral (brain) hemorrhage shortly after a workout session (Herbert, 1999).

You should check the laws in your own state to ensure that you are not violating any of them by advising your clients about food, vitamins, or calorie consumption. You should avoid giving advice on any subject in which you have not received training. Clients with complex dietary concerns should be referred to a registered dietitian.

LEGAL RESPONSIBILITIES

Liability simply means responsibility. Certain obligations and responsibilities arise from the legal relationships between you and your clients, specifically those responsibilities that a court would recognize as part of your employment as a fitness professional. These responsibilities may include facilities, equipment, supervision, instruction, and exercise recommendations and testing. This is clearly illustrated by the claims made in a 1999 case against a personal trainer in Ohio. The case (Markis v. Scandinavian Health Spa, Inc.) alleged that the personal trainer engaged in "negligent training, monitoring, instruction, supervision, and advice."

Facilities

As a personal trainer, you have an obligation to make sure that the facilities you use are free from unreasonable hazards. This may pose a problem if you conduct exercise sessions in your clients' homes or in places of business where you have little control over the setting. You must select the workout area carefully, giving special attention to the following:

✔ Floor surface. Many exercises require floor surfaces that will cushion the feet, knees, and legs from excessive stress.

✔ Adequate free space around workout stations.

✔ Appropriate use of public spaces. Use of public beaches, parks, or public trails for business is illegal in some areas. Check with a local attorney.

✔ Ethical use of other business establishments. Accompanying a client into a fitness center may violate laws as well as ethical business practice. A local attorney can advise you.

Because your primary responsibility is your client's safety, inspect facilities regularly using a safety checklist. If you notice an unsafe facility, you must notify the club management or client. If a club owner does not repair the problem and your client is injured, you are technically responsible. However, juries have often looked favorably on employees who have tried unsuccessfully to persuade management to correct dangerous conditions.

Often, the client may not wish to follow your suggestions for making a safer environment because it does not fit their home's decor. In this case, the client is assuming responsibility for these conditions. Whether a dangerous situation occurs in a club or at a client's home, you must make a professional assessment and decide whether or not to continue.

Equipment

Fitness programs may utilize a variety of equipment, and injuries from the use of exercise equipment give rise to a majority of the litigation in the fitness industry. To protect both you and your clients, all of your equipment should meet the highest safety and design standards. Avoid using homemade equipment because your liability is greater if it causes injury to your client. You must be concerned about the selection, maintenance, and repair of the equipment you use with your clients, and inspect it on a regular basis. Here's why: An injured woman claimed that she had not been properly warned of the risks involved in the use of a given piece of equipment. She further claimed that the equipment had not been properly maintained and that she had not been thoroughly instructed on how to safely use it. The court agreed and she was awarded $20,000.

You may find a conflict between professional practice and legal protection when it comes to equipment owned by a client. A conservative legal stance would be to avoid any contact and adjustment to the client's equipment, but most personal trainers accept some liability by using their expertise to adjust a client's equipment or to recommend maintenance. Here's an example: A personal trainer arrives at a client's home for an initial fitness session

and finds a leg extension machine with a frayed cable. The trainer should inform the client that the equipment needs repairs, suggest that they call the company to order a replacement part, and then conduct sessions without using this equipment until it has been repaired.

The use of automated external defibrillators (AEDs) has gained considerable attention in the last few years. These devices can now be found in many places of public assembly (e.g., airports, shopping malls, amusement parks) and are rapidly becoming standard emergency equipment in health and fitness facilities. The International Health, Racquet & Sportsclub Association (IHRSA), The American College of Sports Medicine (ACSM), and the American Heart Association (AHA) all recommend training for employees in the use of AEDs in sport and fitness settings (Herbert, 2000). The issue is not so clear when it comes to personal trainers. Trainers may want to consider purchasing their own AED for use in client-owned facilities. However, there is no doubt that all personal trainers should be capable of utilizing AEDs in health and fitness facilities. This training can be acquired through most of the first aid certification courses from national agencies. (Please check www.acefitness.org for more information regarding AED training in your area.)

Good Samaritan Laws are in place in all 50 United States to provide protection for caregivers using AEDs. Assuming you are AED-certified and you do not do something negligent (e.g., abandoning the victim before emergency medical personnel arrive), you will be protected. Contact your local American Heart Association chapter to learn more about these laws. For facility owners and supervisors to be protected, they must follow all of the guidelines regarding the use of AEDs, including staff training, the location of the device in the club, care, and maintenance (Anders, 2002).

Recommendations. If a client asks for recommendations about exercise equipment, clothing, or shoes, you should be cautious in giving advice, particularly if you receive payment for endorsing a product or retail store. Before giving advice, you should become completely knowledgeable about the products and equipment available, as well as their advantages and disadvantages. Your other option would be to protect yourself by referring clients to their choice of retail sporting goods stores. Advice based solely on personal experience should be given with that express qualification.

Supervision

Although a group fitness instructor leading a large class may have difficulty ensuring each client's safety, as a personal trainer, you should always be in direct control and in close contact with each client to ensure their safety. You should never leave the client during an exercise session in which direct supervision is needed. If you are working with a couple, position yourself where you can observe both persons during an activity without turning your back on one or the other. If you ask one client to perform an exercise that requires direct supervision, do not ask the other client to perform the same exercise. Instead, engage them in an activity requiring only general observation to ensure safety. For example, you would not ask one client to do squats with a heavy weight while the other is doing a one-rep max on the bench press. You cannot spot both clients at the same time. A safer option would be to have one client stretching or working out on a stationary bike while the other is lifting and being spotted. Proper supervision requires planning to ensure that each client can be monitored at all times.

You also must adequately plan for any emergencies that may arise (see Chapter 17). When training a client, you should always have their emergency medical information with you. This eliminates the need to call back to your office for critical information about your client in the event of an emergency. Determine the availability and location of your client's telephone, as well as the address of your training location. Whether in independent practice or in a club, you should know how to activate the emergency medical system (this is done by calling 911 in most areas).

Instruction

To avoid potential litigation, your instructional techniques should be consistent with current professional practices. If you fail to demonstrate a movement or give proper instructions on how to use a piece of equipment, and your client is injured, you may be found negligent. Legal standards require that you give a client "adequate and proper" instruction before and during an activity. In a courtroom, an expert witness could be asked to assess "proper" or factually correct instruction. Adequate and proper instruction also means avoiding high-risk exercises, or those not recommended by professional peers. Advocating dangerous or controversial exercises puts you at risk for a lawsuit if a client is injured. In one case (Corrigan v. Musclemakers, Inc.), a personal trainer put his client on a treadmill but failed to appropriately adjust the speed for this first-time user, nor did he instruct her on how to adjust the speed or stop the belt. When she could no longer keep up with the pace, she was catapulted backwards and fractured her ankle in the ensuing fall.

A relatively new aspect of instructional liability concerns touching clients. You should avoid touching a client unless it is essential in instruction. Furthermore, you should inform your clients about the purpose of touching; if the client objects, find an alternative. Charges of sexual assault, even if groundless, can have disastrous consequences on your personal training career.

Safety Guidelines

In reference to the above mentioned areas of responsibility, personal trainers should adhere to the following safety guidelines in the conduct of their activities.

- ✔ Be sure that all sessions are well-planned, sequential, and documented.
- ✔ Communicate and enforce all safety rules for equipment use.
- ✔ Be sure that equipment meets or exceeds all industry standards.
- ✔ Inspect all equipment prior to use and document maintenance.
- ✔ Never allow unsupervised activity by the client.
- ✔ Limit participation to those under contract (i.e., no friends).
- ✔ Clearly warn clients about the specific risks of planned activities.
- ✔ Be sure that all activities selected are within the areas of your training.
- ✔ Be sure that clients wear any necessary protective equipment (e.g., athletic supporter or sports bra).
- ✔ Review your emergency plan (access to a phone and 911 for EMS).
- ✔ Stay up-to-date with certifications and education in the field.

Exercise Recommendations and Testing

Many states allow exercise prescriptions to be developed only by licensed doctors. It is important for you to be sure that you are providing exercise programs, not exercise prescriptions. Although the difference between these terms may sound like a technicality, it could become an important issue in a courtroom. To protect yourself, be sure you are following exercise program guidelines recommended by professional organizations such as the American Council on Exercise (ACE), the National Strength and Conditioning Association (NSCA), the American College of Sports Medicine (ACSM), and the American Heart Association (AHA). According to fitness and legal experts Herbert and Herbert (2002), guidelines such as these, while not bearing the same legal impact as a specific law, may well establish an acceptable **standard of care.** Of course, the age,

medical history, and previous activity patterns of each client must be taken into consideration.

Trainers also should be familiar with the position statements (papers) for specific populations developed by these organizations. The NSCA has produced a position paper on weight training for prepubescent youth; the American College of Obstetricians and Gynecologists has produced resource material on pregnant women and exercise; and the ACSM has published numerous position statements regarding various aspects of exercise, fitness, and health.

You may administer fitness assessments if the tests are recognized by a professional organization as appropriate for the intended use and are within the scope of your qualifications and training. For example, ACSM has established protocols for fitness assessments. You should carefully follow ACSM procedures when conducting these tests; never attempt to administer a test that you have not been trained to perform. You can legally administer tests that do not require maximum effort; therefore, you should not hook up electrodes and administer a maximum capacity test, such as a treadmill stress test, unless a qualified physician is present and oversees the test. Any highly specialized testing should be conducted by physicians or exercise physiologists. Some states regulate the administration of tests such as **Graded Exercise Tests (GXTs).** In addition, some professional associations, such as ACSM, the American Heart Association, and the American College of Cardiology, provide guidelines for the role of physicians in GXTs. Even physicians can be sued in the area of testing. In one case, a physician examined a man who wanted to begin an exercise program and gave the man a resting electrocardiogram (ECG), not a GXT. A few days later the man died while jogging, and the courts found in favor of the plaintiff, awarding $500,000 to his estate.

Legal Responsibilities

The development of exercise technology has offered several dilemmas for personal trainers, among them the legal concern over monitoring clients who can attach electrodes to their chests and continuously monitor their heart rates while exercising. You must make every effort to monitor your clients during exercise, with or without the high-tech options currently available. Failure to do so may constitute a breach of legal duty.

LEGAL CONCEPTS AND DEFENSES

It is essential that, as a personal trainer, you conduct your professional activities with the highest standards, not only for your professional competence and training, but also for your ethical and legal position. In court, certain concepts have special meanings that you should be familiar with to protect both yourself and your clients. Some of these concepts have already been discussed. The remainder of this chapter will present several other legal concepts that are important to you.

Standard of Care

Your actions as a personal trainer must be appropriate for the age, condition, and knowledge of the client, as well as for the program selected. To evaluate the standard of care, a court would typically ask an expert witness to describe the current professional standards—what other fitness professionals of similar training would do (or should have done) in the same situation. This manual, for example, constitutes a standard for personal training. With ACE **certification** in personal training, your competence could be verified. In addition, your conduct would be compared to the standards presented in the manual and your ethics would be equated to the ACE **Code of Ethics** located in Appendix A. In a legal dispute, a court would almost certainly look to the practices described in this manual to evaluate the appropriateness of a trainer's actions.

Assumption of Risk

If a client voluntarily accepts the dangers known to be part of an activity, the trainer can use the **assumption of risk** defense. However, the two most important issues here are "voluntarily" and "known danger." If a client's participation was involuntary, this defense cannot be used. Furthermore, if the client was not informed about the specific risks of the program or test, the client cannot be held to have assumed them. Does this defense imply that a trainer must describe every injury that might occur? Yes, in general, but the best way to take care of this issue is to use standard forms for **informed consent** (express assumption of risk) or **waiver** forms.

Known technically as exculpatory agreements, informed consents, warnings, and waivers fall under contract law and are often used by exercise leaders and fitness centers to absolve themselves of liability. Although many fitness professionals have little faith in the value of these documents, the courts have been increasingly willing to uphold them.

Informed Consent. When a client signs an **informed consent** form, he or she is acknowledging to have been specifically informed about the risk associated with the activity in which he or she is about to engage (Figure 18.1). Some personal trainers use an informed consent form in a similar manner to a waiver, but it is primarily intended to communicate the dangers of the program or test procedures to the client (Figure 18.2). You should obtain signed informed consent forms from every person who enters your programs and before every test you administer. Let your clients know that questions about the program or testing are welcome, and that they are free to withdraw consent and discontinue participation at any time. You should inform your clients about:

✔ The exercise program or test, providing a thorough and unbiased explanation of the purpose of each
✔ The risks and possible discomforts involved
✔ The benefits they might expect.

Legal Concepts and Defenses

"I, _____ , have enrolled in a program of strenuous physical activity including, but not limited to, traditional aerobics, weight training, stationary bicycling, and the use of various aerobic-conditioning machinery offered by [name of business]____ . I hereby affirm that I am in good physical condition and do not suffer from any disability that would prevent or limit my participation in this exercise program."

"In consideration of my participation in _____ [name of business]____ exercise program, I, _____ , for myself, my heirs, and assigns, hereby release [name of business]____ (its employees and owners), from any claims, demands, and causes of action arising from my participation in the exercise program."

"I fully understand that I may injure myself as a result of my participation in [name of business]____ exercise program and I, _____ , hereby release [name of business] from any liability now or in the future including, but not limited to, heart attacks, muscle strains, pulls or tears, broken bones, shin splints, heat prostration, knee/lower back/foot injuries, and any other illness, soreness, or injury, however caused, occurring during or after my participation in the exercise program."

_____
Signature

_____
Date

I hereby affirm that I have read and fully understand the above.

_____
Signature

FIGURE 18.1
Sample waiver of liability/informed consent.

This form should not be adopted for use without individual legal review and consultation.

Please note that this waiver is only a guideline, compiled from the forms upheld in Illinois, Minnesota, and Tennessee. The rules vary from state to state, so do not expect this particular waiver to hold up in your state court. See your attorney for advice.

If your attorney discovers that waivers of liability are not upheld in your state, redraft your waiver to comply with these recommendations anyway. You never know when the law may change.

FIGURE 18.2
Sample informed consent form. Reprinted with permission from Herbert, D.L. and Herbert, W.G.(2002). *Legal Aspects of Preventive and Rehabilitative Exercise Programs* (4th ed.). Canton, Ohio: PRC Publishing. All rights reserved.

This form should not be adopted for use without individual legal review and consultation.

Informed Consent for Exercise Testing of Apparently Healthy Adults (without known heart disease)

Name_____

1. Purpose and Explanation of Test

I hereby consent to voluntarily engage in an exercise test to determine my circulatory and respiratory fitness. I also consent to the taking of samples of my exhaled air during exercise to properly measure my oxygen consumption. I also consent, if necessary, to have a small blood sample drawn by needle from my arm for blood chemistry analysis and to the performance of lung function and body fat (skin-fold pinch) tests. It is my understanding that the information obtained will help me evaluate future physical activities and sports activities in which I may engage.

Before I undergo the test, I certify to the program that I am in good health and have had a physical examination conducted by a licensed medical physician within the last_____ months. Further, I hereby represent and inform the program that I have accurately completed the pre-test history interview presented to me by the program staff and have provided correct responses to the questions as indicated on the history form or as supplied to the interviewer. It is my understanding that I will be interviewed by a physician or other person prior to my undergoing the test who will in the course of interviewing me determine if there are any reasons which would make it undesirable or unsafe for me to take the test. Consequently, I understand that it is important that I provide complete and accurate responses to the interviewer and recognize that my failure to do so could lead to possible unnecessary injury to myself during the test.

The test which I will undergo will be performed on a motor driven treadmill or bicycle ergometer with the amount of effort gradually increasing. As I understand it, this increase in effort will continue until I feel and verbally report to the operator any symptoms such as fatigue, shortness of breath, or chest discomfort which may appear. It is my understanding and I have been clearly advised that it is my right to request that a test be stopped at any point if I feel unusual discomfort or fatigue. I have been advised that I should, immediately upon experiencing any such symptoms or if I so choose, inform the operator that I wish to stop the test at that or any other point. My wishes in this regard shall be absolutely carried out.

It is further my understanding that prior to beginning the test, I will be connected by electrodes and cables to an electrocardiographic recorder which will enable the program personnel to monitor my cardiac (heart) activity. During the test itself, it is my understanding that a trained observer will monitor my responses continuously and take frequent readings of blood pressure, the electrocardio-

**Legal Concepts
and Defenses**

gram, and my expressed feelings of effort. I realize that a true determination of my exercise capacity depends on progressing the test to the point of my fatigue.

FIGURE 18.2 continued

Once the test has been completed, but before I am released from the test area, I will be given special instructions about showering and recognition of certain symptoms which may appear within the first 24 hours after the test. I agree to follow these instructions and promptly contact the program personnel or medical providers if such symptoms develop.

2. Risks

It is my understanding and I have been informed that there exists the possibility of adverse changes during the actual test. I have been informed that these changes could include abnormal blood pressure, fainting, disorders of heart rhythm, stroke, and very rare instances of heart attack or even death. Every effort, I have been told, will be made to minimize these occurrences by preliminary examination and by precautions and observations taken during the test. I have also been informed that emergency equipment and personnel are readily available to deal with these unusual situations should they occur. I understand that there is a risk of injury, heart attack, stroke, or even death as a result of my performance of this test, but knowing those risks, it is my desire to proceed to take the test as herein indicated.

3. Benefits to be Expected and Alternatives Available to the Exercise Testing Procedure

The results of this test may or may not benefit me. Potential benefits relate mainly to my personal motives for taking the test, *i.e.*, knowing my exercise capacity in relation to the general population, understanding my fitness for certain sports and recreational activities, planning my physical conditioning program or evaluating the effects of my recent physical habits. Although my fitness might also be evaluated by alternative means, *e.g.*, a bench step test or an outdoor running test, such tests do not provide as accurate a fitness assessment as the treadmill or bike test nor do those options allow equally effective monitoring of my responses.

4. Confidentiality and Use of Information

I have been informed that the information which is obtained form this exercise test will be treated as privileged and confidential and will consequently not be released or revealed to any person without my express written consent or as required by law. I do, however, agree to the use of any information for research or statistical purposes so long as same does not provide facts which could lead to the identification of my person. Any other information obtained however, will be used only by the program staff to evaluate my exercise status or needs.

continued on next page

FIGURE 18.2 continued

5. Inquiries and Freedom of Consent

I have been given an opportunity to ask questions as to the procedure. Generally these requests which have been noted by the testing staff and their responses are as follows:

_____

_____

_____

I further understand that there are also other remote risks that may be associated with this procedure. Despite the fact that a complete accounting of all remote risks is not entirely possible, I am satisfied with the review of these risks which was provided to me and it is still my desire to proceed with the test.

I acknowledge that I have read this document in its entirety or that it has been read to me if I have been unable to read same.

I consent to the rendition of all services and procedures as explained herein by all program personnel.

Date_____   _____

                                    Patient's Signature

_____

Witness' Signature

_____

Test Supervisor's Signature

AGREEMENT AND RELEASE OF LIABILITY

1. In consideration of being allowed to participate in the activities and programs of _____ and to use its facilities, equipment, and machinery in addition to the payment of any fee or charge, I do hereby waive, release, and forever discharge _____ and its officers, agents, employees, representatives, executors, and all others from any and all responsibilities or liability from injuries or damages resulting from my participation in any activities, or my use of equipment or machinery in the above mentioned activities. I do also hereby release all of those mentioned, and any others acting upon their behalf, from any responsibility or liability for any injury or damage to myself, including those caused by the negligent act or omission of any of those mentioned or others acting on their behalf, or in any way arising out of or connected with my participation in any activities of _____ or the use of any equipment at _____ .

(*Please initial _____*)

2. I understand and am aware that strength, flexibility, and aerobic exercise, including the use of equipment, is a potentially hazardous activity. I also understand that fitness activities involve a risk of injury and even death, and that I am voluntarily participating in these activities and using equipment and machinery with knowledge of the dangers involved. I hereby agree to expressly assume and accept any and all risks of injury or death.
(*Please initial _____*)

3. I do hereby further declare myself to be physically sound and suffering from no condition, impairment, disease, infirmity, or other illness that would prevent my participation or use of equipment or machinery except as hereinafter stated. I do hereby acknowledge that I have been informed of the need for a physician's approval for my participation in an exercise/fitness activity or in the use of exercise equipment and machinery. I also acknowledge that it has been recommended that I have a yearly or more frequent physical examination and consultation with my physician as to physical activity, exercise, and use of exercise and training equipment so that I might have his/her recommendations concerning these fitness activities and equipment use. I acknowledge that I have either had a physical examination and been given my physician's permission to participate, or that I have decided to participate in activity and use of equipment and machinery without the approval of my physician and do hereby assume all responsibility for my participation and activities, and utilization of equipment and machinery in my activities.

Date _____ Signature _____

Legal Concepts and Defenses

FIGURE 18.3
Sample waiver of liability. Reprinted with permission from Koeberle, B. E. (1998). *Legal Aspects of Personal Fitness Training* (2nd ed.). Canton, Ohio: PRC Publishing. All rights reserved.

This form should not be adopted for use without individual legal review and consultation.

✔ Alternatives that may be advantageous to them

Warnings. In one Colorado case, a health club's failure to warn a client about the dangers of an activity and piece of equipment was judged "willful and wanton" misconduct. You should obtain signed proof that you have warned your clients about any foreseeable hazards and risks.

Waivers. A voluntary abandonment of the right to file suit, waivers are used to release you from liability for injuries resulting from an exercise program. Waivers must be clearly written and indicate that the client waives all claims for damages, even those caused by the trainer's negligence (Figures 18.1 and 18.3). Occasionally, these documents are so poorly worded that they hold little value in court. However, case law in 45 states clearly supports well-constructed waivers.

Specific to personal trainers, a recent court case addressed the situation in which a member of a health club signed a supplemental contract for personal training services in the club setting. When she was injured in a session with the personal trainer, she contended that the waiver signed with her membership contract did not extend and cover the services of the personal trainer. The courts disagreed and ruled that the services of the personal trainer were part of the activities and benefits offered at the club and were therefore covered by the original waiver (Cotton, 2000a). With the increase in personal training for high school athletes, you should be particularly careful with waivers signed by minors. Some states will not consider these waivers valid, even if signed by a parent, while other states may support such waivers. Another issue regarding waivers can arise when you are working with a couple and only one of the clients signs the waiver. Again, the case law is a bit ambiguous in this area. The prudent practice would be to require signatures from

both clients if you are training a couple (Cotton, 2000b). Courts prefer to deal with these issues on a case-by-case basis. You should consult with attorneys in your own state, providing them with examples to use as a model.

Negligence

Someone who fails to perform as a reasonable and prudent person would under similar circumstances is considered negligent. This definition has two important components: failure to act and appropriateness of the action. A person can be sued both for neglecting something that should have been done, such as not spotting a client in a free-weight bench press, and for doing something that should not have been done, such as programming straight-leg sit-ups for a client with low-back problems. This action may be found inappropriate as compared with what a reasonable and prudent professional would do.

To substantiate a charge of negligence in court, the plaintiff must establish four elements:

✔ The defendant had a duty to protect the plaintiff from injury.
✔ The defendant failed to exercise the standard of care necessary to perform that duty.
✔ Damage or injury to the plaintiff occurred.
✔ This damage or injury was caused by the defendant's breach of duty (proximate causation).

Negligence in personal training could occur, for example, if you agreed to provide instruction and supervision (duties) in weight lifting, and during the first session told the client you would spot them during a lift but failed to do so (breach of duty). Perhaps the client suffered broken ribs and was unable to work for three months, incurring both medical bills and lost wages (damages). The damages would not have occurred if you had not failed to spot for the client during the lift (proximate causation).

Contributory Negligence. If the client played some role in getting injured, a few states prohibit the recovery of damages (check your local state laws). For example, a client might exceed his or her recommended heart rate. It would be important to determine whether the trainer was present when the client was hurt, or whether the client was exercising alone and following the trainer's guidelines. If present, the trainer might have noticed the client's over-taxation and warned them about exceeding the recommendations.

Comparative Negligence. A court may apportion guilt and any subsequent award for damages, measuring the relative fault of both the plaintiff and the defendant. The court or jury then determines the percentage of responsibility of each party to prorate the award. This defense can be useful if a client is somewhat to blame in injuring himself or herself.

LIABILITY INSURANCE

Whether you are a seasoned veteran or a newcomer to the fitness profession, a complete understanding of insurance is essential to your success. Because of the rise in litigation throughout the healthcare industry, purchasing insurance has become one of the best risk-management strategies available to health and fitness professionals. Judgments for millions of dollars are not uncommon, and few could weather such a substantial financial blow. Insurance protection also provides peace of mind; you can be secure in the knowledge that if someone were to be injured as a result of your actions, insurance coverage would be adequate to recompense that individual for his or her losses.

Protection for You

Generally, an insurance policy is a contract designed to protect you and your assets from litigation. There is, however, a sarcastic yet often accurate saying that insurance

---

Table 18.3
Make Sure You Are Covered

General Liability

General liability insurance covers basic trip and fall injuries that occur in a nonbusiness environment. These policies will not provide coverage for accidents that occur at work.

Professional Liability

Professional liability insurance is designed to protect you against a broad spectrum of claims. This includes allegations claiming injury to students or clients as a result of improper supervision of fitness activities, failure to adequately instruct, improper use or recommendation of equipment, and exposure to injury from substandard facilities. This coverage should extend to acts of omission (things you did not do) as well as acts of commission (actual conduct). Most policies also extend coverage for violations of a client's civil rights, such as sexual harassment, an important element to consider in today's sensitive environment. Defense coverage should be extended even if the charges are groundless.

Disability

Disability insurance, which provides income protection should you become injured, may or may not be supplied by your employer. If it is not provided, you may want to consider purchasing this type of insurance for yourself. While worker's compensation covers you when you are injured on or by the job, disability insurance will provide income even if your injury occurs outside of work.

Medical Insurance

Individual medical insurance, which provides hospitalization and major medical coverage, is another type of coverage that may be supplied by your employer. These plans vary widely and, because of increasing costs, many clubs have reduced or eliminated these benefits as a cost-saving measure. Rarely are independent contractors granted benefits.

companies are in the business of collecting premiums and denying claims. Table 18.3 provides a breakdown of the types of coverage available and the provisions of specific policies. It is important to familiarize yourself with these terms before you rush out to purchase an insurance policy.

Independent Contractors

If you are an independent contractor working for clubs or other facilities, you should pay special attention to your coverage. It is imperative that all aspects of any coverage that may be provided for you are understood and included in the written agreements for services. If insurance coverage is not provided by the club, it is in your own best interest, as well as that of your clients, to provide yourself with adequate coverage.

Locating Coverage

Insurance is predicated on a system whereby the risks of financial loss are distributed over policy holders. Therefore, policies available through various professional associations often provide the best value because the risks are spread over a large number of policy holders. Membership in these organizations does not automatically provide this coverage, but these organizations have arrangements that give members the right to purchase policies at a reduced rate. Individual policies are available in the marketplace but are considerably more expensive.

Riders

Some companies offer "business pursuits riders" or "umbrella coverage" that extend current coverage on your residential property or apply a blanket amount to both personal and professional activities. These policies are often less expensive than the policies available through professional associations, but may exclude certain professions. A check with your insurance carrier is certainly warranted.

Words to Choose Your Policy By

The basic tenet of insurance is to obligate the company to defend you as well as to pay for any damages adjudged against you. The following statement, or some version of it, should be included in any basic agreement:

We agree to pay those sums that the insured becomes legally obligated to pay as damages because of bodily injury or property damage to which this insurance applies, and these will include damages arising out of any negligent act, error, or omission in rendering or failing to render professional services described in this policy.

A key provision here indicates that the company will pay even if you fail to provide a service. For example, if an injured person needed first-aid attention and you did not provide it, the policy would still protect you. If "failure to render" or "omission" were not specified, the policy would cover you only if the services you provided were inadequate or improper.

Coverage Where You Need It

When choosing an insurance policy, be sure to describe in detail all of the types of professional services for which you are seeking coverage. If a claim is made, the company will look very closely at the nature of the activity in which the injury occurred. If it was not specified in the policy, the company might deny the claim. Carefully examine the types of services covered to be sure that the ones you provide your clients are included.

Make Sure Legal Fees Are Covered

Another important element of an insurance policy is related to coverage of legal fees, settlements, and defense charges. Look for the following clause before signing on the dotted line:

We will have the right and duty to defend any suit seeking damages under this policy, even if the allegations are groundless, false, or fraudulent and may, at our discretion, make such investigation and settlement of any claim or suit deemed expedient.

The best policies cover the cost of a legal defense and any claims awarded. Policies that only cover an amount equal to awarded damages are not recommended. If you go to court, all of the trial expenses incurred will be your responsibility. A good policy should cover the cost of a legal defense as well as the amount of damages awarded.

Find Out What Is Not Covered

While it is important to identify and understand what is covered, it is also critical to know what is not covered. Most policies delineate specific exclusions. The following liabilities are often excluded in fitness professional policies: abuse, molestation, cancer (resulting from tanning), libel, and slander.

You should also inquire whether your bodily insurance coverage will protect you if a suit is filed alleging mental stress. Most policies differentiate between the two, and a standard bodily injury clause does not include mental injuries. A client filing a suit might claim that you were overly critical and, as a result, they suffered mental injuries. The courts are split on the issue of inclusion. For example, litigation in New York found that bodily injury included mental distress, while a California court said it did not.

Past, Present, and Future Claims

Finally, most policies exclude coverage for acts committed before the policy was purchased. Coverage also might be excluded for claims that occurred during the policy period but are filed after the coverage has been terminated. These issues are related to the "claims-made basis" of a policy. You can purchase "prior acts coverage" from most insurance carriers for an additional cost. An analysis of your past actions should guide your decision in this area. An "extended reporting endorsement" will ensure that claims made in the future for injuries during the policy period will be covered even if you decide to cancel your policy.

As with all business endeavors, you should closely evaluate an insurance company be-fore purchasing a policy. The most reputable insurance carriers have a national affiliation, are licensed, have strong financial backing, and have a reinsurer (corporate policy to ensure that policy holders' claims will be met even if their business collapses). You may also want to check whether or not the company has had complaints filed with state insurance commissions or the Better Business Bureau.

While understanding the language and details of insurance policies can be difficult, keep in mind that your insurance agent works for you. It is their responsibility to give you a complete explanation and answer any questions you may have. By understanding the basic principles outlined here, you will have a head start on finding the insurance coverage to meet your professional needs.

OTHER BUSINESS CONCERNS WITH LEGAL IMPLICATIONS

In addition to your legal responsibilities in the areas of **scope of practice,** facilities, equipment, testing, instruction, and supervision, you must be aware of the legal implications of additional business concerns such as certification and the use of musical recordings.

Certification

Although there are currently no federal laws requiring licensure or certification for personal trainers, certification from a credible professional organization can assist a defendant by providing evidence of **competency.** *Note: It also is important to understand that certification does not protect against findings of negligence.* In fact, some trainers believe that juries will hold certified personal trainers to a higher standard of care than noncertified trainers. In reality, however, negligence is negligence, and a competent attorney can expose a substandard performance in either case. Most legal experts acknowledge that certification demonstrates minimal competency in the fitness profession. It also will help you assure clients that they are receiving instruction from a knowledgeable and recognized professional.

Music

All the popular recordings on radio and television have been protected by artists and studios with copyrights. Any use of this material for profit is a violation of federal law, even if you have purchased the recording. Recordings sold commercially are intended strictly for the private, noncommercial use of the purchaser. Although two groups, ASCAP and BMI, will issue licenses for the commercial use of recordings, their fees are probably prohibitive for most personal trainers. You might find it more economical to use recordings designed and sold for fitness and aerobic programs. Another option is for your clients to purchase their own recordings for use during workouts. In effect, the clients are then using these recordings for their own private, non-commercial enjoyment during exercise.

Bloodborne Pathogens

In special circumstances, you may be involved in situations where a client bleeds. For instance, you may be working with a client who is a boxer or is engaged in other contact sports. In situations where you are exposed to a client's blood, special

precautions must be followed. The Occupational Safety and Health Administration (OSHA) has issued guidelines for handling exposure to blood. Because a variety of maladies can be transmitted through contact with human blood (e.g., human immunodeficiency virus, hepatitis), trainers should have access to protective gloves and exercise caution when exposed to and disposing of any blood-contaminated materials. Trainers involved in contact sports should contact OSHA for more complete details.

Risk Management

Periodically reviewing programs, facilities, and equipment to evaluate potential dangers to clients allows you to decide the best way to reduce costly injuries in each situation. This is called **risk management.**

Most authorities recommend a risk management protocol that consists of the ensuing five steps:

1. Identification of risks—the specification of all risks that may be encountered by the personal trainer in the areas of instruction, supervision, facilities, equipment, contracts, and business structure.

2. Evaluation of each risk—the personal trainer must review each risk with consideration given to the probability that the risk could occur and if so, what would be the conceivable severity. Table 18.4 can be used to assess the identified risks.

3. Selection of an approach for managing each risk—several approaches are available to the personal trainer for managing and reducing the identified risks.

Following are the most common methods of reducing risk:

✔ transfer of risk, as with insurance policies
✔ reduction (through continuing education)
✔ retention (budgeting for minor emergencies)
✔ avoidance of certain activities or equipment

Table 18.4
Evaluating Risk Based on Frequency and Severity

Severity of Injury or Financial Impact	Frequency of Occurrence		
	High or often	Medium or infrequent	Low or seldom
High or vital	Avoid or transfer	Transfer	Transfer
Medium or significant	Transfer	Transfer or retain	Transfer or retain
Low or insignificant	Retain	Retain	Retain

The recommended approach for risks that are extreme is to avoid the activity completely or transfer the risk through appropriate insurance. Risks that fall into one of the high categories can be managed either through insurance or viable actions to reduce the likelihood of occurrence or severity of outcome. Reduction is also the preferred method for addressing risks in the medium category while risks with low impact can be handled through retention.

4. Implementation—putting your plans into practice.

5. Evaluation—assessing the outcome of your risk management endeavors.

You also can manage risk by examining procedures and policies and developing conduct and safety guidelines for your clients' use of equipment. Strict safety guidelines for each activity, accompanied by procedures for emergencies, are particularly important. You must not only develop these policies but become thoroughly familiar with them, mentally practicing your emergency plans. Several lawsuits have resulted in substantial judgments against fitness professionals who failed to respond to the emergency medical needs of clients. Once risks are identified, you should carry out the actions needed to reduce them.

SUMMARY

Although often overlooked when considering the technical aspects of providing quality personalized fitness instruction, the legal, ethical, and business concerns are of paramount importance. You accept a tremendous amount of responsibility when you assume the role of personal trainer. You must always be aware of your scope of practice and, because of the rise in litigation across all aspects of the profession, it is absolutely essential to maintain adequate insurance coverage. This chapter touched on the legal, ethical, and business issues that must be considered. The guidelines offered are not legal advice. Rather, they are a condensed presentation of the technicalities that you, as a responsible trainer, must understand.

References and Suggested Reading

REFERENCES

Anders, M. (2001). The ABCs of AEDs: What you should know about automated external defibrillators in fitness clubs. *ACE Certified News,* 8, 5, 3–5.

Corrigan v. Musclemakers, Inc. 686 N.Y.S. 2d 143 (1999).

Cotton, D.J. (2000a). Carefully Worded Liability Waiver Protects Bally's from Liability for Personal Trainer Negligence. *Exercise Standards and Malpractice Reporter*, 14, 5, p.65.

Cotton, D.J. (2000b). Non-signing Spouses: Are They Bound by a Waiver Signed by the Other Spouse? *Exercise Standards and Malpractice Reporter*, 14, 2, p.18.

Herbert, D.L. (2000). Failure to Defibrillate Litigation Results in Another Defense Verdict. *Exercise Standards and Malpractice Reporter*, 14, 2, p.11.

Herbert, D.L. (1999). $320 Million Lawsuit Filed Against Health Club. *Exercise Standards and Malpractice Reporter*, 13, 3, p.33.

Herbert, D.L. & Herbert, W.G. (2002) *Legal Aspects of Preventive, Rehabilitative and Recreational Exercise Programs* (4th ed.). Canton, Ohio: PRC Publishing, Inc.

SUGGESTED READING

Cotton, D.L. & Cotton, M.B. (1997). *Legal Aspects of Waivers in Sport, Recreation and Fitness Activities.* Canton, Ohio: PRC Publishing, Inc.

International Health, Racquet & Sportsclub Association. (1998). *Know the Law: Legal Issues Affecting Health & Fitness Clubs.* Boston, Mass: International Health, Racquet & Sportsclub Association.

Koeberle, B. E. (1998). *Legal Aspects of Personal Fitness Training*, (2nd ed). Canton, Ohio: PRC Publishing, Inc.

Code
of Ethics

ACE-certified Professionals are guided by the following principles of conduct as they interact with clients, the public, and other health and fitness professionals.

ACE-certified Professionals will endeavor to:

✔ Provide safe and effective instruction

✔ Provide equal and fair treatment to all clients

✔ Stay up-to-date on the latest health and fitness research and understand its practical application

✔ Maintain current CPR certification and knowledge of first-aid services

✔ Comply with all applicable business, employment, and intellectual property laws

✔ Maintain the confidentiality of all client information

✔ Refer clients to more qualified health or medical professionals when appropriate

✔ Uphold and enhance public appreciation and trust for the health and fitness industry

✔ Establish and maintain clear professional boundaries

ACE Code of Ethics

PROVIDE SAFE AND EFFECTIVE INSTRUCTION

Providing safe and effective instruction involves a variety of responsibilities for ACE-certified Professionals. Safe means that the instruction will not result in physical, mental, or financial harm to the client. Effective means that the instruction has a purposeful, intended, and desired effect toward the client's goal. Great effort and care must be taken in carrying out the responsibilities that are essential in creating a positive exercise experience for all participants.

Screening

ACE-certified Professionals should have all potential clients complete an industry-recognized health-screening tool to ensure safe exercise participation. If significant risk factors or signs and symptoms suggestive of chronic disease are identified, refer the client to a physician or primary health-care practitioner for medical clearance and guidance regarding which types of assessments, activities, or exercises are indicated, contraindicated, or deemed high risk. If an individual does not want to obtain medical clearance, have the client sign a legally prepared document that releases you and the facility in which you work from any liability related to any injury that may result from exercise participation or assessment. Once the client has been cleared for exercise and you have a full understanding of the client's health status and medical history, including their current use of medications, a formal risk-management plan for potential emergencies must be prepared and reviewed periodically.

Assessment

The main objective of a health assessment is to establish the client's baseline fitness level in order to design an appropriate exercise program. Explain the risks and benefits of each assessment and provide the client with any pertinent instructions. Prior to conducting any type of assessment, the client must be given an opportunity to ask questions and read and sign an informed consent. The types and order of assessments are dictated by the client's health status, fitness level, symptoms, and/or use of medications. Remember that each assessment has specific protocols and only those within your scope of practice should be administered. Once the assessments are completed, evaluate and discuss the results objectively as they relate to the client's health condition and goals. Educate the client and emphasize how an exercise program will benefit the client.

Program Design

You must not prescribe exercise, diet, or treatment as this is outside your scope of practice and implies ordering or advising a medicine or treatment. Instead, it is appropriate for you to design exercise programs that improve components of physical fitness and wellness while adhering to the limitations of a previous injury or condition as determined by a certified, registered, or licensed allied health professional. Because nutritional laws and the practice of dietetics vary in each state, province, and country, understand what type of basic nutritional information is appropriate and legal for you to disseminate to your client. The client's preferences, and short- and long-term goals as well as current industry standards and guidelines must be taken into consideration as you develop a formal yet realistic exercise program. Provide as much detail for all exercise parameters such as mode, intensity, type of exercise, duration, progression, and termination points.

Program Implementation

Do not underestimate your ability to influence the client on becoming active for a lifetime. Be sure that each class or session is well-planned, sequential, and documented. Instruct the client how to safely and properly perform the appropriate exercises and communicate this in a manner in which the client will understand and retain. Each client has a different learning curve that will require different levels of attention, learning aids, and repetition. Supervise the client closely, especially when spotting or cueing is needed. If supervising a group of two or more, ensure that you can supervise and provide the appropriate amount of attention to each individual at all times. Ideally, the group will have similar goals and will be performing similar exercises or activities. Position yourself so that you do not have to turn your back to any client performing an exercise.

Facilities

Although the condition of a facility may not always be within your control, you are still obligated to ensure a hazard-free environment to maximize safety. If you notice potential hazards in the health club, communicate these hazards to the client and the facility management. For example, if you notice that the clamps that keep the weights on the barbells are getting rusty and loose, it would be prudent of you to remove them from the training area and alert the facility that immediate repair is required.

Equipment

Obtain equipment that meets or exceeds industry standards and utilize the equipment only for its intended use. Arrange exercise equipment and stations so that adequate space exists between equipment, participants, and foot traffic. Schedule regular maintenance and inspect equipment prior to use to ensure it is in proper working condition. Avoid the use of homemade equipment, as your liability is greater if it causes injury to your client.

PROVIDE EQUAL AND FAIR TREATMENT TO ALL CLIENTS

ACE-certified Professionals are obligated to provide fair and equal treatment for each client without bias, preference, or discrimination against gender, ethnic background, age, national origin, basis of religion, or physical disability.

The Americans with Disabilities Act protects individuals with disabilities against any type of unlawful discrimination. A disability can be either physical or mental, such as epilepsy, paralysis, HIV infection, AIDS, a significant hearing or visual impairment, mental retardation, or a specific learning disability. ACE-certified Professionals should, at a minimum, provide reasonable accommodations to each individual with a disability. Reasonable simply means that you are able to provide accommodations that do not cause you any undue hardship that requires additional or significant expense or difficulty. Making an existing facility accessible by modifying equipment or devices, assessments, or training materials are a few examples of providing reasonable accommodations. However, providing the use of personal items or providing items at your own expense may not be considered reasonable.

This ethical consideration of providing fair and equal treatment is not limited to behavioral interactions with clients, but also extends to exercise programming and other business-related services such as communication, scheduling, billing, cancellation policies, and dispute resolution.

STAY UP-TO-DATE ON THE LATEST HEALTH AND FITNESS RESEARCH AND UNDERSTAND ITS PRACTICAL APPLICATION

Obtaining ACE-certification required you to have broad-based knowledge of many disciplines; however, this credential should not be viewed as the end of your professional development and education. Instead, it should be viewed as the beginning or foundation. The dynamic nature of the health and fitness industry requires you to maintain an understanding of the latest research and professional standards and guidelines, and their impact on the design and implementation of exercise programming. To stay informed, make time to review a variety of industry resources such as professional journals, position statements, trade and lay periodicals, and correspondence courses, as well as to attend professional meetings, conferences, and educational workshops.

An additional benefit of staying up-to-date is that it also fulfills your certification renewal requirements for continuing education credit (CEC). To maintain your ACE certification status, you must obtain an established amount of CECs every two years. CECs are granted for structured learning that takes place within the educational portion of a course related to the profession and presented by a qualified health and fitness professional.

MAINTAIN CURRENT CPR CERTIFICATION AND KNOWLEDGE OF FIRST-AID SERVICES

ACE-certified Professionals must be prepared to recognize and respond to heart attacks and other life-threatening emergencies. Emergency response is enhanced by training and maintaining skills in CPR, first aid, and using automated external defibrillators (AEDs), which have become more widely available. An AED is a portable electronic device used to restore normal heart rhythm in a person experiencing a cardiac arrest and can reduce the time to defibrillation before EMS personnel arrive. For each minute that defibrillation is delayed, the victim's chance of survival is reduced by 7 to 10%. Thus, survival from cardiac arrest is improved dramatically when CPR and defibrillation are started early.

COMPLY WITH ALL APPLICABLE BUSINESS, EMPLOYMENT, AND INTELLECTUAL PROPERTY LAWS

As an ACE-certified Professional, you are expected to maintain a high level of integrity by complying with all applicable business, employment, and copyright laws. Be truthful and forthcoming with communication to clients, co-workers, and other health and fitness professionals in advertising, marketing, and business practices. Do not create false or misleading impressions of credentials, claims, or sponsorships, or perform services outside of your scope of practice that are illegal, deceptive, or fraudulent.

All information regarding your business must be clear, accurate, and easy to understand for all potential clients. Provide disclosure about the name of your business, physical address, and contact information, and maintain a working phone number and email address. So that clients can make an informed choice about paying for your services, provide detailed information regarding schedules, prices, payment terms, time limits, and conditions. Cancellation, refund, and rescheduling information must also be clearly stated and easy to understand. Allow the client an opportunity to ask questions and review this information before formally agreeing to your services and terms.

Because employment laws vary between each city, state, province, and country, familiarize yourself with the applicable employment regulations and standards to which your business must conform. Examples of this may include conforming to specific building codes and zoning ordinances or making sure that your place of business is accessible to individuals with a disability.

The understanding of intellectual property law and the proper use of copyrighted materials is an important legal issue for all ACE-certified Professionals. Intellectual property laws protect the creations of authors, artists, software programmers, and others with copyrighted materials. The most common infringement of intellectual property law in the fitness industry is the use of music in an exercise class. When commercial music is played in a for-profit exercise class, without a performance or blanket license, it is considered a public performance and a violation of intellectual property law. Therefore, make sure that any music, handouts, or educational materials are either exempt from intellectual property law, permissible under laws by reason of fair use, or obtain express written consent from the copyright holder for distribution, adaptation, or use. When in doubt, obtain permission first or consult with a qualified legal professional who has intellectual property law expertise.

MAINTAIN THE CONFIDENTIALITY OF ALL CLIENT INFORMATION

Every client has the right to expect that all personal data and discussions with an ACE-certified Professional will be safeguarded and not disclosed without the client's express written consent or acknowledgement. Therefore, protect the confidentiality of all client information such as contact data, medical records, health history, progress notes, and meeting details. Even when confidentiality is not required by law, continue to preserve the confidentiality of such information.

Any breach of confidentiality, intentional or unintentional, potentially harms the productivity and trust of your client and undermines your effectiveness as a fitness professional. This also puts you at risk for potential litigation and puts your client at risk for public embarrassment and fraudulent activity such as identity theft.

Most breaches of confidentiality are unintentional and occur because of carelessness and lack of awareness. The most common breach of confidentiality is exposing or storing a client's personal data in a location that is not secure. This occurs when a client's file or information is left on a desk, or filed in a cabinet that has no lock or is accessible to others. Breaches of confidentiality may also occur when you have conversations regarding a client's performance or medical/health history with staff or others and the client's first name or other identifying details are used.

Post and adhere to a privacy policy that communicates how client information will be used and secured and how a client's preference regarding unsolicited mail and email will be respected. When a client provides you with any personal data, new or updated, make it a habit to immediately secure this information and ensure that only you and/or the appropriate individuals have access to it. Also, the client's files must only be accessed and used for purposes related to health and fitness services. If client information is stored on a personal computer, restrict access by using a protected password. Should you receive any inquiries from family members or other individuals regarding the progress of a client or other personal information, state that you cannot provide any information without the client's permission. If and when a client permits you to release client information to an authorized individual or party, utilize secure methods of communication such as certified mail, sending and receiving information on a dedicated private fax line, or email with encryption.

REFER CLIENTS TO MORE QUALIFIED HEALTH OR MEDICAL PROFESSIONALS WHEN APPROPRIATE

A fitness certification is not a professional license. Therefore, it is vitally important that ACE-certified Professionals who do not also have a professional license (i.e., physician, physical therapist, dietitian, psychologist, and attorney) refer their clients to a more qualified professional when warranted. Doing so not only benefits your clients by making sure that they receive the appropriate attention and care, but also enhances your credibility and reduces liability by defining your scope of practice and clarifying what services you can and cannot reasonably provide.

Knowing when to refer a client is, however, as important as choosing to which professional to refer. For instance, just because a client complains of symptoms of muscle soreness or discomfort or exhibits signs of fatigue or lack of energy is not an absolute indication to refer your client to a physician. Because continual referrals such as this are not practical, familiarize and educate yourself on expected signs and symptoms, taking into consideration the client's fitness level, health status, chronic disease, disability, and/or background as they are screened and as they begin and progress with an exercise program. This helps you better discern between emergent and non-emergent situations and know when to refuse to offer your services, continue to monitor, and/or make an immediate referral.

It is important that you know the scope of practice for various health professionals and which types of referrals are appropriate. For example, some states require that a referring physician first approve visits to a physical therapist, while other states allow you to see a physical therapist directly. Only registered or licensed dietitians or physicians may provide specific dietary recommendations or diet plans; however, a client who is suspected of an eating disorder should be referred to an eating disorders specialist. Refer clients to a clinical psychologist if they wish to discuss family or marital problems or exhibit addictive behaviors such as substance abuse.

Network and develop rapport with potential allied health professionals in your area before you refer clients to them. This demonstrates good will and respect for their expertise and will most likely result in reciprocal referrals for your services and fitness expertise.

UPHOLD AND ENHANCE PUBLIC APPRECIATION AND TRUST FOR THE HEALTH AND FITNESS INDUSTRY

The best way for ACE-certified Professionals to uphold and enhance public appreciation and trust for the health and fitness industry is to represent themselves in a dignified and professional manner. As the public is inundated with misinformation and false claims about fitness products and services, your expertise must be utilized to dispel myths and half-truths about current trends and fads that are potentially harmful to the public.

When appropriate, mentor and dispense knowledge and training to less experienced fitness professionals. Novice fitness professionals can benefit from your experience and skill as you assist them in establishing a foundation based on exercise science, from both theoretical and practical standpoints. Therefore, it is a disservice if you fail to provide helpful or corrective information—especially when an individual, the public, or other fitness professionals are at risk for injury or increased liability. For example, if you observe an individual using momentum to perform a strength-training exercise, the prudent course of action would be to suggest a modification. Likewise, if you observe a fitness professional in your workplace consistently failing to obtain informed consents before clients undergo fitness testing or begin an exercise program, recommend that he or she consider implementing these forms to minimize liability.

Finally, do not represent yourself in an overly commercial or misleading manner. Consider the fitness professional who places an advertisement in a local newspaper stating: Lose 10 pounds in 10 days or your money back! It is inappropriate to lend credibility to or endorse a product, service, or program founded upon unsubstantiated or misleading claims; thus a solicitation such as this must be avoided as it undermines the public's trust of health and fitness professionals.

ESTABLISH AND MAINTAIN CLEAR PROFESSIONAL BOUNDARIES

Working in the fitness profession requires personal trainers to come in contact with many different people. It is imperative that a professional distance be maintained in relationships between trainer and client. Trainers are responsible for setting and monitoring the boundaries between a working relationship and friendship with their clients. To that end, ACE-certified Personal Trainers should

- Never initiate or encourage discussion of a sexual nature.
- Avoid touching your clients unless it is essential to instruction.
- Inform your clients about the purpose of touching and find an alternative if the client objects.
- Discontinue all touching if it appears to make the client uncomfortable.
- Take all reasonable steps to ensure that any personal and social contacts between themselves and their clients do not have an adverse impact on the trainer-client relationship.

If you find yourself unable to maintain appropriate professional boundaries with a client (whether due to your attitudes and actions or those of the client), the prudent course of action is to terminate the relationship and, perhaps, refer the client to another professional. Keep in mind that charges of sexual harassment or assault, even if groundless, can have disastrous effects on your personal training career.

ACE Personal Trainer
Certification Examination
Content Outline

For the most up-to-date version of the
Exam Content Outline please go to
www.acefitness.org/PTexamcontent
and download a free PDF.

PURPOSE

In July 2005, the American Council on Exercise® (ACE®) and CASTLE Worldwide, Inc. conducted a role delineation study to identify the primary tasks performed by personal trainers. The fundamental purpose of this study was to establish and validate appropriate content areas for the ACE Personal Trainer Certification Examination. The result of this process includes this exam content outline, which sets forth the tasks, knowledge, and skills necessary for a personal trainer to perform job responsibilities at a minimum professional level. It is the position of ACE that the recommendations outlined here are not exhaustive to the qualifications of a personal trainer but represent a minimum level of proficiency and theoretical knowledge. Please note that not all knowledge and skill statements listed in the exam content outline will be addressed on each exam administration.

The ACE Personal Trainer Exam includes a Written Simulation portion that is designed to test the decision-making ability of the candidate. The problems in the exam are intended to simulate, as closely as possible, the types of situations that an actual certified personal trainer may encounter in a professional setting. Please visit www.acefitness.org to learn more.

DESCRIPTION

An ACE-certified Personal Trainer works in a health/fitness facility or in another appropriate setting administering individualized physical activity programs to asymptomatic individuals or those who have been cleared by a physician. ACE-certified Personal Trainers will be competent to assess a client's health/medical/fitness status effectively; design safe and effective physical activity programs utilizing goal setting, exercise science principles, and safety guidelines; implement the exercise program safely and effectively; modify the program as necessary to achieve reasonable goals; and adhere to all codes, laws, and procedures applicable within the recognized scope of practice for personal trainers. The ACE Personal Trainer Certification will be granted to those candidates who possess current adult CPR, are at least 18 years of age, and obtain the minimum passing score on an entry-level examination measuring ACE-identified competencies. This certification is appropriate for individuals working one-on-one, with small groups, or as floor staff, etc. The certification will be valid for a two-year period, at which time it may be renewed. Requirements for renewal will be obtaining a pre-determined number of continuing education credits (CECs) and paying the applicable fee.

Attention Exam Candidates!
When preparing for an ACE certification exam, be aware that the material presented in this manual, or any text, may become outdated due to the evolving nature of the fitness industry, as well as new developments in current and ongoing research. These exams are based on an in-depth job analysis and an industry-wide validation survey. By design, these exams assess a candidate's knowledge and application of the most current scientifically based professional standards and guidelines. The dynamic nature of this field requires that ACE certification exams be regularly updated to ensure that they reflect the latest industry findings and research. Therefore, the knowledge and skills required to pass these exams are not solely represented in this or any industry text. *In addition to learning the material presented in this manual, ACE strongly encourages all exam candidates and fitness professionals to keep abreast of new developments, guidelines, and standards from a variety of valid industry sources.*

The Examination Content Outline is essentially a blueprint for the exam. All exam questions are based on this outline, which may also be found in the appendix in the ACE manual.

DOMAINS, TASKS AND KNOWLEDGE AND SKILL STATEMENTS

A Role Delineation Study completed for the Personal Trainer certification first identified the major categories of responsibility for the professional. These categories are defined as Domains and it was determined that the profession could be divided into four Performance domains, or major areas of responsibility. These performance domains are:

- **Domain I: Client Interview and Assessment**
- **Domain II: Program Design and Implementation**
- **Domain III: Program Progression, Modification and Maintenance**
- **Domain IV: Professional Role and Responsibility**

The Personal Trainer, in performing their job, draws upon knowledge from four foundational sciences called Content domains. The content domains include all exercise science topics important to the competence of the Personal Trainer in fulfilling the performance domains. These foundational sciences are:

- Anatomy and Biomechanics
- Physiology
- Nutrition
- Psychology

Within each performance domain are Task Statements that detail the job-related functions under the specific domain. Each task statement is further divided into Knowledge and Skill Statements to further detail the scope of information required and how that information is applied in a practical setting for task statement.

The domains are presented in two dimensions:

- Performance domains that exist vertically for client interview and assessment; program design and implementation; program progression, modification and maintenance; and professional role and responsibility
- Content domains that exist horizontally for anatomy and biomechanics; physiology; nutrition; and psychology

Table 1: Exam Content Outline: Personal Trainer Certification

Applied Exercise Science

Performance Domain	Total Items	Anatomy and Biomechanics (40)	Physiology (33)	Nutrition (20)	Psychology (22)
Client Interview and Assessment	40	14	11	7	8
Program Design and Implementation	41	14	12	7	8
Program Progression, Modification and Maintenance	34	12	10	6	6
Professional Role and Responsibility	10	0	0	0	0
Total:	**125**	**40**	**33**	**20**	**22**

DOMAIN I – CLIENT INTERVIEW AND ASSESSMENT   32%

Task 1 - Establish rapport and program value using effective communication and listening techniques to build trust, confidence, and enthusiasm and to maximize program participation. *(Chapters 13–15)*

Knowledge of:

Psychology *(Chapter 14 & 15)*

1. Communication techniques (e.g., active listening, appropriate eye contact, reflecting and other attending behaviors, nonverbal and verbal communication)
2. Effective interviewing techniques (e.g., open-ended questioning, clarifying, paraphrasing, probing, summarizing)
3. Factors that build and enhance rapport (e.g., empathy, genuineness, nonjudgmental responses, client confidentiality)
4. Cultural, ethnic, and personal differences as they affect communication, lifestyle, dietary habits, and personal and interpersonal behavior (e.g., common assumptions, misconceptions, complicating factors)
5. Environmental factors that affect communication (e.g., location, noise, temperature, distractions, sense of privacy)
6. Psychological factors that influence an individual's self-image and their impact on the communication process
7. Each interaction as an opportunity to enhance or improve an individual's lifestyle
8. Communication technology (e.g., software, email, Website, telephone)

Skill in:

Psychology *(Chapter 14 & 15)*

1. Selecting an appropriate environment for consultation sessions

2. Applying interviewing and communication techniques (e.g., active listening)
3. Respecting the client's personal characteristics (e.g., gender, age, cultural/ethnic background) in all communication
4. Building rapport
5. Avoiding behaviors that are detrimental to building rapport (e.g., prejudicial statements, negative body language, and unproductive assumptions with regard to the client's body size, eating habits, past successes/failures with weight management)
6. Interpreting body language and recognizing incongruities between verbal and nonverbal behaviors
7. Identifying stage of behavioral change
8. Enhancing the perceived value of lifestyle modification for the client
9. Using technology as a communication tool

Task 2 - Assess client attitudes, preferences, motivations, and readiness for behavior change using questionnaires and interviews to set appropriate program goals and to identify potential barriers and unrealistic expectations. *(Chapter 13)*

Knowledge of:

Nutrition *(Chapter 4)*

1. Cultural, ethnic, and personal differences as they affect dietary habits
2. Potential barriers to healthful dietary choices and weight management

Psychology *(Chapter 14 & 15)*

1. Communication techniques (e.g., active listening, appropriate eye contact, reflecting and other attending behaviors, nonverbal and verbal communication)

2. Effective interviewing techniques (e.g., open-ended questioning, clarifying, paraphrasing, probing, summarizing)

3. Factors that build and enhance rapport (e.g., empathy, genuineness, nonjudgmental responses, client confidentiality)

4. Cultural, ethnic, and personal differences as they affect communication, lifestyle, dietary habits, and personal and interpersonal behavior (e.g., common assumptions, misconceptions, complicating factors)

5. Environmental factors that affect communication (e.g., location, noise, temperature, distractions, sense of privacy)

6. Psychological factors that influence an individual's self-image and their impact on the communication process

7. Factors that indicate a client's readiness to change

8. Appropriate forms and assessment tools

Skill in:

Nutrition *(Chapter 4)*

1. Identifying potential barriers to healthful dietary choices and weight management

Psychology *(Chapter 14 & 15)*

2. Applying interviewing and communication techniques (e.g., active listening, empathy)

3. Respecting the client's personal characteristics (e.g., gender, age, cultural/ethnic background) in all communication

4. Interpreting body language and recognizing incongruities between verbal and nonverbal behaviors

5. Avoiding behaviors that are detrimental to building trust (e.g., prejudicial statements, body language, assump-

tions with regard to body size, eating habits, past successes and failures with weight management, activity history, and ability)

6. Identifying stage of behavioral change

7. Using stage-specific strategies for facilitating behavior change

8. Administering appropriate forms and assessment tools

Task 3 - Obtain health and exercise history and lifestyle information (e.g., nutrition habits, activity) using questionnaires, interviews, and available documents to determine risk stratification, to identify the need for medical clearance and referrals, and to facilitate program design *(Chapters 5, 6 & 11)*

Knowledge of:

Anatomy and Biomechanics *(Chapters 2 & 3)*

1. General anatomy (e.g., neuromuscular, musculoskeletal, cardiovascular, respiratory)

2. Anatomical position, muscle actions, functional movements, and planes of motion

3. Normal joint range of motion

4. Physical laws of motion (e.g., inertia, acceleration, momentum, impact and reaction forces, lever classes, muscle and force production)

5. Static postural assessment and movement analysis (e.g., postural and muscle imbalances)

6. Static and dynamic balance (e.g., center of gravity, base of support, proprioception)

Physiology *(Chapters 1 & 12)*

1. General physiology (e.g., neuromuscular, musculoskeletal, cardiorespiratory, cardiovascular, endocrine)

2. General physiology of cardiorespiratory, metabolic, and musculoskeletal diseases and conditions (e.g., diabetes, osteoporosis, cardiovascular disease)

3. Population-specific considerations (e.g., youth, older adults, pregnancy)
4. Cardiovascular risk factors, risk stratification, and industry guidelines
5. Appropriate precautions with respect to prescription and nonprescription drugs

Nutrition *(Chapter 4)*

1. Appropriate allied health professionals to use as referrals (e.g., registered dietitians, physicians)
2. Physical and psychological signs and symptoms that might indicate the need for referral

Psychology *(Chapter 14 & 15)*

1. Communication techniques (e.g., active listening, appropriate eye contact, reflecting and other attending behaviors, nonverbal and verbal communication)
2. Effective interviewing techniques (e.g., open-ended questioning, clarifying, paraphrasing, probing, , summarizing)
3. Factors that build and enhance rapport (e.g., empathy, genuineness, nonjudgmental responses, client confidentiality)
4. Cultural, ethnic, and personal differences as they affect communication, lifestyle, dietary habits, and personal and interpersonal behavior (e.g., common assumptions, misconceptions, complicating factors)
5. Environmental factors that affect communication (e.g., location, noise, temperature, distractions, sense of privacy)
6. Psychological factors that influence an individual's self esteem and body image (e.g., anorexia, bulimia, body dysmorphia) and their impact on the communication process
7. Appropriate data collection forms

Skill in:

Anatomy and Biomechanics *(Chapters 2 & 3)*

1. Applying knowledge of anatomy and biomechanics to the interpretation of health history data

Physiology *(Chapters 1 & 12)*

1. Identifying and taking appropriate precautions with respect to prescription and nonprescription drugs
2. Identifying conditions based on observation and those addressed on the health history and lifestyle questionnaires
3. Stratifying risk and identifying the need for referral

Nutrition *(Chapter 4)*

1. Recognizing physical and psychological conditions that might indicate the need for referral
2. Recognizing the need to refer clients to appropriate allied health professionals

Psychology *(Chapter 14 & 15)*

1. Applying interviewing and communication techniques (e.g., active listening)
2. Respecting the client's personal characteristics (e.g., gender, age, cultural/ethnic background) in all communication
3. Avoiding behaviors that are detrimental to building trust (e.g., prejudicial statements, body language, assumptions with regard to body size, eating habits, past successes and failures with weight management, activity history, and ability)
4. Identifying stage of behavioral change
5. Managing time during the interview and data collection processes

Task 4 - Conduct appropriate baseline assessments (e.g., posture, function, cardiorespiratory fitness, muscular strength and endurance, flexibility, body composition,

heart rate, blood pressure, diet, lifestyle) based on the client interview, questionnaire information, and standardized protocols to establish a safe, effective exercise program and to track changes over time.
(Chapters 5 & 6)

Knowledge of:

Anatomy and Biomechanics *(Chapters 2 & 3)*

1. General anatomy (e.g., neuromuscular, musculoskeletal, cardiovascular, respiratory)
2. Anatomical position, muscle actions, functional movements, and planes of motion
3. Normal joint range of motion
4. Physical laws of motion (e.g., inertia, acceleration, momentum, impact and reaction forces, lever classes, muscle and force production)
5. Static postural assessment and movement analysis (e.g., postural and muscle imbalances)
6. Static and dynamic balance (e.g., center of gravity, base of support, proprioception)

Physiology *(Chapters 1 & 12)*

1. General physiology (e.g., neuromuscular, musculoskeletal, cardiorespiratory, cardiovascular, endocrine)
2. General physiology of cardiorespiratory, metabolic, and musculoskeletal diseases and conditions (e.g., diabetes, osteoporosis, cardiovascular disease)
3. Population-specific considerations (e.g., youth, older adults, pregnancy)
4. Acute physiological responses to exercise testing with consideration for individual differences (e.g., age, gender, disease, environmental conditions)
5. Normal and abnormal responses during physiological assessment
6. Effects of medications on physiological responses during testing

7. Factors that affect body composition
8. Standardized testing protocols, their intended use and limitations
9. Signs indicating the need for test termination

Nutrition *(Chapter 4)*

1. Appropriate dietary assessment protocols and their uses (e.g., 24-hour diet recall, food logs, food frequency questionnaires)
2. Limitations of dietary data (e.g., inaccurate reporting, inaccurate recording)

Psychology *(Chapter 14 & 15)*

1. Communication techniques (e.g., active listening, appropriate eye contact, reflecting and other attending behaviors, nonverbal and verbal communication)
2. Factors that build and enhance rapport (e.g., empathy, genuineness, nonjudgmental responses, client confidentiality)
3. Cultural, ethnic, and personal differences as they affect communication, lifestyle, dietary habits, and personal and interpersonal behavior (e.g., common assumptions, misconceptions, complicating factors)
4. Motivating and demotivating factors of fitness testing

Skill in:

Anatomy and Biomechanics *(Chapters 2 & 3)*

1. Assessing posture and movement
2. Assessing static and dynamic balance
3. Monitoring movement patterns during fitness testing

Physiology *(Chapter 1)*

1. Selecting and administering a variety of physiological assessments (e.g., cardiorespiratory, muscular strength and endurance, body composition, flexibility)

2. Monitoring client responses during test administration (e.g., blood pressure, heart rate, RPE)

3. Measuring and recording exercise testing data accurately

4. Recognizing responses that indicate the need for test termination

5. Terminating exercise tests safely

Nutrition *(Chapter 4)*

1. Administering appropriate dietary assessment protocols

2. Collecting nutrition data

Psychology *(Chapter 14 & 15)*

1. Empathizing with the client's lack of experience, knowledge, or expertise in exercise methods and techniques

2. Modifying communication style and content appropriate to the client (e.g., learning style, sensory limitations, educational background, primary language)

DOMAIN II - PROGRAM DESIGN AND IMPLEMENTATION   33%

Task 1 - Interpret the results of the client interview and assessment by evaluating responses and data to facilitate goal setting and the design of a safe and effective exercise and lifestyle program. *(Chapters 5 & 6)*

Knowledge of:

Anatomy and Biomechanics *(Chapters 2 & 3)*

1. General anatomy (e.g., neuromuscular, musculoskeletal, cardiovascular, respiratory)

2. Anatomical position, muscle actions, functional movements, and planes of motion

3. Normal joint range of motion

4. Physical laws of motion (e.g., inertia, acceleration, momentum, impact and reaction forces, lever classes, muscle and force production)

5. Static postural assessment and movement analysis (e.g., postural and muscle imbalances)

6. Static and dynamic balance (e.g., center of gravity, base of support, proprioception)

Physiology *(Chapters 1 & 12)*

1. General physiology (e.g., neuromuscular, musculoskeletal, cardiorespiratory, cardiovascular, endocrine)

2. General physiology of cardiorespiratory, metabolic, and musculoskeletal diseases and conditions (e.g., diabetes, osteoporosis, cardiovascular disease)

3. Population-specific considerations (e.g., youth, older adults, pregnancy)

4. Data interpretation using standardized norms

5. Relationship between BMI, waist-to-hip ratio, and circumference measures to body weight and determination of appropriate body weight

Nutrition *(Chapter 4)*

1. Methods for interpreting client assessment data in relation to established guidelines

2. Limitations of dietary assessment data

3. Applicable guidelines and standards published by accepted organizations (e.g., American Dietetic Association, US Department of Agriculture, American Heart Association)

Psychology *(Chapter 14 & 15)*

1. Factors that indicate a client's readiness to change

2. Underlying motives that initiate program participation

Skill in:

Anatomy and Biomechanics *(Chapters 2 & 3)*

1. Evaluating musculoskeletal assessment data

Physiology *(Chapter 1)*

1. Interpreting physiological data relative to standardized norms

Nutrition *(Chapter 4)*

1. Evaluating the client's diet history, interview, and observations relative to accepted guidelines
2. Applying relevant standards and guidelines published by accepted organizations
3. Accounting for the limitations of dietary data

Psychology *(Chapter 14 & 15)*

1. Identifying stage of behavioral change
2. Identifying client goals, perceived and unperceived needs, and expectations for change
3. Helping the client to clarify and refine needs and motivations

Task 2 - Establish specific client goals using the interpretation of interview and assessment results and current standards to provide program direction.
(Chapters 13 & 14)

Knowledge of:

Anatomy and Biomechanics *(Chapters 2 & 3)*

1. General anatomy (e.g., neuromuscular, musculoskeletal, cardiovascular, respiratory)
2. Anatomical position, muscle actions, functional movements, and planes of motion
3. Normal joint range of motion
4. Physical laws of motion (e.g., inertia, acceleration, momentum, impact and reaction forces, lever classes, muscle and force production)

5. Static postural assessment and movement analysis (e.g., postural and muscle imbalances)
6. Static and dynamic balance (e.g., center of gravity, base of support, proprioception)

Physiology *(Chapters 1 & 12)*

1. General physiology (e.g., neuromuscular, musculoskeletal, cardiorespiratory, cardiovascular, endocrine)
2. General physiology of cardiorespiratory, metabolic, and musculoskeletal diseases and conditions (e.g., diabetes, osteoporosis, cardiovascular disease)
3. Population-specific considerations (e.g., youth, older adults, pregnancy)
4. Expected physiological adaptations to exercise

Nutrition *(Chapter 4)*

1. Principles of nutrition and weight management for goal setting

Psychology *(Chapter 14 & 15)*

1. Principles of goal setting
2. Potential obstacles and challenges that may interfere with goal setting and goal attainment
3. Psychological and social factors that impact goal setting in the development of safe and effective programs
4. Communication styles and presentation techniques that assure collaborative goal setting based on the client's needs, preferences, and expectations
5. Behavior change principles in goal setting

Skill in:

Anatomy and Biomechanics *(Chapters 2 & 3)*

1. Using musculoskeletal assessment results for goal setting and reinforcement

Physiology *(Chapter 1)*

1. Setting appropriate timeframes for goal attainment in accordance with industry standards

Nutrition *(Chapter 4)*

1. Applying the principles of nutrition and weight management to goal setting

Psychology *(Chapter 14 & 15)*

1. Assisting the client in setting personal goals based on the SMART framework
2. Guiding the goal setting process to address short- and long-term goals
3. Helping the client identify potential barriers to goal attainment
4. Using communication styles and presentation techniques that assure collaborative goal setting based on the client's needs, preferences, and expectations

Task 3 - Apply appropriate exercise principles (e.g., frequency, intensity, duration, type) for cardiorespiratory fitness, muscular strength and endurance, and flexibility using current standards and appropriate techniques to develop a safe and effective exercise program. *(Chapters 7–12)*

Knowledge of:

Anatomy and Biomechanics *(Chapters 2 & 3)*

1. General anatomy (e.g., neuromuscular, musculoskeletal, cardiovascular, respiratory)
2. Anatomical position, muscle actions, functional movements, and planes of motion
3. Normal joint range of motion
4. Physical laws of motion (e.g., inertia, acceleration, momentum, impact and reaction forces, lever classes, muscle and force production)
5. Static postural assessment and movement analysis (e.g., postural and muscle imbalances)

6. Static and dynamic balance (e.g., center of gravity, base of support, proprioception)

Physiology *(Chapter 1)*

1. General physiology (e.g., neuromuscular, musculoskeletal, cardiorespiratory, cardiovascular, endocrine)
2. General physiology of cardiorespiratory, metabolic, and musculoskeletal diseases and conditions (e.g., diabetes, osteoporosis, cardiovascular disease)
3. Population-specific considerations (e.g., youth, older adults, pregnancy)
4. ACSM guidelines for frequency, intensity, duration, and type for cardiorespiratory, muscular strength and endurance, and flexibility programs
5. Principles of fitness (e.g., overload, specificity, diminishing returns, recovery, progression
6. Techniques for measuring and monitoring cardiorespiratory intensity
7. Techniques for developing resistance training programs (e.g., periodization, progression)
8. Techniques for aerobic and anaerobic training programs (e.g., intervals, steady state, tempo, low-intensity long-duration programs)

Skill in:

Anatomy and Biomechanics *(Chapters 2 & 3)*

1. Recognizing muscle functions, weaknesses, and imbalances

Physiology *(Chapters 1 & 12)*

1. Designing individualized programs in accordance with clients' goals for aerobic and anaerobic fitness, muscular strength and endurance, flexibility, and posture consistent recognized standards (e.g., ACSM, ACE, NSCA)
2. Applying principles of fitness to individualized exercise programs

3. Measuring intensity and calculating target training zones for cardiorespiratory fitness

Task 4 - Implement appropriate lifestyle modification strategies (e.g., stress management, nutrition, smoking cessation) using industry standards and best practices to improve quality of life and goal attainment.
(Chapters 11, 12 & 18)

Knowledge of:

Physiology *(Chapters 1 & 12)*

1. General physiology (e.g., neuromuscular, musculoskeletal, cardiorespiratory, cardiovascular, endocrine)
2. General physiology of cardiorespiratory, metabolic, and musculoskeletal diseases and conditions (e.g., diabetes, osteoporosis, cardiovascular disease)
3. Population-specific considerations (e.g., youth, older adults, pregnancy)
4. Physiology of cardiorespiratory and digestive systems
5. Physiological responses to lifestyle changes
6. Physiological changes with age

Nutrition *(Chapter 4)*

1. Appropriate application, safety, and effectiveness of various weight management techniques
2. Safe and effective weight loss methods and quantities
3. Different approaches to weight loss

Psychology *(Chapter 14 & 15)*

1. Communication techniques (e.g., active listening, appropriate eye contact, reflecting and other attending behaviors, nonverbal and verbal communication)
2. Factors that build and enhance rapport (e.g., empathy, genuineness, nonjudgmental responses, client confidentiality)

3. Cultural, ethnic, and personal differences as they affect communication, lifestyle, dietary habits, and personal and interpersonal behavior (e.g., common assumptions, misconceptions, complicating factors)
4. Motivating and demotivating factors of exercise and exercise environments
5. Stress management techniques

Skill in:

Physiology *(Chapter 1)*

1. Educating and communicating about physiological improvements with lifestyle changes

Psychology *(Chapter 14 & 15)*

1. Helping clients identify sources of stress
2. Helping clients identify their reactions to stress
3. Recognizing the motivating and demotivating factors of exercise and exercise environments

Task 5 - Incorporate functional exercise (e.g., balance, agility, and core) in accordance with scientific research to improve movement efficiency, activities of daily living, and overall physical performance.
(Chapters 8, 9 & 12)

Knowledge of:

Anatomy and Biomechanics *(Chapters 2 & 3)*

1. General anatomy (e.g., neuromuscular, musculoskeletal, cardiovascular, respiratory)
2. Anatomical position, muscle actions, functional movements, and planes of motion
3. Normal joint range of motion
4. Physical laws of motion (e.g., inertia, acceleration, momentum, impact and reaction forces, lever classes, muscle and force production)
5. Posture and movement (e.g., postural and muscle imbalances)

6. Static and dynamic balance (e.g., center of gravity, base of support, proprioception)

Physiology *(Chapters 1 & 12)*

1. General physiology (e.g., neuromuscular, musculoskeletal, cardiorespiratory, cardiovascular, endocrine)
2. General physiology of cardiorespiratory, metabolic, and musculoskeletal diseases and conditions (e.g., diabetes, osteoporosis, cardiovascular disease)
3. Population-specific considerations (e.g., youth, older adults, pregnancy)
4. Neuromuscular adaptations to functional exercise
5. Physiological demands of activities of daily living
6. Differences in neuromuscular adaptations to functional training across the lifespan and in chronic disease

Skill in:

Anatomy and Biomechanics *(Chapters 2 & 3)*

1. Selecting and integrating appropriate methods for functional exercise (e.g., balance, agility, core) based on the client's needs
2. Implementing safe and effective exercise programs to address muscle weakness and imbalance

Physiology *(Chapters 1 & 12)*

1. Adapting functional exercises to the individual based on current neuromuscular ability and/or limitations

**Task 6 - Teach safe and effective techniques using a variety of methods and resources to attain desired results and to promote lifestyle modification.
*(Chapter 11)***

Knowledge of:
Anatomy and Biomechanics *(Chapters 2 & 3)*

1. General anatomy (e.g., neuromuscular, musculoskeletal, cardiovascular, respiratory)
2. Anatomical position, muscle actions, functional movements, and planes of motion
3. Normal joint range of motion
4. Physical laws of motion (e.g., inertia, acceleration, momentum, impact and reaction forces, lever classes, muscle and force production)
5. Posture and movement (e.g., postural and muscle imbalances)
6. Static and dynamic balance (e.g., center of gravity, base of support, proprioception)

Physiology *(Chapter 1 & 12)*

1. General physiology (e.g., neuromuscular, musculoskeletal, cardiorespiratory, cardiovascular, endocrine)
2. General physiology of cardiorespiratory, metabolic, and musculoskeletal diseases and conditions (e.g., diabetes, osteoporosis, cardiovascular disease)
3. Population-specific considerations (e.g., youth, older adults, pregnancy)
4. Musculoskeletal injury prevention
5. Physiological effects of overtraining and undertraining
6. Reliable resources to promote desired results and promote lifestyle modification (e.g., authoritative websites, training manuals from respected organizations, textbooks)
7. Physiological effects of lifestyle modification (e.g., smoking cessation, stress management, nutritious eating plan)

Nutrition *(Chapter 4)*

1. Healthful food and beverage selections at home, in restaurants, and at the grocery store based on food guidelines, food labels, methods of preparation, and key words on menus

2. Nutritional requirements during physical activity (e.g., hydration, energy needs)

3. Supplements, weight loss products, and fad diets and the associated risks of each

4. Concepts of energy balance, including dietary intake and expenditure

5. Different approaches to weight management and/or body composition change

6. Dietary guidelines emphasizing balance, variety, and moderation

Psychology (Chapter 14 & 15)

1. Learning styles (e.g., visual, verbal, kinesthetic)

2. Verbal and nonverbal communication

3. Learning theories

Skill in:

Anatomy and Biomechanics (Chapters 2 & 3)

1. Teaching proper use of a variety of equipment and offering appropriate feedback

2. Teaching safe and effective exercise techniques and offering appropriate feedback

Physiology (Chapter 1)

1. Designing safe and effective exercise and lifestyle modification programs that improve physiological systems

Nutrition (Chapter 4)

2. Approximating caloric intake and expenditure

3. Explaining concepts related to nutrition and weight management

4. Selecting healthful foods and beverages at home, in restaurants, and at the grocery store based on food guidelines, food labels, methods of preparation, and key words on menus

5. Implementing appropriate nutritional strategies during physical activity (e.g., hydration, energy needs)

6. Educating clients to supplements, weight loss products, and fad diets and the associated risks of each

7. Applying the concepts of energy balance, including dietary intake and expenditure

8. Applying dietary guidelines emphasizing balance, variety, and moderation

Psychology (Chapter 14 & 15)

1. Empathizing with the client's lack of experience, knowledge, or expertise in exercise methods and techniques

2. Modifying teaching style and content appropriate to the client's personal characteristics

Task 7 - Promote program adherence by applying the principles of motivation to maintain interest in physical activity and achievement of program goals.
(Chapters 13 & 14)

Knowledge of:

Physiology (Chapters 1 & 12)

1. General physiology (e.g., neuromuscular, musculoskeletal, cardiorespiratory, cardiovascular, endocrine)

2. General physiology of cardiorespiratory, metabolic, and musculoskeletal diseases and conditions (e.g., diabetes, osteoporosis, cardiovascular disease)

3. Population-specific considerations (e.g., youth, older adults, pregnancy)

4. Client education about physiology as a tool for motivating clients to work at appropriate levels

Psychology (Chapter 14 & 15)

1. Self efficacy as it relates to exercise participation

2. Common barriers to program compliance (e.g., time, energy, money)

3. Psychological effect of exercise program participation

4. Locus of control as it relates to program adherence and motivation

5. Principles of reinforcement and punishment

Nutrition *(Chapter 4)*

1. Accepted industry standards and weight management planning to educate and motivate clients

Skill in:

Physiology *(Chapter 1)*

1. Educating clients on the response of physiological systems to various levels of training

Nutrition *(Chapter 4)*

1. Using accepted industry standards and weight management planning to educate and motivate clients

Psychology *(Chapter 14 & 15)*

1. Recognizing the client's needs, expectations, fears

2. Identifying barriers that influence program adherence

3. Manipulating factors to maximize adherence

4. Recognizing the personal trainer's influence on the client's adherence

5. Providing appropriate reinforcement

DOMAIN III - PROGRAM PROGRESSION, MODIFICATION, AND MAINTENANCE   27%

Task 1 - Evaluate ongoing progress using assessments, current standards, observation, and client feedback and performance to provide program direction and to optimize program adherence.
(Chapters 6 & 14)

Knowledge of:

Anatomy and Biomechanics *(Chapters 2 & 3)*

1. General anatomy (e.g., neuromuscular, musculoskeletal, cardiovascular, respiratory)

2. Anatomical position, muscle actions, functional movements, and planes of motion

3. Normal joint range of motion

4. Physical laws of motion (e.g., inertia, acceleration, momentum, impact and reaction forces, lever classes, muscle and force production)

5. Static postural assessment and movement analysis (e.g., postural and muscle imbalances)

6. Static and dynamic balance (e.g., center of gravity, base of support, proprioception)

Physiology *(Chapters 1 & 12)*

1. General physiology (e.g., neuromuscular, musculoskeletal, cardiorespiratory, cardiovascular, endocrine)

2. General physiology of cardiorespiratory, metabolic, and musculoskeletal diseases and conditions (e.g., diabetes, osteoporosis, cardiovascular disease)

3. Population-specific considerations (e.g., youth, older adults, pregnancy)

4. Physiological responses to chronic training

5. Principles of progression as it relates to cardiorespiratory, muscular fitness, and flexibility training programs

6. Appropriate frequency for reassessment

7. Standardized testing protocols, their intended use and limitations

8. Signs indicating the need for test termination

9. Current standards for training progression and weight loss

Nutrition *(Chapter 4)*

1. Appropriate dietary assessment protocols, purposes, inherent risks, and ben-

efits (e.g., 24-hour diet recall, food logs, food frequency questionnaires)

2. Methods for interpreting client assessment data as it relates to established guidelines

3. Applicable guidelines and standards published by accepted organizations (e.g., ADA, USDA, AHA, Institute of Medicine)

4. Relationship between BMI, waist-to-hip ratio, and circumference measures to body weight and determination of appropriate body weight

Psychology *(Chapter 14 & 15)*

1. Self efficacy and locus of control as they relate to program adherence

2. Communication and listening techniques

Skill in:

Anatomy and Biomechanics *(Chapters 2 & 3)*

1. Assessing posture and movement in comparison to baseline data

2. Assessing static and dynamic balance in comparison to baseline data

3. Determining appropriate tests for reassessment to compare with baseline results

4. Evaluating data from musculoskeletal reassessment

Physiology *(Chapters 1 & 12)*

1. Identifying physiological responses based on observation and feedback during exercise

2. Selecting and administering a variety of physiological assessments (e.g., cardiorespiratory, muscular strength and endurance, body composition, flexibility)

3. Monitoring client responses during test administration (e.g., blood pressure, heart rate, RPE)

4. Measuring and recording exercise testing data accurately

5. Recognizing responses that indicate the need for test termination

6. Terminating exercise tests safely

7. Determining whether rate of progress is appropriate for the individual based on the expected physiological responses and current standards

Nutrition *(Chapter 4)*

1. Administering appropriate dietary assessment protocols

2. Interviewing and collecting nutrition data

3. Processing the client's diet history, evaluations, and observations, relative to accepted guidelines

4. Gathering, applying, and interpreting applicable standards and guidelines published by accepted organizations

Psychology *(Chapter 14 & 15)*

1. Recognizing the personal trainer's influence on the client's adherence

2. Recognizing client misconceptions about program progress

3. Communicating the results of the reassessments to effectively promote adherence

4. Managing time in the data collection process

Task 2 - Identify lapses and barriers to success by reassessing baseline measures and evaluating compliance to redefine goals and to modify the program.
(Chapter 6, 11 & 14)

Knowledge of:

Anatomy and Biomechanics *(Chapters 2 & 3)*

1. General anatomy (e.g., neuromuscular, musculoskeletal, cardiovascular, respiratory)

2. Anatomical position, muscle actions, functional movements, and planes of motion

3. Normal joint range of motion

4. Physical laws of motion (e.g., inertia, acceleration, momentum, impact and reaction forces, lever classes, muscle and force production)

5. Posture and movement

6. Static and dynamic balance (e.g., center of gravity, base of support, proprioception)

Physiology *(Chapters 1 & 12)*

1. General physiology (e.g., neuromuscular, musculoskeletal, cardiorespiratory, cardiovascular, endocrine)

2. General physiology of cardiorespiratory, metabolic, and musculoskeletal diseases and conditions (e.g., diabetes, osteoporosis, cardiovascular disease)

3. Population-specific considerations (e.g., youth, older adults, pregnancy)

4. Principles of fitness (e.g., overload, specificity, diminishing returns, recovery, reversibility, progression)

5. How to modify the program based on changes in fitness and health status

Nutrition *(Chapter 4)*

1. Cultural, ethnic, and personal differences as they affect dietary habits

2. Potential barriers to healthful dietary choices and weight management

3. Accepted industry standards and weight management planning

Psychology *(Chapter 14 & 15)*

1. Common barriers to program compliance (e.g., time, energy, money)

2. Self efficacy and locus of control as they relate to program participation and adherence

Skill in:

Anatomy and Biomechanics *(Chapters 2 & 3)*

1. Identifying inappropriate movement patterns that may impede progress or adherence

2. Modifying exercise techniques as needed

Physiology *(Chapters 1 & 12)*

1. Modifying program components to accommodate fitness and/or health status

Nutrition *(Chapter 4)*

1. Using accepted industry standards and weight management planning

2. Avoiding prejudicial statements, negative and/or unproductive assumptions with regard to client body size, eating habits, past successes and failures with weight management.

3. Identifying potential barriers to healthful dietary choices and weight management

Psychology *(Chapter 14 & 15)*

1. Identifying barriers and enhancers that influence program adherence

2. Recognizing the client's needs, desires, expectations, and fears

3. Recognizing the personal trainer's influence on the client's adherence

4. Providing appropriate reinforcement

Task 3 - Modify program goals using appropriate educational and motivational techniques to improve compliance and awareness of the benefits of physical activity and a healthful lifestyle.
(Chapters 11–14)

Knowledge of:

Anatomy and Biomechanics *(Chapters 2 & 3)*

1. General anatomy (e.g., neuromuscular, musculoskeletal, cardiovascular, respiratory)

2. Anatomical position, muscle actions, functional movements, and planes of motion

3. Normal joint range of motion

4. Physical laws of motion (e.g., inertia, acceleration, momentum, impact and reaction forces, lever classes, muscle and force production)

5. Posture and movement

6. Static and dynamic balance (e.g., center of gravity, base of support, proprioception)

Physiology *(Chapters 1 & 12)*

1. General physiology (e.g., neuromuscular, musculoskeletal, cardiorespiratory, cardiovascular, endocrine)
2. General physiology of cardiorespiratory, metabolic, and musculoskeletal diseases and conditions (e.g., diabetes, osteoporosis, cardiovascular disease)
3. Population-specific considerations (e.g., youth, older adults, pregnancy)
4. Physiological plateaus in cardiorespiratory, resistance, and weight loss programs

Nutrition *(Chapter 4)*

1. Complexity of issues related to obesity, body size, eating disorders, and related lifestyle factors
2. Safe and effective weight loss and lifestyle change in regard to nutrition
3. Role of nutrition, supplements, weight loss products, and fad diets, their effect on weight management and performance, and the associated risks

Psychology *(Chapter 14 & 15)*

1. Strategies that facilitate behavior change
2. Self efficacy and locus of control as they relate to exercise participation
3. Principles of reinforcement and punishment
4. Principles of goal setting
5. Potential obstacles and challenges that may interfere with goal setting and attainment
6. Biological, psychological, and social factors that impact program compliance

Skill in:

Anatomy and Biomechanics *(Chapters 2 & 3)*

1. Modifying exercise techniques to promote goal attainment

Physiology *(Chapters 1 & 12)*

1. Identifying program components that can be modified to promote a positive training effect
2. Educating clients about the physiological benefits of continued training

Nutrition *(Chapter 4)*

1. Communicating the benefits of healthful nutrition to weight management and performance
2. Applying principles of nutrition to redefine short- and long-term goals

Psychology *(Chapter 14 & 15)*

1. Assisting the client in reevaluating and modifying goals
2. Helping the client recognize potential and actual barriers to adherence
3. Assisting the client in developing coping strategies to overcome barriers
4. Enhancing the client's self efficacy through challenging yet manageable tasks

Task 4 - Implement progressions to the client's program as appropriate using established methods and techniques to facilitate goal achievement and long-term compliance. *(Chapters 7–10)*

Knowledge of:

Anatomy and Biomechanics *(Chapters 2 & 3)*

1. General anatomy (e.g., neuromuscular, musculoskeletal, cardiovascular, respiratory)
2. Anatomical position, muscle actions, functional movements, and planes of motion
3. Normal joint range of motion
4. Physical laws of motion (e.g., inertia, acceleration, momentum, impact and reaction forces, lever classes, muscle and force production)
5. Posture and movement

6. Static and dynamic balance (e.g., center of gravity, base of support, proprioception)

Physiology *(Chapters 1 & 12)*

1. General physiology (e.g., neuromuscular, musculoskeletal, cardiorespiratory, cardiovascular, endocrine)
2. General physiology of cardiorespiratory, metabolic, and musculoskeletal diseases and conditions (e.g., diabetes, osteoporosis, cardiovascular disease)
3. Population-specific considerations (e.g., youth, older adults, pregnancy)
4. Appropriate rate of progression according to established methods and guidelines
5. Various methods of progression for aerobic, anaerobic, muscular strength and endurance, and flexibility training

Skill in:

Anatomy and Biomechanics *(Chapters 2 & 3)*

1. Implementing appropriate exercise technique progressions

Physiology *(Chapters 1 & 12)*

1. Implementing appropriate exercise progressions to facilitate long term success

DOMAIN IV - PROFESSIONAL ROLE AND RESPONSIBILITIES 8%

Task 1 - Maintain a professional trainer-client relationship by adhering to legal requirements, professional boundaries, and standards of care and by operating within the scope of practice, as defined in the ACE Code of Ethics, to protect the client and to limit liability.
(Chapter 18 & Appendices A & F)

Knowledge of:

1. Professional boundaries pertaining to the client-trainer relationship
2. American Council on Exercise Code of Ethics
3. Accepted standards of care
4. Liability issues associated with acting outside the appropriate standard of care, scope of practice, and the American Council on Exercise Code of Ethics
5. Scope of practice
6. Professional ethics regarding technology and communication

Skill in:

1. Assessing areas of risk (e.g., client, facilities, use of technology)
2. Identifying professional boundaries based on professional and ethical obligations

Task 2 - Treat all individuals with respect, empathy, and equality regardless of weight, appearance, ethnicity, nationality, sexual orientation, gender, age, disability, religion, marital status, socioeconomic status, and health status to maintain integrity in all professional relationships.
(Chapters 12, 13 & 18)

Knowledge of:

1. Abilities and limitations of various disabilities
2. Cultural differences related to professional relationships
3. Acceptable and unacceptable behavior related to individual differences
4. Personal issues and biases
5. Qualities of respect, empathy, and equality

Skill in:

1. Demonstrating compassion, empathy, and respect for all individuals
2. Maintaining appropriate behavior patterns regardless of personal issues and biases

Task 3 - Maintain competence and professional growth by staying current with scientifically based research, theories, and practices to provide safe and effective services for clients, the public, and other health professionals. *(Chapter 18 & Appendix A)*

Knowledge of:

1. Available and credible continuing education programs (e.g., conferences, workshops, college/university courses, teleseminars, online courses, in-home study courses) and providers
2. Appropriate and relevant scientifically based consumer and professional publications (e.g., journals, books, texts, videos, DVDs, CDs, online publications and resources)
3. Appropriate agencies and organizations that establish and publish scientifically based lifestyle modification standards and guidelines for the general public and special populations (e.g., ACSM, ACOG, USDA, OSHA, NIH, ADA, NSCA, CDC)
4. American Council on Exercise continuing education requirements and procedures

Skill in:

1. Recognizing credible resources

Task 4 - Exercise leadership by providing direction, motivation, and education and by modeling exemplary behavior to establish an environment for client success and to promote wellness in the community. *(Chapters 17 & 18)*

Knowledge of:

1. General professional and business practices (e.g., time management, organizational skills, appropriate attire, integrity)
2. Educational strategies to promote client safety, program success, and wellness in the community

Skill in:

1. Demonstrating professional business practices
2. Using appropriate educational strategies to promote client safety, program success, and wellness within the community.

Task 5 - Maintain an environment of continual safety by upholding industry standards to reduce the risk of injury and liability. *(Chapters 16, 17 & 18)*

Knowledge of:

1. Cardiopulmonary resuscitation (CPR) and Automated External Defibrillator (AED) procedures
2. Worksite emergency plan
3. Appropriate Emergency Medical Service system activation
4. Basic first aid
5. Occupational Health and Safety Administration guidelines regarding blood borne pathogens
6. Procedures for safe equipment operation (e.g., sizing, usage, inspection)
7. Industry standards for reducing risk of injury
8. Factors that affect liability
9. How to communicate a sense of security and safety to clients

Skill in:

1. Identifying and responding to emergency situations
2. Identifying and responding to hazards in training situations
3. Implementing the emergency plan in a professional manner
4. Communicating the rationale for various techniques that limit the risk of injury
5. Using equipment properly and safely

Task 6 - Develop risk management strategies in accordance with recognized guidelines (e.g.,

IHRSA, ACE, ACSM, OSHA, NSCA, state laws) to protect the client, personal trainer, and other relevant parties.
(Chapter 18)

Knowledge of:

1. Negligence (comparative and contributory) and liability laws as they pertain to personal trainers
2. Intellectual property laws as they apply to video, DVD, written materials, Internet, music, copyright, and trademark
3. Sources for and limitations of waivers and informed consents
4. Appropriate professional and general liability insurance
5. Sexual harassment and discrimination laws
6. Components of a comprehensive risk management program
7. Credible resources for risk management strategies (e.g., McGraw, Wong, ACSM, NSCA, OSHA, IHRSA, ACE, IDEA, Fitness Management, Athletic Business)

Skill in:

1. Complying with business laws and regulations
2. Completing appropriate reports (e.g., incident reports, accident reports, equipment and facility inspection forms, waivers, informed consents)
3. Developing and maintaining an appropriate risk management program for a facility or business
4. Monitoring the client when exercise or fitness assessments have been terminated due to abnormal physiological responses

Task 7 - Document client-related data, communications, and progress using a secure record keeping system in accordance with legal requirements (e.g., HIPAA, FERPA) to main-

tain continuity of care and to minimize liability.
(Chapter 16 & Appendix A)

Knowledge of:

1. Effective and confidential record keeping
2. Confidentiality guidelines
3. Importance of maintaining and implications of breaching client confidentiality
4. All required paperwork and documentation (e.g., waivers, informed consent, medical history, health risk appraisal, client contracts)

Skill in:

1. Maintaining confidentiality
2. Differentiating between confidential and non-confidential documents and information

Task 8 - Participate as a member of a referral network by identifying professional contacts and community resources to ensure the highest quality of service for clients.
(Chapter 18 & Appendix A)

Knowledge of:

1. Appropriate health and allied health professions for outside referral
2. Appropriate forms and documents required when communicating with other health professionals in order to maintain continuity of client care

Skill in:

1. Identifying and networking with appropriate health and allied health professionals
2. Establishing a method for referrals
3. Creating a means of ongoing communication and follow up with appropriate professionals

Mindful Exercise
Overview for
Personal Trainers

Ralph La Forge

Ralph La Forge, M.S., is a physiologist and managing director of the Duke Lipid and Metabolic Disorder Training Program, Duke University Medical Center, Endocrine Division, Durham, N.C. He has worked for 25 years in clinical cardiology/endocrinology and as an instructor of exercise physiology at the University of California, San Diego. La Forge has authored more than 300 consumer and professional publications on cardiovascular disease management, applied exercise science, and preventive cardiology and is the exercise science research editor for IDEA Health & Fitness Source. *He has helped organize and inaugurate cardiovascular disease risk reduction and preventive endocrinology programs for more than 450 healthcare institutions and medical groups throughout the United States, including the Department of Defense.*

INTRODUCTION AND PURPOSE

The advent and growth of complementary exercise programs, specifically those addressing mind-body fitness, have established them as significant players in individual and group exercise programming. Mind-body fitness has been associated with improved muscular strength, flexibility, balance, and coordination, but perhaps most importantly from a health promotion viewpoint, increased mental development and self-efficacy. Mind-body fitness is best acquired by engaging in daily mind-body exercise, or what is also referred to as "mindful exercise."

A mind-body-oriented approach to exercise combines a cognitive or mindful process with physical movement—usually low-to-moderate intensity movements or postures. Although it has eluded a precise universal definition, mindful exercise is defined here as *physical exercise executed with a profound inwardly directed cognitive focus.* This inwardly directed attention is performed in a nonjudgmental fashion on self. Self-focus includes specific attention to breathing and proprioception, or "muscle sense." Clearly, any exercise modality can integrate this inner-attentiveness; however, this is *the* key process in mindful exercise. Mindful exercise prioritizes this meditative state to generate a temporary nonjudgmental self-observation. For example, from the viewpoint of someone who is unfamiliar with yoga, the popular cobra pose may appear to be nothing more than a back extension exercise. However, internally, the yogi's cognition is entirely and deeply entrained on the simple kinesthesis of the pose and breath-centering—nothing more and nothing less. Many of your clients will find these attributes beneficial in managing specific fitness and health concerns including stress-related disorders, deterioration of musculoskeletal health, decreased balance control, hypertension, depression, and decreased self-

confidence. Table 1 is a simple taxonomy of some of the mindful forms of exercise that have gained considerable popularity in the West in recent years. For many, the calming-contemplative states experienced here may confer health benefits precluding the need for higher-intensity exercise for those who either cannot perform or do not require higher-intensity conventional exercise.

There is intuitive neurobiological support for how and why mind-body therapies such as acupuncture and mindful exercise interact with important cognitive functions of the brain and vice versa. The framework for this understanding was achieved in 1972 when G.M. Goodwin, Ian McCloskey, and Peter Matthews at Oxford University carried out careful behavioral studies that demonstrated that **muscle afferents** have direct access to mechanisms of perception, and implied that there must be projections of the muscle afferent pathways to the cortex for this to occur. Recent studies have confirmed the presence of these pathways. Figure 1 simplistically depicts the fundamental mind-body exercise component pathways to various mental processes.

Table 1
A Simple Taxonomy of Mindful Exercise Programs

Classical (>200 year heritage)	Contemporary
Tai chi chuan	Feldenkrais method
Qigong exercise	Alexander technique
Hatha yoga	Pilates
Spiritual and ethnic dance (e.g., Native American, Capioera, Hula)	Laban movement analysis
Some ancient martial arts (e.g., karate, judo, aikido)	Integrative yoga programs (e.g., Integral yoga, Somatic yoga, Yogaflow, Viniyoga)
	Composite mind-body exercise programs (e.g., NIA, E-motion, mind-body circuit programs, BrainGym, Aqua Tai Chi, Chi Ball, Yogarobics)
	Tai chi chih
	Somatics
	Contemporary martial arts (e.g., tae kwon do)
	Meditation walking
	Native American yoga

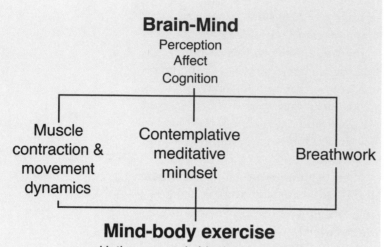

FIGURE 1
Interactive mind-body pathways in mindful exercise.

The purpose of this appendix is to briefly introduce you to the essential tenets of mindful exercise, describe the more influential forms, and provide useful education, training, and research resources. It is not the intent of this appendix to disclose all that is necessary to fully appreciate or competently teach yoga, tai chi, or qigong exercise per se. Each modality addressed here requires hundreds of hours of personal exploration to attain reasonable kinesthetic proficiency and knowledge of that system's tradition. This discussion is limited to the classical and several contemporary forms of mindful exercise.

ROOTS OF CONTEMPORARY MIND-BODY EXERCISE PROGRAMS

The Asian yoga and tai chi disciplines are at the root of most contemporary mindful exercise programs taught today. These two ancient forms have intensively integrated mind and body along with an overt sense of spirituality and groundedness with nature. At the heart of all meditative practice in Asia is what Indians call yoga. Yoga is a complex system of physical and spiritual disciplines that is fundamental to a number of Asian religions (e.g., Hinduism and Buddhism). For example, classical yoga as described in the *Yoga*

Sutra, an ancient text of yogic principles attributed to Patanjali, is composed of eight components, or "limbs": moral principles, observances, posture, breath control, withdrawal of the senses, concentration, meditation, and pure contemplation (Miller, 1995). Here, posture refers to yogic exercises or asanas that originally were used to prepare one for practicing breath control and meditation. In other words, yoga exercise was used as a means to an end—meditation and spiritual freedom. The physical arm of yoga, hatha yoga, when coupled with a meditative-contemplative component is perhaps the most practiced form of mindful exercise in the West today.

Tai chi has a nearly 4,000-year heritage and is derived from the practice of qigong (also called chi kung), which describes the entire tradition of spiritual, martial, and health exercises developed in China. Qigong is the primary Chinese methodology for activating the "medicine within," or the naturally occurring self-healing resource. This ancient practice is a combination of two ideas: qi is the vital energy of the body and gong is the skill of working with the qi (also called chi). Tai chi, the martial art derivative of qigong, is best described as a moving meditation. In some way, most contemporary mind-body exercise programs [e.g., neuromuscular integrative action (NIA), meditation walking, E-Motion] are derived from early yoga and qigong practice.

DIFFERENTIATING CHARACTERISTICS OF MINDFUL EXERCISE

Mindful exercise such as yoga and tai chi is attentive to the present moment and is process-oriented in contrast to many, if not most, forms of conventional exercise that center on body or performance-oriented measures such as fat-burning, body-sculpting, power output, and target heart rate. Mindful exercise generally relies on self-monitoring of perceived effort, breathing, and nonjudgmental self-awareness rather than cuing entirely on an exercise leader or peer-influence experienced in conventional group exercise classes. Unquestionably, conventional aerobic and resistance-training programs can manifest each of these mindful qualities; however, with mindful exercise these cognitive features are both the means and the outcome. Mindful exercise, when appropriately and individually taught, can assist in the management of a number of chronic disease states. Moreover, this form of activity can be readily executed at low-to-moderate exercise intensities adaptable to a wide range of functional capacities.

RESEARCH-SUPPORTED OUTCOMES AND BENEFITS OF MINDFUL EXERCISE

Mindful exercise programs such as tai chi and hatha yoga generally require minimal equipment or exercise materials and they can be performed in the home or outside of fitness facilities. Perhaps most importantly, they are relatively safe and provide a low-impact workout. Specific hatha yoga exercises are particularly helpful for arthritis, asthma, low-back pain, and postural problems, while tai chi is helpful in improving balance and motor coordination. Because of its slow contemplative nature, tai chi can help reduce anxiety, blood pressure, and symptoms of depression.

There is a growing body of scientific evidence supporting various mindful exercise modalities as significant means of improving a variety of health outcomes. Materials on qigong, tai chi, and yoga comprise approximately 95% of the research literature on mind-body exercise. Table 2 depicts research outcomes and benefits of hatha yoga and tai chi practices that have a reasonable volume of research support.

Yoga Research

Approximately 1,600 studies on yoga are listed by Monroe, Ghosh, & Kalish (1989) and many more have been undertaken

Common Components of Mind-body Exercise Programs

For mind-body exercise to be optimally fulfilling, it requires more than merely adding a "cognitive component" to conventional physical activity. The criteria for what constitutes mindful exercise are likely to see a continuing transformation over the next decade as more definitive research is conducted and newer, more relevant interpretations evolve. For now, the following component criteria are recommended for mind-body exercise:

1. Meditative/contemplative. A noncompetitive, present-moment, and nonjudgmental introspective component that is process-centered versus being strictly outcome- or goal-oriented.

2. Proprioceptive awareness. Mindful exercise is generally characterized by relatively low-level muscular activity coupled with mental focus on muscle and movement sense.

3. Breath-centering or breathwork. The breath is frequently cited as the primary centering activity in mind-body exercise. There are many breath-centering techniques in yoga, tai chi, and qigong exercise.

4. Anatomic alignment or proper physical form. Disciplining oneself to a particular movement pattern or spinal alignment is integral to many forms of mind-body exercise such as hatha yoga, Alexander technique, Pilates, and tai chi. It is also important to note that not all mindful exercise forms utilize a set choreography or disciplined anatomical alignment characteristics. Examples include NIA and expressive ethnic dance exercises such as Native American or hula, which exhibit significant free-form movement.

5. Energycentric. The perceptive movement and flow of one's intrinsic energy, vital life force, chi, prana, or other positive energy commonly described in many classical mindful exercise traditions.

since that bibliography was published. Perhaps the most dedicated yoga research repository and publication is the *Yoga Mimamsa,* which is managed and published by the Kaivalyadhama Yoga Institute in Lonavla, India (www.kdham.com). The International Association of Yoga Therapy (www.iayt.org), which is based in California, periodically publishes original investigations on yoga in their *International Journal of Yoga Therapy.*

The majority of the published hatha yoga research suffers from inadequate subject number, low statistical power, subject selection bias, and/or is void of adequate controls. That said, the overall trend of

reported results in most studies is statistically significant with or without controls. There are a growing number of adequately controlled yoga trials demonstrating reasonably clear outcomes (La Forge, 2002). For example, research by Berger and Owen at City University of New York comparing hatha yoga to aerobic exercise demonstrated that exercise does not need to be aerobic to decrease anxiety and anger scores and improve mood (Berger & Owen, 1992). One of the most referenced studies in the West is the Lifestyle Heart Trial conducted by Dr. Dean Ornish and colleagues (Ornish et al., 1990). This study, however, did not isolate hatha yoga

Table 2
Research-supported Outcomes and Benefits of Yoga and Tai Chi

Cardiorespiratory
- Decreased resting blood pressure
  (Murugesan, Govindarajulu, & Bera, 2000; Selvamurthy et al., 1998; Channer et al., 1996; Broota, Varma, & Singh, 1995; Van Montfrans et al., 1990)
- Increased pulmonary function
  (Birkel & Edgren, 2000; Vedanthan et al., 1998; Joshi, Joshi, & Gokhale, 1992)
- Improved respiratory function in patients with asthma
  (Manocha et al., 2002; Khanam, 1996; Fluge, 1994; Jain & Talukdar, 1993)
- Increased parasympathetic tone, increased heart-rate variability
  (Sakakibara, Tekeuchi, & Hayano, 1994; Shannahoff-Khalsa & Kennedy, 1993; Vaananen et al., 2002)
- Improvement in baroreflex function/sensitivity
  (Selvamurthy et al., 1998; Bowman et al., 1997; Bernardi et al., 2002)
- Decreased blood lactate and resting oxygen consumption
  (Raju et al., 1994)
- Enhanced arterial endothelial function
  (Wang, Lan, & Wong, 2001)
- Increased maximum oxygen consumption and physical work capacity
  (Manchanda, 2000; Lan et al., 1998; Lan et al. , 1999; Lai et al., 1993)
- Regression of coronary artery disease
  (Ornish et al., 1990; Manchanda, 2000)
- Improved cardiovascular disease risk factor profile (e.g., blood lipids)
  (Manchanda, 2000; Mahajan et al., 1999; Schmidt, 1997)

Musculoskeletal
- Increased muscular strength and flexibility
  (Lan et al., 1998; Lan et al., 1996; Wolfson et al., 1996)
- Increased balance control
  (Wong et al., 2001; Schaller et al., 1996; Wolfson et al.,1996; Province et al., 1995; Hong,Li & Robinson, 2000)
- Improved posture
  (Wong et al., 2001; Savic et al., 1990)
- Decreased falls in seniors
  (Wolf et al., 1996; Province et al., 1995)

Psychobiological
- Increased cognitive performance
  (Naveen et al., 1997; Jella & Shannahoff-Khalsa, 1993)
- Improved relaxation and psychological well-being
  (Telles et al., 2000; Schell, Allolio, & Schonecke, 1994; Wood, 1993; Berger & Owen, 1992)
- Decreased stress hormones (e.g., cortisol)
  (Kamei et al., 2000)
- Decreased anxiety and depression scores
  (Ray et al., 2001; Sovik, 2000; Tweeddale, Rowbottom, & McHardy, 1993; Jin, 1992; Savic et al., 1990)
- Reduction in frequency of panic episodes
  (Clark, Salkovskis, & Chalkley, 1985)
- Reduced symptoms of insomnia
  (Koch et al., 1998)
- Reduced physiological and psychological responses to threat or stress
  (Sakakibara & Hayano, 1996; Bera, 1995; Cappo & Holmes, 1984; McCaul, Solomon, & Holmes, 1979)
- Decreased symptoms associated with pain, angina, asthma, and chronic fatigue
  (Manchanda, 2000; Nespor, 1991)

Other
- Increased physical functioning in older persons
  (Li et al., 2001; Kutner et al., 1997)
- Improved glucose tolerance
  (Jain et al., 1993)
- Decreased HbA1c (glycosylated hemoglobin) and C-peptide levels in type 2 diabetes
  (Tsujiuchi et al., 2002)
- Decreased obsessive-compulsive disorder symptoms
  (Shannahoff-Khalsa & Beckett, 1996)
- Decreased osteoarthritis symptoms
  (Garfinkel et al., 1994)
- Decreased carpal-tunnel symptoms
  (Garfinkel et al., 1999)

itself as a therapeutic agent. In this study, a blend of a healthy dietary cuisine (10 to 12% fat), social and group support, moderate aerobic exercise (walking), and regular hatha yoga (sequence of 8 to 15 poses) demonstrated a modest regression of atherosclerotic disease in CVD patients as determined by quantitative coronary angiography. More recently, an investigational study by Manchanda demonstrated similar results (Manchanda, 2000). Manchanda evaluated the possible role of lifestyle modification, including hatha yoga, on retardation of coronary atherosclerotic disease. In this prospective, randomized, controlled trial, 42 men with angiographically proven coronary artery disease (CAD) were randomized to control (n = 21) and yoga intervention groups (n = 21) and followed for one year. The active yoga group was treated with a program consisting of hatha yoga, control of risk factors, diet control, and moderate aerobic exercise. The control group was managed by conventional methods (i.e., risk factor control, moderate exercise, and AHA step 1 diet). At one year, the yoga group showed significant reduction in the number of anginal episodes per week, improved exercise capacity, and decreased body weight. Serum total cholesterol, LDL cholesterol, and triglyceride levels also showed greater reductions as compared with the control group. Revascularization procedures (coronary angioplasty or bypass surgery) were less frequently required in the yoga group (one versus eight patients; relative risk = 5.45; $p = .01$). Coronary angiography repeated at one year showed that significantly more lesions regressed (20% versus 2%) and fewer lesions progressed (5% versus 37%) in the yoga group ($p < 0.0001$). Compliance with the total program was excellent and no side effects were observed. One can conclude that the active yoga program was truly an integrated intervention program blending a low-fat diet with meditation and hatha yoga principles.

The Ornish and Manchanda studies show that for a yoga program to either cause regression or at least stop the progression of coronary disease there must be a significant modification of blood lipids and lipoproteins (i.e., LDL cholesterol) primarily by dietary means. In the final analysis, yogic lifestyle intervention, rather than hatha yoga alone, is perhaps the necessary stimulus required for generating significant clinical outcomes as evidenced in these and other trials.

Qigong and Tai Chi Research

In the early 1980s scientists in China began investigating the many potential benefits of qigong and tai chi. Since 1985, approximately 1500 research papers have been published on qigong practice alone (Qigong Database, Academy of East/West Arts, Menlo Park, Calif.). Much of this research has involved qigong exercise and tai chi. A number of these research trials were well-controlled studies that reported statistically significant decreases in the incidence of stroke and stroke mortality, increases in bone mineral density, improved lipid profile, decreased blood pressure, improved effectiveness of cancer therapy, and increased psychological well-being.

Despite all of the interest and perceived benefits of yoga and tai chi in the West, there still remains a great need for more peer-reviewed and adequately controlled research investigating the impact of yoga on chronic disease, musculoskeletal function, and behavioral outcomes. Although there is a considerable international body of research in terms of the total number of research citations, more than 5,000 papers published worldwide, the majority of these trials are statistically underpowered, lack adequate controls, and/or are fraught with selection bias. Still, there are a growing number of well-controlled experimental trials that support the many biological and psychological benefits associated with both classical and contemporary forms of mindful exercise. To be sure, there are a number of well-controlled trials in progress evaluating low-back pain, aging, and multiple sclerosis. Vijay Vad at the Hospital for Special Surgery in Manhattan is studying 50 patients with herniated disks who are suffering from low-back pain and comparing a combination of yoga and Pilates (70% yoga, 30% Pilates exercise) to drug therapy. After three months 80% of the patients in the yoga/Pilates group reported that their pain was reduced by at least 50% versus only 44% of the patients in the drug-treated group reporting reduced pain. The National Institutes of Health (NIH) is currently funding studies evaluating the effect of hatha yoga on insomnia and multiple sclerosis. For more information, go to the NIH Web site (www.clinicaltrials.gov) and enter the search word "yoga." The quantity and quality of this level of research will surely escalate as western graduate schools develop structured course work involving the psychobiology of mindful exercise modalities and students pursue study and investigational projects in these promising forms of contemplative physical activity.

MINDFUL EXERCISE MODALITIES AND PROGRAMS

Hatha yoga, qigong, tai chi, and pranayama (yogic breathing training), all classical forms of mindful exercise, have been practiced by young and old alike for centuries and each has spawned numerous styles perfect for a variety of age groups and functional capacities. More contemporary forms of mindful exercise (e.g., Pilates, NIA, Somatics, E-Motion, Feldenkrais Method, and Alexander Technique) have largely been inspired by these early forms and also deserve consideration in their own right.

Yoga

It is important for personal trainers to know the difference between "yoga" and what much of the fitness industry refers to as yoga exercise or hatha yoga. The word yoga originated from the ancient Sanskrit language spoken by the religious elite of India. Yoga literally means "union," or integration of mind and body disciplines. According to Patanjali's philosophical analyses contained in the *Yoga Sutra,* yoga historically refers to the complex system of physical and spiritual disciplines that are fundamental to Buddhist, Jain, and Hindu religious practice throughout Asia. We must differentiate a "yogic-lifestyle" from participation in hatha yoga classes such as that offered in yoga studios and fitness centers in the United States (e.g., Iyengar yoga and power yoga classes). Those who live yogic lifestyles, while perhaps not in full compliance with the teachings of the *Yoga Sutra,* generally embark upon daily dietary, meditation, and spiritual centering and regular hatha yoga exercise, whereas the routine practice of hatha yoga poses may or may not include dietary or other lifestyle changes. This is an important point because some yoga research outcomes are based on following yogic lifestyle principles that clearly transcend the mere practice of yoga exercise.

All six branches of yoga (Inana, Karma, Mantra, Tantra, Raja, Hatha) attempt to accomplish the same final goal; however, hatha yoga will be the focus of this section as it is perhaps the most relevant branch for personal trainers. Hatha yoga is the physical aspect of yogic disciplines and includes a vast repertoire of physical postures, or asanas, done seated, standing, or lying prone or supine on the floor, and, in some instances, inverted positions. Several basic movement patterns are involved in most asanas: backbends, twists, and forward bends.

The principal challenge of hatha yoga is to become proficient at handling increasingly greater amounts of "resistance" (i.e., complexity and the degree of difficulty) in the various postures and breathing patterns while maintaining a steady and comfortable equilibrium of mind and body. As a general rule, hatha yoga sessions start and end with a relaxation pose (a savasana, or corpse pose) and include a variety of asanas focusing on spinal, postural, and limb muscle groups so that one spends 30 seconds to 1 minute with each pose before transitioning to the next. Optimally, early stages of hatha yoga are taught individually with a certified yoga teacher providing hands-on assessment and guidance through each pose. The use of props (e.g., blankets, blocks, neck and lumbar rolls, and bolsters) is very helpful in early stages of training to help the individual achieve safe and proper alignment, minimizing undue musculoskeletal stress. In virtually all forms of hatha yoga it is paramount that yogic breathing be executed in synchrony with each pose. There are countless yogic breathing techniques [see "Yogic Breathing Training (Pranayama)," page 520]. As a general rule, yogic breathing is combined with yoga exercise in a very logical way. Whenever a yoga movement or pose expands the chest or abdomen, the participant inhales. Conversely, when a movement contracts or compresses your chest or abdomen, the participant exhales.

The following are several methods of hatha yoga that are commonly practiced throughout the United States and Europe:

Iyengar Yoga. Iyengar yoga was originally developed by B.K.S. Iyengar, who systematized more than 200 classical asanas (poses) from very simple to very difficult. Much emphasis is placed on precise anatomical alignment, which over the years has refined the therapeutic aspects of yoga. One preferred form of Iyengar yoga uses standing poses in which the person assumes a stationary position using isometric contractions to attain precise body alignment. As with nearly all styles of hatha yoga, Iyengar places much emphasis on breathing (pranayama). The use of props to assist with attaining appropriate spinal alignment is one of the characteristics of Iyengar

classes. Perhaps the most authoritative and detailed illustrated text on Iyengar yoga is B.K.S. Iyengar's *Light on Yoga.*

Restorative Yoga. This style of hatha yoga is a derivative of the Iyengar yoga tradition and is perhaps most appropriate for those who are just embarking on a yoga program because of the use of props and the elementary nature of the poses. Judith Lasater and others have introduced this form of Iyengar yoga. Restorative yoga is easier and more relaxing for those who are relatively weak, fatigued, or experiencing peak stressful periods in life. Some of the more popular poses in this form are legs-up-the-wall pose, supported half-dog pose, chair forward bend, and half-wall hang (Lasater, 1995).

Ashtanga Yoga. This is the ancient system of hatha yoga currently taught by Pattabhi Jois in Mysore, India. This method synchronizes a progressive series of postures with a specific breathing method (ujjayi pranayama). The asanas in Ashtanga yoga are sequenced in groups of poses that range from moderate to very difficult. The sequence pace and pose difficulty is what often characterizes Ashtanga as "power yoga." Ashtanga places equal emphasis on strength, flexibility, and mental and physical stamina.

Anusara Yoga. Founded by John Friend of Shenandoah, Texas, this form of hatha yoga closely resembles Iyengar and stresses three focus points: attitude, alignment, and action. Participants are taught to be cognizant of their "key power center" or focal point (i.e., the point at which most of the body weight or musculoskeletal force is placed).

Viniyoga. This is a softer and more individualized form of hatha yoga. Emphasis is placed on breathing (pranayama) and coordination of breath and movement and is known for therapeutic application of the classical asanas or poses. Viniyoga is usually taught on a one-on-one basis. Kraftsow's *Yoga for Wellness: Healing with the Timeless Teachings of Viniyoga* and *Yoga for Transformation,* as well as Desikachar's

The Heart of Yoga are consummate descriptive works on Viniyoga.

Kripalu Yoga. This is a three-level style of hatha yoga customized to the needs of western students. The first stage teaches the basic mechanics of the postures, including body alignment and coordination of breath and movement. Stage two includes a prolonged holding of the poses as the student learns to practice a disciplined mental concentration. Stage three involves a spontaneous moving meditation set to the individual's internal awareness and energy. The Kripalu method of teaching and practicing yoga blends the physical postures of Hatha yoga with the contemplative meditation of Raja yoga, the principle tenets of which extend well beyond those of Hatha yoga and include moral discipline, self-restraint, meditation, concentration, breath control, and physical postures.

Integral Yoga. Another yoga form that gently stretches, strengthens, and calms the body and mind, Integral yoga includes comfortable postures, deep relaxation, and breathing practices. This form of yoga emphasizes diet and is employed in Dr. Dean Ornish's heart disease reversal programs around the United States.

Bikram Yoga. Bikram yoga is a vigorous 90-minute, 26-pose series designed to warm and stretch muscles, ligaments, and tendons in a particular sequence. Since most studios are heated to 90 to 105°F (32 to 41°C) each participant needs to have a large towel, a washcloth (sometimes two), and a water bottle for class.

Kundalini Yoga. Also called the yoga of awareness, kundalini yoga's principal purpose is to awaken the serpent power (kundalini, or coiled-up energy) with postures, breath control, chanting, and meditation. Originated by Yogi Bhajan, a kundalini yoga class usually entails a spine and flexibility warm-up, specific asana sequences commensurate with one's "coiled up energy," and relaxation. Each asana is symbolic of life habits and emotion and a specific associated breath (e.g., long-deep breath, segmented breathing, breath of fire).

Sivananda Yoga. A style of classical yoga with traditional poses, breathing exercises, and relaxation, Sivananda teaches 12 postures comprising the Sun Salutation sequence and can be readily adapted to beginners or those who have low functional capacities. The Sivananda Yoga Vedanta Center of New York (see Resources, page 531) has trained more than 10,000 yoga teachers worldwide and is widely respected for teaching authentic hatha yoga.

Somatic Yoga. Eleanor Criswell Hanna of Novato, California, developed this moderate-intensity form of hatha yoga that shares many characteristics of the Feldenkrais and Alexander methods (see pages 527–528). Somatic yoga sessions emphasize contracting particular muscle groups and then relaxing them. Each yoga pose is done slowly and is followed by one minute of deep breathing, self-awareness, and what Hanna refers to as "integration." Classes end with pranayama, guided relaxation (quieting of the senses), and meditation.

Yogic Breathing Training (Pranayama). In the yogic and qigong traditions, breathing functions as an intermediary between the mind and body. The breath itself stands as an independent method of increasing relaxation, reducing anxiety, and improving overall psychological well being (Cappo & Holmes, 1984; Sakakibara, Takeuchi, & Hayano, 1994; Sakakibara & Hayano, 1996). Yogic breathing has also been used as a therapeutic modality in managing chronic heart failure (Bernardi et al., 2002). Yogic breathwork can be either isolated as a training modality itself or function as a necessary component of mindful exercise. The fundamental purpose of breathwork (pranayama) is to develop the ability to: (a) sustain relaxed attention to the flow of the breath, (b) refine and control respiratory movements, and (c) integrate awareness and breathing to reduce stress and enhance psychological functioning. Sovik (2000) characterizes optimal breathwork as

✔ diaphragmatic
✔ nasal (inhalation and exhalation)
✔ deep
✔ smooth
✔ even
✔ quiet
✔ free of pauses

General Precautions with Hatha Yoga Programs.

1. Because many styles of hatha yoga involve acute dynamic changes in body position, it is important to understand the hemodynamic and cardiac ventricular responses to such exercise and how these may alter cardiac function in those with diagnosed cardiovascular disease (CVD), including hypertension or diabetes. Inverted poses in which the head is below the heart (e.g., downward facing dog, headstands) and sequences in which a head-down position is alternated with a head-up pose should be avoided, at least in the early stages of a yoga program. In most cases, those who are initially deconditioned or who have chronic disease should: (a) minimize acute rapid changes in body position (e.g., changes in limbs and trunk in relation to the heart) in early stages of hatha yoga training, and/or (b) use slower transitions from one yoga pose to the next.

2. Ashtanga, Iyengar, and Bikram yoga asanas and sequences require considerable muscular strength and mental concentration. Therefore, they may be more appropriate for higher functional class individuals (i.e., those with >11–12 MET exercise capacity). Some yoga poses may cause significant and rapid changes in blood pressure and may be inappropriate for those with stage two or higher hypertension (i.e., those with blood pressures equal to or greater than 160/105 mmHg). DiCarlo and colleagues (1995) demonstrated significantly greater systolic and diastolic blood pressures in yoga practitioners practicing Iyengar style yoga when compared to mod-

erate treadmill walking (~4 mph). This, however, does not contraindicate Iyengar-style yoga for reasonably conditioned adults with stable cardiovascular disease.

3. Because some yoga programs involve advanced breathing techniques (e.g., breath retentions and breath suspensions), caution must be used with those who have cardiovascular or pulmonary disease. Breath retentions are brief pauses (two to five or more seconds) taken at the end of a controlled inspiration. Breath suspensions are similar pauses taken at the end of controlled expirations. While very brief pauses appear to be relatively safe, those with cardiovascular disease, hypertension, obstructive pulmonary disease, or asthma should avoid retentions or suspensions of greater than four to five seconds and focus on standard breathwork taught in most yoga programs.

Qigong Exercise

Qigong is a system of self-healing exercise and meditation that includes healing postures, movement, self-massage, breathwork, and meditation. Qigong exercise, otherwise known as Chinese health exercise, has a heritage dating back more than 3,000 years. Qigong movements are executed at very low metabolic levels, usually between 2 to 4 METs, and include standing, seated, and supine positions. There are two general categories of qigong: active, or physical, qigong exercise (dong gong) and tranquil, or passive, qigong (jing gong). The active category is what is discussed here, as this is the most popular form of qigong in both China and in the West. There are perhaps many thousands of qigong exercise styles all based on balance, relaxation, breathing, and good posture. Many qigong styles are named after animals whose movements they imitate, (e.g., dragon, crane, snake, wild goose, and animal frolics styles). According to qigong tradition, inhaling brings positive qi into your body and usually accompanies

The Sun Salutation was introduced to the West in the early 1950s and is one of the most popular Hatha yoga sequences. This pose series is an excellent example of how breath is coordinated with yoga pose sequencing. Although this yoga series is for those who are reasonably healthy and fit (e.g., without significant back problems), it exemplifies a method that can improve posture by stretching the spine and strengthening the muscle groups that support it. Coordination and muscular endurance are two additional benefits. There are several styles of sun salutation, including Ashtanga and Shivandana styles.

The following sun salutation 12-step yoga sequence illustrates an intermediate level performance in contrast to a full Ashtanga or Shivandana style, in which greater flexibility is exhibited. This sequence begins and ends with the standing position with the palms together (Tadasana pose).

1. Normal relaxed respiration, standing in prayer pose (Tadasana)

2. Breathe in, back slightly arched

3. Breathe out, bend forward

4. Breathe in, step back with your right leg

5. Breathe out, bring left foot back with the right foot (press-up position)

6. Place knees, chest, and forehead on the floor

7. Breathe in, with upper body raised

8. Breathe out, assume inverted V position

9. Breathe in, bend your right knee and step in between your hands

10. Breathe out, bring your left foot up to meet your right, bend forward

11. Breathe in, reassume pose #2 with back arched

12. Finish by returning to a prayer pose (Tadasana)

an "opening" movement (e.g., arms opening away from the body), while exhaling releases the negative qi and accompanies a "closing" movement (e.g., arms back to the body). One simple qigong series is Taiji qigong (Tse, 1995), which consists of only 18 movements taken from the tai chi and qigong forms (see the four-movement Taiji qigong sequence Pushing the Wave on page 525). Taiji qigong is ideal as a preparation for higher-intensity conditioning exercise or as a cool-down. It is recommended that this series be practiced once or twice a day for 15 to 20 minutes. There are numerous published studies, mostly with small subject numbers, demonstrating many health benefits of qigong exercise (e.g., reduced blood pressure, pain management, anxiety, and tension reduction) (see Table 2). Two resources that describe qigong exercise in good detail are Michael Tse's *Qigong for Health and Vitality* and Kenneth Cohen's *The Way of Qigong*.

Tai Chi

Tai chi (shorthand for tai chi chuan or taijiquan) is only one form of the more ancient practice of qigong. Tai chi chuan is a complex martial arts choreography of 108 flowing graceful movements that can be practiced for health, meditation, and self-defense. There are numerous forms or styles of tai chi chuan, including the original Chen, and the relatively more recent Yang, Chang, and Wu styles. Each form emphasizes a particular aspect, such as breathing, generating power, or relaxation. Some styles have a short form that may be more adaptable to those with disabilities or for seniors. In tai chi, students are taught to allow the practice to evolve into a free-flow exercise such that the movements and breathing become one unified energy flow. As with hatha yoga, it is important that the movements and breathing are coordinated so that the student may derive the energycentric benefits (i.e., unobstructed flow of perceived posi-

tive energy). Another way of looking at tai chi is as a form of inner contemplation choreographed with movement. Students are first taught to be mindful of the postures and movements, then of the coordination of movement with breathing. Finally, students are taught to be "mindful not to be mindful" (i.e., not too become overly focused on the postures, movements, and breathing). Tai chi chih, developed by American Justin Stone, is a simpler form of tai chi chuan and consists of a series of 20 movements and one ending pose. Qigong exercise involves even a simpler set of movements than its martial arts relative tai chi.

It is commonly accepted that all tai chi styles follow similar essential principles: deep synchronous breathing, profound mental concentration, and perceptive and intentional movement of chi. The following is a brief overview of some of the major distinguishable styles of tai chi.

Original Chen Style. The original Chen style (old form) is thought to be the template form from which the more recent Wu and Yang forms descended. The original Chen form contains motions including jumping, leaping, scurrying, bouncing, discharging, and other quick movements that may make it difficult for seniors or those with poor functional capacity. The newer form of Chen style has eliminated many of these movements and involves more circular choreography and is suitable for a broad range of fitness levels.

Yang Style. Originated by Yang Luchan in the 1800s, the Yang form is the most widely practiced form in the West today. The original Yang form consists of 108 movements (Yang Long Form); however, the Yang 24-Short Form is a popular modification practiced today. As with all styles of tai chi, Yang-style movements reflect the principle of opposites commonly called yin and yang, in which offensive and defensive movements unite to form a graceful flow of martial arts choreography and, more importantly, chi.

Pushing the Wave is part of an 18-movement Taiji qigong sequence taught by Michael Tse (1995) and is choreographed to replicate other Taiji forms, dance, and daily life movements. The Pushing the Wave sequence is characterized by a straight front leg with slow but intentional arm and hand movements. The movement coordinates and connects various qi (energy) points throughout the body, particularly the upper extremities, lungs, and stomach. As with yoga's sun salutation the movements are coordinated with the breath.

Chang Style. This is a relatively new style of tai chi developed by Chang Tung-sheng in the 1930s. Chang style consists of more than 100 movements and is based on modifications to the Yang Long Form.

Wu Style. This style of tai chi was developed by Master Wu Chien-chuan and is second in popularity only to Yang-style tai chi. Wu style is an easier form of tai chi, with smaller steps and movements that involve less twisting and impose less stress on the legs and knees. The condensed form of Wu style includes 36 postures, including grasping the sparrow's tail, slant flying, and embrace tiger and push mountain. Other versions of Wu style include 54 movements (e.g., 54 Forms by Master Wu Tai Sin and Sifu Eddie Wu).

Sun Style. Developed by Sun Lu-tang in the late 1800s, Sun-style tai chi combines elements of Wu and Yang-style tai chi. Sun style is characterized by lively steps. When one foot moves forward or backward, the other foot follows. Turns include an opening and closing movement, a very powerful qigong practice. This style also features a high stance, making it easy for older people to learn.

CONTEMPORARY MINDFUL EXERCISE PROGRAMS

Over the last century, numerous mindful exercise derivatives have grown from the classical traditions of qigong, tai chi, and yoga. Pilates, Alexander, Feldenkrais, and various modern hatha yoga styles have matured as respected mindful exercise methods as their techniques have been largely standardized. There are many more contemporary mindful exercise programs that combine attributes from several classical forms, including NIA, Chi Ball, E-Motion, Brain Gym, Yogarobics, Aqua Tai Chi, Yo Chi, Flow Motion, and many ethnic dance routines. The Asian martial arts (e.g., aikido, karate, tae kwon do, kempo, and judo) also clearly employ associative and disassociative cognitive methods to center their attention and direct their movements and strikes.

Pilates

The Pilates Method was developed by German immigrant J. H. Pilates in the early 20th century. Pilates is an orderly system of slow, controlled, distinct movements that demand a profound internal cognitive focus. This method is divided into two modalities, floor/mat work and the work on the Universal Reformer, a piece of resistance equipment developed by Pilates. With either modality, but especially with the Reformer, the principal goal is to achieve efficient functional movement and improved performance. Fundamentally, Pilates is a form of movement re-education in which the exerciser learns to overcome faulty compensatory movement patterns. These inefficient movement patterns are broken down into components by using springs (using a Reformer) and changing the body's orientation to gravity. Pilates exercises are designed to facilitate more efficient movement behavior by allowing the exerciser to be in a position that minimizes undesirable muscle activity, which can cause early fatigue and lead to injury. The Reformer is constructed to adapt to many human anatomic variations. For example, the springs, ropes, and foot bar of the clinical Reformer can be adjusted so that similar properties of movement sequencing can be applied to a variety of body types and limb/torso lengths. Pilates work involves considerable mental focus and coordinated breathwork, particularly during very slow concentric and eccentric muscular contractions. The Pilates method is utilized for rehabilitation, postrehabilitation, and fitness.

There appears to be some variation in technique among contemporary Pilates education and training programs, most of which assert many advantages and benefits of Pilates-style training when compared to conventional strength and muscle re-education training. Pilates is advantageous for

One of many styles of Pilates Reformers similar to Stott's Professional Reformer and Balanced Body's Clinical Reformer. The machine glides forward and backward on rollers, uses springs for resistance, and may include other attachments for a wide variety of movements and positions.

those who desire low-impact exercise to improve posture, flexibility, and functionality. Unfortunately, there remains a paucity of peer-reviewed, published, controlled trials evaluating Pilates, which is somewhat perplexing considering its present growth and popularity. A Medline search from 1990 to 2002 only turned up several small but reasonably well-controlled studies. For example, Hutchinson, Christiansen, and Beitzel (1998) at the University of Illinois demonstrated significant improvements in leap height, explosive power, and reaction time in six elite athletes after one month of Pilates training. Those interested in exploring a reasonably detailed scientific introduction into Pilates-based exercise and rehabilitation are referred to Anderson and Spector's "Introduction to Pilates-Based Rehabilitation," which appeared in *Orthopaedic Physical Therapy Clinics of North America* (2000).

Alexander Technique

The Alexander Technique, as established by Frederick Alexander in the late 19th century, is a method that teaches the transformation of neuromuscular habits by helping an individual to focus on sensory experiences. It corrects unconscious habits of posture and movement that may be precursors to injuries. This method is useful for individuals with disc trouble, sciatica, low-back pain, whiplash injury, shoulder/arm pain, neck pain, or arthritis, and athletes who wish to move with more ease and greater coordination. It is important to remember that this is not an exercise program per se but rather a proprioceptive, postural, and movement technique that is applied to routine day-to-day domestic, recreational, and sports activities. The Alexander technique is taught one-on-one or in small groups by an Alexander-certified teacher.

Feldenkrais Method

The Feldenkrais Method was developed by the Russian Moshe Feldenkrais in 1904 and consists of two interrelated, somatically based educational methods. The first method, Awareness Through Movement (ATM), is a verbally directed technique designed for group work. The second method, Functional Integration, is a nonverbal manual-contact technique designed for people desiring or requiring more individualized attention. The ATM method incorporates active movements, imagery, and other forms of directed attention. These are gentle, nonstrenuous exercises designed to re-educate the nervous system with the emphasis placed on learning from the individual's own kinesthetic feedback. A significant emphasis is placed on posture, breathing, somatically based imagery, and visualization that pertains to perception, cognition, and other aspects of motor function. Functional Integration involves directing and enhancing the efficiency, coordination, grace, and self-possession of a person's movement. Lessons are taught with the practitioner gently touching or moving the student in a variety of ways to facilitate awareness and vitality.

Neuromuscular Integrative Action Technique

The Neuromuscular Integrative Action (NIA) technique, created by Debbie and Carlos Rosas of Portland, Oregon, in 1983, represents a composite of both eastern and western mind-body exercise influences and has grown in popularity in many health clubs and fitness centers throughout the United States. NIA classes blend movements and concepts from a variety of mind-body techniques, including tai chi, yoga, martial arts, and ethnic and modern dance. Unlike other mindful exercise programs, NIA also includes a moderate-level aerobic component to address cardiorespiratory endurance. The aerobic segment is designed to foster creativity and spontaneity rather than strict adherence to standard group movement patterns. NIA movements provide a wide variety in range of motion and numerous choreographed movement choices. Participants are taught to move with self-expression and couple movement tempo with their emotion. E-Motion, developed by Laura Sachs in Northern California, is somewhat similar to NIA and involves a sensory-directed warm-up that uses visualization and tai chi–like low-impact movements.

Native American spiritual dancing and Native American yoga also share common features with NIA and classical forms of

mindful exercise. These unique forms (e.g., hoop dancing) have grown in popularity in recent years, particularly in the Southwestern United States.

A large diabetes and cardiovascular disease prevention project is currently underway with the United States Indian Health Service and Cherokee Nation. Its goal is to reintegrate Native American mindful exercise (e.g., hoop dancing) into daily utilitarian and lifestyle activities. It is hoped that reinstilling the custom of Native American exercise as the centerpiece of tribal physical activity will help reduce the burden of diabetes and cardiovascular disease that is so prevalent in Native American culture.

ASSESSING OUTCOMES

There are a variety of methods, other than muscular strength and flexibility measures, available to objectively measure the response to mindful exercise, particularly for hatha yoga, tai chi, and qigong.

• **Quality of Life.** Quality of life measures, as assessed and scored on a variety of quality of life inventories such as QualityMetric's SF-8 and SF-12 self-report instruments, are reasonably well suited for characterizing the overall functional response (www.qmetric.com). The Centers for Disease Control and Prevention's National Center for Chronic Disease Prevention and Health Promotion is one source of a simple measure of health-related quality of life (Centers for Disease Control and Prevention, 2002).

• **Blood Pressure.** Baseline and serial resting blood pressure measurement is also an accepted outcome measure responsive to four to six weeks of mindful exercise—especially if the participant has a resting blood pressure in the high-normal or higher range (i.e., 135/85–140/90+).

• **Pulmonary Function.** Pulmonary function measures such as FEV-1 (maximum forced expiratory volume in one second) are valid indicators when baseline FEV-1 is less than 80%. Vital capacity itself is not likely to change, but some studies have demonstrated increases in lung volumes and FEV-1 with yoga programs that incorporate significant breathwork.

• **Balance Control.** Balance assessment (e.g., backward tandem walk) is appropriate for evaluating the response to tai chi and qigong exercise or other mindful exercise programs in which balance control is a primary component.

• **Anxiety and Tension.** Anxiety measures may also be helpful in evaluating stress and tension. The Spielberger State Trait Anxiety Inventory (STAI) contains two 20-item self-report scales that assess anxiety-proneness (trait) and report the current level of anxiety (state). The STAI Computer Program (www.mhs.com) is an inexpensive administration and scoring program that is an alternative to paper-and-pencil versions and takes about 10 minutes to administer.

• **Spirituality.** Although very few mindful exercise studies objectively examine spirituality, it is an outcome measure worthy of consideration. There are a number of validated spirituality assessment tools that may be useful for evaluating a client's sense of spirituality before and after a period of mindful exercise training. The following are two examples: *The Spiritual Well-Being Scale* (Paloutzian & Ellison, 1982) is a 20-item self-administered scale with two dimensions: religious and existential; and the *Index of Core Spiritual Experiences,* or *INSPIRIT* (Kass,

1991), which is an 18-item interview scale used in a general population.

INDICATIONS FOR MINDFUL EXERCISE

There are a number of indications for choosing mindful exercise modalities for your clients, including as a complement to conventional aerobic or resistance-training exercise when additional muscular fitness and stress-reduction benefits are desired. Mindful exercise, particularly tai chi, qigong, restorative yoga, and Pilates mat work, may also be appropriate for those with low functional capacity (e.g., deconditioned individuals, seniors, or those with chronic conditions). Many clients are looking for additional balance control; numerous studies have demonstrated improved balance and even reduced falls in seniors who practice tai chi and qigong-type exercise on a regular basis. Mindful exercise is also appropriate for clients with select medical conditions (e.g., high-normal and Stage I hypertension, type 2 diabetes, some anxiety and depression disorders, arthritis, and poor functional capacity) as well as for stable patients requiring cardiac and/or pulmonary rehabilitation, pain management, or anger management. The mindful exercise modality chosen should follow accepted and current pre-exercise assessment and exercise-training guidelines for those with medical conditions (e.g., American College of Sports Medicine, 2000; Fletcher et al., 1995).

PERSONAL TRAINERS AND MINDFUL EXERCISE

You should become familiar with the basic tenets of at least the classical forms of mindful exercise for two reasons. First, this knowledge will reduce the number of unfortunate misconceptions many of us preserve for what we think yoga, tai chi chuan, or qigong are. Many contemporary mindful exercise methods were developed on a platform of qigong, yoga, and Native American culture and exercise. Second, by attaining a better grasp of the cultural, health, and fitness benefits of these unique forms of exercise, you can more confidently refer to qualified mindful exercise teachers, perhaps even inspiring personal interest and participation. Chinese health exercise (i.e., qigong and its countless forms) is practiced by more than two billion people worldwide, yet the majority of fitness professionals in the West would find it difficult to produce even a cursory definition of this time-honored activity. Until recently, these distinctive exercise methods have been ignored and underappreciated by the western fitness culture. Very few contemporary exercise science texts even mention their existence. Moreover, we should avoid the temptation to overly critique, particularly the classical forms of mindful exercise, from a westernized mechanics or target conditioning zone perspective. The central function of most of these methods is to enhance the individual's sense of self-empowerment and personal spirituality while being respectful of their existing faith. Mindful exercise, when genuinely and properly taught, is an opportunity to improve health for those who wish to complement their existing fitness program or who are otherwise sedentary and are looking for some greater purpose in their daily exercise routine.

SUMMARY

Mindful exercise continues to emerge as an effective fitness and health enhancement modality. There is scientific evidence that hypertension, insulin resistance, pain, cardiovascular disease, anxiety, and depression all favorably respond to regular participation in mindful exercise such as tai chi, qigong, and hatha yoga. The core benefits from these programs include increased balance, strength, and flexibility, as well as being an immediate source of relaxation and mental quiescence. Regular and self-regulated mind-body exercise may also be ideal for many of your clients because of its portability and relative low-intensity nature. It is not beyond reason that in the near future the fitness and health promotion industry will benefit from the inclusion of mindful exercise guidelines and professional resources in respected exercise consensus publications that recommend the appropriate quality and quantity of exercise for primary and secondary prevention. The alliance of conventional health promotion programming with mind-body interventions should further reduce healthcare utilization and the unnecessary burden of degenerative disease. Given the present mandate for implementing integrated disease prevention and disease management programs to effectively reduce healthcare costs and inspire self-care in our clients, mindful exercise programs will be a necessary element.

RESOURCES

Yoga, Tai Chi, and Qigong Teacher Training Resources

There are many teacher training and certification programs for prospective tai chi, qigong, and particularly yoga teachers. Unlike many exercise instructor certification programs, most of these programs do not follow a common set of consensus guidelines that cover a core curriculum such as exercise and health assessment, program implementation, and exercise safety. This does not mean that there are not many comprehensively planned and professionally conducted yoga and tai chi teacher training programs; however, historically there have been no central practice guidelines or regulations governing core material in such programs. For yoga, one promising new professional body is the Yoga Alliance. This organization maintains a national registry of yoga teachers and schools who meet the Alliance's recommended educational standards and strongly encourages the inclusion of core competencies.

Select Yoga, Tai Chi, Qigong, and Pilates Education and Training Resources

Yoga Alliance
www.yogaalliance.org
Phone: 877-964-2255

Yoga Research and Education Center
www.yrec.org
Phone: 707-928-9898

International Association of Yoga Therapists
www.iayt.org
Phone: 707-566-9000

Kripalu Center for Yoga and Health
www.kripalu.com
Phone: 800-741-7353

Integrative Yoga Therapy
www.cruzio.com
Phone: 800-750-9642

YogaFit International
www.yogafit.com
Phone: 310-376-1036

Sivananda Yoga Vedanta Center of New York
www.sivananda.org
Phone: 212-255-4560

Yoga for The West Teacher Training Course
by Mara Carrico
www.yogalady.com
Phone: 800-742-1114

Justin Stone's Tai Chi Chih
www.taichichih.com

East West Academy of The Healing Arts (qigong)
www.eastwestqi.com
Phone: 415-285-9400

National Qigong Association USA
www.nqa.org
Phone: 218-365-6330

Qigong Institute
561 Berkeley Avenue
Menlo Park, CA 94025

Qigong Association of America
www.ql.org

Stott Pilates
www.stottpilates.com
Phone: 800-910-0001

PilatesMethod Alliance
www.pilatesmethodalliance.org
Phone: 866-573-4945

Pilates Foundation
www.pilatesfoundation.com
Phone: +44(0) 7071 781-859

Balanced Body
www.pilates.com
Phone: 800-745-2837

NIA Technique
www.nia-nia.com
Phone: 503-245-9886

REFERENCES

American College of Sports Medicine (2006). *ACSM's Guidelines for Exercise Testing and Prescription,* (7th ed.) Philadelphia, Pa.: Lippincott, Williams & Wilkins.

Anderson, B.D. & Spector A. (2000). Introduction to pilates-based rehabilitation. *Orthopaedic Physical Therapy Clinics of North America,* 9, 395–410.

Bera, T.K. (1995). Recovery from stress in two different postures and in Shavasa yogic relaxation positions. *Indian Journal of Physiological Pharmacology,* 42, 473–478.

Berger, B. & Owen, D. (1992). Mood alteration with yoga and swimming: aerobic exercise may not be necessary. *Perceptual and Motor Skills,* 75, 1331–1343.

Bernardi, L. et al. (2002). Slow breathing increases arterial baroreflex sensitivity in patients with chronic heart failure. *Circulation,* 105, 143–145.

Birkel, D.A. & Edgren, L. (2000). Hatha yoga: improved vital capacity in college students. *Alternative Therapies in Health and Medicine,* 6, 55–63.

Bowman, A.J. et al. (1997). Effects of aerobic exercise training and yoga on the baroreflex index in healthy elderly persons. *European Journal of Clinical Investigation,* 27, 443–449.

Broota, A., Varma, R., & Singh, A. (1995). Role of relaxation in hypertension. *Journal of the Indian Academy of Applied Psychology,* 21, 29–36.

Cappo, B.M. & Holmes, D.S. (1984). The utility of prolonged respiratory exhalation for reducing physiological and psychological arousal in non-threatening and threatening situations. *Journal of Psychosomatic Research,* 28, 263–273.

Center for Disease Control (2002). National Center for Chronic Disease Prevention and Health Promotion. Atlanta GA. www.cdc.gov/hrqol/index.htm and go to the Methods and Measures link.

Channer, K.S. et al. (1996). Changes in hemodynamic parameters following tai chi chuan and aerobic exercise in patients recovering from myocardial infarction. *Postgraduate Medicine,* 72, 347–351.

Clark, D.M., Salkovskis, P.M., & Chalkley, A.J. (1985). Respiratory control as a treatment for panic attacks. *Therapeutic and Experimental Psychiatry,* 16, 22–30.

DiCarlo, L.J. et al. (1995). Cardiovascular, metabolic, and perceptual responses to hatha yoga standing poses. *Medicine, Exercise, Nutrition, and Health,* 4, 107–112.

Fletcher, G.A. et al. (1995). Exercise standards: a statement for healthcare professionals from the American Heart Association. *Circulation,* 91, 580—615.

Fluge, T. (1994). Long-term effects of breathing exercises and yoga in patients with bronchial asthma. *Pneumologie,* 48, 484–490.

Garfinkel, M.S. (1994). Evaluation of a yoga-based regimen for treatment of osteoarthritis of the hands. *Journal of Rheumatology,* 21, 2341–2343.

Garfinkel, M.S. et al. (1999). Yoga based intervention for carpal tunnel syndrome: a random trial. *Journal of the American Medical Association,* 281, 2087–2099.

Goodwin, G.M., McCloskey, I., & Matthews, P., (1972). The contribution of muscle afferents to kinesthesia shown by vibration-induced illusions of movement and by effects of paralyzing joint afferents. *Brain,* 95, 705.

Hong, Y., Li, J., & Robinson, P.D. (2000). Balance control, flexibility, and cardiorespiratory fitness among older tai chi practitioners. *British Journal of Sports Medicine,* 34, 29–34.

Hutchinson, M.R., Christiansen, T.L., & Beitzel, J. (1998). Improving leaping ability in elite rhythmic gymnasts. *Medicine and Science in Sports and Exercise,* 30, 1543–1547.

Jain, S.C. & Talukdar, B. (1993). Evaluation of yoga therapy programme for patients with bronchial asthma. *Singapore Medical Journal,* 34, 306.

Jain, S.C. et al. (1993). A study of response pattern of non-insulin dependent diabetics to yoga therapy. *Diabetes Research and Clinical Practice,* 19, 69–74.

Jella, S.A. & Shannahoff-Khalsa, D.S. (1993). The effects of unilateral forced nostril breathing on cognitive performance. *International Journal of Neuroscience,* 73, 61–68.

Jin, P. (1992). Efficacy of tai chi, brisk walking, meditation, and reading in reducing mental and emotional stress. *Journal of Psychosomatic Research,* 36, 361.

Joshi, L.N., Joshi, V.D., & Gokhale, L.V. (1992). Effect of short term pranayama practice on breathing rate and ventilatory functions of the lung. *Indian Journal of Physiology and Pharmacology,* 36, 105–108.

Kamei, T. et al. (2000). Decrease in serum cortisol during yoga exercise is correlated with alpha wave activation. *Perceptual and Motor Skills,* 90(Pt 1), 1027–1032.

Kass, J.J. (1991). INSPIRIT spirituality assessment. *The Scientific Study of Religion.* 30, 203–211.

Khanam, A.A. (1996). Study of pulmonary and autonomic functions of asthma patients after yoga training. *Indian Journal of Physiology and Pharmacology,* 40, 318–324.

Koch, U. et al. (1998). Yoga treatment in psychophysiological insomnia. *Journal of Sleep Research,* 7(Suppl.2), 137.

Kutner, N.G. et al. (1997). Self-report benefits of tai chi practice by older adults. *Journal of Gerontology, Biological Psychology and Social Sciences,* 52, 242–246.

La Forge, R. (2002). Yoga and cardiovascular disease. *ACE Certified News,* 8, 5, 8–11.

Lai, J.S. et al. (1993). Cardiorespiratory responses of tai chi chuan practitioners and sedentary subjects during cycle ergometry. *Journal of the Formosa Medical Association,* 92, 894–899.

Lan, C. et al. (1996). Cardiorespiratory function, flexibility, and body composition assessment of geriatric tai chi chuan practitioners. *Archives of Physical Medicine and Rehabilitation,* 77, 612.

Lan, C. et al. (1998). 12-month tai chi training in the elderly: its effect on health fitness. *Medicine and Science in Sports and Exercise,* 30, 345–351.

Lan, C. et al. (1999). The effect of tai chi on cardiorespiratory function in patients with coronary artery bypass surgery. *Medicine and Science in Sports and Exercise,* 31, 634–638.

Lasater, J. (1995). *Relax and Renew: Restful Yoga for Stressful Times.* Berkeley, Calif.: Rodmell Press.

Li, F. et al. (2001). An evaluation of the effects of tai chi exercise on physical function among older persons: a randomized controlled trial. *Annals of Behavioral Medicine,* 23, 139–146.

Mahajan, A.S. et al. (1999). Lipid profile of coronary risk subjects following yogic lifestyle intervention. *Indian Heart Journal,* 51, 37–40.

Manchanda, S.C. (2000). Retardation of coronary atherosclerosis with yoga lifestyle intervention. *Journal of the Associated Physicians of India,* 48, 687.

Manocha, R. et al. (2002). Sahaja yoga n the management of moderate to severe asthma: randomized controlled trial. *Thorax,* 57, 110–115.

McCaul, K.D., Solomon, S., & Holmes, D.S. (1979). Effects of paced respiration and expectation on the physiological and psychological responses to threat. *Journal of Personality and Social Psychology,* 37, 564–571.

Miller, B.S. (1995). *Yoga Discipline of Freedom: The Yoga Sutra.* New York: Bantam Books.

Monroe, R., Ghosh, A.K., & Kalish, D. (1989). *Yoga Research Bibliography: Scientific Studies on Yoga and Meditation.* Cambridge, England: Yoga Biomedical Trust.

Murugesan, R., Govindarajulu, N., & Bera, T.K. (2000). Effects of selected yoga practices on hypertension. *Indian Journal of Physiological Pharmacology,* 44, 207–210.

Naveen, K.V. et al. (1997). Yoga breathing through a particular nostril increases spatial memory scores without lateralized effects. *Psychology Reports,* 81, 555–561.

Nespor, K. (1991). Pain management and yoga. *International Journal of Psychosomatics,* 38, 76–81.

Ornish, D. et al. (1990). Lifestyle Heart Trial. *Lancet,* 336, 129–133.

Paloutzian, R.F. & Ellison C.W. (1982). Loneliness, spiritual well-being and quality of life. In: Peplau & Perlman (Eds.) *Loneliness: A Sourcebook for Current Therapy.* Hoboken, N.J.: Wiley-InterScience (Book is out of print but in medical and university libraries.)

Province, M.A. et al. (1995). The effects of exercise on falls in elderly patients: A preplanned meta-analysis of the FICSIT Trials. Frailty and injuries. *Journal of the American Medical Association,* 273, 1381.

Raju, P.S. et al. (1994). Comparison of effects of yoga and physical exercise in athletes. *Indian Journal of Medical Research,* 100, 81–86.

Ray, U.S. et al. (2001). Effect of yogic exercises on physical and mental health of young fellowship course trainees. *Indian Journal of Physiological Pharmacology,* 45, 37–53.

Sakakibara, M. & Hayano, J. (1996). Effect of slowed respiration on cardiac parasympathetic response to threat. *Psychosomatic Medicine,* 58, 32–37.

Sakakibara, M., Takeuchi, S., & Hayano, J. (1994). Effects of relaxation training on cardiac parasympathetic tone. *Psychophysiology,* 31, 223–228.

Savic, K. et al. (1990). The effect of hatha yoga on poor posture in children and the psychophysiologic condition in adults. *Med Pregl,* 43, 268.

Schaller, K.J. (1996). Tai chi chih: an exercise for older adults. *Journal of Gerontological Nursing,* 22, 12–17.

Schell, F.J., Allolio, B., & Schonecke, O.W. (1994). Physiological and psychological effects of hatha-yoga exercise in healthy women. *International Journal of Psychosomatics,* 41, 46–52.

Schmidt, T. (1997). Changes in cardiovascular risk factors and hormones during a comprehensive residential three month kriya yoga training program and vegetarian nutrition. *Acta Physiologica Scandinavia Supplement,* 640, 158–162.

Selvamurthy, W. et al. (1998). A new physiological approach to control essential hypertension. *Indian Journal of Physiological Pharmacologyl,* 42, 205.

Shannahoff-Khalsa, D.S. & Beckett, L.R. (1996). Clinical case report: efficacy of yogic techniques in the treatment of obsessive compulsive disorder. *International Journal of Neuroscience,* 85, 1–17.

Shannahoff-Khalsa, D.S. & Kennedy, B. (1993). The effects of unilateral forced nostril breathing on the heart. *International Journal of Neuroscience,* 73, 47–60.

Sovlk, R. (2000). The science of breathing: the yogic view. In: *Progress in Brain Research.* E.A. Mayer & C.B. Sayer (Eds). 491–505. New York: Elsevier Science BV.

Telles, S. et al. (2000). Oxygen consumption and respiration following two yoga relaxation techniques. *Applied Psychophysiology and Biofeedback,* 25, 221.

Tse, M. (1995). *Qigong for Health and Vitality.* New York: St. Martin's Griffin.

Tsujiuchi, T. et al. (2002). The effect of qigong relaxation exercise on the control of type 2 diabetes mellitus. *Diabetes Care,* 25, 241–242.

Tweeddale, P.M., Rowbottom, I., & McHardy, G.J. (1993). Breathing training: effect on anxiety and depression scores n behavioral breathlessness. *J Psychosomatic Research,* 38, 11–21.

Vaananen, J. et al. (2002). Taichiquan acutely increases heart rate variability. *Clinical Physiology and Functional Imaging,* 22, 2–3.

Van Montfrans, G.A. et al. (1990). Relaxation therapy and continuous ambulatory blood pressure in mild hypertension: a controlled study. *British Medical Journal,* 26, 1368–1372.

Vedanthan, P.K. et al. (1998). Clinical study of yoga techniques in university students with asthma: a controlled study. *Allergy and Asthma Prox,* 19, 3–9.

Wang, J.S., Lan, C., & Wong, M.K. (2001). Tai chi chuan training to enhance microcirculatory function in healthy elderly subjects. *Archives of Physical Medicine and Rehabilitation* , 82, 1176–1180.

Wolf, S.L. et al. (1996). Reducing frailty and falls in older persons: an investigation of tai chi and computerized balance training. *Journal of the American Geriatric Society,* 44, 489–497.

Wolfson, L. et al. (1996). Balance and strength training in older adults: intervention gains and tai chi maintenance. *Journal of the American Geriatric Society,* 44, 498–506.

Wong, A.M. et al. (2001). Coordination exercise and postural stability in elderly people: effects of tai chi chuan. *Archives of Physical Medicine and Rehabilitation,* 82, 608–612.

Wood, C. (1993). Mood change and perceptions of vitality: a comparison of the effects of relaxation, visualization, and yoga. *Journal of the Royal Society of Medicine,* 86, 254.

SUGGESTED READING

Carrico, M. (2000). *Fitness Yoga.* San Diego, Calif.: American Council on Exercise.

Chance, J. (1999) *Thorson's Principles of the Alexander Technique.* New York: HarperCollins.

Cohen, K.S. *The Way of Qigong.* (1997). New York: Ballantine Books.

Desikachar, T.K.V. (1999). *The Heart of Yoga.* Rochester, Vt.: Inner Traditions.

Dong, P. & Esser, A. (1990). *Chi Gong: The Ancient Chinese Way to Health.* New York: Marlowe & Co.

Feuerstein, G. & Payne, L. (2000). *Yoga For Dummies.* Indianapolis Ind.: IDG Books.

Gallagher, S.P. & Kryzanowska, R. (1999). *The Pilates Method of Body Conditioning.* Philadelphia, Pa.: BainBridgeBooks.

Huang, A. (1993). *Complete Tai-Chi.* Tokyo: Charles Tuttle Co.

Iknoian, T. (2000). *Mindbody Fitness for Dummies.* Indianapolis, Ind.: IDG Books.

Iyengar, B.K.S. (1977). *Light on Yoga.* New York: Schocken Books.

Khalsa, S.K. (2001). *KISS Guide to Yoga.* New York: Dk Publications.

Kraftsow, G. (1999). *Yoga for Wellness: Healing With The Timeless Teachings of Viniyoga.* New York: Penguin Books.

Kraftsow, G. (2002). *Yoga for Transformation.* New York: Penguin Compass.

Monroe, R., Nagarathma, R., & Nagendra H.R. (1990). *Yoga for Common Ailments.* New York: Simon & Schuster, Inc.

Rosas D. & Rosas C. (1987). *Non-Impact Aerobics: The NIA Technique.* New York: Avon.

Shafarman, S. (1997). *Awareness Heals: The Feldenkrais Method for Dynamic Health.* New York: Addison-Wesley Longman.

Stone, J. (1995). *Tai Chi Chih: New Revised Edition.* Fort Yates, N.Dak.: Good Karma Publishing.

Wilson, S.D. (1997). *Qigong for Beginners: Eight Easy Movements for Vibrant Health.* Portland Oreg.: Rudra Press.

APPENDIX D   *Common*
Medications

Generic and Brand Names of Commonly Prescribed Drugs by Class

Generic Name	Brand Name*

ß-Blockers

Acebutolol	Sectral
Atenolol	Tenormin
Betaxolol	Kerlone
Bisoprolol	Zebeta
Carteolol	Cartrol
Esmolol	Brevibloc
Metoprolol	Lopressor, Toprol
Nadolol	Corgard
Penbutolol	Levatol
Pindolol	Visken
Propranolol	Inderal
Sotalol	Betapace
Timolol	Blocadren

Combination of ß-Blockers + Diuretics

Propranolol + Hydrochlorothiazide	Inderide
Metoprolol + Hydrochlorothiazide	Lopressor HCT
Atenolol + Chlorothalidone	Temoretic
Timolol + Hydrochlorothiazide	Timolide
Nadolol + Bendroflumethiazide	Corzide
Bisoprolol + Hydrochlorothiazide	Ziac

a- and ß-Adrenergic Blocking Agents

Carvedilol	Coreg
Labetalol	Normodyne, Trandate

a_1-Adrenergic Blocking Agents

Doxazosin	Cardura
Prazosin	Minipress
Terazosin	Hytrin

Antiadrenergic Agents Without Selective Receptor Blockade

Clonidine	Catapres
Guanabenz	Wyntensin
Guanadrel	Hylorel
Guanethidine	Ismelin
Guanfacine	Tenex
Methyldopa	Aldomet
Reserpine	Serpasil

Nitrates and Nitroglycerin

Amyl nitrite	Amyl nitrite
Isosorbide mononitrate	Ismo, Monoket, Imdur
Isosorbide dinitrate	Isordil, Sorbitrate, Dilatrate
Nitrogylcerin, sublingual	Nltrostat
Nitrogylcerin, translingual	Nitrolingual
Nitroglycerin, transmucosal	Nitrogard
Nitroglycerin, sustained release	Nitrong, Nitrocine, Nitroglyn, Nitro-Bid
Nitroglycerin, transdermal	Minitran, Nitro-Dur, Transderm-Nitro, Deponit, Nitrodisc, Nitro-Derm
Nitroglycerin, topical	Nitro-Bid, Nitrol

Generic Name	Brand Name*
Calcium Channel Blockers	
Amlodipine	Norvasc
Bepridil	Vascor
Diliazem	Cardizem, Dilacor, Tiazac
Felodipine	Plendil
Isradipine	DynaCirc
Nicardinpine	Cardene
Nifedipine	Adalat, Procardia
Nimodipine	Nimotop
Nisoldipine	Sular
Verapamil	Calan, Isoptin, Covera, Verelan
Cardiac Glycosides	
Digitoxin	Crystodigin
Digoxin	Lanoxin
Peripheral Vasodilators	
Hydralazine	Apresoline
Minoxidil	Loniten
Isoxsuprine	Vasodilan
Papaverine	Pavabid
Angiotensin-Converting Enzyme (ACE) Inhibitors	
Benazepril	Lotensin
Captopril	Capoten
Enalapril	Vasotec
Fosinopril	Monopril
Lisinopril	Zestril, Prinivil
Moexipril	Univasc
Perindopril erbumine	Aceon
Quinapril	Accupril
Ramipril	Altace
Trandolapril	Mavik
ACE Inhibitors + Diuretics	
Captopril and HCTZ	Capozide
Enalapril maleate and HCTZ	Vaseretic
Lisinopril and HCTZ	Prinzine, Zestoretic
Moexipril and HCTZ	Uniretic
Angiotensin II Receptor Antagonists	
Irbesartan	Avapro
Losartan	Cozaar
Valsartan	Diovan
Diuretics	
Thiazides	
Hydrochlorothiazide (HCTZ)	Esidrix
"Loop"	
Bumetanide	Bumex
Ethacrynic acid	Edecrin
Furosemide	Lasix
Potassium-sparing	
Amiloride	Midamor
Spironolactone	Aldactone
Triamterene	Dyrenium
Combinations	
Triamterene and HCTZ	Dyazide, Maxzide
Amiloride and HCTZ	Moduretic
Others	
Metolazone	Zaroxolyn

Generic Name	Brand Name*
Antiarrhythmic Agents	
Class I	
IA	
Disopyramide	Norpace
Moricizine	Ethmozine
Procainamide	Pronestyl, Procan SR
Quinidine	Quinora, Quinidex, Quinaglute, Quinalan, Cardioquin
IB	
Lidocaine	Xylocaine, Xylocard
Mexiletine	Mexitil
Phenytoin	Dilantin
Tocainide	Tonocard
IC	
Flecainide	Tambocor
Propafenone	Rythmol
Class II	
ß-Blockers	
Class III	
Amiodarone	Cordarone
Bretylium	Bretylol
Sotalol	Betapace
Class IV	
Calcium channel blockers	
Antihyperlipidemic Agents	
Atorvastatin	Lipitor
Cerivastatin	Baycol
Cholestyramine	Questran, Cholybar, Prevalite
Clorfibrate	Atromid
Colestipol	Colestid
Fluvastatin	Lescol
Gemfibrozil	Lopid
Lovastatin	Mevacor
Nicotinic acid (niacin)	Nicobid, Nicolar, Slo-Niacin, Niaspan
Pravastatin	Prevachol
Simvastatin	Zocor
Sympathomimetic Agents	
Albuterol	Proventil, Ventolin
Ephedrine	Primatene
Epinephrine	Adrenalin
Isoetharine	Bronkosol
Metaproterenol	Alupent
Terbutaline	Brethine
Others	
Clopidogrel	Plavix
Dipyridamole	Persantine
Pentoxifylline	Trental
Warfarin	Coumadin

*Represent selected brands; these are not necessarily all-inclusive.

Reprinted, with permission, from American College of Sports Medicine (2006). *ACSM's Guidelines for Exercise Testing and Prescription* (7th ed.). Philadelphia: Lippincott Williams & Wilkins.

APPENDIX E

ACE Position Statement on
Nutritional Supplements

It is the position of the American Council on Exercise (ACE) that it is outside the defined scope of practice of a fitness professional to recommend, prescribe, sell, or supply nutritional supplements to clients. Recommending supplements without possessing the requisite qualifications (e.g., R.D.) can place the client's health at risk and possibly expose the fitness professional to disciplinary action and litigation. If a client wants to take supplements, a fitness professional should work in conjunction with a qualified registered dietitian or medical doctor to provide safe and effective nutritional education and recommendations.

ACE recognizes that some fitness and health clubs encourage or require their employees to sell nutritional supplements. If this is a condition of employment, fitness professionals should protect themselves by ensuring their employers possess adequate insurance coverage for them should a problem arise. Furthermore, ACE strongly encourages continuing education on diet and nutrition for all fitness professionals.

GLOSSARY

Abduction Movement of a body part away from the midline of the body; opposite of adduction.

Abrasion A scraping away of a portion of the skin or mucous membrane.

Acclimatization The process whereby the body physiologically adapts to an unfamiliar environment and achieves a new steady state. For example, the body can adjust to a high altitude or a hot climate and gain an increased capacity to work in those conditions.

Acetylcholine A white crystalline neurotransmitter and derivative of choline that is released at the ends of nerve fibers in the somatic and parasympathetic nervous systems and is involved in the transmission of nerve impulses in the body.

Actin Contractile protein in a myofibril.

Active (dynamic) stretching A stretching of muscle and tissue that requires muscle contraction through a range of motion. No outside force is involved.

Active isolated stretching (AIS) A stretching technique modeled after traditional strength-training workouts. Stretches are held very briefly in sets of a specified number of repetitions, with a goal of isolating an individual muscle in each set.

Active recovery Performing stretching exercises or working other body parts to facilitate recovery after intense exercise to allow for more productive use of exercise time.

Acute Descriptive of a condition that usually has a rapid onset and a relatively short and severe course; opposite of chronic.

Adduction Movement of a body part toward the midline of the body; opposite of abduction.

Adenosine triphosphate (ATP) A high-energy phosphate molecule required to provide energy for cellular function. Produced both aerobically and anaerobically, and stored in the body.

Adherence The amount of programmed exercise a client engages in during a specified time period compared to the amount of exercise recommended for that time period.

Adipose tissue Fatty tissue; connective tissue made up of fat cells.

Aerobic With, or in the presence of, oxygen.

Aerobic cross training An individualized combination of numerous training methods characterized by a variety of intensities and modes, primarily for those in the maintenance phase of conditioning. Example: jog 15 minutes to a pool, swim for 20 minutes, and jog home. *See* Cross training.

Aerobic system The metabolic pathway that, in the presence of oxygen, uses glucose for energy production; also known as aerobic glycolysis.

Agonist A muscle that is directly engaged in contraction; opposes the action of an antagonist muscle.

All-or-none principle The principle of muscle contraction that states that when a motor unit is activated, all of the muscle fibers will maximally contract.

Amenorrhea The absence of menstruation.

Amino acids Nitrogen-containing compounds that are the building blocks of proteins.

Anabolic (androgenic) steroids Synthetic derivatives of the male sex hormone testosterone; used for their muscle-building characteristics.

Anaerobic Without the presence of oxygen; not requiring oxygen.

Anaerobic glycolysis The metabolic pathway that uses glucose for energy production without requiring oxygen. Sometimes referred to as the lactic acid system or anaerobic glucose system, it produces lactic acid as a by-product.

Anaerobic threshold The point during high-intensity activity when the body can no longer meet its demand for oxygen and anaerobic metabolism predominates; also called lactate threshold.

Anatomical position Standing erect with the feet and palms facing forward.

Anemic Characterized by a reduction below normal of the number of red blood cells or hemoglobin in the blood.

Angina Pain originating from the heart that is characterized by a substantial "pressure" sensation within the chest, commonly radiating down the arm, up into the jaw, or to another site. Generally caused by decreased blood flow through the coronary arteries supplying oxygen to the myocardium (heart muscle) due to partial occlusion from plaque or clot formation or spasm of the artery itself. Often aggravated or induced by exercise or stress (emotional or environmental); also called angina pectoris.

Angina pectoris *See* Angina.

Anorexia nervosa An eating disorder characterized by an intense fear of becoming obese, a distorted body image, extreme weight loss, and self-starvation. Metabolic abnormalities are commonly associated with this disorder and can sometimes be fatal.

Antagonist The muscle that acts in opposition to the action produced by an agonist muscle.

Antecedent The stimuli that precedes a given behavior; sometimes referred to as a cue or a trigger.

Antecubital space The space just in front of the cubitus (elbow).

Anterior Anatomical term meaning toward the front. Same as ventral; opposite of posterior.

Anthropometric assessments Measurement and analysis of parts of the human body. Examples include skinfold, girth, and body weight.

Antiatherogenic diet A diet designed to minimize atherosclerosis, usually one that is low in cholesterol and saturated fat.

Antioxidants Substances that boost the body's defense against excessive numbers of unstable oxygen molecules (free radicals) to prevent them from causing damage. Five nutrients have been identified as having antioxidant properties: beta carotene, vitamin C, vitamin E, sulfur, and selenium.

Aponeurosis A white, flattened, tendinous expansion that mainly serves to connect a muscle to the parts that it moves.

Arrhythmia Abnormal heart rhythm or beat.

Arteries Vessels that carry oxygenated blood from the heart to the tissues.

Arterioles Smaller divisions of the arteries.

Arthritis Inflammatory condition involving a joint. *See* Osteoarthritis *and* Rheumatoid arthritis.

Articulation Place of union or junction between two or more bones.

Associative stage of learning The second stage of learning a motor skill when performers have mastered the fundamentals and can concentrate on skill refinement.

Assumption of risk A legal defense used to show that a person understood the possible occurrence of known dangers of a specific activity and chose to participate anyway.

Asthma A disease of the pulmonary system characterized by episodes of dyspnea (difficult breathing) due to narrowing of the airways from constriction of bronchial smooth muscle and overproduction of mucous. *See* Chronic obstructive pulmonary disease (COPD).

Asymptomatic Without obvious symptoms.

Atherosclerosis A specific form of arteriosclerosis characterized by the accumulation of fatty material on the inner walls of the arteries, causing them to harden, thicken, and lose elasticity.

ATP *See* Adenosine triphosphate.

ATP-CP energy system *See* Creatine phosphate system.

Atria The two (left and right) upper chambers of the heart (singular: atrium).

Atrium *See* Atria.

Atrophy A decrease in the cross-sectional size of a muscle resulting from inactivity or immobilization following injury.

Attending (behavior) Nonverbal acknowledgments during conversation to encourage the speaker to continue.

Auscultation The act of listening to sounds (through a stethoscope) arising within bodily organs (e.g., the heartbeat).

Autogenic inhibition An automatic reflex relaxation caused by excessive stimulation of Golgi tendon organs (GTOs).

Autonomous stage of learning The third stage of learning a motor skill when the skill has become habitual or automatic for the performer.

Avascular Not vascular; without blood supply.

Avulsion A wound involving forcible separation or tearing of tissue from the body.

Axis of rotation The imaginary line or point about which an object, such as a body or a lever, rotates.

Ballistic High-impact, rapid, jerking movements.

Ballistic stretch A high-force, short-duration stretch using rapid bouncing movements.

Baroreceptors A sensory nerve ending that is stimulated by changes in pressure, as those in the walls of blood vessels.

Basal metabolic rate (BMR) The energy expended by the body while at rest to maintain normal body functions.

Behavioral chain A series of behaviors connected to each other in such a way that the resulting behavior will not occur if any links in the chain of behaviors are broken.

Beta-blockers (beta-adrenergic blocking agents) Medications that "block" or limit sympathetic nervous system stimulation. They act to slow the heart rate and decrease maximum heart rate and are used for cardiovascular and other medical conditions.

Bioelectrical impedance A method of determining body composition by measuring the body's resistance to electrical flow.

Blood pressure The pressure exerted by the blood on the walls of the arteries; measured in millimeters of mercury with a sphygmomanometer.

Body composition The makeup of the body in terms of the relative percentage of fat-free mass and body fat.

Body mass index (BMI) A relative measure of body height to body weight for determining degree of obesity.

Bradycardia Slowness of the heartbeat, as evidenced by a pulse rate of less than 60 bpm.

Bronchioles The smallest tubes that supply air to the alveoli (air sacs) of the lungs.

Bronchitis Acute or chronic inflammation of the bronchial tubes. *See* Chronic obstructive pulmonary disease (COPD).

Bronchodilators Medications inhaled to dilate (enlarge) and relax the constricted bronchial smooth muscle (e.g., Proventil).

Bulimia nervosa An eating disorder characterized by episodes of binge eating followed by self-induced vomiting or the use of diuretics or laxatives.

Bursitis Painful inflammation of a bursa, occurring most often in the knees, hips, shoulders, and elbows.

Calorie The amount of heat required to raise the temperature of one kilogram of water one degree Celsius; also called kilocalorie.

Capillaries The smallest blood vessels that supply blood to the tissues, and the site of all gas and nutrient exchange in the cardiovascular system. They connect the arterial and venous systems.

Carbohydrate (CHO) An essential nutrient that provides energy to the body. Dietary sources include sugars (simple) and grains, rice, and beans (complex). 1 gm CHO = 4 kcals.

Carbohydrate loading Up to a week-long regimen of manipulating intensity of training and carbohydrate intake to achieve maximum glycogen storage for an endurance event.

Cardiac cycle The period from the beginning of

one heart beat to the beginning of the next; the systolic and diastolic movement and the interval in between.

Cardiac output The amount of blood pumped by the heart per minute; usually expressed in liters of blood per minute.

Cardiorespiratory endurance The ability to perform large muscle movements over a sustained period; the capacity of the heart-lung system to deliver oxygen for sustained energy production; also called cardiovascular endurance.

Cardiovascular disease (CVD) General term for any disease of the heart and blood vessels; includes coronary artery disease, hypertension, stroke, congestive heart failure, peripheral vascular disease, and valvular heart disease.

Cardiovascular endurance *See* Cardiorespiratory endurance.

Cartilage A smooth, semi-opaque material providing a "frictionless" surface of a joint.

Cell membrane The enveloping capsule of a cell composed of proteins, lipids, and carbohydrates.

Cerebrovascular accident (CVA) Damage to the brain, often resulting in a loss of function, from impaired blood supply to part of the brain; more commonly known as a stroke.

Certification A credential attesting that an individual or organization has met a specific set of standards.

Cholesterol A fat-like substance found in the blood and body tissues and in animal products; essential for body production of hormones, steroids, and so on. Its accumulation in the arteries leads to narrowing of the arteries (atherosclerosis).

Chronic Descriptive of a condition that persists over a long period of time; opposite of acute.

Chronic disease A disease of long duration and often of gradual onset, involving very slow changes; does not indicate the severity of the disease.

Chronic obstructive pulmonary disease (COPD) A condition, such as asthma, bronchitis, or emphysema, in which there is chronic obstruction of air flow. *See* Asthma, Bronchitis, *and* Emphysema.

Circuit training A form of training that takes the participant through a series of exercise stations, sometimes with brief rest intervals in between; can emphasize muscular endurance, aerobic conditioning, muscular strength, or a combination of all three.

Circumduction The active or passive circular movement of a joint; a combination of flexion, abduction, extension, and adduction movements.

Claudication Cramplike pains in the calves caused by poor circulation of blood to the leg muscles.

Closed-chain exercise (CCE) Exercises that use the body muscles in a weightbearing position; co-contractors, postural stabilizers, and the neuromuscular system are all trained at the same time (e.g., squats and lunges).

Co-contraction The mutual coordination of antagonist muscles (such as flexors and extensors) to maintain a position.

Code of ethics Code, supplementary to other professional standards of practice or legal requirements, developed by professional organizations to govern professional conduct. Adherence to these codes is necessary to maintain professional standing or certification with such organizations.

Cognitions Current thoughts or feelings that can function as antecedents or consequences for overt behaviors.

Cognitive stage of learning The first stage of learning a motor skill when performers make many gross errors and have extremely variable performances.

Collagen The main constituent of connective tissue, such as ligaments, tendons, and muscles.

Competencies Specific skills or knowledge that one must possess to have the capacity to function in a particular way (provide appropriate standard of care) for a specific job.

Complete proteins Foods that contain all eight essential amino acids; most meats and dairy products are considered complete protein foods.

Concentric action *See* Concentric contraction.

Concentric contraction A contraction in which a muscle exerts force, shortens, and overcomes a resistance.

Connective tissue The tissue that binds together and supports various structures of the body (e.g., ligaments and tendons).

Consequence The stimulus that follows a behavior. It may be positive, which increases the possibility of the behavior recurring, or negative, which will have the opposite effect.

Continuous training Conditioning exercise, such as walking, jogging, cycling, or traditional aerobics, in which the intensity is maintained continuously between 50 and 85% of maximal oxygen consumption (functional capacity).

Contract A written agreement signed by the participant and the trainer (and additional third parties as appropriate) that clearly states the exercise goals to be achieved over a given time period. Also, a legally binding agreement stating services, fees, and other pertinent information regarding the trainer/client relationship.

Contracting Systematically providing rewards for positive behavior; stems from the behavioral theory of reinforcement.

Coordination A focus of functional training; the combining of movement pattern, trajectory, speed, and muscle utilization into quality performance.

Coronary artery disease (CAD) The major form of cardiovascular disease; almost always the result of atherosclerosis; also called coronary heart disease (CHD).

Coronary heart disease (CHD) *See* Coronary artery disease (CAD).

Corporation A legal entity, independent of its owners and regulated by state laws; any number of people may own a corporation through shares issued by the business.

Creatine phosphate (CP) A high-energy phosphate molecule that is stored in cells and can be used to immediately resynthesize ATP; one of the phosphagens.

Creatine phosphate system System of transfer of chemical energy for resynthesis of ATP supplied rapidly and without oxygen from the breakdown of creatine phosphate (CP); also called ATP-CP system.

Cross training A method of physical training in which a variety of exercises and changes in body positions or modes of exercise are utilized to positively affect compliance and motivation, and also stimulate additional strength gains or reduce injury risk.

Cyanosis A bluish discoloration, especially of the skin and mucous membranes, due to reduced hemoglobin in the blood.

Deep Anatomical term meaning internal; that is, located further beneath the body surface than the superficial structures.

Defibrillation Termination of atrial or ventricular fibrillation (rapid, randomized contractions of the myocardium), usually by electroshock.

Dehydration A condition of having a less than optimal level of body water.

Delayed onset muscle soreness (DOMS) Muscle soreness that occurs 24 to 48 hours after intense exercise; typically associated with eccentric muscle contractions and thought to be the result of microscopic tears in muscle or connective tissue.

Diabetes A disease of carbohydrate metabolism in which an absolute or relative deficiency of insulin results in an inability to metabolize carbohydrates normally; formerly known as diabetes mellitus.

Diastole The relaxation phase of the cardiac cycle during which blood fills the ventricles.

Diastolic blood pressure The pressure exerted by the blood on the blood vessel walls when the heart relaxes between contractions.

Dichotomous (light-switch) thinking Looking at an event as being all positive or all negative; usually appears in individuals who exclusively link their self-worth to their achievements.

Disability insurance Provides income protection in the case a trainer becomes injured; may or may not be provided by an employer.

Distal Anatomical term meaning away from the attached end of the limb, origin of the structure, or midline of the body; opposite of proximal.

Diuretic Medication that produces an increase in the volume of urine and sodium (salt) that is excreted.

Dorsiflexion Movement of the dorsum (top) of the foot up toward the shin (proximally); opposite of plantarflexion.

Dynamic constant external resistance Strength-training exercises and/or equipment that provide a constant resistance throughout the movement range.

Dynamic flexibility The range of motion about a joint when speed is involved during physical performance; strength, power, neuromuscular coordination, and tissue resistance are all factors.

Dynamic (isotonic) constant resistance equipment *See* Dynamic constant external resistance.

Dynamic (isotonic) variable resistance equipment *See* Dynamic variable external resistance.

Dynamic variable external resistance Strength-training exercises and/or equipment that automatically vary the resistance throughout the movement range.

Dyspnea Shortness of breath, resulting in difficult or labored breathing.

Eccentric action *See* Eccentric contraction.

Eccentric contraction A contraction in which a muscle exerts force, lengthens, and is overcome by a resistance.

Ejection fraction The percentage of the total volume of blood that is pumped out of the left ventricle during the systolic contraction of the heart.

Elasticity Temporary or recoverable elongation of connective tissue.

Electrolytes The minerals sodium, potassium, and chlorine, which are present in the body as electrically charged particles called ions.

Emergency medical services (EMS) system A local system for obtaining emergency assistance from the police, fire department, or ambulance. In the United States, most cities have a 911 telephone number that will automatically set the EMS system in motion.

Empathy The ability to experience another person's world as if it were one's own; understanding another's point of view.

Emphysema A chronic lung disease characterized by loss of air sacs resulting in a decreased ability to exchange gases; carbon dioxide levels are increased and oxygen levels are decreased, causing rapid breathing and dyspnea.

Employee A person who works for another person in exchange for financial compensation. An employee complies by the instructions and directions of their employer and reports to them on a regular basis.

Energy balance theory The principle that body weight will stay the same when caloric intake equals caloric expenditure, and that a positive or negative energy balance will cause weight gain or weight loss, respectively.

Enzymes Proteins necessary to bring about biochemical reactions.

Ergogenic aids Substances thought to enhance energy availability or utilization to improve endurance or strength.

Essential amino acids The eight amino acids needed to make proteins; called essential because they cannot be manufactured by the body and must be obtained from the diet.

Essential fatty acids Fat that cannot be produced by the body and must be supplied by the diet; linoleic acid is the only essential fatty acid; also called essential fat.

Essential nutrient A nutrient that must be supplied by the diet because it cannot be produced by the body.

Eumenorrheic Having normal menstruation.

Eversion Movement of the sole of the foot outward; opposite of inversion.

Excess postexercise oxygen consumption (EPOC) Increased oxygen requirement above resting metabolic rate following a bout of exercise; historically referred to as oxygen debt.

Exercise-induced asthma Intermittent labored breathing precipitated by exertion during exercise. *See* Asthma.

Extension Movement at a joint that brings two parts into or toward a straight line, thereby increasing the angle of the joint, such as straightening the elbow; opposite of flexion.

Fartlek training A form of training similar to interval training, except the work-rest intervals are not systematically measured, but instead are determined by how the participant feels.

Fascia A sheet or band of fibrous tissue that lies deep to the skin or forms an attachment for muscles and organs.

Fast-twitch (Type II) fiber Large muscle fiber characterized by its fast speed of contraction and a high capacity for anaerobic glycolysis.

Fat An essential nutrient that provides energy, energy storage, insulation, and contour to the body. 1 gram fat = 9 kcals.

Fat-free mass That part of the body composition that represents everything but fat—blood, bones, connective tissue, organs, and muscle; is the same as lean body mass.

Fat-free weight *See* Fat-free mass.

Fat soluble Able to be dissolved in fat; relating to vitamins, those that are stored in the body fat, principally in the liver.

Fatty acid The building block of fats; an important nutrient for the production of energy during prolonged, low-intensity exercise.

Feedback Verbal or nonverbal information about current behavior that can be used to improve future performance.

Flat-back posture A position of the spine that minimizes the natural curve by placing the pelvis in a slight posterior tilt.

Flexibility The range of motion possible about a joint.

Flexion Movement about a joint in which the bones on either side of the joint are brought closer to each other; opposite of extension.

Formative evaluation Ongoing tracking of a training program's progress, including effectiveness of trainer strategies, and client's effort level, compliance, and degree of satisfaction.

Frailty The condition of being frail, fragile, easily damaged; the predisposition toward increased risk of injury, illness, disability, and/or death.

Frontal plane An imaginary longitudinal section that divides the body into anterior and posterior halves; lies at a right angle to the sagittal plane.

Fulcrum The support on which a lever rotates when moving or lifting something.

Functional capacity The maximum physical performance represented by maximal oxygen consumption.

Functional training A training model that involves exercises specifically designed to improve a client's performance of activities outside the training environment, including specific movements involved in work, sports, or other activities of daily life.

Gait The manner or style of walking.

General liability insurance Insurance for bodily injury or property damage resulting from general negligence.

Glucose A simple sugar; the form in which all carbohydrates are used as the body's principal energy source.

Glycogen The storage form of glucose found in the liver and muscles.

Golgi tendon organ (GTO) A sensory organ within a tendon that, when stimulated, causes an inhibition of the entire muscle group to protect against too much force.

Graded exercise test (GXT) A treadmill or cycle-ergometer test that measures or estimates maximum aerobic capacity by gradually increasing the intensity until a person has reached a maximal level or voluntary exhaustion.

Grand mal seizure A major motor seizure characterized by violent and uncontrollable muscle contractions.

HDL *See* High-density lipoproteins.

Health Belief Model A model to explain health-related behaviors that suggests that an individual's decision to adopt healthy behaviors is based largely upon their perception of susceptibility to an illness and the probable severity of the illness. The person's view of the benefits and costs of the change are also considered.

Heart disease A structural or functional abnormality of the heart or of the blood vessels supplying the heart that impairs its normal functioning.

Heart-rate (maximum) reserve The result of subtracting the resting heart rate from the maximal heart rate; represents the working heart-rate range between rest and maximal heart rate within which all activity occurs.

Heat cramps A mild form of heat-related illness that generally occurs during or after strenuous physical activity and is characterized by painful muscle spasms.

Heat exhaustion The most common heat-related illness; usually the result of intense exercise in a hot, humid environment and characterized by profuse sweating, which results in fluid and electrolyte loss, a drop in blood pressure, light-headedness, nausea, vomiting, decreased coordination, and often syncope (fainting).

Heat stroke A medical emergency that is the most serious form of heat illness due to heat overload and/or impairment of the body's ability to dissipate heat; characterized by high body temperature (>105° F, or 40.5° C), dry, red skin, altered level of consciousness, seizures, coma, and possibly death.

Hemosiderosis A disorder of iron metabolism in which large deposits of iron are made in the liver; often an effect of the consumption of too many iron supplements.

Hernia A protrusion of the abdominal contents into the groin (inguinal hernia) or through the abdominal wall (abdominal hernia).

Herniated disc A condition in which the disc between two vertebrae of the spine bulges backward, often compressing a nerve root and compromising its function.

High blood pressure A condition in which blood pressure is chronically elevated above levels considered desirable or healthy for a person's age and size.

High-density lipoproteins (HDLs) A plasma complex of lipids and proteins that contains relatively more protein and less cholesterol and triglycerides. High HDL levels are associated with a low risk of coronary heart disease; labeled "good" cholesterol because it removes excess cholesterol from the body.

Homeostasis The tendency toward stability and balance in normal body states.

Hydrostatic weighing An underwater test used to measure body fat and lean body mass percentages based on the relative density of fat and lean tissue.

Hypercalciuric effect The tendency to excrete excessive calcium in the urine; usually caused by leaching of calcium from the bones.

Hypercholesterolemia An excess of cholesterol in the blood.

Hyperextension Extreme or excessive extension of a joint.

Hyperglycemia An abnormally high content of glucose in the blood.

Hyperlipidemia An excess of lipids in the blood.

Hypertension High blood pressure, or the elevation of blood pressure above 140/90 mmHg.

Hyperthermia Abnormally high body temperature.

Hypertrophy An increase in the cross-sectional size of a muscle in response to progressive resistance (strength) training.

Hyperventilation A greater-than-normal rate of breathing that results in an abnormal loss of carbon dioxide from the blood; dizziness may occur.

Hypoglycemia A deficiency of sugar in the blood commonly caused by too much insulin, too little glucose, or too much exercise in the insulin-dependent diabetic.

Hypokalemia A deficiency of potassium in the blood.

Hypokinesis Lack of activity or energy.

Hypothermia Abnormally low body temperature.

Hypotonic A solution having less tonicity (effective osmotic pressure equivalent) than bodily fluids.

Impingement syndrome Reduction of space for the supraspinatus muscle and/or the long head of the biceps tendon to pass under the anterior edge of the acromion and coracoacromial ligament; attributed to muscle hypertrophy and inflammation caused by microtraumas.

Incision A cut in the skin, frequently from a sharp object.

Incomplete proteins Foods that are missing one or more of the essential amino acids.

Independent contractors A person who performs services for another person or business under an expressed or implied agreement and who is not subject to the owner's control or right to control the manner and the means by which the services are performed. The owner is therefore not responsible for the acts or omissions or the insurance of the independent contractor.

Inferior Anatomical term meaning situated below or nearer the soles of the feet in relation to a specific reference point; opposite of superior.

Informed consent Voluntary acknowledgement of the purpose, procedures, and specific risks of an activity in which one intends to engage.

Intensity The physiological stress on the body during exercise; indicates how hard the body should be working to achieve a training effect.

Interdigitate To interlock, like the fingers of folded hands.

Interval training Short, high-intensity exercise periods alternated with periods of rest (e.g.; 100-yard run, one-minute rest, repeated eight times).

Inversion Moving the sole of the foot inward; opposite of eversion.

Ischemia A local deficiency of blood supply caused by the constriction or obstruction of the arteries, which results in a decreased supply of oxygen to the tissues.

Isokinetic Exercises or equipment that provide a fixed speed of movement and vary the resistive force according to the muscle force.

Isokinetic equipment *See* Isokinetic.

Isometric *See* Isometric contraction.

Isometric action *See* Isometric contraction.

Isometric contraction A contraction in which a muscle exerts force but does not change in length.

Isometric (static) equipment Equipment that does not permit joint movement, resulting in static (isometric) muscle contractions.

Isotonic *See* Dynamic constant external resistance *and* Dynamic variable external resistance.

Karvonen formula The mathematical formula that uses maximum heart-rate reserve to determine target heart rate.

Ketone An organic compound (e.g., acetone) with a carbonyl group attached to two carbon atoms. *See* Ketosis.

Ketosis An abnormal increase of ketone bodies in the body; usually the result of a low-carbohydrate diet, fasting, or starvation. *See* Ketone.

Kinesiology The study of the principles of mechanics and anatomy in relation to human movement.

Kinesthetic awareness One's sense of one's position and movement in space during various activities.

Korotkoff sounds Five different sounds created by the pulsing of the blood through the brachial artery; proper distinction of the sounds is necessary to determine blood pressure.

Kyphosis Exaggerated sagittal curvature of the thoracic spine; often accompanied by a forward-head position.

Kyphosis-lordosis An increase in the normal inward curve of the low back and increased outward curve of the thoracic spine.

Laceration A jagged, irregular cut or tear in the soft tissues, usually caused by a blow. Because of extensive tissue destruction, there is a great potential for contamination and infection.

Lactic acid (Lactate) A waste product of anaerobic energy production known to cause localized muscle fatigue.

Lactic acid system *See* Anaerobic glycolysis.

Lacto-ovo vegetarian A person who consumes milk and eggs, but not meat, poultry, or fish.

Lapses The expected slips or mistakes that are usually discreet events and are a normal part of the behavior-change process.

Lateral Anatomical term meaning away from the midline of the body; pertaining to the side, opposite of medial.

Law of acceleration The force (F) acting on a body in a given direction is equal to the body's mass (m) multiplied by the body's acceleration (a) in that direction: $F = ma$, or $a = F/m$.

Law of impact and reaction forces The earth exerts a force against the body that is equal to the force applied to the earth as one moves.

Law of inertia The tendency of all objects and matter to remain at rest, or, if moving, to continue moving in the same straight line unless acted on by an outside force; proportional to body mass.

LDL *See* Low-density lipoproteins.

Leader nutrients Ten nutrients that, if they are consumed in adequate amounts, will ensure that the individual will also be consuming the other nutrients. These nutrients are protein, carbohydrate, fat, vitamins A and C, thiamin, riboflavin, niacin, calcium, and iron.

Lever A rigid bar that rotates around a fixed support (fulcrum) in response to an applied force.

Liability Legal responsibility.

Ligament A connective tissue that functions to connect two bones.

Lipoprotein The vehicle that transports fat throughout the body; made up of protein, fat, and cholesterol.

Lordosis An exaggerated forward curvature of the lumbar spine, often resulting in a protruding abdomen and buttocks; sometimes referred to as a swayback.

Low-density lipoproteins (LDLs) A plasma complex of lipids and proteins that contains relatively more cholesterol and triglycerides and less protein. High LDL levels are associated with an increased risk of coronary heart disease; labeled "bad" cholesterol because it deposits cholesterol on the artery walls.

Macrocycle The longest time frame in a periodized training program, usually a period of six months to a year. The goals of a macrocycle are long-term and require multiple steps to be achieved.

Maximal graded exercise test *See* Graded exercise test (GXT).

Maximal heart rate (MHR) The highest heart rate a person can attain.

Maximal oxygen consumption ($\dot{V}O_2$ max) The highest volume of oxygen a person can consume during exercise; maximum aerobic capacity.

Maximal oxygen uptake *See* Maximal oxygen consumption ($\dot{V}O_2$ max).

Medial Anatomical term meaning toward the midline of the body; pertaining to the center; opposite of lateral.

Medical insurance Provides hospitalization and major medical coverage; may or may not be provided by an employer.

Megadose A dose of a substance that is extremely high compared to the needs of the body.

Menopause Cessation of menstruation in the human female, usually occurring between the ages of 45 and 50.

Mesocycle The mid-length time frame of a periodized training program, usually three to four months long. The goals of a mesocycle are designed to be steps on the way to the overall goal of the macrocycle.

MET *See* Metabolic equivalents (METs).

Metabolic equivalents (METs) A simplified system for classifying physical activities where one MET is equal to the resting oxygen consumption, which is approximately 3.5 milliliters of oxygen per kilogram of body weight per minute (3.5 mL/kg/min).

Microcycle The shortest time frame in a periodized training program, usually one to four weeks long. The goals of a microcycle are short-term and are designed to be steps on the way to the overall goal of the mesocycle.

Minerals Organic substances needed in the diet in small amounts to help regulate bodily functions.

Mirroring Imitating another's behavior or attitudes.

Mitochondria Specialized subcellular structures located within body cells that contain oxidative enzymes needed by the cell to metabolize foodstuffs into energy sources.

Modeling The process of learning by observing and imitating others' behavior.

Monounsaturated fats A type of unsaturated fat (liquid at room temperature) that has one spot available on the fatty acid for the addition of a hydrogen atom. Moderate intake is associated with a lower risk for cardiovascular disease (e.g., oleic acid in olive oil); generally considered to be a "healthy" fat.

Morbidity The disease rate; the ratio of sick to well persons in a community.

Mortality The death rate; the ratio of deaths that take place to expected deaths.

Motive force The force that starts or causes a movement.

Motive muscle contractions An aspect of coordination; eccentric or concentric contractions that produce the actual movement at the joints.

Motor learning effect Improvement in performance during the initial weeks of strength training due to more efficient motor unit utilization.

Motor neurons Nerve cells that conduct impulses from the CNS to the periphery signaling muscles to contract or relax, regulating muscular movement.

Motor unit A motor nerve and all the muscle fibers it stimulates.

Muscle afferents Neurons that conduct impulses from sensory receptors into the central nervous system.

Muscle fiber A muscle cell.

Muscle spindle The sensory organ within a muscle that is sensitive to stretch and thus protects the muscle from being stretched too far.

Muscular endurance The capacity of a muscle to exert force repeatedly against a resistance, or to hold a fixed or static contraction over time.

Muscular strength The maximum force that a muscle can produce against resistance in a single, maximal effort.

Myocardial infarction (MI) Death of a portion of the heart muscle from an interruption of the blood supply; commonly called a heart attack.

Myofibril Contractile protein in a muscle fiber.

Myosin Contractile protein in a myofibril.

Myotatic (stretch) reflex Muscular reflex created by excessive muscle spindle stimulation to prevent potential tissue damage.

MyPyramidFood Guidance System A guide to assist the public with daily food choices that will accomplish dietary goals; published in 2005 by the U.S. Department of Agriculture and the U.S. Department of Health & Human Services.

Negligence Failure of a person to perform as a reasonable and prudent professional would perform under similar circumstances.

Net caloric cost Exercise energy expenditure minus resting energy expenditure during the same period of time.

Neuromuscular junction The site at which a motor neuron transmits information to a muscle fiber; the junction between a nerve fiber and the muscle it supplies.

Neurotransmitters Chemical substances such as acetylcholine or dopamine that transmit nerve impulses across synapses.

Nutrient density Quantitative analysis of the amount of nutrients versus the amount of calories in a given food; nutrient-dense foods provide more nutrients per calorie.

Nutrients Components of food needed by the body. There are six classes of nutrients: water, protein, carbohydrate, fat, minerals, and vitamins.

Obesity An excessive accumulation of body fat. Usually defined as more than 20% above ideal weight, or over 25% body fat for men and over 32% body fat for women; also can be defined as a Body Mass Index of >30 kg/m², or a waist girth of >40 inches (102 cm) in men and >35 inches (89 cm) in women.

One repetition maximum (1 RM) The amount of resistance that can be moved through the range of motion one time before the muscle is temporarily fatigued.

Open-chain exercise (OCE) Exercise in which a muscle or muscle group is isolated to function alone (e.g., seated leg extension).

Orthostatic hypotension A drop in blood pressure associated with rising to an upright position.

Osteoarthritis Degenerative joint disease occurring chiefly in older persons; characterized by degeneration of the articular cartilage, hypertrophy of the bones, and changes in the synovial membrane.

Osteoporosis A disorder in which bone density decreases and susceptibility to fracture increases; primarily affects women past menopause.

Overload principle A principle of human performance that states that beneficial adaptations occur in response to demands applied to the body at levels beyond a certain threshold (overload), but within the limits of tolerance and safety.

Overtraining Constant intense training that does not provide adequate time for recovery; symptoms include increased resting heart rate, impaired physical performance, reduced enthusiasm and desire for training, increased incidence of injuries and illness, altered appetite, disturbed sleep patterns, and irritability.

Overuse injury An injury caused by activity that places too much stress on one area of the body over an extended period.

Oxygen debt *See* Excess postexercise oxygen consumption (EPOC).

Oxygen extraction The amount of oxygen taken from the hemoglobin molecule and used in exercising muscle cells; often referred to as the arterio-venous oxygen difference or a–v̄O_2 diff.

Oxygen uptake reserve (V̇O_2 R) The difference between maximal oxygen uptake and resting oxygen uptake.

Palpation The use of hands and/or fingers to detect anatomical structures or an arterial pulse (e.g., carotid pulse).

Partnership A relationship where two or more people agree to operate a business and share in the profits and losses.

Passive stretch A stretch in which the elastic components of the muscle are relaxed and the portion of muscle most likely to be loaded is the connective tissue (e.g., a static stretch).

Periodization The systematic application of overload through the pre-planned variation of program components to optimize gains in strength (or any specific component of fitness), while preventing overuse, staleness, overtraining, and plateaus.

Peripheral vascular disease A painful and often debilitating condition, characterized by muscular pain caused by ischemia (reduced blood flow) to the working muscles. The ischemic pain is usually due to atherosclerotic blockages or arterial spasms, referred to as claudication.

Peripheral vascular resistance Impedance of blood flow in the peripheral (farthest from the center) blood vessels.

Phosphagens Adenosine triphosphate (ATP) and creatine phosphate (CP), two high-energy phosphate molecules that can be broken down for immediate use by the cells.

Physical working capacity The maximal amount of physical work (cardiorespiratory activity) that can be attained by an individual; also referred to as aerobic capacity or functional capacity. *See* Maximal oxygen consumption ($\dot{V}O_2$ max).

Phytochemicals Plant chemicals that may reduce the risk of cancer and cardiovascular disease if consumed regularly.

Plantarflexion Distal movement of the plantar surface of the foot; opposite of dorsiflexion.

Plyometrics Exercises that maximize the myotatic (stretch) reflex to teach muscles to produce maximum force faster. Plyometrics are usually sport-specific and utilize exercises such as hops, bounds, and depth jumps; may cause overuse tendon injuries in some athletes.

PNF *See* Proprioceptive neuromuscular facilitation.

Polyunsaturated fats A type of unsaturated fat (liquid at room temperature) that has two or more spots on the fatty acid available for hydrogen (e.g., corn, safflower, soybean oils).

Posterior Anatomical term meaning toward the back; opposite of anterior.

Postmenopausal Pertaining to the time after menopause.

Premenopausal Pertaining to the time before menopause.

Primary assessment A rapid examination to identify life- or limb-threatening injuries or illnesses that need immediate attention.

Prime-mover muscle The muscle that contracts concentrically to accomplish the movement in any given joint action.

Principle of Specificity of Training *See* Specificity of training principle.

Probiotics Bacterial cultures that promote the metabolic activity of "good" bacteria, while inhibiting the growth of "bad," or illness-causing, bacteria.

Professional liability insurance Insurance to protect against professional negligence or the failure of a trainer to perform as a competent and prudent professional would under similar circumstances.

Prompts Motivational tools used to improve adherence and remind clients to exercise.

Pronation A triplanar motion at the subtalar joint consisting of abduction, dorsiflexion and eversion; closely resembles eversion (e.g., position of the forearm with the palm facing backward or down).

Proprioception Awareness of the body's position in space; helps the body regulate posture.

Proprioceptive neuromuscular facilitation (PNF) A method of promoting the response of neuromuscular mechanisms through the stimulation of proprioceptors in an attempt to gain more stretch in a muscle; often referred to as a contract/relax method of stretching.

Proprioceptors Specialized nerve endings in muscles, tendons, and joints that are sensitive to changes in tension during activity; gives a body part a sense of where it is in space.

Protein An essential nutrient made up of 20 amino acids that builds and repairs body tissues. 1 gm = 4 kcals.

Protraction Scapular abduction.

Proximal Anatomical term meaning toward the attached end of the limb, origin of the structure, or midline of the body; opposite of distal.

Puncture A piercing wound from a sharp object that makes a small hole in the skin.

Range of motion (ROM) The number of degrees that an articulation (joint) will allow one of its segments to move.

Rapport A relationship of mutual trust, harmony, or emotional affinity.

Rating of perceived exertion (RPE) Developed by Borg, this scale provides a standard means for evaluating a participant's perception of their physical exertion; the original scale rated exertion on a scale of 6–20; the revised scale is 0–10.

Reciprocal innervation (inhibition) Reflex co-acting with stretch reflex to inhibit activity of an opposing muscle group.

Recommended Dietary Allowances (RDA) Recommended vitamin and mineral intake for most people to obtain optimum health.

Residual volume The volume of air left in the lungs after complete expiration.

Resistive force A force that resists the motion of another external force.

Resorption The loss of tissue (e.g., bone) by the breakdown of the tissue, which is soaked up by the blood.

Resting heart rate (RHR) The number of heart beats per minute when the body is completely at rest;

usually counted first thing in the morning before any activity.

Resting metabolic rate (RMR) The number of calories expended per unit time at rest. It is measured early in the morning after an overnight fast and at least 8 hours of sleep. The sleep is at home and the measurement is in the lab.

Retraction Scapular adduction.

Rheumatoid arthritis An autoimmune disease that causes inflammation of connective tissues and joints.

Risk factor A condition, behavior (such as smoking), inherited trait, or a disease that increases one's risk for a given disease.

Risk management Minimizing the risks of potential legal liability.

ROM *See* Range of motion.

RPE *See* Rating of perceived exertion.

Sagittal plane Anatomical term referring to the imaginary longitudinal line that divides the body or any of its parts into right and left sections.

Sarcolemma The membrane surrounding the sarcomere, which is the functional unit of muscle fiber.

Sarcomere Repeating unit of a muscle fiber.

Sarcopenia A loss of skeletal muscle mass that may accompany aging.

Sarcoplasma A gelatin-like tissue surrounding the sarcomere, which is the functional unit of muscle fiber.

Sarcoplasmic reticulum The form of endoplasmic reticulum where calcium is stored to be used for muscle activation; located in striated muscle fibers.

Saturated fats Fatty acids carrying the maximum number of hydrogen atoms; these fats are solid at room temperature and are usually of animal origin.

Saturated fatty acids *See* Saturated fats.

Scoliosis A lateral curvature of the vertebral column, usually in the thoracic area.

Scope of practice The range and limit of responsibilities normally associated with a specific job or profession.

Secondary assessment After immediate life- or limb-threatening injuries/illnesses have been identified, this more thorough evaluation is performed to identify more subtle, yet still important, injuries.

Sedentary Doing or requiring much sitting; not active.

Seizure A disorder originating from the brain in which there is a disturbance of movement, behavior, sensation, or consciousness.

Set-point theory The weight-control theory that states that each person has an established normal body weight. Any deviation from this set point will lead to changes in body metabolism to return to the normal weight.

Shaping The reinforcement of successive approximations of a goal until the result is reached.

Sliding filament theory A generally accepted theory explaining the interaction between actin and myosin proteins and ATP to cause muscle contraction.

Slow-twitch (Type I) fiber A muscle fiber characterized by its slow speed of contraction and a high capacity for aerobic glycolysis.

Sole proprietorship A business owned and operated by one person.

Specificity of training principle A key concept of periodization that states that for an individual to become proficient at any given movement, that movement must be trained and practiced; a specific demand (e.g., exercise) made on the body will result in a specific response by the body.

Sphygmomanometer An instrument for measuring blood pressure in the arteries.

Spondylolisthesis Forward displacement of one vertebra over another; usually occurs at the 4th or 5th lumbar vertebrae.

Spondylolysis Dissolution (dissolving into another) of a vertebra; usually begins with a stress fracture.

Sprain A traumatic joint twist that results in stretching or tearing of the stabilizing connective tissues; mainly involves ligaments or joint capsules, and causes discoloration, swelling, and pain.

Stabilizer muscles Muscles that stabilize one joint so a desired movement can be performed in another joint.

Stabilizing muscle contractions An aspect of coordination; isometric contractions that support the trunk, limit movement in a joint, or control balance.

Stages-of-change model A lifestyle-modification model that suggests that people go through distinct, predictable stages when making lifestyle changes; precontemplation, contemplation, preparation, action, and maintenance. The process is not always linear.

Standard of care Appropriateness of an exercise professional's actions in light of current professional standards and based on the age, condition, and knowledge of the participant.

Static flexibility Range of motion (ROM) about a joint with little emphasis on speed of movement.

Static (passive) stretch A low-force, long-duration stretch that holds the desired muscles at their greatest possible length for 15 to 30 seconds.

Steroids *See* Anabolic (androgenic) steroids.

Strain A stretch, tear, or rip in the muscle or adjacent tissue such as the fascia or tendon.

Stretch weakness The weakening effect on muscles remaining in the elongated position for an extended period of time.

Stroke A sudden and often severe attack due to blockage of an artery into the brain.

Stroke volume The amount of blood pumped from the left ventricle during one heartbeat.

Subluxation A partial dislocation of a joint that usually reduces itself.

Submaximal aerobic exercise test A cardiorespiratory fitness test designed so that the intensity does not exceed 85% of heart-rate reserve or maximal oxygen uptake. This provides an estimation of maximal oxygen uptake without the risks associated with maximal exercise testing.

Superficial External; located close to or on the body surface.

Superior Anatomical term meaning higher or toward the head; opposite of inferior.

Supination A triplanar motion at the subtalar joint consisting of dorsiflexion, adduction, and inversion; looks like inversion (e.g., position of the forearm with the palm facing forward or upward).

Supine The position of the body when lying face upward.

Sway-back posture *See* Lordosis.

Sympathetic nervous system A division of the autonomic nervous system that activates the body to cope with some stressor (i.e., fight or flight response).

Syncope A transient state of unconsciousness during which a person collapses to the floor as a result of lack of oxygen to the brain; commonly known as fainting.

Synergist A muscle that assists another muscle in its function.

Synovial fluid Transparent, viscous lubricating fluid found in joint cavities, bursae, and tendon sheaths.

Systole The contraction phase of the cardiac cycle during which blood leaves the ventricles.

Systolic blood pressure The pressure exerted by the blood on the blood vessel walls during ventricular contractions.

Talk test A subjective method for measuring exercise intensity using observation of respiration effort and the ability to talk while exercising.

Target heart rate (THR) The number of heartbeats per minute that indicate appropriate exercise intensity levels for an individual; also called training heart rate.

Tendinitis Inflammation of a tendon.

Tendon Strong, fibrous connective tissue that attaches a muscle to a bone.

Thrombosis The formation, development, or presence of a blood clot (thrombus).

Torque A force causing rotation about a fixed axis of rotation; the act or process of turning around on an axis.

Training heart-rate range Target heart rate represented as a range of numbers. *See* Target heart rate (THR).

Transient ischemic attack (TIA) Momentary dizziness, loss of consciousness, or forgetfulness caused by a short-lived lack of oxygen (blood) to the brain; usually due to a partial blockage of an artery, it is a warning sign for a stroke.

Transverse plane Anatomical term for the imaginary line that divides the body, or any of its parts, into superior and inferior parts; also known as the horizontal plane.

Triglyceride The storage form of fat consisting of three free fatty acids and glycerol.

Tuberosity A projection or protuberance on a bone usually serving for the attachment of muscles or ligaments.

Type 1 diabetes Form of diabetes caused by the destruction of the insulin-producing beta cells in the pancreas, which leads to little or no insulin secretion; generally develops in childhood and requires regular insulin injections; formerly known as insulin-dependent diabetes mellitus (IDDM) and childhood-onset diabetes.

Type 2 diabetes Most common form of diabetes; typically develops in adulthood, is characterized by a reduced sensitivity of the insulin target cells to available insulin and is usually associated with obesity; formerly known as non-insulin-dependent diabetes mellitus (NIDDM) and adult-onset diabetes.

Valsalva maneuver Increased pressure in the thoracic cavity caused by forced exhalation with the breath held.

Vasoconstriction Narrowing of the opening of blood vessels caused by contraction of the smooth muscle cells in the walls of the vessel.

Vasodilation Increase in diameter of the blood vessels, especially dilation of arterioles leading to increased blood flow to a part of the body.

Vasodilator An agent (motor nerve or drug) that acts to relax (dilate) a blood vessel.

Vegan A pure vegetarian who excludes all animal-derived foods from the diet.

Veins Blood vessels that carry blood, usually deoxygenated, to the heart.

Venous return Return to the heart of the circulatory fluids by way of the veins.

Ventricle One of the two (left and right) lower chambers of the heart. The muscular left ventricle pumps blood to the body; the smaller right ventricle pumps blood to the lungs.

Venule A very small vessel that collects blood from the capillaries and connects to the veins.

Viscoelastic A combination of elastic and plastic properties found in all connective tissue.

Vitamins Organic compounds that function as metabolic regulators in the body; classified as water soluble or fat soluble.

$\dot{V}O_2$ max *See* Maximal oxygen consumption.

Waist-to-hip circumference ratio (WHR) A measure for determining health risk due to the site of fat storage; taken by dividing the abdominal girth (waist measurement) by the hip measurement to form a ratio.

Waiver Voluntary abandonment of a right to file suit; not always legally binding.

Water soluble Dissolvable in water; relating to vitamins, those that require adequate daily intake since the body excretes excesses in the urine.

Wolff's Law (of bone remodeling) Principle stating that bone is capable of adjusting its strength in proportion to the amount of stress placed on it.

INDEX